LABORATORY TESTS FOR THE

ASSESSMENT OF NUTRITIONAL STATUS

SECOND EDITION

Howerde E. Sauberlich

CRC PRESS

Boca Raton   London   New York   Washington, D.C.

Library of Congress Cataloging-in-Publication Data

Catalog record is available from the Library of Congress

Visit the CRC Press Web site at www.crcpresss.com

No claim to original U.S. Government works
International Standard Book Number 0-8493-8506-7
Printed in the United States of America   2 3 4 5 6 7 8 9 0
Printed on acid-free paper

CRC SERIES IN MODERN NUTRITION
Edited by Ira Wolinsky and James F. Hickson, Jr.

Published Titles

Manganese in Health and Disease, Dorothy J. Klimis-Tavantzis

Nutrition and AIDS: Effects and Treatments, Ronald R. Watson

Nutrition Care for HIV-Positive Persons: A Manual for Individuals and Their Caregivers, Saroj M. Bahl and James F. Hickson, Jr.

Calcium and Phosphorus in Health and Disease, John J.B. Anderson and Sanford C. Garner

Edited by Ira Wolinsky

Published Titles

Practical Handbook of Nutrition in Clinical Practice, Donald F. Kirby and Stanley J. Dudrick

Handbook of Dairy Foods and Nutrition, Gregory D. Miller, Judith K. Jarvis, and Lois D. McBean

Advanced Nutrition: Macronutrients, Carolyn D. Berdanier

Childhood Nutrition, Fima Lifschitz

Nutrition and Health: Topics and Controversies, Felix Bronner

Nutrition and Cancer Prevention, Ronald R. Watson and Siraj I. Mufti

Nutritional Concerns of Women, Ira Wolinsky and Dorothy J. Klimis-Tavantzis

Nutrients and Gene Expression: Clinical Aspects, Carolyn D. Berdanier

Antioxidants and Disease Prevention, Harinda S. Garewal

Advanced Nutrition: Micronutrients, Carolyn D. Berdanier

Nutrition and Women's Cancers, Barbara Pence and Dale M. Dunn

Nutrients and Foods in AIDS, Ronald R. Watson

Nutrition: Chemistry and Biology, Second Edition, Julian E. Spallholz, L. Mallory Boylan, and Judy A. Driskell

Melatonin in the Promotion of Health, Ronald R. Watson

Nutritional and Environmental Influences on the Eye, Allen Taylor

Laboratory Tests for the Assessment of Nutritional Status, Second Edition, H.E. Sauberlich

Advanced Human Nutrition, Robert E.C. Wildman and Denis M. Medeiros

Handbook of Dairy Foods and Nutrition, Second Edition, Gregory D. Miller, Judith K. Jarvis, and Lois D. McBean

Nutrition in Space Flight and Weightlessness Models, Helen W. Lane and Dale A. Schoeller

*Eating Disorders in Women and Children: Prevention, Stress Management,
and Treatment,* Jacalyn J. Robert-McComb

Childhood Obesity: Prevention and Treatment, Jana Pařízková and Andrew Hills

Alcohol and Coffee Use in the Aging, Ronald R. Watson

Handbook of Nutrition in the Aged, Third Edition, Ronald R. Watson

Vegetables, Fruits, and Herbs in Health Promotion, Ronald R. Watson

Nutrition and AIDS, Second Edition, Ronald R. Watson

Advances in Isotope Methods for the Analysis of Trace Elements in Man,
Nicola Lowe and Malcolm Jackson

Nutritional Anemias, Usha Ramakrishnan

Handbook of Nutraceuticals and Functional Foods, Robert E. C. Wildman

The Mediterranean Diet: Constituents and Health Promotion, Antonia-Leda Matalas,
Antonis Zampelas, Vassilis Stavrinos, and Ira Wolinsky

Vegetarian Nutrition, Joan Sabaté

Nutrient–Gene Interactions in Health and Disease, Nïama Moustaïd-Moussa
and Carolyn D. Berdanier

Micronutrients and HIV Infection, Henrik Friis

Tryptophan: Biochemicals and Health Implications, Herschel Sidransky

Nutritional Aspects and Clinical Management of Chronic Disorders and Diseases,
Felix Bronner

Forthcoming Titles

Handbook of Nutraceuticals and Nutritional Supplements and Pharmaceuticals,
Robert E. C. Wildman

Insulin and Oligofructose: Functional Food Ingredients, Marcel B. Roberfroid

Dedication

This book is dedicated to my understanding wife, Irene Cartwright Sauberlich,

who was often inconvenienced during the preparation of the manuscript.

Contents

Section I   Introduction

Section II   Vitamins

Water-Soluble Vitamins

Fat-Soluble Vitamins

Semi- or Quasi-Vitamins

Section III   Minerals

Body Electrolytes

Macrominerals

Trace Elements

Ultratrace Elements

Section IV   Protein-Energy Malnutrition

Section V   Essential Fatty Acids Deficiencies

Series Preface

The CRC Series on Modern Nutrition is dedicated to providing the widest possible coverage of topics in nutrition. Nutrition is an interdisciplinary, interprofessional field par excellence. It is noted by its broad range and diversity. We trust the titles and authorship in this series will reflect that range and diversity.

Published for a broad audience, the volumes in the CRC Series in Modern Nutrition are designed to explain, review, and explore present knowledge and recent trends, developments, and advances in nutrition. As such, they will appeal to professionals as well as to the educated layman. The format for the series will vary with the needs of the author and the topic, including, but not limited to, edited volumes, monographs, handbooks, and texts.

Contributors from any bonafide area of nutrition, including the controversial, are welcome. It is a great pleasure to welcome the second edition of *Laboratory Tests for the Assessment of Nutritional Status*, by Howerde E. Sauberlich. The first edition became a standard in the field, without peer, frequently used by both researchers, teachers and students. Over the years, there have been many requests for a second edition of this valuable monograph. We are fortunate to have it as part of the CRC Series on Modern Nutrition. It adds luster to this series.

Ira Wolinsky, Ph.D.
University of Houston
Series Editor

Preface

The U.S. Department of Defense has long had an interest in nutrition in relation to the activities of Quartermaster Research and Development Command. The Surgeon General of the Army was charged with the responsibility of prescribing basic diets for all field conditions. This included the responsibility for providing a nutritive diet to the troops and for the methods used in determining that the troops receive a nutritive diet. However, it was uncertain as to the best methods, techniques, and procedures for determining adequacy of nutrition.

Consequently, in February 1954, the Quartermaster Food and Container Institute sponsored a symposium on "Methods For Evaluation of Nutritional Adequacy and Status" held in Chicago. The symposium presentations were published as a document by the National Academy of Sciences–National Research Council, Washington, D.C., in December 1954. Topics discussed included (a) evaluation of protein adequacy, (b) evaluation of vitamin adequacy, (c) evaluation of mineral adequacy, and (d) evaluation of nutritional status of populations. The document represented the first major effort directed towards evaluating methods then available for the assessment of nutritional status of individuals or population groups.

In 1955, the Interdepartmental Committee on Nutrition for National Defense (ICNND) was organized by Presidential order.[1] The primary objectives of the Committee were to assist developing countries to assess their nutritional status, to define existing problems of malnutrition, and to identify means for solving critical nutrition problems by making maximum utilization of the country's own resources.

In order to perform the ICNND mission, the committee developed the *Manual for Nutrition Surveys*. The manual was published in 1957 and incorporated procedures presented at the earlier noted symposium on "Methods for Evaluation of Nutritional Adequacy and Status."[1] The survey manual was used in nutrition surveys of 18 countries. From these experiences additional methods and guidelines for assessment evolved and were incorporated into the Second Edition of the manual published in 1963. Eventually the manual was used in nutrition assessment in over 35 different countries, in addition to the numerous nutrition studies conducted on various population groups and military personnel of the United States. Even the National Health and Nutrition Examination Surveys (NHANES) incorporated principles used in the ICNND manual.

The present undertaking represents an update of an earlier volume published in 1974 entitled *Laboratory Tests for the Assessment of Nutritional Status*, co-authored by H.E. Sauberlich, J.H. Skala, and R.P. Dowdy. Since that time, remarkable progress has been made on the methodologies applicable to nutrition status assessment and to the expanded number of nutrients that can be evaluated, especially trace elements. Many methods have become easier to use and more sensitive and specific. This has been assisted by the introduction of high-performance liquid chromatography, amperometric detectors, atomic absorption spectrometry, sensitive spectrophotometers, radioassays, radial immunodiffusion assays, microfacilities, autoanalyzers, and many other introductions. Consequently, this volume is a complete rewrite of the earlier edition.

Nutrition is the single most important component of preventive health care. Diet has been associated with heart disease, diabetes, arteriosclerosis, cancer, stroke and hypertension, and cirrhosis of the liver. The ability of the human to respond to stresses, such as heat, trauma, surgery, infection, and altitude can be influenced by nutritional status. Nutritional status is reflected in a variety of metabolic processes that provide the basis for a number of methods for its assessment.

The general public has reduced the consumption of calories. Women consume daily 1500 to 1600 calories and men consume 2300 to 2400 calories. The elderly consume daily 1250 to 1650 calories, while dieting populations consume only 900 to 1200 calories.[1] There is concern as to whether the diets of lower caloric intake supply the required daily allowance of micronutrients. Weight-reducing diets have been reported to be low in B-complex vitamins, calcium, iron, and zinc.

Nutrition assessment should be able to identify undernutrition, overnutrition, specific nutrient deficiencies, and imbalances caused by excessive intakes of required nutrients or of drug nutrient imbalances. Laboratory methods for the assessment nutritional status are important for identifying individuals as well as populations groups with nutritional risks. The assessments can determine the appropriate nutrition intervention and monitor its effects. The intent of this book is to provide a brief outline of the various biochemical techniques that are available in the laboratory to assist in the evaluation of the nutritional status of the human.

Considerable progress has been made in the past 20 years in the development of new approaches and modified techniques for assessing the nutritional status of the human of all ages. The number of nutrients being considered has been expanded to include most of the essential microminerals. Nutritional assessment services have become more available in clinical laboratories. Reliable and validated interpretive guides have become available.

Unfortunately, the scope of this book did not permit a critical review of the individual biochemical methodologies available or a presentation of detailed procedures. The literature citations, although by no means exhaustive, should provide guidance to the readers for the selection of precise methods.

References

1. Schaefer, A. E., Principles and applications of nutrition survey findings, *Int. J. Vit. Nutr. Res.*, 27, 33, 1985.
2. Schaefer, A. E., Surveys, their usefulness and pitfalls, in *Food and Agricultural Research Opportunities to Improve Human Nutrition*, College of Human Resources, University of Delaware, Newark, 1986, C28.

The Author

Howerde E. Sauberlich, Ph.D., is a professor in the Department of Nutrition Sciences, University of Alabama, at Birmingham, Alabama. He received a B.A. degree in physical chemistry, summa cum laude and Phi Beta Kappa, from Lawrence University, Appleton, Wisconsin. He received his M.S. and Ph.D. degrees from the University of Wisconsin in biochemistry and nutrition, with minors in endocrinology and medical sciences. Postdoctoral studies were conducted in the areas of radioisotopes and mineral nutrition at the University of Tennessee, Oak Ridge, and nutritional toxicology at Vanderbilt University, Nashville, Tennessee.

Dr. Sauberlich has served as a Professor of Animal Husbandry and Nutrition, Auburn University, Auburn, Alabama; and as Professor of Animal Nutrition and Microbiology, University of Kentucky, Lexington, and the University of Indonesia, Bogor; Associate Professor of Animal Husbandry and Food Technology, Iowa State University, Ames. He has also served as Chief, Chemistry Division, U.S. Army Medical Research and Nutrition Laboratory, Fitzsimons General Hospital, Denver, Colorado; and as Chief, Division of Nutrition Technology, Letterman Army Institute of Research, Presidio of San Francisco, California. More recently he served as the Acting Director of the Western Human Nutrition Research Center, USDA, Presidio of San Francisco. Dr. Sauberlich has served as an Affiliate Professor at the Colorado State University, Ft. Collins, University of California, Berkeley, and Miami University, Miami, Florida.

Dr. Sauberlich has conducted both basic and applied research encompassing a wide range of topics including cancer research, AIDS research, protein and amino metabolism, microbial nutrition, small animal and livestock nutrition, lipid metabolism, antibiotics, mineral requirements, metabolism and requirements of vitamins by the humans, and nutrition assessment. He has participated in numerous national and international nutrition studies and is the author or co-author of over 300 scientific publications.

Dr. Sauberlich is a member of numerous professional organizations including American Society for Nutritional Sciences, American Society for Clinical Nutrition, American Society for Biochemistry and Molecular Biology, American Association for Cancer Research, Society for Experimental Biology and Medicine, European Academy of Nutritional Sciences, American Chemical Society, American Society for Microbiology, American Society of Animal Science, and New York Academy of Sciences.

Dr. Sauberlich has received numerous fellowships and honors. Included are both the Mead-Johnson Award and Borden Award from the American Society for Nutritional Sciences, Meritorious Civilian Service Award from the Department of the Army; McLester Award for research in human nutrition, Secretary of the Army Research and Study Fellowship Award, Canadian Society for Clinical Chemistry Award; and Outstanding Alumni Achievement Award from Lawrence University. Dr. Sauberlich was elected a Fellow of the American Society for Nutritional Sciences, certified by the American Board of Nutrition, and elected into the Senior Executive Service.

Acknowledgment

I am gratefully indebted to Ms. Janine Smith who labored many long hours in the preparation and typing of the manuscript.

Section I

Introduction

Introduction

Nutrition is the single most important component of preventive health care for diet has been associated with hypertension and stroke, cancer, heart disease, diabetes, artheriosclerosis, and cirrhosis of the liver. Optimum nutrition is the level of intake that should promote the highest level of health. Numerous factors influence nutritional status. Some of these factors are indicated in Tables 1 and 2.

Nutritional assessment should be able to identify undernutrition, overnutrition, specific nutrient deficiencies, and imbalances caused by excessive intakes of essential nutrients or of drug nutrient interactions. The World Health Organization and Food and Agriculture Organization (FAO/WHO) have accepted the concept of "adequacy of all functions that have physiological and/or clinical importance." In 1995, in excess of 300,000 deaths per year in the United States could be attributed to poor diet and insufficient physical activity.[7] Many more suffer from unrecognized subclinical nutritional conditions.

The past 15 years has seen the development of improved laboratory methods for the assessment of nutritional status. The methods have proven to be sensitive, rapid, and reliable and often have been automated. Micromethods have been developed that require only small sample volumes and are particularly applicable to infants and children. This has been enhanced by the application of high-performance liquid chromatography in conjunction with highly sensitive detector systems. The development of sensitive and specific immunodiffusion assays, radioisotope-binding methods, radial diffusion assays, etc., have permitted the measurement of nutrients or metabolites previously difficult or impossible to measure. Commercial assay kits have been developed for many of these measurements which can provide reliable and sensitive analytical capability for the general biochemical laboratory. As an example, serum vitamin B-12 and serum folate analyses are routinely available in hospital clinical laboratories.

Various non-biochemical procedures have been used that can provide a functional evaluation of nutritional status. Included in these procedures are electroretinography, dark adaptation tests, electroencephalography, capillary fragility measurements, taste tests, neurological changes and behavioral or psychological changes. Although these procedures have low invasiveness, they are time-consuming, or involve the use of expressive equipment, and have often poor sensitivity and specificity.

In medicine, diagnosis is the forerunner of treatment and prognosis. With respect to nutrition, diagnosis can be equated with nutritional assessment.[1] The assessment techniques must be specific and sensitive. For many of the vitamins and essential minerals, the available tests have a high specificity and sensitivity. Biochemical evaluations have the potential of being objective and quantitative indicators of nutritional status. Clinical signs may not be apparent in a mild degree of nutritional deficiency but may be evident from biochemical measurements. Nutritional assessments may identify patients with excessive intakes such as of retinol, selenium, or vitamin B-6.

When intakes of nutrients are inadequate, body stores are gradually depleted. For most nutrients, the body stores are limited, and frequently capable of depletion in a few weeks (e.g., vitamins B-1, B-6, and C). Eventually with depletion, clinical and physiological signs are manifested in a nonspecific fashion such as loss of appetite, weight loss, behavioral changes, malaise, irritability, or skin lesions.

TABLE 1
Phases in the Development of a Nutrient Deficiency

Phase	I	II	III	IV	V
Biochemical alterations	Normal pool size and concentration in tissues, blood, urine. Normal metabolite levels and enzyme activities.	Reduction in body pool size.	Lowering of nutrient concentration in blood, urine and tissues; lowering of metabolite levels in urine, blood, etc.	Lowering of activity of vitamin- or mineral-dependent enzymes; early signs of metabolic disturbances.	Severe metabolic disturbances, abnormal metabolites present in urine or blood, anemia.
Clinical changes	Normal	Normal	Normal	CNS changes, behavioral changes, hyperirritability, etc.	Eye lesions, seborrheic dermatitis, cheilosis, glossitis, angular stomatitis, etc.
Morphological changes	Normal	Normal	Normal	CNS changes, behavioral changes, hyperirritability, etc.	Eye lesions, seborrheic dermatitis, cheilosis, glossitis, angular stomatitis, etc.
Functional changes	Normal	Normal	Normal	Abnormal electro-encephalograms, abnormal EKG, impaired dark adaptation, etc.	Convulsive seizures, hyperacusis, hypogeusia, weakness, etc.

Increasing Severity or Duration of Deficiency →

TABLE 2
Factors Influencing Nutritional Status

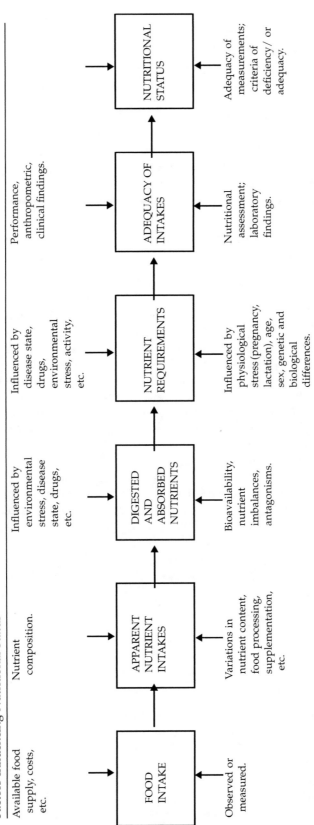

Nutritional status is reflected in a variety of metabolic processes, which provide a basis for laboratory tests. These tests can provide specific nutrition information as well as identify borderline nutritional conditions prior to the appearance of perceptible symptoms. Some of the various types of biochemical tests that may be useful for nutritional status assessment are summarized as follows:

1. Static measurement of nutrient under study in blood, plasma, leukocytes, urine, and other biological samples (e.g., iodine, vitamin C, vitamin B-6, folate, riboflavin).

2. Measurement of a metabolite of the nutrient in blood or urine (e.g., 4-pyridoxic acid, N'-methylnicotinamide, 4-pyridone).

3. Functional tests (e.g., erythrocyte enzyme activity: transaminase, transketolase, glutathione reductase).

4. Abnormal metabolites (e.g., homocysteine, methymalonate, FIGLU, xanthurenic acid).

5. Product of nutrient under study (e.g., hemoglobin, albumin).

6. Load or saturation test (e.g., transferrin saturation, thiamin, vitamin C).

7. Other procedures (e.g., stable isotopes, body composition measurements).

Some investigators consider that subjects with vague symptoms, such as irritability, insomnia, lethargy, and difficulty in concentrating may reflect on underlying physiological condition that may be related to nutritional status. It is commonly recognized that detecting and treating disease at the early stage of cellular biochemical abnormality, rather than delay for clinical signs, is highly beneficial. Laboratory biochemical tests can provide an early detection of a compromised nutritional status. The phases in the development of a nutrient deficiency are presented in Tables 1 and 2.

Functional laboratory measurements can provide specific information on nutritional status. For example, Wada and King[6] found that men achieved zinc balance when fed 5.5 mg of zinc/day; however, laboratory measurements revealed that the men's circulating concentrations of serum albumin, transthyretin, retinol-binding protein, thyroid-stimulating hormone, and free thyroxine declined significantly. A subclinical zinc nutritional deficiency existed.

Guidelines and Interpretation of Data

For many nutrients adequate information is not available to establish reliable guidelines.[3,4] Hence, caution must be applied in their use. Guidelines used for evaluating nutritional status must consider the influence of factors such as age, sex, lactation, pregnancy, inflammation, infection, and trauma.

Often guidelines or cut-offs are derived from laboratory measurement of the nutrient of interest in blood, serum, or other biological samples, from a group of "healthy" individuals, often young healthy adults.[4] Sometimes it is more appropriate to use other population groups, such as elderly, infants, or pregnant women.[2,4]

Biochemical assessment measurements can be of considerable value in the identification of nutritional problems in population groups and in the evaluation of the effectiveness of nutritional intervention programs, and provide surveillance and monitoring.[5] This has been exemplified in the U.S. Ten-State Nutrition Survey and in the National Health and Nutrition Examination Surveys (NHANES-I, -II, -III).[5]

Interpretation of biochemical results may use a statistical approach. The result may be classified into three states of risk; high, borderline or moderate, and low. Subjects with values below the 2.5 percentile would be classified at high risk; the 2.5 to 30th percentile range would consider those subjects to have possibly abnormal values or to have a subclinical deficiency; and subjects above the 30th percentile would be considered at low risk or with acceptable values.

Quality Assurance and Quality Control

Urinary excretion measurements can provide guidance concerning the adequacy of dietary intakes of certain vitamins and minerals. Iodine, zinc, copper, selenium, calcium, phosphorus, and magnesium have been evaluated in this manner. For many years, urinary iodine concentrations have been used as an index of adequacy of iodine in the diet. Urinary concentrations of thiamin, riboflavin, and vitamin B-6 have been used to assess the nutritional adequacy of these nutrients. When urine is used for nutritional assessment measures, 24-hr urine samples are preferred. However, it must be recognized that obtaining such samples is often difficult and the completeness of the collection unreliable. If creatinine values are used as a reference of collection completeness, it must be recognized that a large variation in individual creatinine excretion occurs.

Barring improper sample collection and handling or contamination,[2] trace element analyses are capable of providing accurate results that are in agreement between laboratories.[4] Certified quality controls and reference samples are available for standardizing methods and results between laboratories. For the measurement of vitamins and other biological components or enzyme activities, suitable reference standards are not always available. It is the essential for the laboratory to establish their own quality controls.

Quality controls can be prepared by various procedures. For example, two quantities of plasma are obtained for preparation of quality controls. One quantity of plasma is abnormal or deficient in the nutrient to be analyzed and the other quantity of plasma is normal or high in content. The controls are aliquoted into small vials, stabilized if necessary, and stored at −72°C. Repeated analysis of the controls for the nutrient of interest is performed to establish a mean value and a standard deviation value. These two quality controls are included in a routine manner with each batch of samples analyzed. Similar preparations can be prepared for urine, blood, and erythrocytes samples. These preparations can be shipped in dry ice to other laboratories for comparison of analytical results. Analytical sources of error relate largely to the accuracy and precision of the laboratory. A quality-control program can improve the performance of the laboratory and give reliability and validity to the analytical results.

References

1. Sauberlich, H. E., Implications of nutritional status on human biochemistry, physiology, and health, *Clin. Biochem.*, 17, 132, 1984.

2. Garry, P. J., Hunt, W. C., VanderJagt, D. J., and Rhyne, R. L., Clinical chemistry reference intervals for healthy elderly subjects, *Am. J. Clin. Nutr.*, 50, 1219, 1989.
3. Malvy, D. J. M., Biomarkers in nutrition epidemiology and prevention: the path between the laboratory and the population, *Int. J. Vit. Nutr. Res.*, 66, 282, 1996.
4. Van Den Berg, H., Heseker, H., Lamand, M., Sandstrom, B., and Thurnham, D., Flair concerted action No. 10 status papers: introduction, conclusions, and recommendations, *Int. J. Vit. Nutr. Res.*, 63, 247, 1993.
5. Executive summary from the Third Report on Nutrition Monitoring in the United States, Life Sciences Research Office Report, *J. Nutr.*, 126, 1907S, 1996.
6. Wada, L. and King, J. C., Effect of low zinc intake on basal metabolic rate, thyroid hormones, and protein utilization in adult men, *J. Nutr.*, 116, 1045, 1986.
7. Satcher, D. (Director of the Centers for Disease Control and Prevention, Atlanta, GA), *International Life Science Institute News*, 13, 3, 1995.

Section II

Vitamins

Water-Soluble Vitamins

Fat-Soluble Vitamins

Semi- or Quasi-Vitamins

Vitamin C (Ascorbic Acid)

Ascorbic acid: hydroascorbic acid
   molecular weight: 176.1

Oxidized ascorbic acid: dehydroascorbic acid
   molecular weight: 174.1

Converting metric units to System International (SI) units:
   $\mu g/mL \times 5.679 = \mu mol/L$
   $\mu mol/L \times 0.1762 = \mu g/mL$

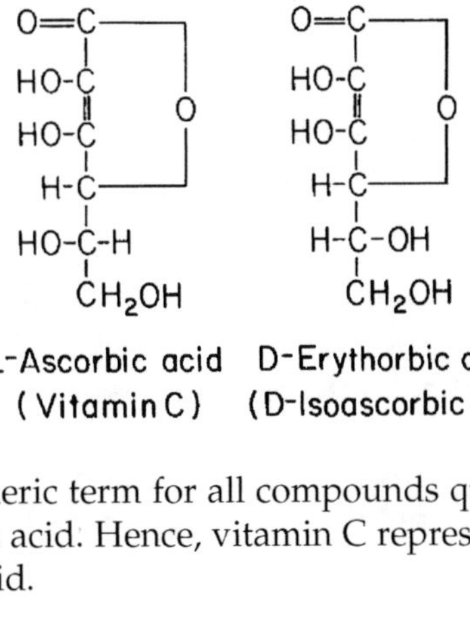

FIGURE 1
Structures of L-ascorbic acid and D-erythorbic acid.

L-Ascorbic acid   D-Erythorbic acid
(Vitamin C)   (D-Isoascorbic acid)

Vitamin C is used as a generic term for all compounds qualitatively exhibiting the biological properties of ascorbic acid. Hence, vitamin C represents the sum of hydroascorbic acid and dehydroascorbic acid.

History of Vitamin C and Scurvy

Over the centuries, vitamin C deficiency, in the form of scurvy, has inflicted enormous misery and tragedy worldwide. The conquest of scurvy represents a high mark in the history of nutrition. The writings and documents on scurvy dating back to the Thebes Ebers Papyrus of circa 1500 B.C. are extensive. Several overviews of the long and tragic history of scurvy are available and provide interesting reading.[3-6,31,48] Scurvy was the scourge of seafarers and explorers of yore. Over a million seamen have been estimated to have died of scurvy during the seventeenth and eighteenth centuries alone. Scurvy was not however, confined to seafarers, but also took a heavy toll on land, particularly in association with wars, sieges, and famines.

By the end of the 1800s, it was recognized that citrus fruits could cure scurvy, but the concept that the disease was caused by the lack of a nutrient in the diet was not accepted. This concept changed in 1907 when Holst and Frolich of Norway reported that they could experimentally produce scurvy in the guinea pig with a simple diet of wheat, rye, oats, and barley. They found that the disease could be prevented by feeding the guinea pigs fresh potatoes, cabbage, and apples, or fresh lemon juice.

With the availability of this guinea pig bioassay, the antiscorbutic factor was isolated in 1932 essentially simultaneously in the laboratories of Albert Szent-Gyorgy at the University of Szeged, in Hungary and of Charles Glen King, at the University of Pittsburgh in Pennsylvania. Originally, the antiascorbutic compound was called vitamin C. When the structure of vitamin C proved to be that of hexuronic acid, Haworth and Szent-Gyorgy renamed it *ascorbic acid.*

Vitamin C Deficiency

A deficiency of vitamin C leads to scurvy. Scurvy is characterized by hemorrhagic disorders such as petechiae (pinpoint hemorrhages around hair follicles) and ecchymoses (large areas of dermal hemorrhage). Scurvy may be associated with loosening of the teeth, gingivitis, and anemia. Swollen or bleeding gums may occur early in a vitamin C deficiency.

In controlled metabolic studies on ascorbic acid metabolism in women, depletion of the vitamin for less than 30 days resulted in scorbutic-type changes including inflammation of the gums, red and tender gums, and bleeding gums; petachia developed on the upper chest, abdomen, and upper back.[74]

Similar metabolic studies were conducted in adult men with the use of radioisotopically labeled ascorbic acid.[76-79] After feeding the subjects vitamin C-deficient diets for 38 days, symptoms of scurvy appeared. The principle signs and symptoms observed included follicular hyperkeratosis, hemorrhagic manifestations, swollen or bleeding gums, and aching limbs. At this point, the normal vitamin C body pool of 1500 to 2000 mg had fallen to less than 300 mg. Plasma ascorbic acid concentrations were less than 11.4 µmol/L (0.20 mg/dL).[76] Their initial plasma ascorbic acid concentration was 68.1 µmol/L (1.2 mg/dL). Daily vitamin C supplements of 66.5 mg produced a slow increase in the plasma ascorbate concentration to 39.8 µmol/L (0.7 mg/dL).[76]

Garry et al.[75] observed in elderly men that a daily intake of 60 mg of ascorbic acid (U.S. Recommended Dietary Allowance) maintained a median plasma vitamin C concentration of 25 µmol/L (0.44 mg/dL). In men, whole blood ascorbic acid concentrations of < 28 µmol/L were associated with signs of scurvy.[46]

In the Nutrition Survey National Canada,[118] a serum ascorbic acid concentration of ≥ 23 µmol/L was considered necessary for both women and men to be classified as at a low risk with respect to vitamin C status.

In the National Health and Nutrition Examination Survey (NHANES-II), only 3% of the overall population (3 to 74 years) had low plasma vitamin C concentrations.[147] However, 16% of black males 55 to 74 years of age had low plasma vitamin C concentrations.

Occurrence of Vitamin C Deficiency

Although overt scurvy is rare in industrialized countries, low plasma vitamin C concentrations are commonly noted.[177,178] In a study conducted in Finland, Scotland, and Italy; 5% of the adult men had low plasma vitamin C concentrations (e.g., below 10 µmol/L; 0.176 mg/dL).[98]

Food programs have been initiated to provide relief to refugee, displaced, or famine-affected populations. Because of inadequate levels of vitamin C and lack of diversity of food sources, outbreaks of scurvy have occurred in these populations. Cooking losses of about 70% of the vitamin C originally present enhanced the problem.[124]

Dietary Sources of Vitamin C

Vitamin C is present in relatively large amounts in most fruits, including citrus fruits, tomatoes, and strawberries, and in various vegetables including cabbage, turnip greens, broccoli, brussel sprouts; cauliflower; and green peppers. The vitamin C content of several foods is summarized in the following table.

Major Contributions (Sources) of Vitamin C in the United States Diets

Food Item	Vitamin C Content (mg/100 g)
Orange juice	50
Potatoes, baked	20
Tomatoes, fresh	24
Oranges, fresh	50
Grapefruit, fresh	38
Turnip greens, cooked	60
Coleslaw and cabbage, raw	46
Broccoli, cooked	110
Lemon juice, fresh	53
Brussel sprouts, cooked	85
Strawberries, fresh	60
Cauliflower, cooked	55
Bananas, fresh	10
Cantaloupe, fresh	33
Green pepper, raw	128
Green beans, cooked	13
Cranberry juice, canned	40
Rutabagas, cooked	26

References 10, 56–58, 60, 61.
mg/100 g $\times$ 56.8 = µmol/L.

The amount of vitamin C present in foods may vary considerably due to the influence of numerous factors.[58,59] These factors include postharvest storage, maturation, and varietal differences; cooking preparation and food handling losses.[56-59]

Vitamin C Functions and Metabolism

The chemistry, metabolism, and functions of ascorbic acid have been the subject of numerous reviews.[9-12,30,31,37,38,42,45-48,87,92,194]

During the past 25 years, numerous biological functions of ascorbic acid have been established. It has long been recognized that vitamin C has a primary role in the formation of collagen.[194] However, only more recently has its specific function in collagen synthesis been elucidated. As a result, the role of ascorbic acid in wound healing and in the formation and maintenance of cartilage, teeth, gums, bones, muscles, and skin is now appreciated.[42,87]

Thus, these vitamin C participates in the hydroxylation of lysine to hydroxylysine and hydroxylation of proline to hydroxyproline.[174,194] Vitamin C also participates in the synthesis of tyrosine, carnitine, adrenal hormones, vasoactive amines, microsomal drug metabolism, leucocyte functions, and wound healing.[87,90] As a consequence a number of enzymes have been recognized that require ascorbic acid for their maximal activity.[9,10,42,87,92,194] They include the following:

Lysine hydroxylase (EC 1.14.11.4)

Proline hydroxylase (EC 1.14.11.2)

Procollagen-proline 2-oxoglutarate 3-dioxygenase (EC 1.14.11.7)

Trimethyllysine-2-oxoglutarate dioxygenase (EC 1.14.11.8)

Dopamine β-monooxygenase (EC 1.14.17.1)

4-Hydroxyphenylpyruvate dioxygenase (EC 1.13.11.27)

γ-Butyrobetaine, 2-oxoglutarate 4-dioxygenase (EC 1.14.11.1)

Ascorbic acid is an excellent antioxidant and as a free-radical scavenger to protect cells from damage by oxidants.[157,175,194] Ascorbic acid is absorbed very efficiently from the diet.[9,24,31,103,194] Plasma concentrations of ascorbic acid are linearly related to the intake of ascorbic acid up to 140 mg/day.[29,108]

The overall half-life was calculated to be 10 to 20 days.[31,85] The body pool of ascorbic acid was approximately 20 mg/kg body weight at a plasma ascorbate concentration of 50.0 μmol/L (0.9 mg/dL).[25,77,79,195] Kallner et al.[24,25,31] found that an apparent linear relationship existed between body stores and plasma ascorbic acid concentrations. Thus, plasma ascorbic acid concentrations provide a measure of vitamin C body stores.

Oral contraceptive agents may reduce the plasma concentration of vitamin C and increase its requirement.[104,105] The effects appear variable and the significance of these observations is uncertain. Treatment of rheumatoid arthritis with aspirin may reduce the concentrations of vitamin C in plasma and platelets. Supplements of vitamin C can prevent the reduction.[106]

Proline and Hydroxyproline and Vitamin C Deficiency

The role of vitamin C in collagen metabolism has been reviewed by Berg and Kerr.[180] Collagens represent the major extracellular proteins found in the body. Collagen represents about one-third of the total body protein. Several types of collagens are present in most tissues and organs. An extensive collagen turnover occurs in the body. From 3 to 5% of the skin collagen may turn over per day. Ascorbic acid is a required cofactor for the prolyl hydroxylase in the hydroxylation of prolyl residues in the synthesis of collagen. In vitamin

C deficiency, underhydroxylated collagen is formed. This defective collegen is subject to intracellular degradation.[180,182]

The increased metabolism of collagen results in an increased urinary excretion of hydroxyproline. Hevia et al.[181] investigated the urinary excretion of hydroxyproline in 11 healthy adult males placed in a metabolic unit and fed a vitamin C-deficient diet for a period of 14 weeks. The urinary excretion of hydroxproline increased during the vitamin C deficiency period. However, the increase was not extensive. The investigators considered the effect inadequate to serve as a reliable indicator of a mild vitamin C deficiency.[181]

Potential Pharmacological Benefits of Vitamin C

The extensive consumption of vitamin C has been stimulated by claims of various benefits derived from its use. Vitamin C is the most commonly available single supplement used in the United States.[7-9,69] An intake of approximately 140 mg/day of ascorbic acid appears necessary to saturate the total body vitamin C pool.[40] Ascorbic acid has been considered the most effective antioxidant in the plasma of the human.[122,123]

The potential pharmacological use of vitamin C was the topic of an extensive review.[9] Related reviews have also been published in recent years.[11,12,19,30,42,81-87,94,112,122] Numerous potential pharmacological benefits of vitamin C have been indicated in these reviews. Evidence exists for an association of vitamin C with cataracts reduction,[42,82,83,93,119-121,196] diabetes mellitus,[9] blood pressure reduction,[89,90,97,122] lipoproteins and coronary heart disease,[30,65,88,91,122] cancer incidence,[11,12,94-96] iron metabolism,[9] Parkinson's disease,[9] respiratory symptoms,[9] immunity,[9,85,86] sickle cell anemia,[9] and asthma.[128,129,197]

Vitamin C Interactions

Vitamin C and Iron Nutrition

Ascorbic acid may enhance the availability and absorption of iron from non-heme sources.[48-54,62,63] Heme iron, provided mainly as hemoglobin and myoglobin in meats, has a high bioavailability. In most developing countries, the consumption of heme iron is low or negligible. Instead, non-heme iron is the main source of dietary iron (wheat, rice, maize, cassava, and millet). Hence, the importance of vitamin C in the diet for the enhancement of iron absorption from these foods and in the prevention of iron deficiency.[49,51]

The influence of ascorbic acid on iron absorption by the human is exemplified by the report of Davidson et al.[130] Their study was conducted with the use of stable isotopic iron (^{57}Fe and ^{58}Fe). The addition of ascorbic acid to an iron-fortified chocolate-flavored milk drink enhanced the iron absorption from 1.6 to 5.1%. The ascorbic acid was added at a level of 25 mg per serving of the chocolate-flavored milk. When 50 mg of ascorbic acid was used, iron absorption increased to 7.7%.

For the normal individual, excessive iron absorption does not appear to occur with elevated intakes of ascorbic acid.[64] However, subjects with hemochromatosis or other iron storage diseases should avoid large doses of ascorbic acid.

Vitamin C Status and Cigarette Smoking

Smokers are at an increased risk of developing atherosclerosis and cardiac ischemic disease.[13-17,28,44] An association between plasma levels of vitamin C to ischemic heart disease have been reported from a number of laboratories.[13,18-21,28,30] A number of investigators have also observed that the plasma concentration of vitamin C in smokers was lower than that of nonsmokers.[18,22-36,41,43,45,198,199] Plasma vitamin C concentrations for smokers were consistently lower than nonsmokers by about 11.4 µmol/L (0.2 mg/dL).[22,45-48] It has been estimated that smokers would need to ingest an additional 59 mg/day of vitamin C to maintain an equivalent plasma vitamin C concentration as nonsmokers.[22,29,31]

Lyhkesfeldt et al.[138] found 1.8 ± 4.2% of the total ascorbic acid was present as dehydroascorbic acid in the plasma of smokers. Only trace amounts were present in plasma of nonsmokers. Total plasma ascorbic acid levels were higher in nonsmokers, with women having higher concentrations than men. Evaluation of the vitamin C data collected in the Second National Health and Nutrition Examination Survey (NHANES-II; 1976–1980) indicated that smokers would need to consume over 200 mg of ascorbic acid per day to maintain a serum ascorbate concentrations equivalent to that of the nonsmoker meeting the Recommended Dietary Allowance (60 mg/day ascorbic acid).[32,33] Even passive smokers (i.e., chronic smoke exposure) may have reduced plasma vitamin C concentrations.[36]

Vitamin C Status and the Elderly

A number of studies have found that the plasma vitamin C concentrations are higher in elderly women than those of elderly men.[70,71,75] The differences, although not apparent, may be the result of higher intakes of vitamin C by the women. The median plasma ascorbic acid concentration increased rapidly with vitamin C intakes above 45 mg/day in both elderly males and females.[75] Jacob et al.[70] studied the vitamin C status in 677 healthy, non-institutionalized elderly people from the Boston area (60 to 98 years old). Only 6% of the males and 3% of females were found to have a marginal vitamin C status (plasma ascorbic acid concentrations of < 23 µmol/L). The mean plasma ascorbic acid concentrations were higher in women than in men.

In a controlled ascorbic acid intake experiment with healthy elderly subjects, plasma vitamin C concentrations were measured.[71] With an intake of about 80 mg/day of ascorbic acid, the women had a plasma acorbate concentration of about 56.78 µmol/L (1.0 mg/dL). In men, an intake of 60 mg/d of ascorbic acid resulted in plasma vitamin C concentrations of about 22.71 µmol/L (0.4 mg/dL). In France, a study was conducted on 756 institutionalized elderly men and women whose vitamin C status was poor.[72] Very low plasma concentrations of vitamin C were reported for 56% of the men and 41% of the women. In another study conducted in Paris, France on elderly institutionalized subjects, low plasma vitamin C concentrations were also observed.[73]

Determination of Vitamin C in Biological Specimens

Plasma Sample Preparation and Stability of Ascorbic Acid

Earlier studies demonstrated that ascorbic acid in plasma could be stabilized with the use of metaphosphoric acid. The ascorbic acid in the treated sample was stable for at least 21 days when stored at –70°C.[183] Unstabilized frozen plasma lost nearly 50% of the ascorbic acid content in 13 days.[141] Samples of freshly separated serum were stable for 6 hours under refrigeration, but were found to have a continuous loss of ascorbic acid when held at room temperature.[184]

Margolis and Davis[172] conducted extensive studies on stability of ascorbic acid in plasma. With the use of metaphosphoric acid and dithiothreitol as an antioxidant, ascorbic acid in plasma, when stored at –80°C, was stable for as long as 57 weeks. The dithiothreitol reduces any dehydroascorbic acid present to ascorbic acid permitting the measurement of total ascorbic acid in plasma.

Subsequently in an interlaboratory study,[185] total ascorbic acid (ascorbic acid plus dehydroascorbic acid) in properly prepared plasma was stable when stored at –70°C for at least 6 years. Total ascorbic acid in serum or plasma preserved with metaphosphoric acid degraded at a rate of no more than 1% per year.

Colormetric, Fluorometric, and Ultraviolet Methods

Methods that have been used to measure ascorbic acid in plasma include: 2,6-dichlorophenolindophenol color reduction (DCI),[37,115,139-141,161] dinitrophenylhydrazine procedure (DNPH),[115,173,179] O-phenylenediamine fluorometry (PDA),[37,115,142] α, α'dipyridyl complex (ADPYR),[115,139,143] ferrozine reaction (FERR),[127] ascorbic acid oxidase action,[144] and HPLC.[98,110,179,188] In a comparative study, DNPH, PDA, FERR, and HPLC provided results that were not significantly different from each other when erythorbic acid was not present in the sample.[74] HPLC analysis is suitable for samples that contain erythorbic acid.[74,99-102,109,110]

High-Performance Liquid Chromatography (HPLC)

HPLC is the method of choice for the determination of vitamin C in blood components. Over 200 publicatons have appeared on this sensitive, specific, and rapid analytical procedure. It is the procedure recommended by World Health Organization (WHO), Geneva, Switzerland. The general analytical procedure is as follows:

1. Blood samples, with EDTA added, were obtained from the subject in a fasting state. The plasma and leucocytes are immediately separated. If necessary, the leucocytes can be separated into mononuclear leucocytes (monocytes) and polymorphonuclear leucocytes (polycytes) fractions with the procedure of Schaus et al.[109] and Omaye et al.[110,111]

2. Plasma and leucocyte preparations are stablized immediately with metaphosphoric acid and held frozen at –70°C. Vitamin C samples prepared and stored in this manner are stable for at least 1 year.

3. Preparation of samples for HPLC analysis.

   a. To 100 μL plasma, 100 μL cold metaphosphoric acid (0.44 mol/L) was added, mixed, and centrifuged at 5000 × g for 5 minutes.

   b. To 50 μL of the supernatant, 950 μL of a solution containing 1.04 nmol L-cysteine/L and 0.54 mmol sodium EDTA/L was added and mixed gently.

   c. Then 20 μL of the preparation was injected onto the HPL chromatographic column.

4. The HPLC system of Kutnink et al.[99] has been a simple, reliable, specific, fast and sensitive procedure to measure both ascorbic acid and erythorbic acid in

blood samples. The procedure involves the use of a paired-ion, reversed-phase HPLC system in conjunction with amperometric detection.

D-Erythorbic acid (isoascorbic acid) is an epimer of L-ascorbic acid, but without antiscorbutic activity.[74,100] Erythorbic acid is used extensively in the United States as a food additive.[102] Items such as ham, bacon, frankfurters, beef bologna, and some soft drinks may contain 0.15 to 0.58 mg of erythorbic acid/gram.[101,102] Consequently, significant amounts of the additive are consumed in diet and may appear in the blood.[101] The HPLC procedure described above quantitates both ascorbic acid and erythorbic acid. Other nonchromatographic analytical procedures cannot distinguish between the two compounds.[74,100] Erythorbic acid clears rapidly from the body and hence, fasting morning blood samples are usually cleared of erythorbic acid.[100,101] If the samples being analyzed are known to be free of erythrobic acid, erythrobic acid may be used as an internal standard. Other quality controls are included routinely that are prepared from plasma aliquots with low, medium, or high vitamin C concentrations.

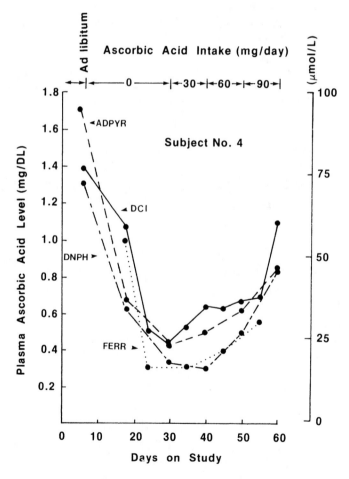

FIGURE 2
The effect of ascorbic acid intake on plasma ascorbic acid concentrations. Four different analytical methods were compared: FERR, ferrozine; DCI, dichlorophenolindophenol; ADPYR, α, α'-dipyridyl; DNPH, 2,4-dinitrophenylhydrazine.[74] (With permission.)

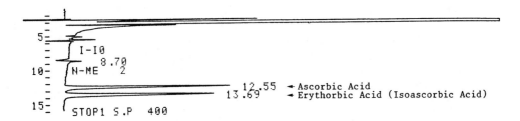

FIGURE 3

HPLC chromatogram of serum from a human subject receiving both ascorbic acid and erythorbic acid in the diet using the procedure of Kutninck et al.[99]

Any dehydroascorbic acid present in the sample may be converted to ascorbic acid by treatment of the sample with homocysteine, glutathione, cysteine, or dithiothreitol. This permits total ascorbic acid measurement by HPLC or by the FERR method.[127] The DNPH method and PDA fluorometric method can also measure total ascorbic acid. With each procedure, frozen aliquots of a stabilized control plasma can be included for ascorbic acid analysis to serve as a quality control for evaluating the validity of the analytical values.[179] Plasma samples prepared in metaphosphoric acid and held at –70°C are very stable and suitable for this purpose.[185]

Other Methods for Measuring Vitamin C in Biological Specimens

Several methods have been described for measuring ascorbic acid in blood or serum with the use of ascorbate oxidase.[144,189,190] The assay could detect in plasma about 1 μmol/L of ascorbic acid.[189] The procedure is capable of measuring both ascorbic acid and dehydroascorbic acid in plasma.[189]

HPLC with ultraviolet detection (248 to 265 nm) has been used to measure ascorbic acid human serum and urine.[192-194] A disadvantage of the ultraviolet detection methods for measuring ascorbic acid is the relatively low level of sensitivity. Washko et al.[187] used HPLC with coulometric electrochemical detection to measure ascorbic acid in biological samples. The procedure was highly sensitive and could detect less than 1 pmol of ascorbic acid. Tsao and Salimi[188] used HPLC with electrochemical detection to measure ascorbic acid concentrations in plasma and leucocytes.

Dehydroascorbic Acid

Some studies have indicated that part of the ascorbic acid in plasma and leucocytes was in the dehydroascorbic acid form.[39] Several reports indicate that about 5 to 10% of the vitamin C in leucocytes was as the oxidized form, L-dehydroascorbic acid.[135-137] In the investigation of Schaus et al.,[109] leucocyte ascorbic acid concentrations were measured by both the 2,4-dinitrophenylhydrazine method and by HPLC, with amperometric detection. With these methods, approximately 87% of the ascorbate was in the reduced state. Lee et al.[163] found less than 5% of the total ascorbic acid in plasma was present as dehydroascorbic acid. However, the presence of dehydroascorbic acid in plasma and leucocytes has been controversial since its presence has not always been observed. Hence, some consider the presence of dehydroascorbic acid may be an artifact of inappropriate specimen handling whereby vitamin C is oxidized.[71,161-164]

More recent studies indicate that little, if any, dehydroascorbic acid is present when the samples are properly handled.[109,151-153] Nevertheless, reduction of dehydroascorbic acid to asorbic acid is accomplished in tissues by GSH-dependent dehydroascorbate reductase and by NADPH-dependent selenoenzyme thioredoxin reductase. Methods are available for the measurement of dehydroascorbic acid in plasma and other blood fractions.[37,52,71,138,152,161-171,187] However, the HPLC methods with an amperometric detector measures total ascorbic acid.[99] This is accomplished with the use of a reducing agent in the sample preparation (i.e., cysteine, dithiothreitol).[100,172]

Assessment of Vitamin C Status

Assessment of vitamin C status can be performed only by static measurements of plasma and leucocyte ascorbic acid concentrations. Functional methods are not available. The measurement of the body pool size of ascorbic acid would provide meaningful information as to status but these procedures can be considered only in special research situations. Controlled vitamin C depletion and repletion studies have provided relationships of plasma and leucocyte ascorbic acid concentrations and dietary vitamin C intakes and to the occurrence of clinical manifestations of a vitamin C deficiency.

Plasma or serum ascorbic acid concentrations are considered more reflective of recent intakes of ascorbic acid than of body stores.[158] Blood leucocyte ascorbic acid concentrations are more reflective of tissue stores of ascorbic acid.[159,160] The body pool of vitamin C can be depleted rather rapidly when subjects are maintained on a vitamin C-deficient diet.[77,79] Within one month, plasma ascorbic acid concentrations decreased to $10.2 \pm 2.3\,\mu mol/L$ with scorbutic-type changes occurring.[74,76] In men, plasma ascorbic acid concentrations of < 23 $\mu mol/L$ (0.40 mg/dL) have been considered to indicate a marginal vitamin C status.[40,118]

Various analytical procedures have been used to measure ascorbic acid concentrations in blood components.[10,37,38,74,109,110,113,115,117] Without the availability of a suitable functional biochemical procedure that relates to vitamin C status, information concerning inadequacies in this nutrient has been derived mainly from measuring concentrations of ascorbic acid in serum, blood, erythrocytes, leucocytes, and urine.[112,113,115]

The biochemical evaluation of vitamin C status in the human has been conducted usually through the determination of serum (plasma) ascorbate concentrations.[179] Within a relatively limited range, serum (plasma) concentrations of ascorbic acid show a linear relationship with the intake of vitamin C.[186] In controlled human studies, a deprivation of vitamin C resulted in a rapid decrease in the plasma ascorbic acid concentrations.[74,76-79,100] With a given intake of the vitamin, the plasma ascorbic acid concentration will plateau at a given level.[74,76,100] The maximum plasma ascorbic acid concentration appears to be about 1.6 mg/dL at which point renal clearance of the vitamin rises abruptly.[114] However, higher plasma ascorbic acid concentration can be attained temporarily following the ingestion of a large dose of the vitamin.

Hodges et al.[76,77] conducted a study with adult men receiving controlled intakes of ascorbic acid and with their body pools of ascorbic acid labeled with isotopic ascorbic acid. They observed that plasma or serum and whole blood concentrations of vitamin C fell rapidly with a diet free of ascorbic acid.[76,77] Plasma ascorbic acid fell to concentrations lower than those of whole blood. Ascorbic acid disappeared from the urine early in depletion.

The first signs of scurvy appeared when the plasma ascorbic acid level ranged from 7 to 14 $\mu mol/L$ (0.13 to 0.24 mg/dL), and the pool size had been depleted to a range of 96 to 490

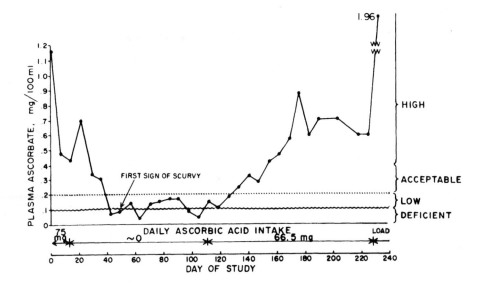

FIGURE 4

The influence of ascorbic acid intake on the plasma ascorbic acid concentrations of adult men maintained in a metabolic unit.[76,77] (With permission.)

mg from an average initial pool of 1,500 mg.[76-79] There was also a definite relationship between whole blood ascorbic acid values and the body reserves of the vitamin. Signs of scurvy appeared when the whole blood ascorbate concentration fell below 17 μmol/L (0.30 mg/dL). Nevertheless, low serum concentrations of ascorbic acid (<0.30 mg/dL) do indicate low or inadequate intakes of the vitamin with only partial reserves present. For maximum saturated body reserves or pools of ascorbic acid, higher intakes of vitamin C are required (> 100 mg/day) which will be reflected in serum ascorbic acid concentrations in excess of 1.0 mg/dL.

Sauberlich et al.[74] studied the metabolism and requirement of adult women maintained in a metabolic unit and fed a formula diet that provided controlled amounts of ascorbic acid. After 24 days of vitamin C depletion, the subjects received increasing supplements of ascorbic acid. Plasma ascorbic acid concentrations were determined in plasma, red cells, whole blood, and leucocytes.[74] The depletion period resulted in a marked decrease in ascorbic acid in all blood indices. During the study scorbutic signs developed in some of the subjects. When this occurred, plasma vitamin C concentrations were 10.2 μmol/L. The effects of ascorbic acid depletion and repletion on the whole blood ascorbic acid concentrations were very similar to those observed for plasma ascorbic acid in the same subjects.[74] However, the whole blood ascorbic acid concentrations were somewhat higher than those obtained for the plasma samples, probably a reflection of the generally higher concentrations of ascorbic acid observed for red blood cells.[40,74,76] In this study, the whole blood ascorbic acid concentrations of the subjects was 18 ± 3 μmol/L with an intake of 30 mg/day of ascorbic acid. Whole blood ascorbic acid concentrations of less than 20 μmol/L may be associated with signs of scurvy.[74,76,139]

The measurement of the ascorbic acid concentrations in whole blood or red blood cells appeared to provide no advantage over plasma ascorbic acid measurements for evaluating vitamin C status. Moreover, the measurement of ascorbic acid in red cell or whole blood is somewhat more difficult. Similarly, the concentrations of ascorbic acid in leucocytes are affected by ascorbic acid depletion and repletion in a manner similar to that observed for plasma ascorbic acid.[74] Hence, the leucocytes ascorbic acid concentrations did not appear

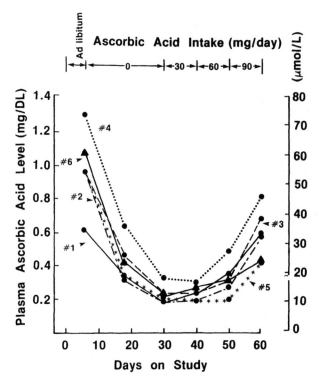

FIGURE 5
The effect of ascorbic acid intake on the plasma ascorbic acid concentrations of adult women.[74] (With permission.)

to be anymore sensitive or responsive than plasma ascorbate concentrations to changes in dietary ascorbic acid. Moreover, the procedure to measure leucocyte ascorbic acid concentrations is more tedious to perform.[38,40] Leucocyte ascorbic acid concentrations may be expressed in 10^8 cells, mL of sample, DNA level, or unit of protein. Hence, it has been difficult to make comparisons between laboratories or to establish guidelines regarding vitamin C status.

Smith and Hodges[29] found a positive linear relationship between vitamin C dietary intake and mean serum level for each intake range when intake was below 140 mg/day for nonsupplemented nonsmokers. Little risk of vitamin C deficiency exists with plasma ascorbic acid concentrations of 34 μmol/L (0.60 mg/dL). For the adult, a daily intake of 60 mg of vitamin C can maintain this plasma concentration of the vitamin. Signs of a vitamin C deficiency were observed in young women when their plasma concentrations of ascorbic acid fell below 17 μmol/L (0.30 mg/dL).[74] Ascorbic acid supplements of 30 mg/day for 10 days failed to increase plasma ascorbate concentrations (10 to 11 μmol/L); 60 mg/day for 10 days produced a small increase (13 to 15 μmol/L); 90 mg/day intake resulted in a mean ascorbic acid concentration of 29 μmol/L.[74]

Vitamin C Concentrations in Whole Blood, Red Cells and Leucocytes and Plasma

Controlled human studies have been useful to investigate the relationship of ascorbic acid intake to ascorbic acid concentrations in blood components and to the occurrence of clinical manifestation of vitamin C deficiency.[24,25,38,40,74,76–79,100,110,111,113,140]

Whole Blood and Red Blood Cells Ascorbic Acid

Whole blood ascorbic acid concentrations obtained in the ascorbate study with adult women[74] are presented in Figure 6. The effects of ascorbic acid depletion and repletion on the whole blood concentrations were very similar to those observed for plasma ascorbic acid in the same subjects. However, the whole blood ascorbic acid concentrations were somewhat higher than those obtained for the plasma samples and probably reflect the generally higher concentrations of ascorbic acid observed for the red blood cells (see Table 3). The ascorbic acid concentrations of whole blood and red blood cells appeared to reflect the vitamin C status of the subject. As noted previously, whole blood and red blood cell ascorbic acid measurements do not appear to be superior to plasma ascorbic acid measurements for evaluating vitamin C status.[116,117] Ascorbic acid can be analyzed in whole blood and red blood cells with the use of the DNPH method.[115] The measurement of ascorbic acid in whole blood and red blood cells is more difficult than in plasma.

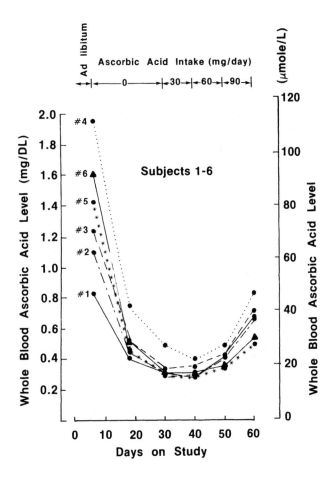

FIGURE 6
Ascorbic acid concentrations in whole blood obtained from adult women maintained on controlled intakes of ascorbic acid. Analyses were performed using the 2,4-dinitrophenylhydrazine method.[74] (With permission.)

Plasma and Leucocyte Vitamin C Concentration

In the past, the measurement of ascorbic acid in leucocytes was time-consuming, cumbersome, frequently inaccurate, and required a relatively large blood sample.[140] However,

TABLE 3
Guidelines for the Interpretation of Vitamin C Biochemical Data (All Ages)

1. Population Surveys

| | Serum Ascorbic Acid | | | |
| | Deficient (High Risk) μmol/L | Low (Moderate Risk) μmol/L | Acceptable (Low Risk) μmol/L | |
Survey				References
NHANES -II (all ages)	< 11	11–23	> 23	32
ICNND (all ages)	< 5.7	5.7–11	> 11	117,126,140
Ten-State (all ages)	< 5.7	5.7–11	> 11	117,126,140,200
Canada Nutrition Survey				118,140
0–19 years (M–F)	< 11	11–34	> 34	
20+ years (M–F)	< 11	11–23	> 23	

2. Guidelines Suggested by Jacob [38,126]

| | Plasma | | Leucocytes | |
Status	μmol/L	μg/mL	nmol/10⁸ cells	μg/10⁸ cells
Deficient	< 11.4	< 2.0	< 57	< 10
Low	11.4–23	2–4	57–114	10–20
Adequate	> 23	> 4.0	> 114	> 20

3. Other Suggested Guidelines*

| | Plasma/Serum | | Whole Blood | |
Status	μmol/L	μg/mL	μmol/L	μg/mL
Deficient	< 11	< 2.0	< 17	< 3.0
Low	11–18	2–3.2	17–28	3.0–4.9
Acceptable	> 18	> 3.2	> 28	≥ 5.0

4. Leucocyte Ascorbic Acid Concentrations in Normal Women

Analytical Method	Concentrations	References
DNPH	90 nmol/10⁸ cells (mean; n = 11 women)	74
DNPH	102 nmol/10⁸ cells (mean; n = 6 women)	109
HPLC	99 nmol/10⁸ cells (mean; n = 6 women)	109

NHANES-II = National Health and Nutrition Examination Survey-II.
ICNND = Interdepartmental Committee on Nutrition for National Defense.
* References: 74, 126, 140.

despite these problems, various procedures for the isolation of plasma leucocytes and platelets have been utilized.[40,109-111,134,135,145-147,149,150,155,156] The ascorbic acid concentrations in the leucocytes decreased with ascorbate depletion and paralleled that observed for plasma ascorbic acid.[74] Leucocyte ascorbic acid concentrations decreased approximately 33% with the 24 days of depletion (Figure 7).[74] The initial mean leucocyte ascorbic acid concentration for the 11 women was 90 nmol/10⁸ cells (Table 4). Schaus et al.[109] reported 102 nmol/10⁸ cells for 6 women. For these adult women, leucocyte ascorbic acid measurements did not appear to be anymore sensitive or responsive than plasma to changes in dietary ascorbic acid intakes. Leucocyte ascorbic acid concentrations of about 50 nmol/10⁸ cells were associated with the occurrence of scorbutic-type changes.

Lee et al.[145] measured ascorbic acid concentrations in plasma, mononuclear leucocytes, and polymorphonuclear leucocytes. The separations were accomplished with the use of Ficoll/Plaque variable-density solutions. No more than 2 mL of whole blood were required. The ascorbic acid concentrations were determined by high performance liquid chromatography and amperometric detection.[154]

Normal subjects were found to have ascorbic acid concentrations in the mononuclear leucocytes of 0.3 to 0.6 mmol/L (1.0 to 2.0 mg/g protein).[145] This was ten-fold the ascorbic

TABLE 4

Relationship of Dietary Intakes of Ascorbic Acid to Plasma and Leucocyte
Ascorbate Concentrations[74]

Days Subjects in Study	Dietary Ascorbic Acid Intakes (Mg/d)	Ascorbic Acid Concentrations		
		Plasma		Leucocytes
		PDA Method (μmol/L)	HPLC Method (μmol/L)	HPLC Method (μmol/10^8 cells)
6	Ad libitum	63.1 ± 21.6	63.0 ± 19.9	90 ± 11
18	0	26.7 ± 9.7	21.6 ± 7.9	66 ± 13
30	0	10.2 ± 2.3	10.2 ± 2.8	60 ± 14
40	30	10.2 ± 3.4	10.8 ± 2.8	58 ± 8
50	60	14.8 ± 5.7	13.1 ± 4.0	70 ± 11
60	90	32.9 ± 10.8	29.0 ± 8.0	76 ± 14

χ ± SD.
Measured by HPLC (99) or PDA methods (115).

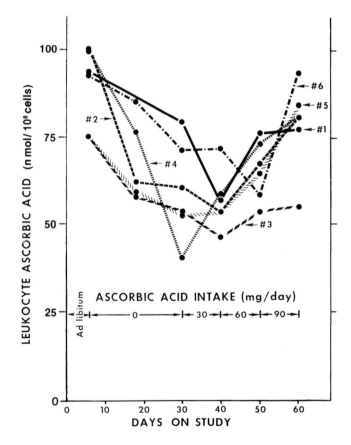

FIGURE 7

The effect of ascorbic acid intake on the leucocyte ascorbic acid concentrations of adult women.[74] (With permission.)

acid concentration of serum and twice that in polymorphonuclear leucocytes. They noted
that both mononuclear and polymorphonuclear leucocytes were saturated with ascorbic
acid at 2.5 and 1.2 mg/g of protein, respectively. With hospitalized patients, 60% had very
low ascorbic acid concentrations in serum and leucocytes. Their mean serum concentrations of ascorbic acid were 1.67 mg/L (reference mean 7.0 mg/L), while their mononuclear

and polynuclear leucocytes had mean ascorbic acid concentrations of 1.02 and 0.40 mg/g protein, respectively.

In another study, young women were fed diets that provided only 10 mg of ascorbic acid per day. After 30 days on these diets, their plasma ascorbic acid concentrations had fallen from an original mean 25.4 μmol/L to a mean of 8.0 ± 2.5 μmol/L.[100] During this period of time, the ascorbic acid concentrations in the mononuclear leucocytes (monocytes) of these young women fell from 13.3 ± 3.2 mmol/g protein to 10.2 ± 3.1 mmol/g protein.[100] The ascorbic acid concentrations in the polymorphonuclear leucocytes (polycytes) remained constant at a level of 2.2 ± 1.2 mmol/g protein.[100] The leucocytes were isolated and separated into mononuclear leucocytes and polymorphonuclear leucocytes by the procedure of Schaus et al.[109] and Omaye et al.[110,111]

Comparable differences in ascorbic acid concentrations between mononuclear leucocytes and polymorphonuclear leucocytes were found by Omaye et al.[110] They reported for their study of 6 young men mean ascorbic acid concentrations of the following:

Polymorphonuclear leucocytes (μg/10^8 cells)	2.97 ± 1.78
Mononuclear leucocytes (μg/10^8 cells)	15.8 ± 6.44
Platelets (μg/10^8 cells)	0.253 ± 0.054
Plasma (mg/dL)	0.98 ± 0.36
Plasma (μmol/L)	55.7 ± 2.0

Other investigators have reported platelet ascorbic acid concentration of 0.03 ± 0.013 μmol/L/10^8 cells.[135,156] Jacob et al.[40] concluded from a controlled vitamin C diet study on eleven young men that plasma, erythrocyte, and leucocyte ascorbic acid concentrations all reflected ascorbic acid intakes. Plasma ascorbic acid concentrations of < 22.7 μmol/L (< 0.4 mg/dL) reflected reliably low ascorbic acid intakes. Plasma ascorbic acid concentrations showed less variability than erythrocyte ascorbic acid concentrations and were considerably easier to determine than leucocyte ascorbic acid concentrations.

In another study, Jacob et al.[148] reported that in individuals plasma ascorbic acid concentrations correlated strongly with lymphocyte ascorbic acid concentrations. These findings are in agreement with the observations of Sauberlich et al.[74] whose subjects were young women. Blanchard et al.[150] found in their study with women that the average plasma ascorbic acid concentration was reflected in changes in the mean mononuclear leucocytes ascorbic acid concentrations. But for an individual, plasma levels of ascorbic acid were not considered reliable for predicting the mononuclear or polymorphonuclear leucocytes ascorbic acid concentrations. Ikeda[146] has made comparable measurements of the ascorbic acid concentrations in cellular fractions.

Urinary Excretion of Vitamin C

Ascorbic acid is rapidly and efficiently absorbed. Excess ascorbic acid is cleared rapidly from the body by excretion into the urine. Urinary excretion of ascorbic acid declines rapidly to undetectable levels when a subject is placed on a vitamin C-deficient diet.[78,79,100] In fact, when the body pool size of ascorbic acid drops to only slightly below normal, the urinary excretion of ascorbic acid ceases. Consequently, the measurement of urinary levels of ascorbic acid has limited value. Urinary ascorbic acid levels often reflect recent dietary intakes of the vitamin. A saturation or loading test of ascorbic acid can provide information on the vitamin C body pool size and thus may provide diagnostic guidance.[115,133,134] This test is useful for evaluating vitamin C status of an individual, but not practical for use in nutrition surveys.

Potential New Assessment Methods

Studies with the guinea pig have indicated that methacetin metabolism is related to the vitamin C status.[131] It has been suggested that a vitamin C functional breath test could be developed for evaluating vitamin C status in the human based on the participation of ascorbic acid in the metabolism of methacetin.[132] A preliminary study was not successful.[132]

Vitamin C Toxicity and Safety

Numerous reviews have considered the safety of high intakes of ascorbic acid.[48,65,66] Ascorbic acid is probably the most effective and least toxic antioxidant found in the human body. Reports on the safety of vitamin C up until 1993 were reviewed by Bendich and Langseth.[66] Subsequent reports up to 1996 were evaluated in depth by Bendich.[65] From the examined literature, it was concluded that vitamin C was safe at an intake level ten times the current U.S. Recommended Dietary Allowance of 60 mg.[65] Ascorbic acid is readily absorbed by the body, normally 80 to 90% of the vitamin C in the diet. However, when the body pool of vitamin C is saturated, the excess absorbed ascorbic acid is either metabolized or excreted into the urine. The upper limit of plasma ascorbic acid concentrations has been considered to be 1.69 mg/dL for females and 1.68 mg/dL for males. This would indicate that the renal threshold for ascorbic acid is the same for males and females.[1,2]

Earlier reports of adverse effects from the ingestion of elevated amounts of ascorbic acid have not been substantiated.[67,68,107] Rather, subjects with higher intakes of vitamin C have a lower risk for cancer or cardiovascular disease and other diseases.[9,11,12,18,30,65] Ascorbic acid intakes of up to 10 g/day for up to 3 years have been without any observed adverse side effects in clinical trials.[66] Earlier studies reported that high doses of ascorbic acid (> 4 g/day) resulted in an elevation of urinary oxalate.[80] Subsequent investigations established that the apparent increased urinary oxalate associated with an increased ascorbic acid intake can be the result of oxalate production during the analytical procedure.[80]

Summary

In comparison with measurements of ascorbic acid in leucocytes, red blood cells, or whole blood, plasma ascorbic acid analysis remains the most feasible procedure for evaluating vitamin C nutritional status in individuals or population groups. The preferred method of ascorbic acid analysis utilizes HPLC with either amperometric or electrochemical detection. In conjunction with an automatic sampler, large numbers of samples can be quickly analyzed. leucocyte concentrations of ascorbic acid can provide information about the body stores of the vitamin, but the measurement is technically difficult to perform.

Standardized methods and suitable guidelines for the interpretation of data need further development. Nevertheless, correlations have been observed between the ascorbic acid concentrations in plasma (serum) or whole blood and the concentrations in leucocytes.

References

1. Garry, P. J., Goodwin, J. S., Hunt, W. C., and Gilbert, B. A., Nutritional status in a healthy elderly population: vitamin C, *Am. J. Clin. Nutr.*, 36, 332, 1982.
2. Garry, P. J. and Hunt, W. C., Letter to the editor, *Am. J. Clin. Nutr.*, 37, 332, 1983.
3. Sauberlich, H. E., A history of scurvy and vitamin C, in *Vitamin C in Health and Disease*, Packer, L. and Fuchs, J., Eds., Marcel Dekker, New York, 1997, 1.
4. Carpenter, K. J., *The History of Scurvy and Vitamin C*, Cambridge University Press, Cambridge, 1986.
5. Stare, F. J. and Stare, I. M., Charles Glen King, 1896–1988, *J. Nutr.*, 118, 1272, 1988.
6. Jukes, T. H., The identification of vitamin C: a historical summary, *J. Nutr.*, 118, 1290, 1988.
7. Park, Y. K., Kim, I., and Yetley, E. A., Characteristics of vitamin and mineral supplement products in the United States, *Am. J. Clin. Nutr.*, 54, 750, 1991.
8. Subar, A. F. and Block, G., Use of vitamin and mineral supplements: demographics and amounts of nutrient consumed, *Am. J. Epidemiol.*, 132, 1091, 1990.
9. Sauberlich, H. E., Pharmacology of vitamin C, *Annu. Rev. Nutr.*, 14, 371, 1994.
10. Sauberlich, H. E., Ascorbic acid, in *Present Knowledge in Nutrition*, Brown, M. L., Ed., 6th edition, International Life Science Institute, Washington D.C., 1990, 132.
11. Sauberlich, H. E., Evaluation of publicly available scientific evidence regarding certain nutrient-disease relationship: 8B. *Vitamin C and Cancer*, Life Sciences Research Office, Bethesda, MD, *Fed. Am. Soc. Exp. Biol.*, 1991, 53.
12. Sauberlich, H. E., Vitamin C and cancer, in *Nutrition and Disease Update: Cancer*, Kritchevsky, D. and Carroll, K., Eds., chap. 3, *J. Am. Oil Chem. Soc.*, 1994, 61.
13. Mezzetti, A., Lapenna, D., Pierdomenico, S. D., Calafiore, A. M., Constantini, F., Riario-Sforza, G., Imbastaro, T., Neri, M., and Cuccurullo, F., Vitamins E, C, and lipid peroxidation in plasma and arterial tissue of smokers and non-smokers, *Atherosclerosis*, 112, 91, 1995.
14. Duthie, G. G., Arthur, J. B., and Beattie, J. A., et al., Cigarette smoking, antioxidants, lipid peroxidation, and coronary heart disease, *Ann. N.Y. Acad. Sci.*, 686, 120, 1993.
15. Ball, K. and Turner, R., Smoking and the heart: the basis for action, *Lancet*, 2, 822, 1974.
16. Kannel, W. B., Update on the role of cigarette smoking in coronary artery disease, *Am. Heart J.*, 101, 319, 1981.
17. Lakier, J. B., Smoking and cardiovascular disease, *Am. J. Med.*, 93, 88, 1992.
18. Gey, K. F., Stahelin, H. B., Puska, P., and Evans, A., Relationship of plasma level of vitmain C to mortality from ischemic heart disease, *Ann. N.Y. Acad. Sci.*, 498, 110, 1987.
19. Frei, B., Vitamin C as an antiatherogen: mechanisms of action, in *Vitamin C in Health and Disease*, Packer, L. and Fuchs, J., Eds., Marcel Dekker, New York, 1997, 163.
20. Jialal, I. and Grundy, S. M., Influence of antioxidant vitamins on LDL oxidation, *Ann. N.Y. Acad. Sci.*, 669, 237, 1992.
21. Gaziano, M. M., Manson, J. E., Buring J. E., and Hennekens, C. H., Dietary antioxidants and cardiovascular disease, *Ann. N.Y. Acad. Sci.*, 669, 249, 1992.
22. Smith, J. L. and Hodges, R. E., Serum levels of vitamin C in relation to dietary and supplemental intake of vitamin C in smokers and nonsmokers, *Ann. N.Y. Acad. Sci.*, 498, 144, 1987.
23. Norkus, E. P., Hsu, H., and Cehelsky, M. R., Effect of cigarette smoking on the vitamin C status of pregnant women and their offspring, *Ann. N.Y. Acad. Sci.*, 498, 500, 1987.
24. Kallner, A., Requirement for vitamin C based on metabolic studies, *Ann. N.Y. Acad. Sci.*, 498, 418, 1987.

25. Kallner, A. B., Hartman, D., and Hornig, D. H., On the requirement of ascorbic acid in man: steady-state turnover and body pool in smokers, *Am. J. Clin. Nutr.*, 34, 1347, 1981.

26. Pelletier, O., Vitamin C status of cigarette smokers and non-smokers, *Am. J. Clin. Nutr.*, 23, 520, 1970.

27. Jarvinen, R. and Knekt, P., Vitamin C, smoking, and alcohol consumption, in *Vitamin C in Health and Disease*, Packer, L. and Fuchs, J., Eds., Marcel Dekker, New York, 1997, 425.

28. Salonen, J. T., Nyyssonen, K., and Parviaminen, M. T., Vitamin C, lipid peroxidation, and the risk of myocardia infarction: epidemiological evidence from Eastern Finland, in *Vitamin C in Health and Disease*, Packer, L. and Fuchs, J., Eds., Marcel Dekker, New York, 1997, 457.

29. Smith, J. L. and Hodges, R. E., Serum levels of vitamin C in relation to dietary and supplemental intake of this vitamin by smokers and non-smokers (personal communication).

30. Simon, J. A., Vitamin C and cardiovascular disease: a review, *J. Am. Coll. Nutr.*, 11, 107, 1992.

31. Kallner, A., Hornig, D., and Hartman, D., Kinetics of ascorbic acid in humans, in *Ascorbic Acid: Chemistry, Metabolism and Uses*, Seib, P. A. and Tolbert, B. M., Eds., Advances in Chemistry Series, No. 200, American Chemical Society, Washington D.C., 1982, 335.

32. Schectman, G., Byrd, J. C., and Hoffman, R., Ascorbic acid requirements for smokers: analysis of a population survey, *Am. J. Clin. Nutr.*, 53, 1466, 1991.

33. Schectman, G., Byrd, J. C., and Gruchow, H. W., The influence of smoking on vitamin C status in adults, *Am. J. Public Health*, 79, 158, 1989.

34. Anderson, R., Assessment of the roles of vitamin C, vitamin E, and β-carotene in the modulation of oxidant stress mediated by cigarette smoke-activated phagocytes, *Am. J. Clin. Nutr.*, 53, 358S, 1991.

35. Pamuk, E. R., Byers, T., Coates, R. J., Vann, J. W., Sowell, A. L., Gunter, E. W., and Glass, D., Effect of smoking on serum nutrient concentrations in African-American women, *Am. J. Clin. Nutr.*, 59, 891, 1994.

36. Tribble, D. L., Giuliano, L. J., and Fortmann, S. P., Reduced plasma ascorbic acid concentrations in non-smokers regularly exposed to environmental tobacco smoke, *Am. J. Clin. Nutr.*, 58, 886, 1993.

37. Sauberlich, H. E., Green, M. D., and Omaye, S. T., Determination of ascorbic acid and dehydroascorbic acid, in *Ascorbic Acid: Chemistry, Metabolism, and Uses*, Seib, P. A., and Tolbert, B. M., Eds., Advances in Chemistry Series, No. 200, American Chemical Society, Washington D.C., 1982, 199.

38. Jacob, R. A., Vitamin C, in *Modern Nutrition in Health and Disease*, Shils, M. E., Olson, J. A., and Shike, M., Eds., 8th edition, Lea & Febiger, Philadelphia, 1994, 432.

39. Jacob, R. A., Assessment of human vitamin C status, *J. Nutr.*, 120, 1480, 1990.

40. Jacob, R. A., Skala, J. H., and Omaye, S. T., Biochemical indices of human vitamin C status, *Am. J. Clin. Nutr.*, 46, 818, 1987.

41. Benton, D., Haller, J., and Fordy, J., The vitamin status of young British adults, *Int. J. Vit. Nutr. Res.*, 67, 34, 1997.

42. England, S. and Seifter, S., The biochemical functions of ascorbic acid, *Annu. Rev. Nutr.*, 6, 365, 1986.

43. Chow, C. K., Vitamin C and cigarette smoke exposure, in *Vitamin C in Health and Disease*, Packer, L. and Fuchs, J., Eds., Marcel Dekker, New York, 1997, 413.

44. Eiserich, J. P., Cross, C. E., and van der, Vliet, A., Nitrogen oxides are important contributors to cigarette smoke-induced ascorbate oxidation, in *Vitamin C in Health and Disease*, Packer, L. and Fuchs, J., Eds., Marcel Dekker, New York, 1997, 399.

45. Horning, D. H. and Glatthaar, B. E., Vitamin C and smoking: increased requirements of smokers, *Int. J. Vit. Nutr. Res.*, (Suppl.) 27, 139, 1985.

46. Ball, G. F. M., *Water-Soluble Vitamin Assays in Human Nutrition*, Chapman & Hall, New York, 1994, 416.

47. Ball, G. F. M., *Bioavailability and Analysis of Vitamins in Foods*, Chapman & Hall, New York, 1998, 569.

48. Horning, D. H., Moser, U., and Glatthaar, B. E., Ascorbic acid, in *Modern Nutrition in Health and Disease*, Shils, M. E. and Young, V. R., Eds., 7th edition, Lea & Febiger, Philadelphia, 1988, 417.

49. Hallberg, L., The role of vitamin C in improving the critical iron balance situation in women, *Int. J. Vit. Nutr. Res.*, 27 (Suppl.), 177, 1985.
50. Hallberg, L., Bioavailability of dietary iron in man, *Annu. Rev. Nutr.*, 1, 123, 1981.
51. Gershoff, S. N., Vitamin C (ascorbic acid): new roles, new requirements, *Nutr. Revs.*, 51, 313, 1993.
52. Monsen, E. R., Iron nutrition and absorption: dietary factors which impart iron bioavailability, *J. Am. Diet. Assoc.*, 88, 786, 1988.
53. Hallberg, L., Brune, M., Rossander-Hulthen, L., Is there a physiological role of vitamin C in iron absorption? *Ann. N.Y. Acad. Sci.*, 498, 324, 1987.
54. Hunt, J. R., Gallagher, S. K., and Johnson, L. K., Effect of ascorbic acid on apparent iron absorption by women with low iron stores, *Am. J. Clin. Nutr.*, 59, 1381, 1994.
55. Horning, D., Metabolism and requirements of ascorbic acid in man, *S. Afr. Med. J.*, 60, 818, 1981.
56. Leveille, G. A., Zabik, M. E., and Morgan, K. J., *Nutrients In Foods, The Nutrition Guild*, Cambridge, U.K., 1983, 291.
57. Bauernfeind, J. C., Ascorbic acid technology in agricultural, pharmaceutical, food, and industrial applications, in *Ascorbic Acid: Chemistry, Metabolism, and Uses*, Seib, P. A. and Tolbert, B. M., Eds., Advances in Chemistry Series, No. 200, American Chemical Society, Washington D.C., 1982, 395.
58. Erdman, J. W., Jr. and Klein, B. P., Harvesting, processing, and cooking influences on vitamin C in foods, in *Ascorbic Acid: Chemistry, Metabolism, and Uses*, Seib, P. A. and Tolbert, B. M., Eds., Advances in Chemistry Series, No. 200, American Chemical Society, Washington D.C., 1982, 499.
59. Vanderslice, J. T. and Higgs, D. J., Vitamin C content of foods: sample variability, *Am. J. Clin. Nutr.*, 54, 1323S, 1991.
60. Paul, A. A. and Southgate, D. A. T., McCance and Widdowson's, *The Composition of Foods*, Elsevier/North-Holland, New York, 1978, 418.
61. Handbook No. 8 Series, United States Department of Agriculture, Agricultural Research Service, U.S. Government Printing Office, Washington D.C.
62. Hunt, J. R., Mullen, L. M., Lykken, G. I., Gallager, S. K., and Nielsen, F. H., Ascorbic acid: effect on ongoing iron absorption and status in iron-depleted young women, *Am. J. Clin. Nutr.*, 51, 649, 1990.
63. Hallberg, L., Brune, M., and Rossander, L., The role of vitamin C in iron absorption, in *Elevated Dosages of Vitamins: Benefits and Hazards*, Walter, P., Brubacher, G. and Stahelin, H., Eds., Hans Huber Publication, Toronto, Canada, 1989, 103.
64. Bendich, A. and Cohen, M., Ascorbic acid safety: analysis of factors affecting iron absorption, *Toxicol. Lett.*, 51, 189, 1990.
65. Bendich, A., Vitamin C safety in humans, in *Vitamin C in Health and Disease*, Packer, L. and Fuchs, J., Eds., Marcel Dekker, New York, 1997, 367.
66. Bendich, A. and Langseth, L., The health effects of vitamin C supplementation: a review, *J. Am. Coll. Nutr.*, 14, 124, 1995.
67. Hathcock, J. N., Vitamins and minerals: efficacy and safety, *Am. J. Clin. Nutr.*, 66, 427, 1997.
68. Marks, J., *Vitamin Safety*, Human Nutrition and Health Pharma Industry Unit, F. Hoffmann-La Roche and Company, Basle, Switzerland, 1989, 25.
69. Bendich, A., Safety issues regarding the use of vitamin supplements, *Ann. N.Y. Acad. Sci.*, 669, 300, 1992.
70. Jacob, R. A., Otradovec, C. L., Russell, R. M., Munro, H. N., Hartz, S. C., McGandy, R. B., Morrow, F. D., and Sadowski, J. A., Vitamin C status and nutrient interactions in a healthy elderly population, *Am. J. Clin. Nutr.*, 48, 1436, 1988.
71. VanderJagt, D. J., Garry, P. J., and Bhagavan, H. N., Ascorbic acid intake and plasma levels in healthy elderly people, *Am. J. Clin. Nutr.*, 46, 290, 1987.
72. Monget, A. L., Galan, P., Preziosi, P., Keller, H., Bourgeois, C., Amaud, J., and Hercherg, S., Micronutrient status of elderly people, *Int. J. Vit. Nutr. Res.*, 66, 71, 1996.
73. Birlouez-Argon, I., Girard, F., Ravelontscheno, L., Bourgeois, C., Belliot, J. –P., and Abitbol, G., Comparison of two levels of vitamin C supplementation on antioxidant vitamin status in elderly institutionalized subjects, *Int. J. Vit. Nutr. Res.*, 65, 261, 1995.

74. Sauberlich, H. E., Kretsch, M. J., Taylor, P. C., Johnson, H. L., and Skala, J. H., Ascorbic acid and erythorbic acid metabolism in nonpregnant women, *Am. J. Clin. Nutr.*, 50, 1039, 1989.

75. Garry, P. J., VanderJagt, D. J., and Hunt, W. C., Ascorbic acid intakes and plasma levels in healthy elderly, *Ann. N.Y. Acad. Sci.*, 498, 90, 1987.

76. Hodges, R. E., Hood, J., Canham, J. E., Sauberlich, H. E., and Baker, E. M., Clinical manifestations of ascorbic acid deficiency in man, *Am. J. Clin. Nutr.*, 24, 432, 1971.

77. Baker, E. M., Hodges, R. E., Hood, J., Sauberlich, H. E., March, S. C., and Canham, J. E., Metabolism of ^{14}C- and ^{3}H-labeled L-ascorbic acid in human scurvy, *Am. J. Clin. Nutr.*, 24, 444, 1971.

78. Hodges, R. E., Baker, E. M., Hood, J., Sauberlich, H. E., and March, S. C., Experimental scurvy in man, *Am. J. Clin. Nutr.*, 22, 535, 1969.

79. Baker, E. M., Hodges, R. E., Hood, J., Sauberlich, H. E., and March, S. C., Metabolism of ascorbic -1-^{14}C acid in experimental human scurvy, *Am. J. Clin. Nutr.*, 22, 549, 1969.

80. Wandzilak, T. R., D'Andre, S. D., Davis, P. A., and Williams, H. E., Effect of high dose vitamin C on urinary oxalate levels, *J. Urol.*, 151, 834, 1994.

81. Bendich, A., Machlin, L. J., Scandurra, O., Burton, G. W., and Wayner, D. M., The antioxidant role of vitamin C, *Adv. Free-Radical Biol. Med.*, 2, 419, 1986.

82. Bunce, G. E., Nutritional factors in cataract, *Annu. Rev. Nutr.*, 10, 233, 1990.

83. Taylor, A., Role of nutrients in delaying cataracts, *Ann. N.Y. Acad. Sci.*, 669, 111, 1992.

84. Gaby, S. K. and Singh, V. N., Vitamin C, in *Vitamin Intake and Health: A Scientific Review*, Gaby, S. K., Bendich, A., Singh, V. N., and Machlin, L. J., Eds., Marcel Dekker, New York, 1991, 103.

85. Gross, R. L. and Newberne, P. M., Role of nutrition in immunologic functions, *Physiol. Rev.*, 60, 188, 1980.

86. Hemila, H., Vitamin C and the common cold, *Br. J. Nutr.*, 67, 3, 1992.

87. Padh, H., Vitamin C newer insight into its biochemical functions, *Nutr. Revs.*, 49, 65, 1991.

88. Trout, D. L., Vitamin C and cardiovascular risk factors, *Am. J. Clin. Nutr.*, 53, 322S, 1991.

89. Moran, J. P., Cohen, L., Greene, J. M., Xu, G., Feldman, E. B., Hames, C. G., and Feldman, D. S., Plasma ascorbic acid concentrations relate inversely to blood pressure in human subjects, *Am. J. Clin. Nutr.*, 57, 213, 1993.

90. Jacques, P. F., Relationship of vitamin C status to cholesterol and blood pressure, *Ann. N.Y. Acad. Sci.*, 669, 205, 1992.

91. Enstrom, J. E., Kanim, L. E., and Klein, M. A., Vitamin C intake and mortality among a sample of the United States population, *Epidemiology*, 3, 194, 1992.

92. Levine, M., New concepts in the biology and biochemistry of ascorbic acid, *N. Engl. J. Med.*, 314, 892, 1986.

93. Jacques, P. F. and Taylor, A., Micronutrients and age-related cataracts, in *Micronutrients in Health and in Disease Prevention*, Bendich, A. and Butterworth, C. E., Jr., Eds., Marcel Dekker, New York, 1991, 359.

94. Block, G., Henson, D. E., and Levine, M., Ascorbic acid: biological functions and relation to cancer, *Am. J. Clin. Nutr.*, 54, 1113S, 1991.

95. Glatthaar, B. E., Horning, D. H., and Moser, U., The role of ascorbic acid in carcinogenesis, *Adv. Exp. Med. Biol.*, 206, 357, 1986.

96. Block, G., Vitamin C and cancer prevention: the epidemiologic evidence, *Am. J. Clin. Nutr.*, 53, 270S, 1991.

97. Hemila, H., Vitamin C and lowering of blood pressure: need for intervention trial? *J. Hypertens.*, 9, 1076, 1991.

98. Riemersma, R. A., Oliver, M., Elton, R. A., Alfthan, G., Vartianen, E., Salo, M., et al., Plasma antioxidants and coronary heart disease: vitamin C and E, and selenium, *Eur. J. Clin. Nutr.*, 44, 143, 1990.

99. Kutnink, M. A., Skala, J. H., Sauberlich, H. E., and Omaye, S. T., Simultaneous determination of ascorbic acid, isoascorbic acid (erythorbic acid) and uric acid in human plasma by high-performance liquid chromatography with amperometric detection, *J. Liquid Chromatogr.*, 8, 31, 1985.

100. Sauberlich, H. E., Tamura, T., Craig, C. B., Freeberg, L. E., Liu, T., Effects of erythorbic acid on vitamin C metabolism in young women, *Am. J. Clin. Nutr.*, 64, 336, 1996.

101. Sauberlich, H. E., Wood, S. M., Tamura, T., and Freeberg, L. E., Influence of dietary intakes of erythorbic acid on plasma vitamin C analyses. *Am. J. Clin. Nutr.*, 54, 1319S, 1991.

102. Kutnink, M. A. and Omaye, S. T., Determination of ascorbic acid, erythrobic acid, and uric acid in cured meats by high-performance liquid chromatography, *J. Food Sci.*, 52, 53, 1987.

103. Kallner, A., Hartmann, D., and Horning, D., On the absorption of ascorbic acid, *Int. J. Vit. Nutr. Res.*, 47, 383, 1977.

104. McLeroy, V. J. and Schendel, H. E., Influence of oral contraceptives on ascorbic acid concentrations in healthy, sexually mature women, *Am. J. Clin. Nutr.*, 26, 191, 1973.

105. Rivers, J. M., Oral contraceptives and ascorbic acid, *Am. J. Clin. Nutr.*, 28, 550, 1975.

106. Sahud, M. A. and Cohen, R. J., Effect of aspirin ingestion on ascorbic acid levels in rheumatoid arthritis, *Lancet*, 1, 937, 1971.

107. Curhan, G. C., Willett, W. C., Rimm, E. B., and Stampfer, M. J., A prospective study of the intake of vitamins C and B_6, and risk of kidney stones in men, *J. Urol.*, 155, 1847, 1996.

108. Payette, H. and Gray-Donald, K., Dietary intake and biochemical indices of nutritional status in an elderly population, with estimates of the precision of the 7-d food record, *Am. J. Clin. Nutr.*, 54, 478, 1991.

109. Schaus, E. E., Kutnink, M. A., O'Connor, D. K., and Omaye, S. T., A comparison of leukcyte ascorbate levels measured by the 2,4-dinitrophenylhydrazine method with high-performance liquid chromatography using electrochemical detection, *Biochem. Med. Metab. Biol.*, 36, 369, 1986.

110. Omaye, S. T., Schaus, E. E., Kutnink, M. A., and Hawkes, W. C., Measurement of vitamin C in blood components by high-performance liquid chromatography, *Ann. N.Y. Acad. Sci.*, 498, 389, 1987.

111. Omaye, S. T., Skala, J. H., and Jacob, R. A., Plasma ascorbic acid in adult males: effects of depletion and supplementation, *Am. J. Clin. Nutr.*, 44, 257, 1986.

112. Weber, P., Bendich, A., and Schalch, W., Vitamin C and human health: a review of recent data relevant to human requirement, *Int. J. Vit. Nutr. Res.*, 66, 19, 1996.

113. Maiani, G., Azzini, E., and Ferro-Luzzi, A., Vitamin C, *Int. J. Vit. Nutr. Res.*, 63, 289, 1993.

114. Friedman, G. J., Sherry, S., and Ralli, E. P., The mechanism of the excretion of vitamin C by the human kidney at low and normal plasma levels of ascorbic acid, *J. Clin. Invest.*, 19, 685, 1940.

115. Omaye, S. T., Turnbull, J. D., and Sauberlich, H. E., Selected methods for the determination of ascorbic acid in animal cells, tissues, and fluids, McCormick, D. B. and Wright, L. D., Eds., Academic Press, New York, *Methods Enzymol.*, 62, 3, 1979.

116. Schorah, C. J., The level of vitamin C reserves required in man: towards a solution to the controversy, *Proc. Nutr. Soc.*, 40, 147, 1981.

117. Manual for Nutrition Surveys, Interdepartmental Committee on Nutrition for National Defense, 2nd edition, Superintendent of Documents, Washington D.C., 1963.

118. Information Canada, Nutrition Canada National Survey, Canadian Government Publishing Centre, Ottawa, 1973.

119. Jacques, P. F., Taylor, A., Hankinson, S. F., Willett, W. C., Mahnken, B., Lee, Y., Vaid, K., and Lahav, M., Long-term vitamin C supplement use and prevalence of early age-related lens opacities, *Am. J. Clin. Nutr.*, 66, 911, 1997.

120. Dickinson, A., Optimal Nutrition for Good Health: The Benefits of Nutritional Supplements, Council for Responsible Nutrition, Washington D.C., 1998.

121. Rose, R. C., Ricker, S. P., and Bode, A. M., Ocular oxidants and antioxidant protection, PSEBM, 217, 397, 1998.

122. Jacob, R. A., The integrated antioxidant system, *Nutr. Res.*, 15, 755, 1995.

123. Nyyssonen, K., Parviainen, M. T., Salonen, R., Tuomilehto, J., Salonen, J., Vitamin C deficiency and risk of myocardial infarction: prospective population study of men from Eastern Finland, *Br. Med. J.*, 314, 634, 1997.

124. Richard Jally, United Nations Development Programs, United Nations, New York, Sub-Committee on Nutrition, *SCN News*, 15, 2, 1997.

125. Stahelin, H. B., Gey, K. F., and Brubacher, G., Plasma vitamin C and cancer death: the prospective Basel study, *Ann. N.Y. Acad. Sci.*, 498, 124, 1987.

126. Sauberlich, H. E., Dowdy, R. P., and Skala, J. H., *Laboratory Tests for the Assessment of Nutritional Status*, CRC Press, Boca Raton, FL, 1974.

127. McGown, E. L., Rusnak, M. G., Lewis, C. M., and Tillotson, J. A., Tissue ascorbic acid analysis using ferrozine compared with the dinitrophenylhydrazene method, *Anal. Biochem.*, 119, 55, 1982.

128. Cohen, H. A., Neuman, I., and Nahum, H., Blocking effect of vitamin C in exercise-induced asthma, *Arch. Pediatr. Adolesc. Med.*, 151, 367, 1997.

129. Bielory, L. and Gandhi, R., Asthma and vitamin C, *Annu. Allergy*, 73, 89, 1994.

130. Davidson, L., Walczyk, T., Morris, A., and Hurrell, R. F., Influence of ascorbic acid on iron absorption from an iron-fortified, chocolate-flavored milk drink in Jamaican children, *Am. J. Clin. Nutr.*, 67, 873, 1998.

131. Powers, H. J., The potential of a ^{13}C-methacetin breath test for estimating ascorbic acid requirements, *Int. J. Vit. Nutr. Res.*, 57, 455, 1987.

132. Powers, H. J., Whitehead, J., Downes, R., Dighton, D., and Perry, M., An investigation into the effect of different intakes of vitamin C on drug metabolism in Gambian men, *Int. J. Vit. Nutr. Res.*, 61, 135, 1991.

133. Neale, R. L., Lim, H., Turner, J., Freeman, C., and Kemm, J. R., The excretion of large vitamin C loads in young and elderly subjects: and ascorbic acid tolerance, *Age and Aging*, 17, 35, 1988.

134. Blanchard, J., Conrad, K. A., Mead, R. A., and Garry, P. J., Vitamin C disposition in young and elderly men, *Am. J. Clin. Nutr.*, 51, 837, 1990.

135. Evans, R. M., Currie, L., and Campbell, A., The distribution of ascorbic acid between various cellular components of blood, in normal individuals, and its relation to the plasma concentrations, *Br. J. Nutr.*, 47, 473, 1982.

136. Rose, R. C., Transport of ascorbic acid and other water-soluble vitamins, *Biochem. Biophy. Acta*, 947, 335, 1988.

137. Willson, C. W. N., Ascorbic acid metabolism and the clinical factors which effect tissue saturation with ascorbic acid, *Acta Vit. Enzymol*, 31, 35, 1977.

138. Lykkesfeldt, J., Loft, S., Nielsen, J. B., and Poulsen, H. E., Ascorbic acid and dehydroascorbic acid as biomarkers of oxidative stress caused by smoking, *Am. J. Clin. Nutr.*, 65, 959, 1997.

139. Sauberlich, H. E., Ascorbic acid (vitamin C), *Clin. Lab. Med.*, 1, 673, 1981.

140. Sauberlich, H. E., Vitamin C status: methods and findings, *Ann. N.Y. Acad. Sci.*, 258, 438, 1975.

141. Sauberlich, H. E., Goad, W. C., Skala, J. H., and Waring, P. P., Procedure for mechanized (continuous-flow) measurement of serum ascorbic acid (vitamin C), *Clin. Chem.*, 22, 105, 1976.

142. Deutsch, M. J. and Weeks, C. E., Microfluorometric assay for vitamin C., *J. Assoc. Off. Anal. Chem.*, 48, 1248, 1965.

143. Zannoni, V., Lynch, M., Goldstein, S., and Sato, P., A rapid method for the determination of ascorbic acid in plasma and tissue, *Biochem. Med.*, 11, 41, 1974.

144. Liu, T. Z., Chin, N., Kiser, M. D., and Bigler, W. N., Specific spectrophotometry of ascorbic acid in serum or plasma by use of ascorbate oxidase, *Clin. Chem.*, 28, 2225, 1982.

145. Lee, W., Hamernyik, P., Hutchinson, M., Raisys, V. A., and Labbe, R. F., Ascorbic acid in lymphocytes: cell preparation and liquid chromatography assay, *Clin. Chem.*, 28, 2165, 1982.

146. Ikeda, T., Comparison of ascorbic acid concentrations in granulocytes and lymphocytes, *Tohoku J. Exp. Med.*, 142, 117, 1984.

147. Yetley, E. and Johnson, C., Nutritional applications of the Health and Nutrition Examination Surveys (HANES), *Annu. Rev. Nutr.*, 7, 441, 1987.

148. Jacob, R. A., Pianalto, F. D., and Agee, R. E., Cellular ascorbate depletion in healthy men, *J. Nutr.*, 122, 1111, 1992.

149. Kutnink, M. A., Hawkes, W. C., Schaus, E. E., and Omaye, S. T., An internal standard method for the unattended high-performance liquid chromatographic analysis of ascorbic acid in blood components, *Anal. Biochem.*, 166, 424, 1987.

150. Blanchard, J., Conrad, K. A., Watson, R. R., Barry, P. J., and Crawley, J. D., Comparison of plasma, mononuclear and polymorphonuclear leukocyte vitamin C levels in young and elderly women during depletion and supplementation, *Eur. J. Clin. Nutr.*, 43, 97, 1990.

151. Washko, P., Rotrosen, D., Levine, M., Ascorbic acid in human neutrophils, *Am. J. Clin. Nutr.*, 54 (Suppl.), 1221S, 1991.

152. Dhariwal, K. R., Hartzell, W. O., and Levine, M., Ascorbic acid and dehyroascorbic acid measurements in human plasma and serum, *Am. J. Clin. Nutr.*, 54, 712, 1991.

153. Wang, Y.-H., Dhariwal, K. R., and Levine, M., Ascorbic acid bioavailability in humans: ascorbic acid in plasma, serum, and urine, *Ann. N.Y. Acad. Sci.*, 669, 383, 1992.
154. Pachla, L. A. and Kissinger, P. T., Analysis of ascorbic acid by liquid chromatography with amperometric detection, *Methods Enzymol.*, 62, 15, 1979.
155. Kalmar, J. R., Arnold, R. R., Warbington, M. L., and Gardner, M. K., Superior leukocyte separation with a discontinuous one-step Ficoll-Hypoque gradient for the isolation of human neutrophils, *J. Immunol. Methods*, 110, 275, 1988.
156. McCullock, R. K. and Vandongen, R., Measurement of ascorbic acid in platetets and its relationship to polymorphonuclear leukocytes levels, *Clin. Chim. Acta.*, 213, 15, 1992.
157. Macklin, L. and Bendich, A., Free radical tissue damage: protective role of antioxidant nutrients, *FASEB J.*, 1, 441, 1987.
158. Tillotson, J. A. and O'Connor, R. J., Ascorbate requirements in the trained monkey as determined by blood ascorbate levels, *Int. J. Vit. Nutr. Res.*, 50, 171, 1980.
159. Turnbull, J. D., Sudduth, J. H., Sauberlich, H. E., and Omaye, S. T., Depletion and repletion of ascorbic acid in the Rhesus monkey: relationship between ascorbic acid concentration in blood components with total body pool and liver concentration of ascorbic acid, *Int. J. Vit. Nutr. Res.*, 51, 47, 1981.
160. Omaye, S. T., Tillotson, J. A., and Sauberlich, H. E., Metoblism of L-ascorbic acid in the monkey, in *Ascorbic Acid: Chemistry, Metabolism, and Uses*, Seib, P. A. and Tolbert, B. M., Eds., Advances in Chemistry Series No. 200, American Chemical Society, Washington D.C., 1982, 317.
161. VanderJagt, D. J., Garry, P. J., and Hunt, W. C., Ascorbate in plasma as measured by liquid chromatography and by dichlorophenolindophenol colorimetry, *Clin. Chem.*, 32, 1004, 1986.
162. Dhariwal, K. R., Hartzell, W. O., and Levine, M., Ascorbic acid and dehydroascorbic acid measurements in human plasma and serum, *Am. J. Clin. Nutr.*, 54, 712, 1991.
163. Lee, W., Davis, K. A., Rettmer, R. L., and Labbe, R. F., Ascorbic acid status: biochemical and clinical consideration, *Am. J. Clin. Nutr.*, 48, 286, 1988.
164. Vanderslice, J. T., Higgs, D. J., Beecher, G. R., Higgs, H. E., and Bouma, J., On the presence of dehydroascorbic acid in human plasma, *Int. J. Vit. Nutr. Res.*, 62, 101, 1992.
165. Farber, C. M., Kanengiser, S., Stahl, R., Liebes, L., and Silber, R., A specific high-performance liquid chomatography assay for dehydroascorbic acid shows an increased content in CLL lymphocytes, *Anal. Biochem.*, 134, 355, 1983.
166. Cammack, J., Oke, A., and Adams, R. N., Simultaneous high-performance liquid chromatographic determination of ascorbic acid and dehydroascorbic acid in biological samples, *J. Chromatog. Biomed. Appl.*, 565, 529, 1991.
167. Schorah, C. J., Downing, C., Piripitsi, A., Gallivan, L., Al-Hazaa, A. H., Sanderson, M. J., and Bodenham, A., Total vitamin C, ascorbic acid, and dehydroascorbic acid concentrations in plasma of critically ill patients, *Am. J. Clin. Nutr.*, 63, 760, 1996.
168. Tessier, F., Birlouez-Aragon, I., Ijani, C., and Guilland, J.-C., Validation of a micromethod for determining oxidized and reduced vitamin C in plasma by HPLC-fluorescence, *Int. J. Vit. Nutr. Res.*, 66, 166, 1996.
169. Okamura, M., An improved method for determination of L-ascorbic acid and L-dehydroascorbic acid in blood plasma, *Clin. Chim. Acta*, 103, 259, 1980.
170. Margolis, S. A., Ziegler, R. G., and Helzlsouer, K. J., Ascorbic acid and dehydroascorbic acid measurement in human serum and plasma, *Am. J. Clin. Nutr.*, 54, 1315S, 1991.
171. Margolis, S. A., Paule, R. C., and Ziegler, R. G., Ascorbic and dehydroascorbic acids measured in plasma preserved with dithiothrentol or metaphosphoric acid, *Clin. Chem.*, 36, 1750, 1990.
172. Margolis, S. A. and Davis, T. P., Stabilization of ascorbic acid in human plasma, and its liquid-chromatographic measurement, *Clin. Chem.*, 34, 2217, 1988.
173. Schuep, W., Vuilleumier, J. P., Gysel, D., and Hess, D., Determination of ascorbic acid in body fluids, tissues and feedstuffs, in *Ascorbic Acid in Domestic Animals*, Wegger, I., Tagwerker, F. J., and Moustgaard, J., Eds., Royal Danish Agricultural Society, Copenhagen, 1984, 50.
174. Peterkofsky, B., Ascorbate requirement for hydroxylation and secretion of procollagen: relationship to inhibition of collagen synthesis in scurvy, *Am. J. Clin. Nutr.*, 54, 1135S, 1991.
175. Padh, H., Cellular functions of ascorbic acid, *Biochem. Cell Biol.*, 68, 1166, 1990.
176. Rebouche, C. J., Ascorbic acid and carnitine biosynthesis, *Am. J. Clin. Nutr.*, 54, 1147S, 1991.

177. Reuler, J. B., Broudy, V. C., and Cooney, T. G., Adult scurvy, *JAMA*, 253, 805, 1985.
178. Brubacher, G., Horning, D., Rettenmaier, R., and Vuilleumier, J. P., Borderline vitamin deficiency and the assessment of vitamin status in man, *Ernehrung Nutrition*, 3, 4, 1979.
179. Bates, C. J., Plasma vitamin C assays: a European experience, *Int. J Vit. Nutr. Res.*, 64, 283, 1994.
180. Berg, R. A. and Kerr, J. S., Nutritional aspects of collagen metabolism, *Annu. Rev. Nutr.*, 12, 369, 1992.
181. Hevia, P., Omaye, S. T., and Jacob, R. A., Urinary hydroxyproline excretion and vitamin C status in healthy young men, *Am. J. Clin. Nutr.*, 51, 644, 1990.
182. Bates, C. J., Proline and hydroxyproline excretion and vitamin C status in elderly human subjects, *Clin. Sci. Mol. Med.*, 52, 535, 1977.
183. Bradley, D. W., Emery, G., and Maynard, J. E., Vitamin C in plasma: a comparative study of the vitamin stabilized with trichloroacetic acid or metaphosphoric acid and the effects of storage at $-70°C$, $-20°C$, $4°C$, and $25°C$ on the stabilized vitamin, *Clin. Chim. Acta*, 44, 47, 1973.
184. Butts, W. C. and Mulvihill, H. J., Centrifugal analyzer determination of ascorbate in serum or urine with Fe^{3+}/Ferrozine, *Clin. Chem.*, 21, 1493, 1975.
185. Margolis, S. A. and Duewer, D. L., Measurement of ascorbic acid in human plasma and serum: stability, intralaboratory repeatability, and interlaboratory reproducibility, *Clin. Chem.*, 42, 1257, 1996.
186. Finglas, P. M., Bailey, A., Walker, A., Loughridge, J. M., Wright, A. J. A., and Southon, S., Vitamin C intake and plasma ascorbic acid concentration in adolescents, *Br. J. Nutr.*, 69, 563, 1993.
187. Washko, P. W., Hartzell, W. O., and Levine, M., Ascorbic acid analysis using high-performance liquid chromatography with coulometric electrochemical detection, *Anal. Biochem.*, 181, 276, 1989.
188. Tsao, C. S. and Salimi, S. L., Ultramicromethod for the measurement of ascorbic acid in plasma and white blood cells by high-performance liquid chromatography with electrochemical detection, *J. Chromatogr. Biomed. Appl.*, 224, 477, 1981.
189. Wunderling, M., Paul, H.–H., and Lohmann, W., Evaluation of a direct spectrophotometric method for the rapid determination of ascorbate and dehydroascorbate in blood using ascorbate oxidase, *Biol. Chem. Hoppe-Seyler*, 367, 1047, 1986.
190. Samyn, W., 'True' ascorbic acid in plasma and serum: investigation of a new method, *Clin. Chim. Acta*, 133, 111, 1983.
191. Hatch, L. L. and Sevanian, A., Measurement of uric acid, ascorbic acid, and related metabolites in biological fluids, *Anal. Biochem.*, 138, 324, 1984.
192. Kah, E. V., Bissell, M. G., and Ito, R. K., Measurement of vitamin C by capillary eletrophoresis in biological fluids and fruit beverages using a stereoisomer as an internal standard, *J. Chromatogr.*, 633, 245, 1993.
193. Manoharan, M. and Schwille, P. O., Measurement of ascorbic acid in human plasma and urine by high-performance liquid chromatography. Results in healthy subjects and patients with idiopathic calcium urolithiasis, *J. Chromatogr. Biomed. Appl.*, 654, 134, 1994.
194. Tsao, C. S., An overview of ascorbic acid chemistry and biochemistry, in *Vitamin C in Health and Disease*, Packer, L. and Fuchs, J., Eds., Marcel Dekker, New York, 1997, 25.
195. Kallner, A., Hartmann, D., and Horning, D., Steady-state turnover and body pool of ascorbic acid in man, *Am. J. Clin. Nutr.*, 22, 530, 1979.
196. Taylor, A., Dorey, C. K., and Nowell, T., Oxidative stress and ascorbate in relation to risk of cataract and age-related maculopathy, in *Vitamin C in Health and Disease*, Packer, L. and Fuchs, J., Eds., Marcel Dekker, New York, 1997, 205.
197. Hatch, G. E., Vitamin C and asthma, in *Vitamin C in Health and Disease*, Packer, L. and Fuchs, J., Eds., Marcel Dekker, New York, 1997, 279.
198. Chow, C. K., Vitamin C and cigarette smoke exposure, in *Vitamin C in Health and Disease*, Packer, L. and Fuchs, J., Eds., Marcel Dekker, New York, 1997, 413.
199. Jarvinen, R. and Knekt, P., Vitamin C, smoking, and alcohol consumption, in *Vitamin C in Health and Disease*, Packer, L. and Fuchs, J., Eds., Marcel Dekker, New York, 1997, 425.
200. O'Neal, R. M., Johnson, O. C., and Schaefer, A. E., Guidelines for classification and interpretation of group blood and urine data collected on part of the National Nutrition Survey, *Pediatr. Res.*, 4, 103, 1970.

Vitamin B-1 (Thiamin)

Converting metric units to International System units (SI):

ng/mL × 2.69 = nmol/L

nmol/L × 0.3373 = ng/mL

molecular weight (thiamin hydrochloride): 337.28

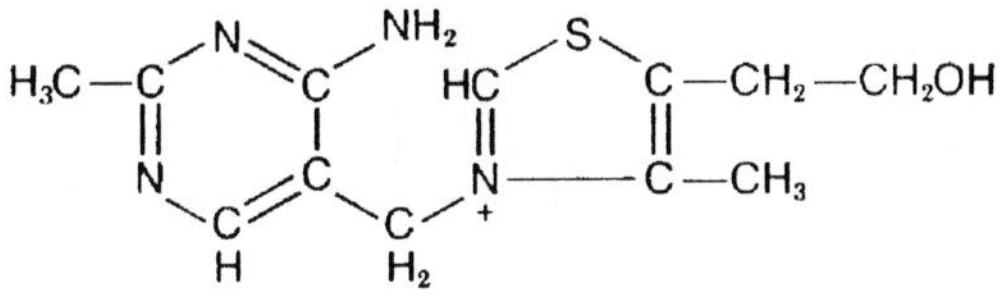

FIGURE 8
Structure of thiamin (vitamin B-1).

Thiamin

History of Thiamin

Beriberi, now known to result from a deficiency of thiamin (vitamin B-1, thiamine), varies widely in its clinical features.[130-132] Usually it manifests three main features: (1) those of cardiac insufficiency; (2) those of peripheral neuritis; and (3) a generalized tendency to edema. Many instances have been reported of prisoners and soldiers suffering from beriberi suddenly while performing their usual duties. The disease was also the scourge of seafarers.[130-132] Patients often become numb, weak, and unable to stand or walk.

Infantile beriberi occurs usually in an acute form in breast-fed infants of mothers who reveal signs of a thiamin deficiency. In the infant, beriberi is usually associated with generalized edema, dyspnea, anorexia, vomiting, cardiac disturbances, oliguria, and aphonia or "beriberi cry".[37,130]

Beriberi has been mainly associated with populations where rice is the main staple. With the increased use of milled or polished rice in the mid-1800s, the incidence and severity of beriberi increased.

Beriberi was long considered to be caused by a toxin in rice. However, in 1896, Christian Eijkman, a Dutch army surgeon, was sent to Indonesia to study the cause of beriberi. He reported in 1897 that fowls fed a diet of milled (polished) rice developed a disease that closely resembled human beriberi.[130,133] After additional studies, Eijkman concluded that a diet of over-milled rice was the main cause of the paralysis in fowls and of beriberi in humans. Subsequently, through the efforts of Col. E. B. Veder of the U.S. Army and R. R. Williams and colleagues, thiamin was isolated, characterized, and synthesized.[130] The availability of synthetic thiamin permitted the fortification of flour and rice, which has virtually eliminated beriberi.

Sources of Thiamin

Pork, ham, beef liver, green peas, whole grain wheat, corn meal, oatmeal, brown rice, and whole-grain rye, are good sources of thiamin.[135,136]

It is estimated that 25% of our thiamin intake is provided by thiamin-fortified foods. Consequently, thiamin fortification has an essential role in nutrition and public health.[105,118,119]

Function of Thiamin

In the human, thiamin pyrophosphate catalyzes two general types of reactions:[37,44,101,103] (1) the formation of ketoses as catalyzed by transketolase and (2) the oxidative decarboxylation of α-keto acids catalyzed by dehydrogenase complexes.

The body storage of thiamin is small (30 mg) with a rapid turnover. Consequently, a thiamin deficiency can be induced in the human rather rapidly when thiamin is withheld from the diet.[43,45-48,99,100]

Thiamin Deficiency

Most Americans receive ample thiamin in the diet, but impaired thiamin status exists in about 5% of the population over 60 years of age.[75] This occurs particularly among the poor and the institutionalized. Similar findings were reported for Finland,[72] North Ireland,[73] the Netherlands,[74] and elsewhere.[49] Occasionally, outbreaks of beriberi occur.[110-113,139]

Elderly subjects have been reported to have lower erythrocyte thiamin pyrophosphate concentrations than younger subjects.[40,78,83] In a study conducted in Canada, evidence of inadequate thiamin intakes was observed in a group of 60 independently-living elderly subjects (≥ 65 y).[127] Thiamin deficiency is often observed in malnourished alcoholic patients.[37,40,75] Alcohol impairs thiamin absorption and may also effect intermediary metabolism of thiamin and thereby increase its requirement.

Thiamin deficiency may occur in some areas of Thailand as a result diets high in unfortified milled rice, which may be aggravated by the consumption of foods containing antithiamin factors.[71] Thiamin deficiency may occasionally occur in infants and children and during pregnancy.[113-117,120]

Alcohol and Thiamin Status

The role of thiamin in alcoholism has attracted considerable study since up to 80% of the alcoholics are thiamin deficient.[13,14,35,94,100-103] This deficiency may progress to the life-threatening Wernicke's encephalopathy or to Wernicke-Korsakoff syndrome.[103,128,129] A severe thiamin deficiency may result in Wernicke-Korsakoff syndrome.[11,13,94] Although the syndrome

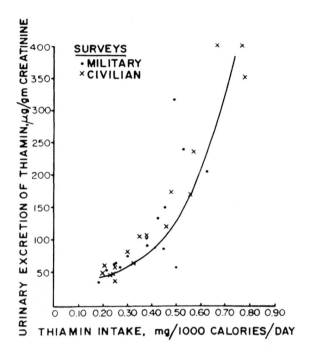

FIGURE 9

Relationship between thiamin intake and the urinary excretion of thiamin in adults as observed in nutrition surveys conducted in 18 countries by the Interdepartmental Committee on Nutrition for National Defense (ICCNND).[8,141]

occurs in the alcoholic population, an abusive intake of alcohol is not essential to the induction of the condition.

Wernicke's encephalopathy is characterized by numerous abnormalities including mental symptoms, nystagmus, ataxia, disorientations, global confusion, apathy, indifference, and drowsiness. The erythrocyte transketolase activity stimulation ranged from 28 to 67% in patients (*n* = 18) suffering from Wernicke's encephalopathy.[39] In a group of healthy subjects (*n* = 54), the stimulation effect ranged from 8.3 to 18.5% (mean = 13.5%).

Thiamin deficiency in alcoholics is generally due to a decreased intake of the vitamin, but may be aggravated by malabsorption, impaired utilization, or by increased metabolism and excretion.[101-108] The incidence of thiamin deficiency in the aging nonalcoholic population has been estimated to be less than 1%.[105]

The majority of alcoholics with neuropathy have low levels of blood thiamin.[14] However, alcoholics without neuropathy commonly have lowered blood levels of thiamin. Erythrocyte transketolase activity is reduced in alcoholics, but responds to thiamin adminstration.[12]

Assessment of Thiamin Nutritional Status

Various biochemical procedures have been developed which have been useful for detecting thiamin deficiency or assessing thiamin nutritional status.[37,38,41,134] Currently, the most common procedures to assess thiamin nutritional status are the measurement of erythrocyte transketolase activity, thiamin concentrations in the blood, and urinary excretion of thiamin (see Tables 5 to 11).

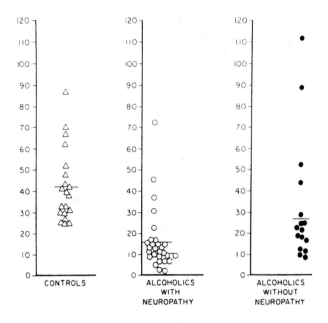

FIGURE 10
Blood thiamin concentrations (ng/mL) in alcoholic subjects with or without neuropathy.[14] (With permission.)

TABLE 5
Guidelines Used for Interpretation of
Erythrocyte Transketolase Thiamin
Pyrophosphate Stimulation Assay
(same for both sex and age)

Classification[1]	TPP Effect or Stimulation
Normal (acceptable)	0–15%
Low (marginally deficient)	16–24%
Deficient (high risk)	> 25%

References 32, 33, 36, 37, 39, 45, 134.

TABLE 6
Tentative Guide for Evaluating Erythrocyte Thiamin
Pyrophosphate Concentrations

Classification	Erythrocyte Thiamin Pyrophosphate (nmol/L)
Normal (acceptable)	> 150
Low (marginally deficient)	120–150
Deficient (high risk)	< 120

References 51 and 81.

TABLE 7
Thiamin Concentrations in Whole Blood of Infants
and Children

Age	Phosphorylated (nmol/L)	Nonphosphorylated (nmol/L)
< 0–3 mo (n = 64)	177 ± 48	81 ± 26
3–12 mo (n = 100)	148 ± 33	66 ± 20
> 12 mo (n = 159)	120 ± 31	67 ± 21

Adapted from Reference 114.

TABLE 8
Literature Values for Thiamin Pyrophosphate
Concentrations

Subjects	Thiamin Pyrophosphate (nmol/L)	References
Adults (n = 33)		95
Whole blood	115 ± 25	
Erythrocytes	233 ± 60	
Adults (n = 48)		80
Erythrocytes	132–284	

TABLE 9
Literature Values for Serum Thiamin Concentrations

Subjects	Total Thiamin (nmol/L)	Thiamin Monophosphate (nmol/L)	References
Adults (n = 50)	11.2 ± 3.5		96
Adults (n = 20)	19.4 ± 7.0		98
Adults (n = 40)	12.7 ± 4.2	4.0 ± 1.5	1, 2

TABLE 10
Literature Values for Whole-Blood Thiamin Concentrations

| Subjects | Thiamin mean ± SD or range | | |
	Total (nmol/L)	Phosphorylated (nmol/L)	Nonphosphorylated (nmol/L)
Whatt et al.[5]			
(n = 140)	191 ± 32	130 ± 24	62 ± 17
Schrijver et al.[50]			
Adults (n = 94)	115 (70–85)		
Kimura et al.[53]			
Adults (n = 20)	137		
Wielders and Mink[68]			
Adults (n = 56)	117 (71–185)		
Laschi-Loquerie et al.[96]			
Adults (n = 50)			
Microbiological (*L. viridescens*)	157 ± 31		
HPLC method	101 ± 15		
Bottcher and Bottcher[98]			
Adults (n = 20)	184 ± 61		

TABLE 11
Guidelines for the Interpretation of Urinary Excretion of Thiamin

| Subjects | Less Than Acceptable (At Risk) | | Acceptable (Low Risk) |
| | Deficient (High Risk) | Low (Medium Risk) | |
	μg/g creatinine		
1–3 years	< 120	120–175	≥ 176
4–6 years	< 85	85–120	≥ 121
7–9 years	<70	70–180	≥ 181
10–12 years	< 60	60–180	≥ 181
13–15 years	< 50	50–150	≥ 151
Adults	< 27	27–65	≥ 66

References: 8, 56, 88.

Erythrocyte Transketolase Assay

The classical studies of Brin et al.[15-19,36] introduced the use of erythrocyte transketolase activity to assess thiamin nutritional status. Transketolase is an enzyme that requires thiamin pyrophosphate for activity. Erythrocyte transketolase measurement represents a functional test of thiamin adequacy.[25,36,39]

The relative enhancement of erythrocyte transketolase activity by *in vitro* saturation with thiamin pyrophosphate has proven to be a sensitive and specific measure for the detection and evaluation of thiamin deficiency in the human.[32,34,41,45] This measurement is referred to as the "TPP effect" (in percent), or as the "erythrocyte thiamin transketolase activity coefficient."

Values obtained without the addition of thiamin pyrophosphate represent the absolute enzyme activity and are dependent upon the coenzyme available in the erythrocytes. The addition of thiamin pyrophosphate permits an estimation of the amount of apoenzyme uncomplexed as well as the maximum potential transketolase activity. A thiamin deficiency results in a reduction in the thiamin pyrophosphate available and, in some instances, may result in a reduction of the apotransketolase as well.[36,37]

Numerous procedures have been proposed for the measurement of erythrocyte transketolase (EC 2.2.1.1) activity.[20-33,39,41] Several reports have evaluated this measurement in detail.[22,25,29] Finglas[82] has summarized a few of the factors that need to be considered in the interpretation of erythrocyte transketolase results.

Basu et al.[23] have described a simplified colorimetric procedure for the determination of transketolase in blood. Erythrocyte transketolase activity could be measured in as little as 50 μL of whole blood. This is a modification of the procedure of Schouten et al.[24] The micromethod permits the measurement of erythrocyte transketolase activity in blood of children since only a single finger prick is required.

Transketolase catalyzes the following two reactions in the pentose phosphate pathway:

1. xylulose-5-phosphate + ribose-5-phosphate $\rightleftarrows$ sedoheptulose-7-phosphate + glyceraldehyde-3-phosphate.

2. xylulose-5-phosphate + erythrose-4-phosphate $\rightleftarrows$ fructose-6-phosphate + glyceraldehyde-3-phosphate.

The glyceraldehyde-3-phosphate produced is coupled with an NADH indicator reaction. This procedure developed by Smeets et al.,[28] has been used successfully in numerous laboratories.[21,25,29,31] Waring et al.[22] modified the manual method of Smeets et al.[28] to a simple and rapid semi-automated assay for erythrocyte transketolase activity. The use of dialysis eliminated hemoglobin interference and increased the reproducibility and sensitivity of procedure. The author has used this procedure extensively for evaluating thiamin nutritional status.

Automated procedures for the assessment of thiamin have been developed. Mak and Swaminathan[26] have used a centrifugal analyzer (Cobas Bio centrifugal analyzer) to measure erythrocyte transketolase activity. Both basal transketolase activity and percentage of activation by thiamin pyrophosphate are obtained. The automated procedure needs further validation with the use of subjects known to have a vitamin B-1 deficiency. Duffy et al.[42] used an Abbott ABA-100 biochromatic analyzer to provide a semi-automated measurement of the stimulation of erythrocyte transketolase by thiamin pyrophosphate.

Earlier, Stevens et al.[27] measured erythrocyte transketolase activity with a continuous-flow (Auto-Analyzer) procedure based on the pentose-utilization method of Brin et al.[17] Although the procedure was used in a few studies, the method was abandoned because the acid reagents required produced a rapid deterioration of equipment.

Bailey et al.[86] investigated the thiamin status of a group of adolescents (13 to 14 years; $n = 54$). Although thiamin intake appeared largely adequate by United Kingdom dietary recommendations, some subjects had erythrocyte transketolase activity coefficients that were associated with a marginal or severe thiamin deficiency. However, a statistically significant relationship between total erythrocyte thiamin concentrations, determined by HPLC, and erythrocyte transketolase activity was not observed. This is in contrast to the reports of other investigators.[35,40,51,87]

Takeuchi et al. studied erythrocyte transketolase activity[34] and found that the thiamin pyrophosphate stimulation effect reflects the saturation status of transketolase with coenzyme.[35] Kaufmann and Guggenheim[92] found in a study with 109 elderly people that there was an inverse correlation of –0.33 between erythrocyte transketolase activity coefficient and the urinary excretion of thiamin expressed as μg/g creatinine.

Sample Preparation and Storage

If the plasma is carefully removed, washing of the erythrocytes was not essential. The use of packed erythrocytes permits the availability of the plasma for other measurements. The transketolase procedure appears not to be influenced by age or sex of the subject and fasting samples are not essential.[70]

Red blood cells stored –72° for over a year retained their transketolase activity. Cells stored at –20°C retained their activity for over 8 months. Packed in with dry ice the frozen erythrocyte samples can be shipped to distant laboratories for assay. No differences have been observed between males and females.

Rarely, a very malnourished subject may be encountered with low transketolase activity. If a thiamin deficiency is involved, the *in vitro* addition of thiamin pyrophosphate in the transketolase assay will still result in a high "TPP" effect.

Erythrocyte transketolase thiamin pyrophosphate activity and stimulation effects methodology may be followed with the use of quality control samples. These may be prepared from blood obtained from several volunteers with different activity coefficients. The erythrocytes are stored in small aliquots at –72°C or colder. In our experience, the coefficient of variations of the activation coefficient ranges from 2 to 5% for within and between day analyses.

Guides for Interpretation of Erythrocyte Transketolase Activity

Guides used have been developed from studies with human volunteers maintained on controlled intakes of thiamin.[36,45-48,91] Erythrocyte transketolase activity and urine excretion of thiamin correlated with the level of dietary thiamin intake (Figure 11).[45,46] As a result of these studies and from general use of the procedure, thiamin pyrophosphate stimulation effects of less than 15% are generally considered acceptable or normal. A stimulation of 15 to 25% indicates a low or marginal thiamin status, while stimulation effects of greater than 20 to 25% are deficient and usually respond quickly to thiamin supplementation.[134]

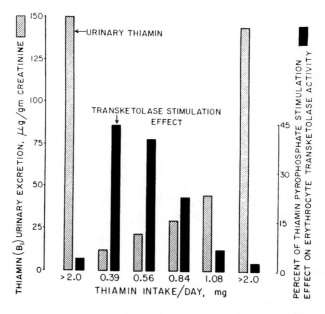

FIGURE 11

Relationship of erythrocyte transketolase activity to urinary excretion of thiamin in adult male subjects during controlled intakes of thiamin. Subjects received 3600 kcal per day.[45] (With permission.)

Herbeth et al.[89] in study of 360 adult men and women found a mean erythrocyte transketolase activity coefficient of 1.13 ± 7.4. This value is similar to that observed by other investigators.[21,22,25,87,90,91] For example, Vuilleumier et al.[91] studied the erythrocyte transketolase activity coefficient for 75 men and 75 women. The mean activity coefficient was 1.08 ± 0.5 for the men and 1.07 ± 0.05 for the women.

The erythrocyte transketolase activity coefficient represents the ratio of transketolase activity of the sample with and without added thiamin pyrophosphate. Erythrocyte transketolase activity may be expressed also as mU/g hemoglobin where 1 mU = 1 nmole NADH consumed per unit of time. The measurement of enzyme activity may assist in determining if the deficiency is due to a lack of apoenzyme or to a lack of the coenzyme, thiamin pyrophosphate (Table 5).

Blood Thiamin Measurements

Early studies concluded that blood thiamin concentrations did not appear to be useful for the evaluation of thiamin status in the human.[9] However, with the development of new methods, with improved sensitivity and reduced variability, blood measurements of thiamin have been useful for the evaluation of thiamin status.[78,106] HPLC methods with fluorescent detection have been particularly useful.[78,79,82]

The HPLC procedure of Warnock[79] has been useful for the measurement of erythrocyte thiamin pyrophosphate concentrations.[78] Other similar HPLC methods are available for the measurement of thiamin and thiamin phosphates in plasma, erythrocytes, and other tissues.[80,81,87,90,91,95-97,109]

Various attempts have been made to improve methods used to measure thiamin and its phosphorylated forms in serum or blood samples.[41,51,53,55] Most of these methods are variations of the long-used fluorimetric thiochrome method, but assisted with the use of HPLC.[53] Thus, Schrijver et al.[50] reported on a semiautomated HPLC procedure for measuring total thiamin in plasma and whole blood. The thiamin was converted to thiochrome and detected fluorometrically. They found that erythrocytes contained approximately 80% of the thiamin present in whole blood.

Baines and Davies[40] found that erythrocyte thiamin diphosphate concentrations correlated with erythrocyte transketolase activity measurements. Kuriyama et al.[52] found a correlation between blood thiamin pyrophosphate concentrations and with erythrocyte transketolase activity. They reported that the total thiamin level in whole blood and erythrocyte transketolase activity were significantly lower in beriberi patients than in normal subjects. However, the investigators noted that the thiamin pyrophosphate stimulation effect on erythrocyte transketolase activity was the most useful parameter in distinguishing between normal subjects from beriberi patients.[52]

The whole blood thiamin levels of normal subjects were reported by Kawai et al. to be 6.96 ± 1.26 µg/dL blood in contrast to 2.29 ± 1.06 µg/dL blood of beriberi patients.[49] This is similar to an early report that the mean thiamin level in whole blood of beriberi patients was 3.2 µg/dL.[54]

Wilkinson et al.[78] studied the erythrocyte thiamin pyrophosphate concentrations in a group of 222 subjects aged 65 years or older. Of this group, 35 subjects (16%) had erythrocyte thiamin pyrophosphate concentrations of less than 140 nmol/L. The thiamin pyrophosphate concentrations increased when the subjects were supplemented with thiamin. The supplements enhanced their quality of life. Similar effects were reported by Smidt et al.[84]

Erythrocyte thiamin pyrophosphate concentrations above 140 nmol/L were considered acceptable. This cutpoint was derived from a study conducted on a healthy blood donor population.[78] A cutoff value of above 150 nmol/L of erythrocyte thiamin pyrophosphate was suggested by Warnock et al.[51] and by Bailey and Finglas (Table 6).[81]

Urinary Excretion of Thiamin

In the past, the most commonly used procedure to assess thiamin nutritional status has been the measurement of the urinary levels of thiamin.[8,10,56] Measurement of urinary thiamin excretion has limitations, particularly when applied to individuals,[126] but has been useful when applied to populations groups. Urinary excretion of thiamin provides an indication of recent dietary intake of the vitamin but only a limited reflection of body stores of thiamin.[47,93]

Thiochrome Method

The thiochrome method has been most commonly used to measure urinary levels of thiamin.[3,7,8,10,56,66,125,126] Early spectophotometric and colorimetric methods to measure thiamin in biological materials proved unsatisfactory. This was overcome with the development of the thiochrome procedure.[6] In this procedure, thiamin is oxidized to thiochrome, which fluoresces instantly in ultraviolet light.[3,4,6] The method is sensitive, simple, and highly reproducible. Various modifications of the method have been reported that relate to the oxidant used, sample purification, and quantitation.[5,6,66,67] An automated method for the determination of urinary thiamin concentrations has been described.[126] More recently, thiamin has been determined in urine with the use of a HPLC system.[63,64]

Samples for thiamin analyses were found stable for at least two years when held frozen at –20°C.[5] The samples were even stable for two days when held at room temperature. Hence, the thiochrome assays for the measurement of thiamin concentrations in urine have proven useful for population surveys. The procedure of Michelsen et al.[7] with some modification was used extensively in the population surveys conducted by Interdepartmental Committee on Nutrition for National Defense.[89]

Microbiological Assay

Urinary levels of thiamin may be determined by microbiological assay or the use of the thiochrome method. The microbiological assay has most commonly used *Lactobacillus viridescens*[45,135] as the assay organism although *Lactobacillus fermenti* and *Ochromonas danica* have been used.[121-124] An automated microbiological assay for thiamin has been described.[123] Cultures of the organisms may be obtained from the American Type Culture Collection, Rockville, MD. Culture media and assay procedures are outlined in the Supplementary Literature of Difco Laboratories, Detroit, MI.

The urinary excretion procedure to assess thiamin nutritional status evolved as a result of findings from various investigations that established the existence of a reasonably close correlation between the development of a thiamin deficiency and the decreasing excretion of thiamin in the urine.[9,45-48,56,83,88]

Urinary excretion of thiamin decreases proportionately with thiamin intake to a critical point after which further lowering of intake results in only minor and variable changes in urinary excretion. Tissue stores of thiamin will be depleted with intakes of the vitamin below the critical point and, if continued, will result in symptoms of a deficiency.

The thiamin requirement of adult human has generally been considered to be about 0.30 to 0.35 mg/1,000 calories.[45,138] Approximately 40 to 90 μg of thiamin are excreted in the urine daily on intakes of 0.30 to 0.36 mg thiamin/1,000 calories, while 100 μg and above are excreted when the intake of thiamin is increased to 0.50 mg/1,000 calories.[45,88] When the daily intake of thiamin is reduced to only about 0.2 mg/1,000 calories, urinary excretions fall to only 5 to 25 μg of thiamin per day.[45,88,130] In cases of beriberi, 24-hr urinary excretions of 0 to 15 μg of thiamin have been reported.[130] As a result of these observations, measurement of the 24-hr urinary excretion of thiamin has been useful in evaluating thiamin nutriture. Under survey conditions, however, it is usually not feasible to collection 24-hr urine samples.

Consequently, as a matter of expedience, random urine samples are obtained, preferably during fasting state, and the thiamin content related to creatinine content.[8,9,56,139] A correlation between the urinary excretion of thiamin per gram of creatinine and thiamin intake has been observed.[45,140,141] Interpretive guidelines commonly used for adults are indicated in Table 11.[8,56,142]

The evaluations of Pearson[143] revealed that children have a markedly higher level of thiamin excretion when expressed on a creatinine basis than adults. This was also exemplified in the findings of the Ten-State Nutrition Survey.[142] In view of this age variable, Pearson developed adjusted sliding scale interpretive guides for thiamin excretion values for children of various ages (Table 11).

Occasionally, when patients with signs or symptoms of a thiamin deficiency have been encountered, a thiamin retention test (load test), has been applied.[143,144] For the test, commonly 5 mg of thiamin is administrated and the urinary excretion followed in the following 4-hr period. Subjects deficient in thiamin will usually excrete less than 20 μg of the dose during this period. Although the test may not specifically identify clinical thiamin deficiency, or indicate the severity of a deficiency, it can be useful as an indicator of low intakes and tissue deficits of the vitamin.

Toxicity

Thiamin is considered to be a generally recognized safe (GRAS) food ingredient.[76] Only with an exceedingly high intake of thiamin (e.g., 50 mg/kg or in excess of 3 g/day) have toxic effects been reported.[77]

Summary

Measurement of erythrocyte transketolase activity with and without the *in vivo* addition of thiamin pyrophosphate is the preferred means to evaluate thiamin nutritional status. The transketolase test represents a sensitive, specific, and biochemical functional measurement. Measurement of erythrocyte thiamin pyrophosphate concentrations by high performance liquid chromatography have also been useful for the evaluation of thiamin status. Although blood thiamin pyrophosphate concentrations correlate with erythrocyte transketolase activity, erythrocyte transketolase assays were more sensitive and reliable. Formerly, urinary excretion analysis was the only practical means available to assess thiamin nutriture. Such analyses will provide information as to thiamin intake levels, particularly with respect to the immediate intakes. However, the measurements do not provide the desired information regarding the state of deficiency or the degree of depletion of thiamin tissue reserves.

References

1. Tallaksen, C. M. E., Bohmer, T., and Bell, H., Concentration of the water-soluble vitamins thiamin, ascorbic acid, and folic acid in serum and cerebrospinal fluid of healthy individuals, *Am. J. Clin. Nutr.*, 56, 559, 1992.

2. Tallaksen, C. M. E., Bohmer, T., Bell, H., and Karlsen, J., Concomitant determination of thiamin and its phosphate esters in human blood and serum by high-performance liquid chromatography, *J. Chromatogr.*, 564, 127, 1991.
3. Freed, M., *Methods of Vitamin Assay*, Interscience Publications, New York, 1966.
4. Ball, G. F. M., *Water-Soluble Vitamin Assays in Human Nutrition*, Chapman & Hall, New York, 1994.
5. Wyatt, D. T., Lee, M., and Hillan, R. E., Factors affecting cyanogen bromide-based assay of thiamin, *Clin. Chem.*, 35, 2173, 1989.
6. Burch, H. B., Bessey, O. A., Love, R. H., and Lowry, O. H., The determination of thiamin and thiamin phosphates in small quantities of blood and blood cells, *J. Biol. Chem.*, 198, 477, 1952.
7. Mickelsen, O., Condiff, H., and Keys, A., The determination of thiamin in urine by means of the thiochrome technique, *J. Biol. Chem.*, 160, 361, 1945.
8. Interdepartmental Committee on Nutrition for National Defense, Manual for Nutrition Surveys (2nd edition), U.S. Government Printing Offices, Washington D.C., 1963.
9. Bessey, O. A., Blood levels, Methods for Evaluation of Nutritional Adequacy and Status, Committee on Foods, National Academy of Sciences–National Research Council, Washington D.C., 1954, 59.
10. Unglaub, W. G., Goldsmith, G. A., Urinary excretion tests, Methods for Evaluation of Nutritional Adequacy and Status, Committee on Foods, National Academy of Sciences National Research Council, Washington D.C., 1954, 69.
11. Charness, M. E., Simon, R. P., and Greenberg, D. A., Ethanol and the nervous system, *N. Engl. J. Med.*, 321, 442, 1989.
12. Dreyfus, P. M., Clinical application of blood transketolase activity, *N. Engl. J. Med.*, 267, 596, 1962.
13. Dreyfus, P. M. and Seyal, M., Diet and nutrition in neurological disorders, in *Modern Nutrition in Health and Disease*, Shils, M. E., Olson, J. A., and Shike, M., Eds., Lea & Febiger, Philadelphia, 1994, 1349.
14. Leevy, C. M., Thiamin deficiency and alcoholism, *Ann. N.Y. Acad. Sci.*, 378, 316, 1982.
15. Brin, M., Erythrocyte transketolase in early thiamin deficiency, *Ann. N.Y. Acad. Sci.*, 98, 528, 1962.
16. Wolfe, S. J., Brin, M., and Davidson, C. S., The effect of thiamin deficiency on human erythrocyte metabolism, *J. Clin. Invest.*, 37, 1476, 1958.
17. Brin, M., Tai, M., Ostachever, A. S., and Kalinsky, H., The effect of thiamin deficiency on the activity of erythrocyte hemolysate transketolase, *J. Nutr.*, 71, 273, 1960.
18. Brin, M., Erythrocyte as a biopsy tissue for functional evaluation of thiamin adequacy, *JAMA*, 187, 762, 1964.
19. Brin, M., Thiamin deficiency and erythrocyte metabolism, *Am. J. Clin. Nutr.*, 12, 107, 1963.
20. Warnock, L. G., A new approach to erythrocyte transketolase measurement, *J. Nutr.*, 100, 1057, 1970.
21. Warnock, L. G., Transketolase activity of blood hemolysate a useful index for diagnosing thiamin deficiency, *Clin. Chem.*, 21, 432, 1975.
22. Waring, P. P., Fisher, D., McDonnell, J., McGown, E. L., and Sauberlich, H. E., A continuous-flow (AutoAnalyzer II) procedure for measuring erythrocyte transketolase activity, *Clin. Chem.*, 28, 2206, 1982.
23. Basu, T. K., Patel, D. R., and Williams, D. C., A simplified microassay of transketolase in human blood, *Int. J. Vit. Nutr. Res.*, 44, 319, 1974.
24. Schouten, H., Statius van Epps, L. W., and Struykes Boudier, A. M., Transketolase in blood, *Clin. Chim. Acta*, 10, 474, 1964.
25. Bayoumi, R. A. and Rosalki, S. B., Evaluation of methods of coenzyme activation of erythocyte enzymes for detection of deficiency of vitamin B_1, B_2, and B_6, *Clin. Chem.*, 22, 327, 1976.
26. Mak, Y. T., and Swaminathan, R., Assessment of vitamin B_1, B_2, and B_6 status by coenzyme activation of red cell enzymes using a centrifugal analyzer, *J. Clin. Chem. Clin. Biochem.*, 24, 213, 1988.
27. Stevens, C. O., Sauberlich, H. E., and Long., J. L., An automated assay for transketolase determination, in *Automation in Analytical Chemistry*, Technicon Symposium 1967, Mediad Inc., White Plains, NY, 1968, 553.

28. Smeets, E. H. J., Muller, H., and DeWael, J., A NADH-dependent transketolase assay in erythrocyte hemolysates, *Clin. Chim. Acta*, 33, 379, 1971.
29. Rosalki, S. B., Detection of vitamin B deficiency by red cell enzyme activation tests, in *Quality Control in Laboratory Medicine*, Henry, J. B., and Giegel, J. L., Eds., Mason Publications, U.S.A., Inc., New York, 1977, 121.
30. Williams, D. G., Methods of the estimation of three vitamin dependent red cell enzymes, *Clin. Biochem.*, 9, 252, 1976.
31. Graudal, N., Torp-Pederson, K., Hanel, H., Kristensen, M., Thomsen, A. C., and Norgard, G., Assessment of the thiamin nutritional status, *Int. J. Vit. Nutr. Res.*, 55, 399, 1985.
32. Lonsdale, D. and Shamberger, R. J., Red cell transketolase as an indicator of nutritional deficiency, *Am. J. Clin. Nutr.*, 33, 205, 1980.
33. Massod, M. F., McGuire, S. L., and Werner, K. R., Analysis of blood transketolase activity, *Am. J. Clin. Pathol.*, 55, 465, 1971.
34. Takeuchi, T., Nishino, K., and Itokawa, Y., Improved determination of transketolase activity in erythrocytes, *Clin. Chem.*, 30, 658, 1984.
35. Takeuchi, T., Jung, E. H., Nishino, K., and Itokawa, Y., The relationship between the thiamine pyrophosphate effect and the saturation status of the transketolase with its coenzyme in human erythrocytes, *Int. J. Vit. Nutr. Res.*, 60, 112, 1990.
36. Brin, M., Functional evaluation of nutritional status: thiamin, in *Newer Methods of Nutritional Biochemistry*, Albanese, A. A., Ed., Volume III, Academic Press, New York, 1967, 407.
37. Sauberlich, H. E., Biochemical alterations in thiamin deficiency — their interpretation, *Am. J. Clin. Nutr.*, 20, 528, 1967.
38. Sauberlich, H. E., Dowdy, R. P., and Skala, J. H., *Laboratory Tests for the Assessment of Nutritional Status*, CRC Press, Boca Raton, FL, 1974.
39. Boni, L., Kieckens, L., and Hendrikx, A., An evaluation of a modified erythrocyte transketolase assay for assessing thiamin nutritional adequacy, *J. Nutr. Sci. Vitaminol.*, 26, 507, 1980.
40. Baines, M. and Davis, G., The evaluation of erythrocyte thiamin diphosphate as an indicator of thiamin status in man, and its comparison with erythrocyte ttransketolase activity measurements, *Annu. Clin. Biochem.*, 25, 698, 1988.
41. Sauberlich, H. E., Newer laboratory methods for assessing nutriture of selected B-complex vitamin, *Annu. Rev. Nutr.*, 4, 377, 1984.
42. Duffy, P., Morris, H., and Neilson, G., Thiamin status of a Melanesian population, *Am. J. Clin. Nutr.*, 34, 1584, 1981.
43. Ariaey-Nejad, M. R., Balaghi, M., Baker, E. M., and Sauberlich, H. E., Thiamin metabolism in man, *Am. J. Clin. Nutr.*, 23, 764, 1970.
44. Tanphaichitr, V., Thiamin, in *Modern Nutrition in Health and Disease*, Shils, M.E., Olson, J. A., and Shike, M., Eds., 8th edition, Lea & Febiger, Philadelphia, 1994, 359.
45. Sauberlich, H. E., Herman, Y. F., Stevens, C. O., and Herman, R. H., Thiamin requirement of the adult human, *Am. J. Clin. Nutr.*, 32, 2237, 1979.
46. Wood, B., Gijsbers, A., Goode, A., Davis, S., Mulholland, J., and Breen, K., A study of partial thiamin restriction in human volunteers, *Am. J. Clin. Nutr.*, 33, 848, 1980.
47. Ziporin, Z. Z., Nunes, W. T., Powell, R. C., Waring, P. P., and Sauberlich, H. E., Thiamin requirement in the adult human as measured by urinary excretion of thiamin metabolites, *J. Nutr.*, 85, 297, 1965.
48. Ziporin, Z. Z., Nunes, W. T., Powell, R. C., Waring, P. P., and Sauberlich, H. E., The excretion of thiamin and its metabolites in the urine of young adult males receiving restricted intakes of the vitamin, *J. Nutr.*, 85, 287, 1965.
49. Kawai, C., Wakabayashi, A., Matsumur, T., and Yui, Y., Reappearance of beriberi heart disease in Japan, A study of 23 cases, *Am. J. Med.*, 69, 383, 1980.
50. Schrijver, J., Speek, A. J., Kolsse, J. A., Van Rijn, H. J., and Schreurs, W. H., A reliable semiautomated method for the determination of total thiamin in whole blood by the thiochrome method with high-performance liquid chromatography, *Annu. Clin. Biochem.*, 19, 52, 1982.
51. Warnock, L. G., Prudhomme, C. R., and Wagner, C., The determination of thiamin pyrophosphate in blood and other tissues, and its correlation with erythrocyte transketolase activity, *J. Nutr.*, 108, 421, 1979.

52. Kuriyame, M., Yokomine, R., Arima, H., Hamada, R., and Igats, A., Blood vitamin B$_1$, transketolase and thiamin pyrophosphate (TPP) effect in beriberi patients, with studies employing discriminate analysis, *Clin. Chim. Acta*, 108, 159, 1980.

53. Kimura, M., Fujita, T., and Itokawa, Y., Liquid-chromatographic determination of the total thiamin content of blood, *Clin. Chem.*, 28, 29, 1982.

54. Burch, H. B., Salcedo, J., Jr., Carasco, E. O., Intengen, C. L., and Caldwell, A. B., Nutrition survey and tests in Bataan, Philippines, *J. Nutr.*, 42, 9, 1950.

55. Sanemori, H., Ueki, H., and Kawasaki, T., Reversed-phase high-performance liquid chromatographic analysis of thiamin phosphate esters at subpicomole levels, *Anal. Biochem.*, 107, 451, 1980.

56. O'Neal, R. M., Johnson, O. C., and Schaefer, A. E., Guidelines for classification and interpretation of group blood and urine data collected as part of the National Nutrition Survey, *Pediatr. Res.*, 4, 103, 1970.

57. Hilker, D. M. and Clifford, A. J., Thiamin analysis and separation of thiamin phosphate esters by high-performance liquid chromatography, *J. Chromatogr.*, 10, 433, 1982.

58. Echols, R. E., Harris, J., and Miller, R. H., Jr., Modified procedure for determining vitamin B$_1$ by gas chromatography, *J. Chromatogr.*, 193, 470, 1980.

59. Ryan, M. A. and Ingle, J. D., Jr., Fluorometric reaction rate method for the determination of thiamin, *Anal. Chem.*, 52, 2177, 1980.

60. Park, J. Y., Comparative study of colorimetric and fluorometric determination of thiamin (vitamin B$_1$) by automated discrete-sampling technique, *Anal. Chem.*, 47, 452, 1975.

61. Patrini, C. and Rindi, G., An improved method for the electrophoretic separation and fluorometric determination of thiamin and its phosphates in animal tissues, *Int. J. Vit. Nutr. Res.*, 50, 10, 1980.

62. Penttinen, H. K., Determination of thiamin and its phosphate esters by electrophoresis and fluorometry, *Acta Chem. Scand.*, B32, 609, 1978.

63. Dong, M. G., Green, M. D., and Sauberlich, H. E., Determination of urinary thiamin by the thiochrome method, *Clin. Biochem.*, 14, 16, 1981.

64. Roser, R. L., Andrist, A. H., Harrington, W. H., Naito, H. K., and Lonsdale, D., Determination of urinary thiamin by high-performance liquid chromatography utilizing the thiochrome fluorescent method, *J. Chromatogr.*, 146, 43, 1978.

65. Cheng, C. H., Koch, M., and Shank, R. E., Leukocyte transketolase activity as an indicator of thiamin nutriture in rats, *J. Nutr.*, 106, 1678, 1976.

66. Leveille, G. A., Modified thiochrome procedure for the determination of urinary thiamin, *Am. J. Clin. Nutr.*, 25, 273, 1972.

67. Edwin, E. E., Jackman, R., and Hebert, N., An improved procedure for the determination of thiamin, *Analyst*, 100, 689, 1975.

68. Wielders, J. P. M. and Mink, C. J. K., Quantitative analysis of total thiamin in human blood, milk and cerebrospinal fluid by reversed-phase ion-pair high-performance liquid chromatography, *J. Chromatogr.*, 277, 145, 1983.

69. Zempleni, J., Link, G., and Kubler, W., The transport of thiamin, riboflavin and pyridoxal 5'-phosphate by human placenta, *Int. J. Vit. Res.*, 62, 165, 1992.

70. Makkanen, T., Heikinketmo, R., and Dahl, M., Transketolase activity of red blood cells from infancy to old age, *Acta Haematolog.*, 42, 148, 1969.

71. Sauberlich, H. E., Antithiamins — their biochemical and nutritional importance, in Present and Future Problems of Nutrition Research; Symposium held March 3, 1993, Zurich, Switzerland, Swiss Nutrition Society, Bern, 1994, 15.

72. Roine, P., Koivula, L., and Pekkarinen, M., Plasma vitamin C level and erythrocyte transketolase activity compared with vitamin intakes among old people in Finland, *Nutrition*, 4, 116, 1972.

73. Vir, S. C. and Love, A. H. G., Nutritional status of institutionalized and noninstitutionalized aged in Belfast, Northern Ireland, *Am. J. Clin. Nutr.*, 32, 1934, 1979.

74. Hoorn, R. K. J., Flikweert, J. P., and Westerink, D., Vitamin B-1, B-2, and B-6 deficiencies in geriatric patients, measured by coenzyme stimulation of enzyme activities, *Clin. Chim. Acta*, 61, 151, 1975.

75. Iber, F. L., Blass, J. P., Brin, M., and Leevy, C. M., Thiamin in the elderly – relation to alcoholism and to neurological degenerative disease, *Am. J. Clin. Nutr.*, 36, 1067, 1982.
76. Scientific literature reviews on generally recognized as safe (GRAS) for ingredients: thiamin, U.S. Food and Drug Administration, Washington D.C., 1974.
77. Mills, C. A., Thiamin overdosage and toxicity, *J. Am. Med. Assoc.*, 116, 2101, 1941.
78. Wilkinson, T. J., Hanger, H. C., Elmslie, J., George, P. M., and Sainsbury, R., The response to treatment of subclinical thiamin deficiency in the elderly, *Am. J. Clin. Nutr.*, 66, 925, 1997.
79. Warnock, L. G., The measurement of erythrocyte thiamin pyrophosphate by high-performance liquid chromatography, *Anal. Biochem.*, 126, 394, 1982.
80. Baines, M., Improved high performance liquid chromatographic determination of thiamin diphosphate in erythrocytes, *Clin. Chim. Acta*, 153, 43, 1985.
81. Bailey, A. L. and Finglas, P. M., A normal phase high-performance liquid chromatographic method for the determination of thiamin in blood and tissue samples, *J. Micronutr. Anal.*, 7, 147, 1990.
82. Finglas, P. M., Thiamin, *Int. J. Vit. Nutr. Res.*, 63, 270, 1993.
83. O'Rourke, N., Bunker, V. W., Thomas, A. J., Finglas, P. M., Bailey, A. L., and Clayton, B. E., Thiamin status of healthy and institutionalized elderly subjects: analysis of dietary intake and biochemical indices, *Age and Aging*, 19, 325, 1990.
84. Smidt, L. J., Cremin, F. M., Grivetti, E. E., and Clifford, A. J., Influences of thiamin supplementation on the health and general well-being of an elderly Irish population with marginal thiamin deficiency, *J. Gerontol.*, 46, M16, 1991.
85. Horwitt, M. K. and Kreisler, O., The determination of early thiamin-deficient status by estimation of blood lactic and pyruvic acids after glucose administration, *J. Nutr.*, 33, 411, 1949.
86. Bailey, A. C., Finglas, P. M., Wright, A. J. A., and Southon, S., Thiamin, erythrocyte transketolase (EC 2.2.1.1) activity and total erythrocyte thiamin in adolescents, *Br. J. Nutr.*, 72, 111, 1994.
87. Fidanza, F., Simonetti, M. S., Floridi, A., Codini, M., and Idanze, R., Comparison of methods for thiamin and riboflavin nutriture in man, *Int. J. Vit. Nutr. Res.*, 59, 40, 1989.
88. Pearson, W. N., Blood and urine vitamin levels as potential indices of body stores, *Am. J. Clin. Nutr. Res.*, 20, 514, 1967.
89. Herbeth, B., Zitloun, J., Mirarret, L., Bourgeay-Causse, M., Carre-Guery, G., Delacoux, E., LeDevehat, C., Lemoine, A., Mareschi, J. P., Martin, J., Potier de Courcy, G., and Sancho, J., Reference intervals for vitamins B_1, B_2, E, D, retinol, beta-carotene, and folate in blood: usefulness of dietary selection criteria, *Clin. Chem.*, 32, 1756, 1986.
90. Delacoux, E., Santho, J., Evstignuff, T., Determination de l'activite de la transcetolase erythrocytaire, *Clin. Chim. Acta*, 108, 483, 1980.
91. Vuilleumier, J. P., Keller, H. E., Rettenmaier, R., and Hunziker, F., Clinical chemical methods for the routine assessment of the vitamin status in human populations. Part II: The water-soluble vitamins B_1, B_2, and B_6, *Int. J. Vit. Nutr. Rev.*, 53, 359, 1983.
92. Kaufmann, N. A. and Guggenheim, K., The validity of biochemical assessment of thiamin, riboflavin and folacin nutrition, *Int. J. Vit. Nutr. Res.*, 47, 40, 1977.
93. Bhuvaneswaran, C. and Sreenivaran, A., Problems of thiamin deficiency status and their amelioration, *Ann. N.Y. Acad. Sci.*, 98, 576, 1962.
94. *The Surgeon General's Report on Nutrition and Health*, Chapter 17: Alcohol, U.S. Department of Health and Human Services, Washington D.C., 1988, 629.
95. Floridi, A., Pupita, M., Palmerini, C. A., Fini, C., and Fidanza, A. A., Thiamin pyrophosphate determination in whole blood and erythrocytes by high performance liquid chromatography, *Int. J. Vit. Nutr. Res.*, 54, 165, 1984.
96. Laschi-Loquerie, A., Vallas, S., Viollet, J., Leclercq, M., and Fayol, V., High performance liquid chromatographic determination of total thiamin in biological and food products, *Int. J. Vit. Nutr. Res.*, 62, 248, 1991.
97. Botticher, B. and Botticher, D., Simple rapid determination of thiamin by a HPLC method in foods, body fluids, urine and faeces, *Int. J. Vit. Nutr. Res.*, 56, 155, 1986.
98. Botticher, B. and Botticher, D., A new HPLC-method for the simultaneous determination of B_1, B_2, and B_6 vitamins in serum and whole blood, *Int. J. Vit. Nutr. Res.*, 57, 273, 1987.
99. Anonymous, Beriberi can complicate TPN, *Nutr. Rev.*, 45, 239, 1987.

100. Baumgartner, T. G., What the practicing nurse should know about thiamin, *J. Intravenous Nursing*, 14, 130, 1991.
101. Martin, P. R., McCool, B. A., and Singleton, C. K., Molecular genetics of transketolase in the pathogenesis of the Wernick-Korsakoff syndrome, *Metab. Brain Dis.*, 10, 45, 1995.
102. McLaren, D. S., Docherty, M. A., and Boyd, D. H. A., Plasma thiamin pyrophosphate and erythrocyte transketolase in chronic alcoholism, *Am. J. Clin. Nutr.*, 34, 1031, 1981.
103. Haas, R. H., Thiamin and the brain, *Annu. Rev. Nutr.*, 8, 483, 1988.
104. Tomasulo, P. A., Kater, R. M. H., and Iber, F. L., Impairment of thiamin absorption in alcoholism, *Am. J. Clin. Nutr.*, 21, 1341, 1968.
105. Baum, R. A. and Iber, F. L., Thiamin — the interaction of aging, alcoholism and malabsorption in various populations, *World Rev. Nutr. Diet.*, 44, 85, 1984.
106. Herve, C., Beyne, P., Letteron, P., Delacoux, E., Comparison of erythrocyte transketolase activity with thiamin and thiamin phosphate ester levels in chronic alcoholic patients, *Clin. Chim. Acta*, 234, 91, 1995.
107. Molina, J. A., Bermejo, F., de Sen, T., Jimenez-Jimenez, F. J., Herranz, A., Fernadez-Calle, P., Ortuno, B., Villanueva, C., and Sainz, M. J., Alcoholic congnitive deterioration and nutritional deficiencies, *Acta Neurol. Scand.*, 89, 384, 1994.
108. Devgun, M. S., Fiabane, A., Patterson, C. R., and Zarembski, P., Vitamin and mineral nutrition in chronic alcoholics including patients with Korsakoff's psychosis, *Br. J. Nutr.*, 45, 469, 1981.
109. Bontemps, J., Philippe, P., Betendorff, Lombet, J., Dadrifosse, G., and Schoffeniels, E., Determination of thiamin and thiamin phosphates in excitable tissues and thiochrome derivatives by reversed-phase high-performance liquid chromatography on octadecyl silica, *J. Chromatogr.*, 307, 283, 1984.
110. Tang, C. M., Wells, J. C., Rolfe, M., and Cham, K., Outbreak of beri-beri in the Gambia, *Lancet*, 206, 1989.
111. Djoenaidi, W., Notermans, S. L. H., and Dunda, G., Beriberi cardiomyopathy, *Eur. J. Clin. Nutr.*, 46, 227, 1991.
112. Macias-Matos, C., Rodriguez-Ojea, A., Chi, N., Jimenez, S., Zulueta, D., and Bates, C. J., Biochemical evidence of thiamin depletion during the Cuban neuropathy epidemic, 1992–1993, *Am. J. Clin. Nutr.*, 64, 347, 1996.
113. Changbumrung, S., Pashakrishana, P., Vudhival, N., Hontong, K., Pongpaew, P., and Migasena, P., Measurement of B_1, B_2, and B_6 status in children and mothers attending a well-baby clinic in Bangkok, *Int. J. Vit. Nutr. Res.*, 54, 149, 1984.
114. Wyatt, D. T., Nelson, D., and Hillman, R. E., Age-dependent changes in thiamin concentrations in whole blood and cerebrospinal fluid in infants and children, *Am. J. Clin. Nutr.*, 53, 530, 1991.
115. Wethuilt, H., Ackurt, F., Brubacher, G., Okan, B., Aktas, S., and Turdu, S., Blood vitamin and mineral levels in 7–17 year old Turkish children, *Int. J. Vit. Nutr. Res.*, 62, 21, 1992.
116. Pongpanich, B., Srikrikkrich, N., Dhanamitta, S., and Valyasevi, A., Biochemical detection of thiamin deficiency in infants and children in Thailand, *Am. J. Clin. Nutr.*, 27, 1399, 1974.
117. Butterworth, R. F., Maternal thiamin deficiency: a factor in intrauterine growth retardation, *Ann. N.Y. Acad. Sci.*, 678, 325, 1993.
118. Anderson, S. H., Vickery, C. A., and Nicol, A. D., Adult thiamin requirements and the continuing need to fortify processed cereals, *Lancet*, 85, 1986.
119. Carroll, M. D., Abraham, S., and Dressu, C. M., National Center for Health Statistics: Dietary Intake Source Data, United States 1976–1980, Vital and Health Statistics Series II (Public Health Service, DHHS, U.S. Government Printing Office, Hyattsville, 1982.
120. Heller, S., Salkeld, R. M., and Korner, W. F., Vitamin B_1 status in pregnancy, *Am. J. Clin. Nutr.*, 27, 1221, 1974.
121. Olkowski, A. A. and Gooneratne, S. R., Microbiological methods of thiamin measurement in biological material, *Int. J. Vit. Nutr. Res.*, 62, 34, 1992.
122. Icke, G. C. and Nicol, D. J., Thiamin status in pregnancy as determined by direct microbiological assay, *Int. J. Vit. Nutr. Res.*, 63, 33, 1993.
123. Icke, G. C. and Nicol, D., Automated microbiological assay of thiamin in serum and red cells, *J. Clin. Pathol.*, 47, 639, 1994.

124. Deibel, R. H., Evans, J. B., Niven, C. F., Jr., Microbiological assay for thiamin using *Lactobacillus viridescens*, *J. Bacteriol.*, 74, 818, 1957.
125. Muiruri, K. L., Romos, D. R., and Kirk, J. R., A simple automated method for the determination of urinary thiamin, *Am. J. Clin. Nutr.*, 27, 837, 1974.
126. van Dokkum, W., Schrijver, J., and Wesstra, J. A., Variability in man of the levels of some indices of nutritional status over a 60-day period on a constant diet, *Eur. J. Clin. Nutr.*, 44, 665, 1990.
127. Nichols, H. K. and Basu, T. K., Thiamin status of the elderly: dietary intake and thiamin pyrophosphate response, *J. Am. Coll. Nutr.*, 13, 57, 1994.
128. Wood, B., Currie, J., and Brun, K., Wernicke's encephalopathy in a metropolitan hospital, *Med. J. Aust.*, 144, 12, 1986.
129. Yellowlees, P. M., Thiamin deficiency and prevention of the Werniche-Korsakoff syndrome, *Med. J. Aust.*, 145, 216, 1986.
130. Williams, R. R., *Toward the Conquest of Beriberi*, Harvard University Press, Cambridge, U.K., 1961.
131. Major, R. H., *Classic Descriptions of Disease*, Thomas Publication, Springfield, CT, 1932, 575.
132. McCollum, E. V., *A History of Nutrition*, Houghton Mifflin Co., Boston, MA, 1957.
133. Eijkman, C. von, Eine beri beri-ahnliche Krankheit des Huhner, *Virchow Arch. Pathol. Anat. Physiol.*, 148, 523, 1987.
134. Sauberlich, H. E., Assessment of vitamin B_1, vitamin B_2, niacin, and pantothenic acid, in *Nutritional Assessment of the Individual*, Livingston, G. F., Ed., Food and Nutrition Press, Trumbull, 1989, 295.
135. Dong, M. H., McGown, E. L., Schwenneker, B. W., and Sauberlich, H. E., Thiamin, riboflavin, and vitamin B_6 contents of selected foods as served, *J. Am. Diet. Assoc.*, 76, 156, 1980.
136. Paul, A. A. and Southgate, D. A. T., *The Composition of Foods*, Elsevier/North-Holland Biomedical Press, New York, 1978.
137. Isaeva, V. A., Sakolnikov, E. A., Alekseeva, I. A., Aleinik, S. I., Blazheevich, N. V., and Spirichev, V. B., Providing with vitamins of different population groups in Sverdlovsk, *Vop. Pitan.*, May–June (3), 65, 1992.
138. Food and Nutrition Board, Recommended Dietary Allowances, 10th edition, National Research Council, National Academy Press, Washington D.C., 1989.
139. Louhi, H. A., Yu, H. H., Hawthorne, B. E., and Storvick, C. A., Thiamin metabolism on women in controlled diets. I. Daily urinary thiamin excretion and its relation to creatinine excretion, *J. Nutr.*, 48, 297, 1952.
140. Plough, I. C. and Bridgefort, E. B., Relation of clinical and dietary findings in nutrition surveys, *Public Health Rep.*, 75, 699, 1960.
141. Requirements of vitamin A, thiamin, riboflavin and niacin, Report of a Joint FAO/WHO Expert Group, *FAO Nutrition Meeting Report* Series No. 41, Food and Agriculture Organization of the United Nations, Rome, 1967.
142. *Ten-State Nutrition Survey Reports*, I–V, Centers for Disease Control and Prevention, Atlanta, GA, 1972.
143. Pearson, W. H., Biochemical appraisal of the vitamin nutritional status in man, *JAMA*, 180, 49, 1962.
144. Lossy, F. T., Goldsmith, G. A., and Sarett, H. P., A study of test dose excretion of five B complex vitamins in man, *J. Nutr.*, 45, 213, 1951.

Vitamin B-2 (Riboflavin)

Converting metric units to International System units (SI):

μg/mL × 2.66 = μmol/L

μmol/L × 0.376 = μg/mL

molecular weight: 376.4

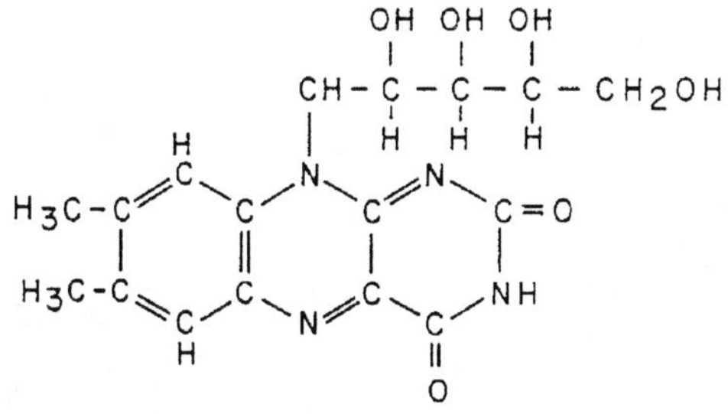

FIGURE 12
Structure of riboflavin.

D-Riboflavin

History of Riboflavin

The presence of a growth factor in yeast was first reported by Emmett and Luros in 1920.[3] In 1932, Warburg and Christian in Germany isolated a yellow enzyme from yeast.[2,4] The yellow color was determined to be due to the presence of an alloxazine derivative which was characterized as riboflavin by Kuhn et al. in 1933.[5,6] The vitamin was synthesized for the first time in 1935 by Karrer et al.[2,7,8]

Suboptimal dietary intakes of riboflavin occur in many third-world countries, including Thailand, Gambia, India, Nigeria, and China.[30-33,94] Biochemical evidence of a riboflavin deficiency are often observed in the United States, particularly among the adolescent population.[34]

Riboflavin Functions

Riboflavin is a component of flavin mononucleotide (riboflavin-5′-phosphate; FMN) and flavin adenine dinucleotide (riboflavin-5′-adenosyldiphosphate; FAD). These compounds serve as coenzymes of the flavoproteins that participate in tissue oxidation and respiration processes.[2,14-16] This includes oxygen and monooxygen reductases, pyridine and nonpyridine-dependent dehydrogenases, disulfide reductases, and one-electron transfers.

55

This yellow vitamin is stable in dry form, but in solution the vitamin activity is rapidly destroyed by exposure to visible light and ultraviolet lighting. Light-protected solutions are stable in a pH range of 2 to 5. At an alkaline pH, riboflavin is converted rapidly to mainly lumiflavin, a highly fluorescing compound.

Riboflavin Metabolism

The body stores little riboflavin as such. Consequently urinary excretion of riboflavin reflects the dietary intake of the vitamin. Normally, 60 to 70% of the urinary flavins present are in the form of riboflavin. The remaining flavins present are accounted for mainly as 7-hydroxymethyl-riboflavin (10 to 15%), 8α-sulfomylriboflavin (5 to 10%), 8-hydroxymethyl-riboflavin (4 to 7%), and riboflavinyl peptide (5%).[2,15,38]

Riboflavin Deficiency

Individuals who regularly consume a diet low in dairy products and animal protein foods are prone to the development of a riboflavin deficiency.[2] Worldwide, riboflavin deficiency is thought to be one of the most common dietary-related disorders.[17]

The clinical manifestations of a riboflavin deficiency include cheilosis, glossitis, seborrheic dermatitis (face and scrotum), corneal vascularization, photophobia, visual impairment, burning of the eyes, and pruritus.[17] Clinical manifestations must be evaluated with caution as many of the signs or symptoms noted are not always specific to only a riboflavin deficiency. Hence, a clinical suspicion of a riboflavin deficiency requires conformation by laboratory tests.

Riboflavin deficiency has been observed in both institutionalized and non-institutionalized elderly.[27,28,53,93] Riboflavin supplements promptly corrected the deficiency.[93] Good dietary sources of riboflavin include milk, dairy products, liver, kidney, eggs, and some green leafy vegetables, such as broccoli.[9] In the United States, cereals and breads are generally enriched with riboflavin.

A marked riboflavin deficiency may impair the conversion of vitamin B-6 to pyridoxal phosphate.[25,36] This has been demonstrated in the study of Madigan et al.[113] with free-living elderly subjects ($n = 83$). Of their subjects, 49% had a suboptimal riboflavin status and 39% had a suboptimal vitamin B-6 status. A suboptimal status for both vitamins was observed in 21% of the subjects. Supplementation with riboflavin corrected the riboflavin deficiency in the groups as well as corrected the low plasma pyridoxal-5'-phosphate concentrations. This appears to confirm the interdependency of these two nutrients.

Patients in a negative nitrogen status excrete increased amounts of riboflavin in the urine.[12,68] Increased excretion of riboflavin may occur with the use of certain antibiotics and phenothiazine drugs.[10,11] Riboflavin metabolism may be impaired by various other types of drugs, including chlorpromezine, imipromine, amitriptyline, adriomycin, alcohol, and quinocrine.[16,18]

Riboflavin excretion may also be increased by additional factors such as heavy physical work, heat stress, and enforced bed rest. Exercise training may increase the excretion of riboflavin in the urine and increase the erythrocyte glutathione reductase activity coefficient.[69] Oral contraceptive use did not influence riboflavin status.[70,88]

When riboflavin is withdrawn from the diet, the urinary excretion of riboflavin promptly falls.[63] Hence, rapid changes in riboflavin excretions may not provide accurate information about the riboflavin status of the body.

In contrast, erythrocyte glutathione reductase measurements are not influenced by such effects and represent a more long-term assessment of riboflavin status. The measurement can be considered a "functional" procedure.[118] The measurement is more sensitive to changes in riboflavin status than erythrocyte riboflavin measurement.[87] Erythrocyte glutathione reductase assay results are usually expressed in terms of "activity coefficients" (AC).[53]

Riboflavin Nutritional Assessment

Riboflavin (vitamin B-2) nutritional status has usually been assessed by (a) urinary excretion of riboflavin, (b) plasma and blood concentrations of riboflavin, and (c) erythrocyte glutathione reductase activities.[118,119] Other less used procedures for the assessment of riboflavin nutrition have been summarized elsewhere.[37,39,112] A comprehensive review of vitamin B-2 analytical procedures has been published by Russell and Vanderslice.[97]

Urinary Excretion of Riboflavin

Since little storage of riboflavin occurs, riboflavin in excess of requirement is excreted in the urine. When riboflavin intakes are below those that achieve tissue saturation, the urinary excretion rate increases very slowly with increasing intake (Figure 13).[13] However, at the point where tissue saturation is reached, there is a sharp increase in the excretion rate, which approximately equals the rate of riboflavin absorption. Urinary excretion of riboflavin by an adult of less than 100 µg in a 24-hr urine collection is indicative of an inadequate intake of the vitamin. When 24-hr urine collections are not practical, random urine samples may be obtained and analyzed for riboflavin and the results expressed in terms of urine creatinine levels.[20-23] Riboflavin load tests have been reported but they have seldom been used because of the cumbersomeness of the test procedures.[19]

Clinical signs of a riboflavin deficiency and dietary intake of the vitamin have been shown to correlate with urinary riboflavin levels in controlled adult human studies.[13] From these studies, guidelines for interpreting urinary riboflavin excretion data have been extrapolated.[29]

Riboflavin Analytical Methods

High-Performance Liquid Chromatography

Urinary riboflavin levels may be measured by HPLC procedures.[72,73] Untreated urine samples were injected directly onto the column and quantitated by fluorometric detection. The procedures are sensitive, specific, and rapid.

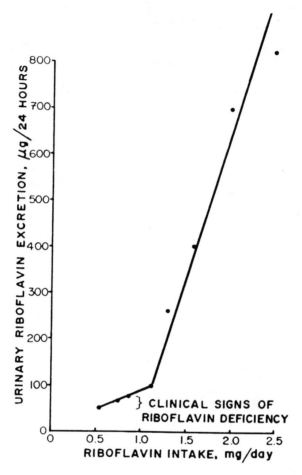

FIGURE 13

Relationship of riboflavin intakes to urinary excretion of riboflavin as observed in the studies of Horwitt et al.[13] (With permission.)

Guide to Interpretation of Urinary Riboflavin Excretion

Adults	Urinary Excretion of Riboflavin (Vitamin B-2)	
	µg/24 hr	µg/g Creatinine
Deficient (high risk)	< 40	< 27
Marginal (moderate risk)	40–119	27–79
Acceptable (low risk)	≥ 120	≥ 80

From References 39, 92, and 104.

Competitive Binding Protein Assays

Competitive binding protein procedures have also been reported for measuring riboflavin in urine.[35,74] The procedures require the isolation of the competitive binding protein from chicken egg white. The procedure of Tillotson and Bashor was rapid and sensitive and the urine sample required no treatment prior to analysis.[35] The radioisotope competitive binding assay of Lotter et al.[74] requires the availability of [2-^{14}C] riboflavin. The sensitivity of the method depended upon the specific activity of the radioactive riboflavin used.

Microbiological Assays

Riboflavin concentration in whole blood and plasma may be measured by microbiological assay using *Lactobacillus rhamnosus*, formerly *L.casei*, (ATCC 7469) as the test organism.[18,97] Whole blood levels of riboflavin for young athletes were reported as 327 ± 69 nmol/L.[86] Urinary excretion of riboflavin was 2.10 ± 1.52 µmol/g creatinine.[86] Microbiological assays have been useful for the routine analysis of riboflavin where a large number of samples are involved. The protozoan, *Tetrahymena pyriformis*, has also been used to assay riboflavin levels in biological samples.[95]

In a study involving 504 military personnel, urinary riboflavin excretion levels had a modest correlation with dietary riboflavin intake data ($r = 0.60$).[40,41] Fasting urine samples were used which helped reduce variation in excretion that may follow a meal. A microbiological assay was used.[111] In another study a correlation of -0.33 was reported between erythrocyte glutathione reductase activities and urinary riboflavin excretion.[45]

Fluorometric Procedures

Several fluorometric procedures have been developed and used to analyze riboflavin levels in urine and blood. Most fluorometric procedures are based on the method of Slater and Morell.[82,96] In principle, riboflavin is measured fluorometrically after some interfering substances have been destroyed by oxidation and others have been eliminated by extraction of the riboflavin into a butanol-pyridine solution. An internal standard is used and the blank determined by destruction of the riboflavin by irradiation.[82] An automated fluorometric method for the determination of urinary riboflavin concentration was reported by Mellor and Maass.[107]

Pregnancy

During pregnancy, urinary excretion of riboflavin has been reported to increase during the second trimester and fall during the third trimester.[42,43] Although measurements of urinary riboflavin excretion during pregnancy are seldom conducted, a reference guide has been proposed.

Guide to Interpretation of Urinary Riboflavin Excretion in Pregnant Women[43]

	µg/g Creatinine		
Trimester	Deficient	Low	Acceptable
1st	< 27	27–65	66–129
2nd	< 23	23–54	55–109
3rd	< 21	21–49	50–99

Riboflavin Load Test

Occasionally a riboflavin load test has been used to evaluate riboflavin status.[83,85] The procedure commonly used consists of measuring the urinary excretion of riboflavin in the 4-hr period following the oral administration of a 5-mg test dose of the vitamin.[80-82]

High activity coefficients of EGR assays were associated with low excretion levels in the 4-hr urinary excretion test.[83]

Interpretation of Riboflavin Load Test

Urinary Return in Adults of a 5 mg Riboflavin Dose		
mg in 4 hr:	< 1.00	(Deficient/high risk)
	1.00 to 1.40	(Low/marginal risk)
	≥ 1.40	(Acceptable/low risk)

From Reference 81.

Blood Riboflavin Analyses

Most of the flavins present in blood is located in the erythrocytes. FAD is the predominant form present. Two FAD-requiring enzymes are found in the erythrocyte: (a) glutathione reductase (EGR), which ensures the maintenance of proper levels of reduced glutathione and (b) methemoglobin reductase.[24]

Red blood cell riboflavin is not a very sensitive index of riboflavin status due to the small magnitude of change noted with large variations in dietary riboflavin intake.[13,44] However, red blood cell riboflavin concentrations have been considered an index of riboflavin stores.[44] Erythrocyte riboflavin concentrations of less than 15 µg/dL cells indicate a low riboflavin nutritional status.[44,82]

Both microbiological assays and fluorometric procedures have been used to estimate the riboflavin concentrations of red blood cells.[37,46-49] Human red blood cells were reported to contain 18.3 ± 1.58 µg/dL cells by fluorometric assay and 17.4 ± 1.47 µg/dL of cells by microbiological assay. The difference observed was not significant.

A micro spectrofluorimetric method has been described for measuring riboflavin levels in the blood of newborn babies and their mothers.[51] The procedure required a purification step with the use of a chromatographic column. The riboflavin levels of blood from women were 14.2 ± 2.5 µg/dL blood (hematocrit = 39.4). The riboflavin levels of newborn babies was 17.1 ± 2.4 µg/dL (hematocrit = 53.6).

Erythrocyte Glutathione Reductase Assays

Erythrocyte glutathione reductase (EGR) (EC 1.6.4.2) is a flavoprotein which is sensitive to the riboflavin status of the subject. Glutathione reductase measurements (EGR) provide a functional test for riboflavin status. Since this is an NADPH-dependent reaction, a simple spectrophotometric assay can be conducted on a small amount of blood.[37,39] With the use of a centrifugal analyzer, an automated method of measuring erythrocyte glutathione reducatase activity has been reported.[100] A similar procedure also using a centrifugal analyzer has been published by Mount et al.[108] Garry et al. have also used an automated procedure to measure EGR activity.[75,78,79,105] For those planning to conduct EGR assays may find the reports of Thurnham and Rathankette[76] and of Bayoumi and Rosalki[52,106] helpful.

Erythrocyte glutathione reductase catalyzes the reduction of oxidized glutathione (GSSG) in the following manner:

$$NADPH (NADH) + H^+ + GSSG \rightarrow NADP^+ (NAD^+) + 2GSH$$

Erythrocyte gluatathione reductase measurements represent the preferred method for evaluating riboflavin status (vitamin B-2).[37] The general procedure is to determine the

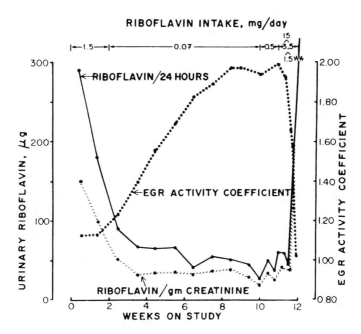

FIGURE 14

Relationship of riboflavin intake to urinary riboflavin excretion and erythrocyte glutathione reductase activity coefficients. Mean values for six young adult males. (Adapted from Tillotson and Baker.[63] (With permission.)

degree of activation of erythrocyte glutathione reductase by *in vitro* addition of flavin-adenine dinucleotide (FAD). Thus, the *in vitro* addition of FAD provides a measure of the undersaturation of glutathione reductase apoenzyme with respect to its coenzyme.

Erythrocyte glutathione reductase assay results are usually expressed in terms of "activity coefficients" (AC) or "percent of stimulation" resulting from the *in vitro* addition of FAD (Figure 14).[53,62,63] The activity coefficient may be expressed as follows:

$$AC = \frac{\text{Reduction of absorbance with added FAD/12 min}}{\text{Reduction of absorbance without added FAD/12 min}}$$

In normal subjects, an AC of approximately 1.00 to 1.10 (0 to 10%) is obtained indicating little or no stimulation. With an inadequate intake of riboflavin, a marked stimulation occurs. An activity coefficient AC value of 1.20 (20% stimulation) and above has been considered as indicative of an inadequate riboflavin nutriture.[53,62,63,119] Values above 1.40 are at high risk and usually respond promptly to riboflavin supplementation.[53,61,62,93,94,99,109]

Guide for the Interpretation of Erythrocyte Glutathione Reductase

Subjects	Activity Coefficients		
	Deficient (high risk)	Marginal (medium risk)	Acceptable (low risk)
All ages	1.40 (40%)	1.20–1.40 (20–40%)	<1.20 (20%)

Erythrocyte glutathione reductase assays can be readily performed spectrophotometrically requiring only a small quantity of blood. The early assay procedures of Glatzle et al.,[53-55] Thurnham et al.,[56] Beutler,[24,57-59] and Bamji[50,60] have received extensive use for evaluating riboflavin nutritional status.[37,53,56,64,65,67,71,78,83,84,86,93,109,110]

It has been suggested that in a severe riboflavin deficiency, the erythrocyte glutathione reductase apoenzyme may be reduced as well as the flavin coenzyme. In such an instance, a low activation coefficient could occur resulting in an erroneous assessment of riboflavin status. Availability of information on the basal level of activity may identify such a possibility.[53] In practice, we have not encountered this problem. Subjects with a low erythrocyte glutathione reductase apoenzyme level, due to a riboflavin deficiency, have always had a marked response to the *in vitro* addition of FAD (i.e., elevated activity coefficient value). (This is in agreement with Brubacher.[101]) The validity of EGR activity measurements to assess riboflavin status in individuals with low erythrocyte glucose-6-phosphate dehydrogenase activity had been questioned.[77,115,116] Approximately 10% of the Black population have this condition.[117]

Lakshmi and Bamji [61] studied a group of subjects with evidence of a riboflavin deficiency based on the presence of angular stomatitis and glossitis. All of the subjects were found to have a high activity coefficient, which fell to normal values with riboflavin supplementation. Erythrocyte riboflavin concentrations were low but improved also with riboflavin supplementation (0.20 ± 0.006 µg/mL cells vs. 0.28 ± 0.01 µg/mL cells after supplements; $n = 13$).

In a National Nutrition Survey of Korea, conducted in 1953 and in 1982–83, 11.98% of the subjects studied had angular stomatitis.[102,114] Elevated erythrocyte glutathione reductase coefficient were common. Supplements of 5 mg of riboflavin for one week resulted in normal coefficients.[103] Based on elevated erythrocyte glutathione reductase activity coefficients, a poor riboflavin status was reported for infants and children of India.[109,110] Because of the high incidence of elevated EGR activity coefficients in the Indian children, Prasad et al. suggested that a cut-off value for acceptable riboflavin status might be < 1.50.[109] In view of other reports, the justification for this criterion requires further investigation.

Red Blood Cell Glutathione Reductase Activity Coefficient Determination

In order to simplify the procedure and to reduce the time required to perform the determination, we have modified our procedure to employ 96 well plates and a plate reader. Basic studies for the development of the procedure were conducted by P.E. Cornwell, Ph.D., Department of Nutrition Sciences, University of Alabama at Birmingham (personal communication). The following is a description of the procedure.

Materials Needed:

- Disposable glass culture tubes (13 × 100 mm)
- Pipettes (285 µl)
- Repeater pipette
- Multi-channel pipettor (15 µl)
- Vortex
- Incubator (37°C)
- Plate reader (340 nm)

- 96-Well plates
- Kim wipes
- Analytical balance
- Weighing paper
- Weighing spatula
- Reagent reservoirs

Reagents

FAD: Flavin adenine dinucleotide (Sigma F-6625)

2 mg FAD to 92 mL dH_2O. Prepare fresh each day.

NADPH: β-Nicotinamide adenine dinucleotide phosphate, reduced form (Sigma N-6505)

3.6 mg NADPH to 2.0 mL 1% $NaHCO_3$. Prepare fresh each day.

Glutathione (Sigma G-4626)

40 mg glutathione to 2.5 mL .01 N NaOH. Prepare fresh each day.

EDTA: (K-salt)

1.6 g EDTA to 50 mL dH_2O. Prepare as needed and store at room temperature.

1% $NaHCO_3$

1 g $NaHCO_3$ to 100 mL dH_2O. Prepare as needed and store at 2 to 8°C.

0.01N NaOH

1 mL of 50% NaOH solution (12.5 N) to 12.5 mL dH_2O (1 N).

Dilute 1 N solution 1:100 for 0.01 N solution. Prepare as needed and store at 2 to 8°C.

Phosphate Buffer (0.1M, pH 7.4)

0.1 M monobasic: 13.61 g to 1000 mL with dH_2O.

0.1M dibasic: 22.82 g to 1000 mL with dH_2O.

Titrate dibasic with monobasic to a pH of 7.4. Prepare as needed and store at room temperature.

Hemolysate Preparation

Dilute red blood cells

1. 100 µl RBC to 1.9 mL dH_2O
2. Vortex.

Sample Preparation and Assay

1. Label 13 × 100 mm glass test tubes; unstimulated in front row and stimulated in back.
2. Add in the following order to each tube:

   2.0 mL buffer

   100 µL hemolysate

   50 µL EDTA

   100 µL glutathione

3. To the unstimulated tubes only add 100 μL dH$_2$O.

4. To the stimulated tubes only add 100 μL FAD.

5. Vortex all tubes well.

6. Remove 285 μL of sample to the corresponding wells.

7. Incubate at 37°C for 30 minutes.

8. Turn on Plate Reader for 10 to 15 minutes to allow for warm-up (wavelength 340 nm).

9. Add 15 μL NADPH to all wells quickly and mix.

10. Read at 340 nm immediately for the initial reading (= T$_0$).

11. Incubate plate at 37°C for 12 minutes.

12. Read plate for final reading at 340 nm (= T$_{12}$).

Calculations

Transfer absorbance values to the worksheet and calculate the activity coefficient (AC).

Unstimulated: T$_0$ – T$_{12}$ = TA

FAD stimulated: T$_0$ – T$_{12}$ = TB

Divide as follows to yield AC

$$\frac{TB}{TA} = \text{Activity Coefficient}$$

Erythrocyte glutathione reductase apoenzyme and holoenzyme are both stable in erythrocytes stored at –72°C for over a year. Quality-control samples may be prepared from blood samples with different EGR activity coefficients. The erythrocytes are stored in small aliquots at –72°C or colder.

Riboflavin Toxicity

No riboflavin toxicity has been reported for the human. Doses of up to 20 mg daily were without toxicity.[1] Hence, the toxicity of riboflavin is considered very low.[26]

Summary

Riboflavin nutritional status has been assessed through measurements of erythrocyte glutathione reductase activity coefficient, erythrocyte riboflavin concentrations, and urinary riboflavin excretion.

The activity coefficient of erythrocyte glutathione reductase provides a sensitive functional indicator of riboflavin nutritional status in the human. This measurement is the method of choice. In contrast, urinary measurements of riboflavin reflect recent dietary intakes of riboflavin and do not provide a reliable measure of the severity of a riboflavin deficiency. If blood samples can not be obtained for glutathione reductase measurements, information on urinary riboflavin excretion may be of use.

References

1. Cumming, F., Briggs, M., and Briggs, M., Clinical toxicology of vitamin supplements, in *Vitamins in Human Biology and Medicine*, Briggs, M. H., Ed., CRC Press, Boca Raton, FL, 1981, 187.
2. McCormick, D. B., Riboflavin, in *Modern Nutrition in Health and Disease*, Shils, M. E., Olson, J. A., and Shike, M., Eds., 8th edition, Lea & Febiger, Philadelphia, 1994, 366.
3. Emmett, A. D. and Luros, G. O, Water-soluble vitamins. I. Are the antineuritic and the growth-promoting water-soluble B vitamins the same, *J. Biol. Chem.*, 43, 265, 1920.
4. Warburg, O. and Christian, W., The yellow enzyme and its functions, *Biochem. Z.*, 254, 438, 1932.
5. Kuhn, R., Reinemund, K., and Kaltschnitt, H. et al., *Naturwissinschaften*, 23, 260, 1935.
6. Kuhn, R., Reinemund, K., Weygand, F., and Storobele, R., Über die synthese de lactoflavins (Vitamin B_4), *Chem. Ber.*, 68, 1765, 1935.
7. Karrer, P., Schopp, K., and Benz, F., Synthesen von flavinen IV, *Helv. Chim. Acta*, 18, 426, 1935.
8. Karrer, P., Salomon, H., and Schopp, K. et al., Synthetische flavine VII, *Helv. Chim. Acta*, 18, 1143, 1935.
9. Watt, B. K. and Merrill, A. L., Composition of food: raw, processed, prepared, in Agriculture Handbook No. 8, U.S. Department of Agriculture, Washington D.C., 1963.
10. Goldsmith, G. A., Vitamin B complex, thiamin, riboflavin, niacin, folic acid (folacin), vitamin B_{12}, biotin (Review), *Prog. Food Nutr. Sci.*, 1, 559, 1975.
11. Pinto, J., Huang, Y. P., and Rivlin, R. S., *Clin. Res.*, 27, 444A, 1979.
12. Bro-Rasmussen, F., The riboflavin requirements of animals and man and associated metabolic relations. 1. Technique of estimating requirement, and modifying circumstances. 2. Relation of requirement to the metabolism of protein and energy, *Nutr. Abstr. Revs.*, 28, 1, 1-23; 3696, 1985.
13. Horwitt, M. K., Harvey, C. C., Hills, O. W., and Liebert, E., Correlation of urinary excretion with dietary intake and symptoms of ariboflavinosis, *J. Nutr.*, 41, 247, 1950.
14. Rivlin, R. S., Medical progress: riboflavin metabolism, *N. Engl. J. Med.*, 283, 463, 1970.
15. Merrill, A. H., Jr., Lambeth, J. D., Edmondson, D. E., and McCormack, D. B., Formation and mode of action of flavoproteins, *Annu. Rev. Nutr.*, 1, 281, 1981.
16. Rivlin, R. S. and Dutta, P., Vitamin B-2 (Riboflavin), *Nutr. Today*, 30, 62, 1995.
17. Sauberlich, H. E., Other water-soluble vitamins, in *Tropical and Geographical Medicine*, Warren, K. S., and Mahmond, A. A. F., Eds., McGraw-Hill, New York, 1984.
18. Nicholalds, G. E., Riboflavin, *Clin. Lab. Med.*, 1, 685, 1981.
19. Lossy, F. T., Goldsmith, G. A., Sarett, H. P., A study of test dose excretion of five B-complex vitamins in man, *J. Nutr.*, 45, 213, 1951.
20. Horwitt, M. K., Nutritional requirements of man with special reference to riboflavin, *Am. J. Clin. Nutr.*, 18, 458, 1966.
21. Plough, I. C. and Consolazio, F. C., The use of casual urine specimens in the evaluation of the excretion rates of thiamin, riboflavin, and N'-methylnicotinamide, *J. Nutr.*, 69, 365, 1959.
22. Lowry, O. H., Biochemical evidence of nutritional status, *Physiol. Rev.* 32, 431, 1952.
23. Hegsted, D. M., Gershoff, S. N., and Trulson, M. F. et al., Variation in riboflavin excretion, *J. Nutr.*, 60, 581, 1956.
24. Beutler, E., The effect of flavin coenzymes on the activity of erythrocyte enzymes, *Experientia*, 25, 804, 1969.
25. Sauberlich, H. E., Interactions of thiamin, riboflavin, and other B-vitamins, *Ann. N.Y. Acad. Sci.*, 355, 80, 1980.
26. Life Sciences Research Office, Federation of American Societies for Experimental Biology, *Evaluation of the Health Aspects of Riboflavin and Riboflavin-5'-Phosphate as Food Ingredients*, Prepared for Bureau of Foods, Food and Drug Administration, Washington D.C., 1979.
27. Vir, S. C. and Love, A. H. G., Nutritional evaluation of B groups of vitamins in institutionalized aged, *Int. J. Vit. Nutr. Res.*, 47, 211, 1977.
28. Vir, S. C. and Love, A. H. G., Riboflavin status of institutionalized and non-institutionalized aged, *Int. J. Vit. Nutr. Res.*, 47, 336, 1977.

29. Tillotson, J. A. and Baker, E. M., An enzymatic measurement of the riboflavin status in men, *Am. J. Clin. Nutr.* 25, 425, 1972.
30. Bates, C. J., Prentice, A. M., Watkinson, M., Morrell, P., Foord, F. A., Watkinson, A., Cole, T. J., and Whitehead, R. G., Efficacy of a food supplement in correcting riboflavin deficiency in pregnant Gambian women, *Hum. Nutr.: Clin. Nutr.*, 38C, 363, 1984.
31. Bates, C. J., Prentice, A. M., Sharkey, K. A., Murphy, P. K., Villard, L., and Prentice, A., Physiological tests during an improvement in riboflavin status in lactating Gambian women, *Int. J. Vit. Res.*, 52, 14, 1982.
32. Ajayi, O. A. and James, O. A., Effect of riboflavin supplementation on riboflavin nutriture of a secondary school population in Nigeria, *Am. J. Clin. Nutr.*, 39, 787, 1984.
33. Lo, C. S., Riboflavin status of adolescents in southern China, Average intake of riboflavin and clinical findings, *Med. J. Aust.*, 141, 635, 1984.
34. Lopez, R., Schwartz, J. V., and Copperman, J. M., Riboflavin deficiency in an adolescent population in New York City, *Am. J. Clin. Nutr.*, 33, 1283, 1980.
35. Tillotson, J. A. and Bashor, M. M., Fluorometric apoprotein titration of urinary riboflavin, *Anal. Biochem.*, 107, 214, 1980.
36. Anderson, B. B., Saary, M., Stephens, A. D., Perry, G. M., Lersudi, I. C., and Horn, J. E., Effect of riboflavin on red-cell metabolism of vitamin B_6, *Nature*, 264, 574, 1976.
37. Sauberlich, H. E., Newer laboratory methods for assessing nutriture of selected B-complex vitamins, *Annu. Rev. Nutr.*, 4, 377, 1984.
38. Chastain, J. L. and McCormick, D. B., Flavin catabolites: identification and quantitation in human urine, *Am. J. Clin. Nutr.*, 46, 830, 1987.
39. Sauberlich, H. E., Skala, J. H., and Dowdy, R. P., *Laboratory Tests for the Assessment of Nutritional Status*, CRC Press, Inc., Boca Raton, FL, 1974.
40. Sauberlich, H. E., Limitation in the assessment of nutrient status, in *Food and Agricultural Research Opportunities to Improve Human Nutrition*, Doberenz, A. R., Milner, J. A., and Schweigert, B. S., Eds., College of Human Resources, University of Delaware, Newark, 1986.
41. Kretsch, M. J., Sauberlich, H. E., and Skala, J. H., Nutritional status assessment of marines before and after the installation of the "Multi-Restaurant" food service system at the Twentynine Palms Marine Corps Base, California, Institute Report No. 192, Letterman Army Institute Research, Presidio of San Francisco, December 1984.
42. Darby, W. J., Densen, P. M., Cannon, R. O. et al., The Vanderbilt cooperative study of maternal and infant nutrition. I. Background. II. Methods. III. Description of the samples and data, *J. Nutr.*, 51, 539, 1953.
43. Darby, W. J., McGanity, W. J., Martin, M. P. et al., The Vanderbilt cooperative study of maternal and infant nutrition. IV. Dietary, laboratory and physical findings in 2,129 delivered pregnancies, *J. Nutr.*, 51, 565, 1953.
44. Bessey, O. A., Horwitt, M. K., and Love, R. H., Dietary deprivation of riboflavin and blood riboflavin levels in man, *J. Nutr.*, 58, 367, 1956.
45. Kaufmann, N. A. and Guggenheim, K., The validity of biochemical assessment of thiamine, riboflavin and folacin nutriture, *Int. J. Vit. Nutr. Res.*, 47, 40, 1977.
46. Bamji, M. S., Sharada, D., and Naidu, A. N., A comparison of the fluorometric and microbiological assay for estimating riboflavin content of blood and liver, *Int. J. Vit. Nutr. Res.*, 43, 351, 1973.
47. Clegg, K. M., Kodicek, E., and Mistry, S. P., A modified medium for *Lactobacillus casei* for the assay of B vitamins, *Biochem. J.*, 50, 326, 1952.
48. Strong, F. M., Feeney, R. E., and Moore, B., The riboflavin content of blood and urine, *J. Biol. Chem.*, 137, 363, 1941.
49. Burch, H. B., Bessey, O. A., and Lowry, O. H., Fluorometric measurement of riboflavin and its natural derivatives in small quantities of blood, serum and cells, *J. Biol. Chem.*, 175, 457, 1948.
50. Bamji, M. S., Glutathione reductase activity in red blood cells and riboflavin nutritional status in humans, *Clin. Chim. Acta*, 26, 263, 1969.
51. Knobloch, E., Hodr, R., Janda, J., Herzmann, J., and Houdkova, V., Spectrofluorimetric micromethod for determining riboflavin in blood of new-born babies and their mothers, *Int. J. Vit. Nutr. Res.*, 49, 144, 1979.

52. Bayoumi, R. A. and Rosalki, S. B., Evaluation of methods of coenzyme activation of erythrocyte enzymes for detection of deficiency of vitamins B_1, B_2, and B_6, *Clin. Chem.*, 22, 327, 1976.
53. Glatzle, D., Korner, W. F., Christeller, S., and Wise, O., Method for the detection of a biochemical riboflavin deficiency, *Int. J. Vit. Nutr. Res.*, 40, 166, 1970.
54. Glatzle, D., Weber, F., and Wiss, O., Enzymatic test for the detection of a riboflavin deficiency, *Experientia*, 24, 1122, 1968.
55. Glatzle, D., Dependency of the glutathione reductase activity on the riboflavin status, *Clin. Enzymology*, S. Karger, Basel, 2, 89, 1970.
56. Thurnham, D. I., Migasena, P., and Pavapootanon, N., The ultramicro red-cell glutathione reductase assay for riboflavin status: its use in field studies in Thailand, *Microchim. Acta (Wien)*, 5, 988, 1970.
57. Beutler, E., The correction of glutathione reductase deficiency by riboflavin administration, *J. Clin. Invest.*, 48, 7a, 1969.
58. Beutler, E., Effect of flavin compounds on glutathione reductase activity: *in vivo* and *in vitro* studies, *J. Clin. Invest.*, 48, 1957, 1969.
59. Beutler, E., Glutathione reductase: stimulation in normal subjects by riboflavin supplementation, *Science*, 165, 613, 1969.
60. Scharada D., and Bamji, M. S., Erythrocyte glutathione reductase activity and riboflavin concentration in experimental deficiency of some water soluble vitamins, *Int. J. Vit. Nutr. Res.*, 42, 43, 1972.
61. Lakshmi, A. V. and Bamji, M. S., Tissue pyridoxal phosphate concentration and pyridoxaminephosphate oxidase activity in riboflavin deficiency in rats and man, *Br. J. Nutr.*, 32, 249, 1974.
62. Sauberlich, H. E., Judd, J. H., Nichoalds, G. E., Broquist, H. P., and Darby, W. J., Application of the erythrocyte glutathione reductase assay in evaluating riboflavin nutritional status in a high school student population, *Am. J. Clin. Nutr.*, 25, 756, 1972.
63. Tillotson, J. A. and Baker, E. M., An enzymatic measurement of the riboflavin status in man, *Am. J. Clin. Nutr.*, 25, 425, 1972.
64. Flatz, G., Population study of erythrocyte glutathione reductase activity. I. Stimulation of the enzyme by flavin adenine dinucleotide and by riboflavin supplementation, *Humangenetik*, 11, 269, 1971.
65. Thurnham, D. L., Migasena, P., Vudhivai, N., and Supawan, V. A longitudinal study on dietary and social influences on riboflavin status in pre-school children in Northeast Thailand, *South-East Asian J. Tropical Med. Public Health*, 2, 552, 1971.
66. Glatzle, D., Vuillenmier, J. P., Weber, F., and Decher, K., Glutathione reductase test with whole blood, a convenient procedure for the assessment of the riboflavin status in humans, *Experientia*, 30, 665, 1974.
67. Bates, C. J., Prentice, A. M., and Prentice, A., Physiological test during an improvement in riboflavin status in lactating Gambian women, *Int. J. Vit. Nutr. Res.*, 52, 14, 1982.
68. Pollock, H. and Bookman, J. J., Riboflavin excretion as a function of protein metabolism in the normal, catabolic, and diabetic human being, *J. Lab. Clin. Med.*, 38, 561, 1951.
69. Winters, L. R. T., Yoon, J.-S., Kalkwarf, H. J., Davies, J. C., Berkowitz, M. G., Hass, J., and Roe, D. A., Riboflavin requirements and exercise adaptation in older women, *Am. J. Clin. Nutr.*, 56, 526, 1992.
70. Roe, D. A., Boqusz, S., Sheu, J., and McCormick, D. B., Factors affecting riboflavin requirements of oral contraceptive users and nonusers, *Am. J. Clin. Nutr.*, 35, 495, 1982.
71. Cooperman, J. M., Cole, H. S., Gordon, M., and Lopez, R., Erythrocyte glutathione reductase as a measure of riboflavin nutritional status of pregnant women and newborns, *Proc. Soc. Exptl. Biol. Med.*, 143, 326, 1972.
72. Gatautis, V. J. and Naito, H. K., Liquid-chromatographic determination of urinary riboflavin, *Clin. Chem.*, 27, 1672, 1981.
73. Smith, M. D., Rapid method for determination of riboflavin in urine by high-performance liquid chromatography, *J. Chromatogr.*, 182, 285, 1980.
74. Lotter, S. E., Miller, M. S., Bruch, R. C., and White, H. B., III., Competitive binding assays for riboflavin and riboflavin-binding protein, *Arch. Biochem.*, 125, 110, 1982.

75. Garry, P. J. and Owen, G. M., An automated flavin adenine dinucleotide-dependent glutathione reductase assay for assessing riboflavin nutriture, *Am. J. Clin. Nutr.*, 28, 663, 1976.

76. Thurnham, D. I. and Rathakette, P., Incubation of NAD(P)H$_2$: glutathione oxidoreductase (EC 1.6.4.2) with flavin adenine dinucleotide for maximal stimulation in the measurement of riboflavin status, *Br. J. Nutr.*, 48, 459, 1982.

77. Prentice, A. M., Bates, C. J., Prentice, A., Welch, S. G., Williams, K., and McGregor, I. A., The influence of G-6-PD activity on the response of erythrocyte glutathione reductase to riboflavin deficiency, *Int. J. Vit. Nutr. Res.*, 51, 211, 1981.

78. Garry, P. J., Goodwin, J. S., and Hunt, W. C, Nutritional status in a healthy elderly population: riboflavin, *Am. J. Clin. Nutr.*, 36, 902, 1982.

79. La Rue, A., Koehler, K. M., Wayne, S. J., Chiulli, S. J., Haaland, K. Y., and Garry, P. J., Nutritional status and cognitive functioning in a normally aging sample: a 6-y assessment, *Am. J. Clin. Nutr.*, 65, 20, 1997.

80. Lossy, F. T., Goldsmith, G. A., and Sarett, H. P., A study of test dose excretion of five B complex vitamins in man, *J. Nutr.*, 45, 213, 1951.

81. Unglaub, W. G. and Goldsmith, G. A., Evaluation of vitamin adequacy: Urinary excretion tests, in *Methods for Evaluation of Nutritional Adequacy and Status – A Symposium*, Advisory Board on Quartermaster Research and Development, Committee on Foods, National Academy of Sciences, National Research Council, Washington D.C., 1954, 69.

82. *Manual for Nutrition Surveys*, 2nd edition, Interdepartmental Committee on Nutrition for National Defense, Superintendent of Documents, U.S. Government Printing Office, Washington D.C., 1963.

83. Brun, T. A., Chen, J., Campbell, T. C., Boreham, J., Feng, Z., Parpia, B., Shen, T. F., and Li, M., Urinary riboflavin excretion after a load test in rural China as a measure of possible riboflavin deficiency, *Eur. J. Clin. Nutr.*, 44, 195, 1989.

84. Bates, C. J. and Thurnham, D. I., Human requirements for riboflavin, *Am. J. Clin. Nutr.*, 53, 574, 1991.

85. Roughead, Z. K. and McCormick, D. B., Urinary riboflavin and its metabolites: effects of riboflavin supplementation in healthy residents of rural Georgia (USA), *Eur. J. Clin. Nutr.*, 45, 299, 1991.

86. Rokitzki, L., Sagredos, A., Keck, E., Sauer, B., and Keul, J., Assessment of vitamin B$_2$ status in performance of athletes of various types of sports, *J. Nutr. Sci. Vitaminol.*, 40, 11, 1994.

87. Van Dokkum, W., Schrijver, J., and Wesstra, J. A., Variability in man of the levels of some indices of nutritional status over a 60-d period on a constant diet, *Eur. J. Clin. Nutr.*, 44, 665, 1990.

88. Carrigan, P. J., Machinist, J., and Kershner, R. P., Riboflavin nutritional status and absorption in oral contraceptive users and nonusers, *Am. J. Clin. Nutr.*, 32, 2047, 1979.

89. Ajayi, O. A. and James, O. A., Effect of riboflavin supplementation on riboflavin nutriture of a secondary school population in Nigeria, *Am. J. Clin. Nutr.*, 39, 789, 1984.

90. Beach, R. S., Mantero-Atienza, E., Shor-Posner, G., Javier, J. J., Szapocznik, J., Morgan, R., Sauberlich, H. E., Cornwell, P. E., Eisdorfer, C., and Baum, M. K., Specific nutrient abnormalities in asymptomatic HIV-1 infection, *AIDS*, 6, 701, 1992.

91. Dror, Y., Stern, F., and Komarnitsky, M., Optimal and stable conditions for the determination of erythrocyte glutathione reductase activation coefficient to evaluate riboflavin status, *Int. J. Vit. Nutr. Res.*, 64, 257, 1994.

92. Becker, K., Krebs, B., and Shirmer, R. H., Protein-chemical standardization of the erythrocyte glutathione reductase activation test (EGRAC test), Application to hypothyroidism, *Int. J. Vit. Nutr. Res.*, 61, 180, 1991.

93. Boisvert, W. A., Castoneda, C., Mendoza, I., Langeloh, G., Solomons, N. W., Gershoff, S. N., and Russell, R. M., Prevalence of riboflavin deficiency among Guatemalan elderly people and its relationship to milk intake, *Am. J. Clin. Nutr.*, 58, 85, 1993.

94. Bates, C. J., Prentice, A. M., Watkinson, M., Morrell, P., Sutcliffe, B. A., Foord, F. A., and Whitehead, R. G., Riboflavin requirements of lactating Gambian women: a controlled supplementation trial, *Am. J. Clin. Nutr.*, 35, 701, 1982.

95. Baker, H., Frank, O., Feingold, S., Gellene, R. A., Leevy, C. M., and Hutner, S. H., A riboflavin assay suitable for clinical use and nutritional surveys, *Am. J. Clin. Nutr.*, 19, 17, 1966.
96. Slater, E. C. and Morell, D. B., A modification of the fluorimetric method of determining riboflavin in biological materials, *Biochem. J.*, 40, 644, 1946.
97. Russell, L. F. and Vanderslice, J. T., A comprehensive review of vitamin B_2 analytical methodology, *J. Micronutr. Anal.*, 8, 257, 1990.
98. Mohammed, H. V., Veening, H., and Dayton, D. A., Liquid chromatographic determination and time-concentration studies of riboflavin in hemodialysate from uremic patients, *J. Chromatogr.*, 226, 471, 1981.
99. Vuilleumier, J. P., Keller, H. E., Rettenmaier, R., Hunziker, F., Clinical chemical methods for the routine assessment of the vitamin status in human populations. II. The water-soluble vitamins B_1, B_2, and B_6, *Int. J. Vit. Nutr. Res.*, 53, 359, 1983.
100. Mak, Y. T. and Swaminathan, R., Assessment of vitamin B_1, B_2, and B_6 status by coenzyme activation of red cell enzymes using a centrifugal analyser, *J. Clin. Biochem.* 26, 213, 1988.
101. Brubacher, G., Biochemical studies for assessment of vitamin status, *Bibl. Nutr. Diet.*, 20, 31, 1974.
102. *Ministry of Health and Social Welfare*; National Nutrition Survey, 1982–1983, Seoul, Korea, 1984.
103. Lee, I. E. and Paik, H. Y., A study on the riboflavin nutritional status by biochemical tests in healthy female college students in Korea, *Korean J. Nutr. Soc.*, 18, 272, 1985.
104. O'neal, R. M., Johnson, O. C., and Schaefer, A. E., Guidelines for classification and interpretation of group blood and urine data collected as part of the National Nutrition Survey, *Pediatr. Res.*, 4, 103, 1970.
105. Garry, P. J. and Hunt, W. C., Biochemical assessment of vitamin status in the elderly: effects of dietary and supplemental intakes, in *Nutrition and Aging*, Hutchinson, M. L. and Munro, H. N., Eds., Academic Press, New York, 1986.
106. Rosalki, S. B., Detection of vitamin B deficiency by red cell enzyme activation tests, in *Quality Control In Laboratory Medicine*, Henry, J. B. and Giegel, J. L., Eds., Masson Publications USA, New York, 1977, 121.
107. Mellor, N. P. and Maass, A. R., An automated fluorometric method for the determination of riboflavin in human urine, *Advances in Automated Analyses*. 9. Pharmaceutical Science, Medical Inc., Tarrytown, NY, 1973.
108. Mount, J. N., Heduan, E., Herd, C., Jupp, R., Kearney, E., and Marsh, A., Adaptation of coenzyme stimulation assays for the nutritional assessment of vitamins B_1, B_2, and B_6 using the Cobas Bio centrifugal analyzer, *Annu. Clin. Biochem.*, 24, 41, 1987.
109. Prasad, A. P., Lakshmi, A. V., and Bamji, M. S., Interpretation of erythrocyte glutathione reductase activation tests values for assessing riboflavin status, *Eur. J. Clin. Nutr.*, 46, 753, 1992.
110. Bamji, M. S., Chowdhury, N., Ramalakshmi, B. A., and Jacob, C. M., Enzymatic evaluation of riboflavin status of infants, *Eur. J. Clin. Nutr.*, 45, 309, 1991.
111. Difco Supplementary Literature, Difco Laboratories, Detroit, 1972.
112. Freed, M., *Methods of Vitamin Assay*, Interscience Publications, New York, 1966.
113. Madigan, S. M., Tracey, F., McNulty, H., Eaton-Evans, J., Coulter, J., McCarney, H., and Strain, J. J., Riboflavin and vitamin B-6 intakes and status and biochemical response to riboflavin supplementation in free-living elderly people, *Am. J. Clin. Nutr.* 68, 389, 1998.
114. Sandstead, H. R. and Koehn, C. J., Nutrition of Korean Army. Field studies: May–June 1953, *Am. J. Clin. Nutr.*, 13, 25, 1963.
115. Flatz, G., Enhanced binding of FAD to glutathione reductase in G6PD deficiency, *Nature*, 226, 755, 1970.
116. Thurnham, D. I., Influence of glucose-6-phosphate dehydrogenase deficiency on the glutathione reductase test for ariboflavinosis, *Annu. Trop. Med. Parasitol.*, 66, 505, 1972.
117. Frischer, H., Bowman, J. E., Carson, P. E. et al., Erythrocyte glutathione reductase, glucose-6-phosphate dehydrogenase, and 6-phosphogluconic dehydrogenase deficiencies in populations of the United States, South Vietnam, Iran, and Ethiopia, *J. Lab. Clin. Med.*, 81, 603, 1973.
118. Bates, C., Riboflavin, *J. Int. Vit. Nutr. Res.*, 63, 274, 1993.
119. Benton, D., Haller, J., and Fordy, J., The vitamin status of young British adults, *Int. J. Vit. Nutr. Res.*, 67, 34, 1996.

Vitamin B-6 (Pyridoxine)

Vitamin B-6 exists in a number of related forms. The following are the major forms.

Form	Molecular Weight	Conversion Factors
Pyridoxine	169.18	ng/mL × 5.91 = nmol/L
Pyridoxal	167.16	ng/mL × 5.98 = nmol/L
Pyridoxamine	168.20	ng/mL × 5.95 = nmol/L
Pyridoxine 5′-phosphate	249.16	ng/mL × 4.01 = nmol/L
Pyridoxal 5′-phosphate	247.14	ng/mL × 4.046 = nmol/L
Pyridoxamine 5′-phosphate	248.18	ng/mL × 4.03 = nmol/L
4-Pyridoxic acid	183.16	ng/mL × 5.46 = nmol/L

Molecular weights are for the anhydrous, salt-free, non-hydrochloride form.[83]

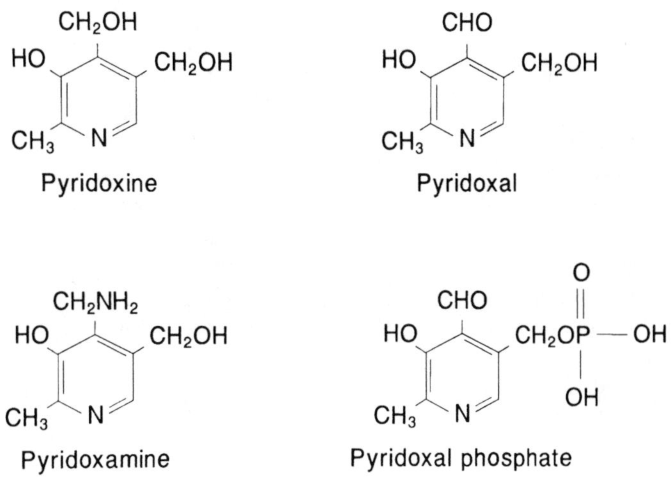

Pyridoxine

Pyridoxal

Pyridoxamine

Pyridoxal phosphate

FIGURE 15
Structure of commonly occurring forms of vitamin B-6.

Introduction

Gryörgy[77,131-133] established in 1934 that vitamin B-6 was a nutritional factor required to prevent rat acrodynia. Subsequently the vitamin was isolated, characterized, and called pyridoxine.[137,138] Pyridoxine is the form commonly used for food fortification and pharmaceutical preparations.

The discovery of vitamin B-6 and its three forms, pyridoxine, pyridoxal, and pyridoxamine, has been detailed in a review by Snell.[124] Subsequently, the phosphorylated forms were recognized.[124] Vitamin B-6 is commonly used as a collective term for these various biologically active forms. Pyridoxal 5'-phosphate and pyridoxamine 5'-phosphate were established as essential coenzymatic forms in transamination reactions.[94,124]

Because of the widespread availability of vitamin B-6 in foods, serious outbreaks of vitamin B-6 deficiency have not been observed. Nevertheless, considerable interest exists in vitamin B-6 nutriture of the human because of its (a) ease of depletion to produce deficiency symptoms, (b) participation in numerous metabolic functions, (c) association with immunity and with brain metabolism and development, (d) participation in homocysteine metabolism and cardiovascular disease, (e) marked losses in food processing, and (f) antagonisms by certain drugs and hormones. Consequently, various biochemical procedures have been developed and used in the evaluation of vitamin B-6 nutritional status.[88,171]

Bioavailability and Source of Vitamin B-6

Bioavailability of vitamin B-6 represents that proportion of the vitamin that undergoes intestinal absorption and metabolic utilization.[10-15] Vitamin B-6 is present in foods primarily in the form of pyridoxine, pyridoxal 5'-phosphate, and pyridoxamine phosphate. Most of the phosphorylated forms at physiological levels are hydrolyzed by intestinal phosphatases before absorption. The bioavailability of vitamin B-6 does not appear to be altered with aging.[24] However, bound forms of vitamin B-6 such as pyridoxine-5'-β-D-glucoside are found in plant foods.[11-13,15-20,258] Human studies indicate that the glucoside has bioavailability of approximately 58%.[17,19]

Vitamin B-6 losses are high in cooking and in the processing and canning of meats and vegetables. The milling of wheat into flour may result in a 70 to 90% loss in vitamin B-6 content, while frozen vegetables may experience a loss of 35 to 55% of the vitamin.[10,11] Kant and Bock[21] have provided data on the vitamin B-6 content of 50 food items, while Dong et al.[22] have reported on the vitamin B-6 of content of 81 food items "as served". Table 12 lists the vitamin B-6 content of selected foods items from these reports.[21-23] Meats provide about 40% of the daily intake of vitamin B-6.[23,125] The bioavailability of vitamin B-6 in the average American diet has been estimated to range from 61 to 81%.[10,12-14]

Clinical Vitamin B-6 Deficiency

Human subjects suffering from vitamin B-6 deficiency are rarely encountered. Clinically, however, a vitamin B-6 deficiency in the human is manifested often as central nervous system changes.[134] Abnormal electroencephalograms may occur and have been produced in adult human vitamin B-6 depletion studies.[77,103,134,136,200] Hyperirritability and convulsive seizures may occur in children.[77,134] Seborrheic dermatitis and eczema have been reported to occur in the regions of the mouth, nose, and ears.[77] Angular stomatitis, glossitis, and cheilosis may be observed. On occasion, hypochromic, microcytic anemia may occur in children as well as adults.[77,134,135]

TABLE 12
Vitamin B-6 Contents of Edible Portions
of Selected Food Items as Consumed[21-23]

Description	Vitamin B-6 Content (mg/100 g)
Meats, Poultry, Fish	
Beef steak and roasts	0.35
Pork chops and roasts	0.33
Fried chicken	0.48
Fried fish (haddock)	0.35
Hamburger	0.24
Ham steak, fried	0.27
Chili	0.18
Eggs and Dairy	
Whole milk	0.04
Eggs	0.14
Fruits	
Bananas	0.58
Cantaloupe	0.12
Grapes, raw	0.13
Vegetables	
French fries	0.19
Sweet potatoes	0.28
Green peppers, stuffed	0.22
Peas, green, boiled	0.11
Potatoes, baked	0.14
Tomato, juice	0.13
Miscellaneous	
Spaghetti with tomato sauce	0.12
Pizza, all kinds	0.41
Macaroni and cheese, baked	0.02
Pancakes	0.02
Bread, white	0.04
Rice	0.18

Although overt clinical deficiency of vitamin B-6 occurs only rarely, nutrition surveys indicate that vitamin B-6 intakes may be marginal or inadequate in segments of the American population. Consequently, the presence of a subclinical deficiency may be fairly widespread.

Vitamin B-6 Metabolism and Utilization

Vitamin B-6 metabolism, requirements, and utilization have been the subject of a number of reviews.[75,77,82-88,94,95,128,145,182,198,199] Orally ingested pyridoxine appears to be rapidly metabolized in the liver and its products released into circulation in the form of pyridoxal 5'-phosphate, pyridoxal and 4-pyridoxic acid.[25,128,129,186,188]

As a coenzynme, pyridoxal 5'-phosphate participates in over 100 different enzyme systems.[94,124,128,130] The majority of the enzyme systems that require pyridoxal 5'-phosphate are concerned with protein and amino acid metabolism. Several important roles of the vitamin are in transamination reactions, biosynthesis of delta-aminolevulinic acid essential for hemoglobin synthesis, formation of serotonin from 5-OH-tryptophan, and in the metabolism of homocysteine to cystathionine and its further conversion to cysteine. Pyridoxal 5'-phosphate is the predominant form of vitamin B-6 in the human plasma.[127]

Assessment of Vitamin B-6 Nutritional Status

Procedures used for the assessment of vitamin B-6 status have developed over a number of years. Using these procedures, numerous studies have been reported on the vitamin B-6 status of different populations and age groups.[42,204,208,211,234,235,246-250]

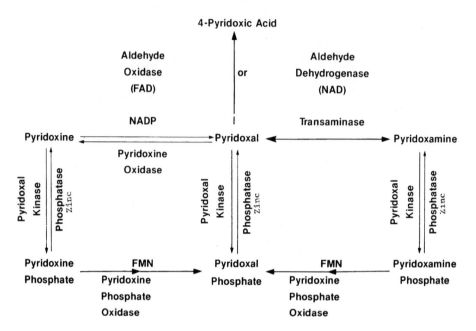

FIGURE 16
Participation of niacin, riboflavin, and zinc in the formation and metabolism of pyridoxal 5'-phosphate.[130]

Laboratory methods used for the assessment of vitamin B-6 nutritional status include the following:

1. Plasma pyridoxal 5'-phosphate concentrations
2. Blood concentrations of other vitamin B-6 vitamins (e.g., pyridoxal)
3. Activities and activity coefficients of plasma or erythrocyte AST and GPT enzymes
4. Urinary excretion of xanthurenic acid following a load dose of tryptophan
5. Urinary excretion of 4-pyridoxic acid
6. Urinary excretion of "free" or total vitamin B-6
7. Methionine load

Human Studies on Vitamin B-6 Nutritional Assessment Methods

A number of controlled human studies on the effect of vitamin B-6 depletion and repletion has permitted the development and evaluation of various methods that may be used to assess vitamin B-6 status.[77,82,84,86-89,94,96,99,103-105] Earlier studies with men and women on vitamin B-6 requirements and assessment methods have been summarized in several reports.[77,82,84,87,88,90,94,99,209]

Hansen et al.[206] studied the response of vitamin B-6 status indicators to varying levels of vitamin B-6 intake in young women. The investigators found the indicators that responded significantly were urinary excretion of 4-pyridoxic acid and total vitamin B-6; in plasma, total vitamin B-6 and pyridoxal 5'-phosphate; and urinary excretion of xanthurenic acid following a tryptophan load. In addition, they reported significant correlations existed between vitamin B-6 intake and plasma pyridoxal 5'-phosphate, total plasma vitamin B-6, urinary 4-pyridoxic acid, total urinary vitamin B-6, erythrocyte alanine aminotransferase activity coefficient, and post-loading xanthurenic acid excretion.[206]

In a vitamin B-6 depletion and repletion study on vitamin B-6 requirement of young women fed a high protein diet, Huang et al.[210] used a battery of vitamin B-6 status indicators. The indicators used included the measurement of urinary 4-pyridoxic acid excretion, plasma concentrations of pyridoxal-5'-phosphate, erythrocyte pyridoxal 5'-phosphate levels, and erythrocyte alanine and aspartate aminotransferase activity coefficients. The eight subjects were provided for 27 days only 0.45 mg of vitamin B-6 per day. All of the vitamin B-6 status indicators became abnormal during the depletion period. Following the vitamin B-6 depletion, the subjects were repleted over a period of 35 days with incremental amounts of vitamin B-6. The amount of dietary vitamin B-6 required to normalize the vitamin B-6 status indicators was considered to be 1.94 mg per day (0.019 mg/g protein) (Table 13).[210]

TABLE 13
Assessment of Vitamin B-6 Status in Eight Young Women on Controlled Diets

Parameter	Initial 1.60 mg/day of Vitamin B-6	Depletion of 27 Days 45 µg/day of Vitamin B-6	Repletion with Vitamin B-6	
			1.66 mg/day for 21 Days	2.06 mg/day for 14 Days
Plasma (nmol/L)				
Pyridoxal 5'-phosphate	58.2	32.4	45.4	53.6
Pyridoxal	22.1	3.8	2.3	4.9
Erythrocyte (nmol/L)				
Pyridoxal 5'-phosphate	53.9	28.0	39.6	62.0
Pyridoxal	3.2	0.6	3.5	5.3
Pyridoxamine phosphate	15.2	8.4	11.1	11.5
EAST–AC	1.43	2.41	1.63	1.52
EALT–AC	1.21	3.23	1.36	1.30

Adapted from Huang et al.[210]

Of interest, the investigators found a significant relation between vitamin B-6 intake and erythrocyte pyridoxal 5'-phosphate and erythrocyte pyridoxal concentrations. Moreover, plasma and erythrocyte pyridoxal 5'-phosphate determinations were equivalent measures of vitamin B-6 status. A dietary intake of vitamin B-6 of 1.66 mg per day was associated with a plasma pyridoxal 5'-phosphate concentration of 30 nmol/L.[96,99,198,210]

Similar observations were reported by Kretsch et al.[96] in a vitamin B-6 depletion and repletion study conducted also with young women residing in a metabolic unit (Figure 17). Multiple vitamin B-6 nutritional status measures were evaluated under controlled experimental conditions. The study also provided information as to the daily requirement for vitamin B-6. The criterion used to assess requirement was restoration of clinical, functional, and biochemical indexes to baseline values after a period of vitamin B-6 depletion. Abnormal electroencephalograms were observed for two of the eight subjects during the vitamin

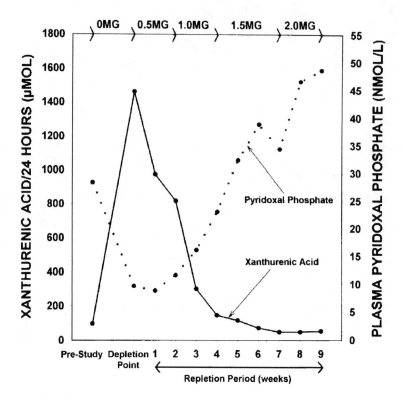

FIGURE 17

Relationship of vitamin B-6 intake in young women to plasma pyridoxal-5'-phosphate concentrations and xanthurenic acid excretion following a 4-g L-tryptophan load.[96] (With permission.)

B-6 depletion period.[136] During the vitamin B-6 repletion period this condition was quickly corrected.

All of the functional and biochemical indexes used became abnormal during the vitamin B-6 depletion periods. Mean responses to controlled intakes of vitamin B-6 for the urine and blood markers are shown in the Table 14. Xanthurenic acid excretion after a tryptophan load was the most sensitive biochemical test for evaluating vitamin B-6 status under controlled conditions. The mean low point for all other measures lagged behind the maximum excretion point for xanthurenic acid. The mean low point occurred 1 week later than maximum xanthurenic acid excretion for plasma pyridoxal 5'-phosphate, urinary 4-pyridoxic acid, total urinary vitamin B-6, and free urinary vitamin B-6, and 2 to 3 weeks later for the erythrocyte aminotransferases. Based on the response of these functional and biochemical measures to vitamin B-6, the vitamin B-6 requirements for young women of 0.020 mg/g dietary protein intake appears justified.

In an unpublished study conducted in this laboratory (Sauberlich, H.E. and Tamura, T.), six young women were placed on a vitamin B-6 deficient diet for 3 weeks followed by 1 week with the diet providing 1.60 mg vitamin B-6 per day. Initially and the end of each week, an L-methionine load was given with the breakfast meal (80 mg/kg body weight). Blood samples were obtained at 0, 2, and 4 hours after the ingestion of the L-methionine. Analyses were performed on the fasting plasma samples for homocysteine and pyridoxal 5'-phosphate and erythrocyte EAST. Homocysteine analyses were performed also on the plasma samples obtained at 2 hours and 4 hours after the methionine load.

TABLE 14
Response of Vitamin B-6 Assessment Parameters to Controlled Intakes of Vitamin B-6 in Eight Young Women[4]

				Experimental Period		
	I	II	III	IV	V	VI
	Control	Depletion (11–28 days)	Repletion (14 days)	Repletion (14 days)	Repletion (21 days)	Repletion (14 days)
				Vitamin B-6 Intake (mg/day)		
Assessment Parameter	2.0	0.05	0.5	1.0	1.5	2.0
Plasma pyridoxal 5-phosphate (nmol/L)[1]	25.4	9.1	8.7	18.7	30.4	42.3
Erythrocyte AST activity coefficient (EAST-AC)[3]	1.53	1.84	2.06	2.01	1.72	1.60
Erythrocyte ALT activity coefficient (EALT-AC)[3]	1.35	1.71	2.05	1.69	1.38	1.37
Urinary 4-pyridoxic acid (μmol/d)	5.50	1.26	0.91	1.95	3.80	5.74
Free urinary vitamin B-6 (μmol/d)	0.49	0.13	0.14	0.26	0.35	0.48
Total Urinary vitamin B-6 (μmol/d)	0.92	0.24	0.22	0.35	0.52	0.61
Xanthurenic acid excretion (μmol/d)[2]	82	1423	851	284	98	83

1 Measured by the method of Sloger and Reynolds.[119]
2 Net 24-hr xanthurenic acid excretion after a 4-g L-tryptophan load.
3 Measured by the method of Skala et al.[117]
4 Adapted from Kretsch et al.[96] With permission.

After 3 weeks on the vitamin B-6 deficient diet, the plasma pyridoxal 5′-phosphate decreased from an average initial concentration of 58.8 nmol/L to 23.6 nmol/L. During this time period, the erythrocyte EAST activity coefficient increased from 1.77 to 2.07. The average plasma homocysteine concentration, without the methionine load, was 8.6 µmol/L. Vitamin B-6 deficiency had little effect on the plasma homocysteine concentrations present 4 hours after the methionine load. Thus, after 3 weeks of vitamin B-6 deficiency, the average homocysteine concentration 4 hours after the load was 23.9 µmol/L. The response to the methionine load was variable for some subjects. It is doubtful that a methionine load will enhance the usefulness of plasma homocysteine measurements for evaluating vitamin B-6 status, but may have application in folate studies.

From a controlled vitamin B-6 deficiency study involving 11 elderly subjects, Miller et al.[162] concluded that fasting plasma homocysteine concentrations were not a reliable indicator of vitamin B-6 status. Only one of the 11 subjects on the vitamin B-6 deficient for 20 days had elevated plasma homocysteine concentrations. However, all of the subjects had high urinary xanthurenic acid excretion after a 5 gram L-tryptophan load.

Pyridoxal 5′-phosphate and Vitamin B-6 Assessment

The earlier procedures to measure pyridoxal 5′-phosphate were unsatisfactory, lacked sensitivity and values obtained were wide in range.[112] Currently, the quantitative determination of pyridoxal 5′-phosphate in plasma is commonly performed with procedures that utilize tyrosine apodecarboxylase (EC 4.1 1.25).[25,84,96,99,119,139-143,146,147,171,175,176,198]

The general reactions are as follows:[147]

1. Tyrosine apodecarboxylase + pyridoxal 5′-phosphate → holoenzyme.
2. L-tyrosine-1-^{14}C $\xrightarrow{\text{tyrosine decarboxylase}}$ tyramine + $^{14}CO_2$.
3. The radioactive carbon dioxide is trapped and counted in a scintillation counter.
4. An alternative method utilizes L-tyrosine labeled with tritium on the ring structure.[142] This reaction results in the formation of tritiated tyramine, which is extracted and counted in a scintillation counter.

In the authors' experiences, the procedures provide the same analytical results. Both were specific and sensitive. The use of the tyramine extraction procedure avoids the need for special reaction flasks. Tyrosine apodecarboxylase preparations suitable for these reactions are available from Sigma, St. Louis, MO. An apotryptophanase assay for pyridoxal phosphate is available but has seldom been used.[144]

High-performance liquid chromatogram cation-exchange procedures have been reported for the measurement of vitamin B-6 compounds in biological samples.[127,147,164,257] Extraction requirements, lack of sensitivity, technical problems, and long analytical times, have limited the use of many of the HPLC procedures. Ideally for the assessment of vitamin B-6 status, information on the plasma concentrations of both pyridoxal and pyridoxal 5′-phosphate would be useful. However, the procedures of Coburn and Mahuren,[127] Lui et al.,[147] Sampson and O'Connor,[213] and Kamp et al.[214] have received limited use for the determination of vitamin B-6 vitaminers. Schrijver et al.[243,251] have used a semi-automatic fluorometric method with HPLC for separation and measurement of pyridoxal 5′-phosphate in whole blood samples.

Various approaches have been reported used in attempts to separate and quantitative the various forms of vitamin B-6.[171-174,239-243,251,257] The HPLC procedure of Coburn and Mahuren[127] has been used successfully and is relatively simple. The procedure requires a single column and one fluorometer. Pyridoxal phosphate, pyridoxamine phosphate, pyridoxine phosphate, pyridoxal, pyridoxamine, pyridoxine, and 4-pyridoxic acid can be measured with 0.25 mL of serum. The complete analysis of each sample required 40 minutes. Chauhan and Dakshinamurti[172,173] separated pyridoxal 5'-phosphate, pyridoxamine 5'-phosphate, pyridoxal, pyridoxamine, and pyridoxine by ion-exchange chromatography. The cynohydrin derivatives of the separated compounds were quantitated fluorometrically. However, the procedure required 5 mL of serum and 6 hours to complete an analysis.

A similar analytical procedure was described by Smith et al.[241] and applied to the measurement of pyridoxal and pyridoxal 5'-phosphate concentrations in neutrophils. The neutrophils were found to have a mean concentration pyridoxal of 7.6 ± 2.5 pmol per mg of protein and a pyridoxal 5'-phosphate concentration of 13.4 ± 8.1 pmol per mg of protein. Hess and Vuilleimier[240] measured pyridoxal 5'-phosphate and pyridoxal in plasma by oxidizing these vitamin B-6 vitaminers to their corresponding acids. The acids were separated by HPLC and quantitated by fluorometric detection.

Ubbink et al.[164,239] used precolumn semicarbazone formation of pyridoxal and pyridoxal 5'-phosphate. The semicarbazones were separated by high-performance liquid chromatography and quantitated by fluorescence detection. The semicarbazone forms are very stable and are not affected by exposure to light. Gregory[252] reviewed the methods available for the determination of vitamin B-6 in foods and biological materials.

Long-term stability of pyridoxal phosphate in human plasma was investigated by R.D. Reynolds (personal communication). Pyridoxal 5'-phosphate was measured by the tyrosine decarboxylase method in a pooled plasma sample held at –20°C. The concentrations of pyridoxal 5'-phosphate were determined on 113 separate occasions over a 700-day period. Approximately 2.2% per year of loss in pyridoxal 5'-phosphate occurred in the plasma sample. Capillary blood plasma samples obtained by finger-prick are suitable for plasma pyridoxal 5'-phosphate determinations.[236] A commercial kit is available for the determination of plasma pyridoxal 5'-phosphate based on the procedure of Camp et al.[142] (American Laboratory Products Company, Windham, NH 03087). Its use has been published as an abstract.[238]

Determination of Plasma Homocysteine

Various methods have been described for the measurement of homocysteine. Most of the procedures utilize HPLC separation and either fluorescence detection[149,156,157,163] or electrochemical (amperometric) detection.[72,73,150-152]

Occasionally automated amino analyzers are utilized[153,154,158] as well as capillary gas chromatography-mass spectrometry.[155] Radioenzymatic procedures have also been used to determine plasma homocysteine concentrations.[161] Similar enzymatic methods have been reported by others.[169,170] The author has utilized HPLC in conjunction with electrochemical[150,151] or fluorescence detection[165] with equal satisfaction and comparable results in the determination of plasma homocysteine concentrations. The relative simplicity, stability, and speed of the assays have facilitated the analysis of large population groups.

In the European project, plasma homocysteine was studied in 800 control men and women and in 750 cases of with atherosclerotic vascular disease.[168] The measurement performed included the effect of a methinine loading test on plasma homocysteine, plasma concentration of pyridoxal 5'-phosphate, red blood cell folate, and vitamin B-12. The methionine load test identified an additional 24% of at risk cases from the controls.

An elevated plasma homocysteine concentration was defined as $\geq 12\ \mu mol/L$ fasting, and $\geq 38\ \mu mol/L$ after the standardized methionine load test. Plasma pyridoxal 5'-phosphate concentrations were significantly lower in the cases than in the controls (cases: 26.32 nmol/L vs. 31.11 nmol/L for the controls). The 156 cases with peripheral vascular disease had a mean plasma pyridoxal 5'-phosphate concentrations of only 22.73 nmol/L.[168]

Determination of Transaminase Activities

General

The automated procedure of Skala et al.[117,118] provides for a rapid, reproducible, and satisfactory method to measure erythrocyte transaminase activities. Only a relatively small quantity of packed erythrocytes is required (0.25 mL) for the determination of the activities and the activity coefficient. The procedure permits the use of quality-control samples prepared from a pool of erythrocytes that are aliquoted and stored at –70°C or lower. Such samples are quite stable. Unfortunately, most laboratories do not have available automation facilities and must depend upon manual procedures.[93,106,114,116,120,177,178,180] Erythrocyte aspartic acid transaminase activity coefficients (EAST-AC) have been also determined with the use of Cobas-Bio analyzer instrumentation.[223]

The most commonly used colorimetric methods have been based on the procedure of Reitman and Frankel,[121] and the generally used spectrophotometric methods are modifications of the procedures of Karmen,[122] Babson et al.,[179] Wroblewski and LaDue,[123] or Sax and Moore.[192] Packed erythrocytes for transaminase activity measurements are stable for over 60 days when stored at –70°C or colder.

Rosalki and Bayoumi[253,254] investigated in detail the optimum conditions for the erythrocyte aspartate transaminase assay. The method utilized ultraviolet specrophotometric measurements.

Blood Transaminase Activities and Vitamin B-6 Status

Transaminase measurements represent a biochemical functional test which possesses the possibility of providing information regarding the state of deficiency or degree of depletion of vitamin B-6 reserves. Controlled human vitamin B-6 depletion studies have demonstrated that pyridoxal 5'-phosphate-dependent transaminases such as aspartate aminotransferase (AST) (formerly GOT) (EC 2.6.1.1) and alanine aminotransferase (ALT) (formerly GPT) (EC 2.6.1.2) activities fall in erythrocytes, leucocytes and plasma (serum).[86,87,89,93,96,106,113,115,212]

Plasma (serum) contains considerable less transaminase activities than do the erythrocytes.[96,116] Moreover, serum transaminase activities observed in normal individuals show a wide range. As a consequence, serum or plasma AST and ALT activity measurements are of limited use for assessing vitamin B-6 nutriture.[87,96,113,116] Plasma transaminase activity measurements are used as indicator enzymes for the diagnosis of various diseases such as myocardial infarction.

The measurement of AST and ALT activities in erythrocytes are of value in detecting and evaluating human deficiencies of vitamin B-6.[96,206-208,210,212] Erythrocyte transaminase activities provide a much closer reflection of vitamin B-6 status than serum transaminase activities.[115,116] Considerably more AST enzyme activity than ALT enzyme activity is present in erythrocytes.[96] Nevertheless, both enzyme activities decline with inadequate intakes of vitamin B-6 and both are accompanied by increases in the percentage stimulation produced by *in vitro*-supplied pyridoxal 5'-phosphate.[96,116]

The measurement of the stimulation of erythrocyte AST (EAST) and erythrocyte ALT (EALT) activities induced by the *in vitro* addition of pyridoxal 5'-phosphate (PLP) to the assay reaction appears to provide a reasonable satisfactory indication of vitamin B-6 status.[96] In order to overcome some of the differences in methods of measurement and in erythrocyte transaminase activities between normal healthy individuals, an erythrocyte transaminase index has been useful:[88,96]

$$\text{EAST activity coefficient } (\alpha \text{ EAST}) = \frac{\text{EAST} + \text{pyridoxal 5'-phosphate}}{\text{EAST} - \text{pyridoxal 5'-phosphate}}$$

$$\text{EALT activity coefficient } (\alpha \text{ EALT}) = \frac{\text{EALT} + \text{pyridoxal 5'-phosphate}}{\text{EALT} - \text{pyridoxal 5'-phosphate}}$$

Based on extensive experience involving large numbers of samples, the following criteria have been applied to erythrocyte transaminase activity data to evaluate vitamin B-6 status. The procedure Skala et al.[117,118] was used for these determinations.

Erythrocyte AST Activity Coefficient Value (αEAST)

Acceptable	< 1.70
Marginal	1.70 –1.85
Deficient	> 1.85

The values have been applied also to erythrocyte ALT activity values (αEALT). Erythrocyte ALT has been found to be a somewhat more sensitive measure of vitamin B-6 insufficiency than erythrocyte AST.[96,114] Because of the lower level of erythrocyte ALT enzyme activity, the measurement of the activity of this enzyme has been more difficult to reliability measure.[217] In addition, the use of erythrocyte ALT as a measure of vitamin B-6 insufficiency may be influenced by the genetic polymorphism of the erythrocyte alanine aminotransferase.[217]

Leucocyte Transaminase Activity

Little information is available on transaminase activities in leucocytes. Racia and Sauberlich[116] measured aspartate aminotransferase (AST) activity in leucocyte isolates obtained from a human vitamin B-6 deficiency study. The AST activities of the leucocytes seemed to reflect the subject's vitamin B-6 status. However, the changes over the 7-week vitamin B-6 deficiency period were not dramatic. The transaminase activity fell about 35%. There appeared to be a 3- to 4-week lag period before the levels fell. Technical difficulties in isolating the leucocytes along with their instability have made this assessment technique impractical for routine vitamin B-6 assessment.

Tryptophan Load and Xanthurenic Acid Excretion

In 1943, Lepkovsky and associates[78] noted that animals deprived of vitamin B-6 excreted abnormal metabolites of tryptophan which were enhanced following a load of this amino acid. A green pigment was found in the urine collected in rusty metabolism cages. The green pigment was established to be a reaction product between xanthurenic acid and ferric ammonium sulfate.

The xanthurenic acid was found to originate from the dietary tryptophan. Thus, the tryptophan load test evolved for evaluating vitamin B-6 status and requirements. In 1949, Greenberg et al.[79] utilized the test for the first time on the human. In subsequent years, the test has been often utilized in the numerous experimental vitamin B-6 deficiency studies that have been conducted.[77] The tryptophan load test has been evaluated extensively.[80,93] Brown and associates also attempted to develop a kynurenine load test.[80,81] This test, however, has seen little use primarily because of the high expense of the L-kynurenine sulfate load.

Various amounts of L-tryptophan have been used in the tryptophan load test such as 2 or 3 grams.[100-102,106] In our investigations, we have used a 4-g L-tryptophan load. In other studies it was found that a 2-g L-tryptophan load does not always produce a sufficient challenge to the tryptophan metabolic pathways to provide an early detection of vitamin B-6 inadequacy.[88,96] The xanthurenic acid present in the urine can be measured with the use of a colorimetric procedure[93] or by HPLC.[195]

Under controlled conditions, xanthurenic acid excretion after a tryptophan load was the most sensitive biochemical test for evaluating vitamin B-6 status.[96] This included comparisons with plasma pyridoxal 5′-phosphate, urinary 4-pyridoxic acid excretion, total and free urinary vitamin B-6 excretion, and erythrocyte transaminases.

Methionine Load Test

A methionine loading test has also been studied as a possible indicator of vitamin B-6 status.[82,90,91] Increased excretion of cystathionine was the only methionine metabolite which increased significantly in the urine during vitamin B-6 deficiency.[90] The excretion was increased following a 3 g L-methionine load. Little use has been made of the methionine load test primarily do to the lack of available convenient and sensitive analytical methods of measure methionine metabolites. More recently a standardized methionine load test has been successfully used.[168] The general procedure involves the administration of 100 mg of L-methionine per kilogram of body weight. Blood samples are obtained from the subjects fasting and 6 hours after the administration of the methionine load. Concentrations of plasma homocysteine and pyridoxal 5′-phosphate are measured in the samples. The increases in homocysteine concentrations that results are evaluated in terms of the vitamin B-6 status.[168]

Urinary Excretion of 4-Pyridoxic Acid

The main catabolite of pyridoxine metabolism is 4-pyridoxic acid.[182,183] When vitamin B-6 is omitted from the diet, the excretion of 4-pyridoxic acid falls rapidly, but increases promptly with the readministration of the vitamin. Thus, the excretion of 4-pyridoxic acid depends upon the amount of vitamin B-6 ingested.[77,96,99] When 24-hr urine collections are not feasible, random urine samples have been used and the 4-pyridoxine acid excretion expressed on a creatinine ratio basis.[77,205] The HPLC method of Gregory and Kirk[98] has been reliable and satisfactory for the measurement of 4-pyridoxic in urine. Other procedures have been described that provide comparable results.[210,211,216] Under controlled experimental conditions, 4-pyridoxic acid excretion correlated reasonably well with vitamin B-6 intakes, urinary excretion of vitamin B-6, and plasma pyridoxal 5'-phosphate levels.[96]

An acceptable level of 4-pyridoxic acid was reported as > 5.0 µmol/24-hr for adults.[99] Kretsch et al.[96] observed in a controlled vitamin B-6 intake study that the excretion of 4-pyridoxic acid by the control adult women was 5.5 ± 3.4 µmol/d, which fell to 0.91 ± 0.48 µmol/d when the subjects received only 0.5 mg of vitamin B-6 per day in the diet.

Lui et al.[186] considered from their study with four young men that urinary excretion of 4-pyridoxic acid was a better indicator of vitamin B-6 intake than plasma pyridoxal 5'-phosphate concentrations. However, plasma pyridoxal 5'-phosphate concentrations were a better indicator of the body stores of the vitamin.

Urinary Excretion of Vitamin B-6

Vitamin B-6 is present in the urine in a "free" form and a "bound" form.[77,96,99] To obtain the total amount vitamin B-6 excreted into the urine requires an acid hydrolysis treatment of the urine sample.[96,98] The vitamin B-6 levels present in the urine samples can be measured by microbiological assay using the yeast, *Saccharomyces uvarum (Sach. Carlsbergenis)*, ATCC No. 9080, as the test organism.[93,106-108,174] The excretion of "free" and "total" vitamin B-6 paralleled each other. Hence, the measurement of the total vitamin B-6 excretion is unnecessary for evaluating vitamin B-6 intake status. Approximately 50 to 75% of the vitamin B-6 present in the urine is in the "free" form.

In controlled studies with adult subjects, the urinary excretion of free vitamin B-6 correlated closely with the level of intake of the vitamin.[84,86-88,96,99,103-106] As an alternative to the collection of 24-hr urine samples, random fasting urine collections have been employed and the urinary excretion of vitamin B-6 expressed in terms of per gram of creatinine. Based on information obtained from the controlled adult vitamin B-6 excretion studies, a urinary excretion level of "free" vitamin B-6 above 20 µg/g creatinine has been considered an indication of an acceptable vitamin B-6 intake.[77] Although the urinary level of vitamin B-6 may be of limited value per se as an indicator of the severity of a vitamin B-6 deficiency in an individual, it is useful as a reflection of the individual's recent dietary intakes of vitamin B-6.

Schultz and Leklem[99] considered a 24-hr total vitamin B-6 urinary excretion of above > 0.60 µmol for men and > 0.64 for women as an acceptable level of vitamin B-6 excretion. These values are comparable to the findings of Kretsch et al.[96]

Vitamin B-6 Status

TABLE 15
Comparison of Guidelines for Vitamin B-6 Status Assessment with Experimental Observation

Assessment Parameter	Guidelines Derived from Reports of Leklem et al.[99,198,206] Acceptable Levels	Actual Mean Values for Subjects Receiving 1.5 mg Vitamin B-6 Daily for 21 Days (Kretsch et al.[96])* Observed Levels
Plasma pyridoxal 5'-phosphate	>30 nmol/L	30.4 ± 14.7 nmol/L
Urinary 4-pyridoxic acid	>3.0 μmol/d	3.8 ± 0.41 μmol/d
Urinary total vitamin B-6	>0.5 μmol/d	0.52 ± 0.08 μmol/d
Erythrocyte AST activity coefficient**	<1.80	1.72 ± 0.08
Erythrocyte ALT activity coefficient	<1.25	1.38 ± 0.10

* A daily intake of 1.5 mg of vitamin B-6 is considered marginal.
** Erythrocyte AST activity level is approximately 15-fold higher than that of erythrocyte ALT.[96]
n = 8 young women.

TABLE 16
Vitamin B-6 Guidelines for Adolescent Girls

Subjects	Plasma Pyridoxal 5'-phosphate Concentration (nmol/L)
Adolescent girls (*n* = 186)	
Mean	45.2
Marginal vitamin B-6 deficient	28.3–40.4
Vitamin B-6 deficient	<28.3

Adapted from Driskell and Moak.[245]

TABLE 17
Plasma Pyridoxal 5'-Phosphate Concentrations in Adult Men

Adult Men	Plasma pyridoxal 5'-phosphate
Without vitamin B-6 supplements (*n* = 414)	49.8 ± 1.2 nmol/L (12.3 ± 0.3 ng/mL)
Receiving vitamin B-6 supplement (2.5 mg/day average) (*n* = 203)	82.9 ± 4.0 nmol/L (20.5 ± 1.0 ng/mL)
Marginal vitamin B-6 status	< 34 nmol/L (8.5 ng/mL)

Adapted from Rose et al.[237]

TABLE 18

Concentrations of Vitamin B-6 Compounds in Plasma
and Erythrocytes

Compound	Plasma (nmol/L)	Erythrocyte (nmol/L)
Pyridoxal-5′-phosphate	80.4 ± 21.5	86.0 ±19.3
Pyridoxamine-5′-phosphate	1.8 ± 3.6	3.0 ± 5.3
Pyridoxal	28.3 ± 19.5	11.5 ± 9.0
Pyridoxine	34.0 ± 23.3	4.5 ± 4.7
Pyridoxamine	11.9 ± 27.0	0.5 ± 1.0
4-Pyridoxic acid	15.2 ± 35.5	2.8 ± 5.4

n = 11 nonsmokers.
From Giraud et al.[233]

TABLE 19

Guidelines for Evaluating Vitamin B-6, Folate,
and Vitamin B-12 Plasma Concentration

Nutrient	Acceptable Concentration
Pyridoxal 5′-phosphate	≥30 nmol/L
Folate	≥5 nmol/L
Cobalamin	≥200 pmol/L

From Ubbink et al.[44]

TABLE 20

Evaluation of Urinary Excretion of Vitamin B-6

Age Group (Years)	Urinary Excretion of Vitamin B-6 Acceptable Levels (μg/g creatinine)
1–3+	≥90
4–6+	≥80
7–9+	≥60
10–12+	≥40
13–15+	≥30
≥16	≥20

Free vitamin B-6: unhydrolyzed samples.[88,112,244]

TABLE 21

Relation of Plasma Homocysteine Concentrations to Plasma Vitamin B-6, Folate,
and Vitamin B-12 Concentrations

Subjects	Plasma pyridoxal 5′-phosphate (nmol/L)	Plasma Folate (nmol/L)	Plasma Cobalamin (pmol/L)
Group I (*n* = 274)			
Homocysteine concentrations ≤ 16.3 μmol/L	83 ± 76	6.7 ± 3.6	275 ± 148
Group II (*n* = 44)			
Homocysteine concentrations > 16.3 μmol/L	56 ± 50	5.5 ± 2.9	202 ± 61

Adapted from the report of Ubbink, et al.[44]
Moderate hyperhomocysteinemia considered when plasma homocysteine concentration was > 16.3 μmol/L.
See also Robinson et al.[71] for similar observations.

TABLE 22
Biochemical Tests for Assessment of Vitamin B-6 Status

Measurement	Reference Values
Plasma pyridoxal 5′-phosphate	20–86 nmol
Erythrocyte aspartate aminotransferase (EAST)	8.4 –18.9 μkat/L
Erythrocyte aspartate aminotransferase activation coefficient (α EAST)	1.42–2.05
Urinary 4-pyridoxic acid	128–680 nmol/nmol creatinine

From Bitsch.[95]

TABLE 23
Guidelines for Evaluation of Vitamin B-6 Status in Adults

Metabolite	Marginally Deficient Concentration
Plasma pyridoxal 5′-phosphate	
Male (*n* = 35)	< 36.8 nmol/L
Female (*n* = 41)	< 31.5 nmol/L
Urinary 4-pyridoxic acid (μmol/24 hr)	
Male (*n* = 35)	< 5.0–5.7
Female (*n* = 41)	< 4.6–5.2
Urinary Total Vitamin B-6 (μmol/24 hr)	
Male (*n* = 35)	< 0.6–0.7
Female (*n* = 41)	< 0.6–0.7

Values from Shultz and Leklem.[99]

TABLE 24
Summary of Guidelines for Evaluating Vitamin B-6 Status

Parameter	Acceptable Value
Plasma pyridoxal 5′-phosphate	> 30 nmol/L
Plasma total vitamin B-6	> 40 nmol/L
Urinary 4-pyridoxic acid	> 3.0 μmol/d
Urinary total vitamin B-6	> 0.5 μmol/d
Urinary xanthurenic acid excretion	< 65 μmol/d
(2 g L-tryptophan load)	
Erythrocyte AST–AC (αEAST)	< 1.80 (< 80%)
Erythrocyte ALT–AC (αEALT)	< 1.25 (< 25%)

Adapted from Hansen et al.,[206] Leklem,[198] and Shultz and Leklem.[99]

TABLE 25
Effect of Age on the Concentrations of Blood Vitamin B-6 Components

Component	Age Group (*n* = 12/group)		
	25–35 yr (nmol/L)	45–55 yr (nmol/L)	65–75 yr (nmol/L)
Plasma pyridoxal 5′-phosphate	76	48	42
Plasma total vitamin B-6	128	71	78
Erythrocyte pyridoxal 5′-phosphate	85	72	76
Erythrocyte total vitamin B-6	85	88	91

Adapted from Kant et al.[211]

Pregnancy, Infants, and Children

Low plasma pyridoxal 5'-phosphate levels are reported for infants and during pregnancy.[121,122] The values require careful evaluation since the plasma pyridoxal concentration is higher in these subjects. Consequently, the total amount of pyridoxal plus pyridoxal 5'-phosphate does not differ between pregnant and non-pregnant women.[109,110]

Heiskanen et al.[219,220] have published reference ranges for erythrocyte pyridoxal 5'-phosphate and for erythrocyte aspartate transaminase activity coefficients (EAST-AC) for lactating mothers and for infants and children, at birth through 11 years. Vitamin B-6 status, high in infancy, fell with age. Abnormal plasma pyridoxal 5'-phosphate concentrations may be encountered in numerous inborn errors of metabolism and organic diseases.[75,83]

Vitamin B-6 status was assessed in a study of term and preterm infants.[191,218] Status was based on plasma pyridoxal 5'-phosphate determinations, measurements of vitamin B-6 vitaminers found in plasma and erythrocytes, and by erythrocyte alanine aminotransferase coefficient determinations. The plasma and erythrocyte measurement values of the infants correlated with their intakes of vitamin B-6. In the infant, plasma pyridoxal 5'-phosphate represented over 65% of the vitamin B-6 active forms present (40 nmol/L plasma pyridoxal 5'-phosphate; 9 nmol/L plasma pyridoxal; 77 nmol/L erythrocyte pyridoxal 5'-phosphate).[191]

Adults and Elderly

Joosten et al.[42] found serum vitamin B-6 (pyridoxal phosphate) concentrations were low in 9% of the healthy young subjects studied, while 51% were low in the elderly population. Plasma pyridoxal phosphate concentrations of > 40 nmol/L were considered normal.[42] The studied involved 350 elderly subjects and 99 healthy young people. The subjects were recruited from Belgium, Germany, and The Netherlands. Lowik et al.[204] found approximately 9% of a Dutch elderly population ($n = 476$) had a marginal vitamin B-6 status. Status was based on plasma pyridoxal 5'-phosphate concentrations and erythrocyte AST activity coefficients (EAST-AC). In the Euronut SENECA Study of 2,500 elderly subjects in 11 European countries, a widespread prevalence of biochemical vitamin B-6 deficiency was observed.[259]

Cardiovascular Disease and Atherosclerosis

Studies have been conducted for some time on the role of vitamin B-6 in the development of atherosclerosis.[255] Rinehart and Greenberg were the first to note that a vitamin B-6 deficiency may be a contributory factor in the development of atherosclerosis.[32] Subsequently, McCully made the observation that linked plasma homocysteine concentrations with arteriosclerotic vascular disease.[33] He proposed that hyperhomocysteinemia resulted in arteriosclerotic disease. This association between plasma homocysteine concentrations and atherosclerosis has since been demonstrated in a number of studies.[45,46,71,72,167]

Some subsequent reports did not support the contention that a vitamin B-6 deficiency may be a risk factor for ischemic heart disease.[34-37] However, numerous other studies supported an association of vitamin B-6 status with the risk of coronary heart disease.[38,39,41-44] More recently Selhub et al.[40] evaluated the plasma homocysteine status in the elderly men ($n = 418$) and women ($n = 623$) from the Framingham Heart Study. From their detailed study, they concluded that high plasma homocysteine concentrations and low concentrations of folate and vitamin B-6, via their role in homocysteine metabolism, were associated with an increased risk of extracranial carotid-artery stenosis in the elderly.[40] In the Framingham Heart Study, 21% of the subjects had plasma homocysteine concentrations of over 15.8 μmol/L. Elevated plasma homocysteine concentrations have been defined as > 15.8 μmol/L by Sampfer et al.;[47] > 13.9 μmol/L by Joosten et al.,[42] and > 14 μmol/L by Selhub et al.[41] In the Framingham Heart Study, it was observed that the risk of stenosis was elevated in individuals with homocysteine concentrations between 11.4 and 14.3 μmol/L.[40]

In a study of 304 patients with coronary disease and of 231 healthy controls, Robinson et al.[71] from the Cleveland Clinic, found that 10% of the heart disease patients had low plasma pyridoxal 5′-phosphate concentration. Only 2% of the controls had low concentration. Plasma homocysteine concentrations were higher in the patients than in the controls (14.4 ± 15.4 μmol/L compared to the controls [10.9 ± 3.4 μmol/L]). The plasma homocysteine concentrations were lower in the female controls (10.1 ± 4.7 μmol/L) when compared to the male controls (11.2 ± 2.9 μmol/L). Plasma pyridoxal 5′-phosphate concentrations < 20 nmol/L were considered low.[71]

In a study conducted in Belfast, Northern Ireland, male subjects (aged 30 to 49) had a median plasma homocysteine concentration of 7.18 μmol/L.[48] Subjects with a plasma homocysteine concentration of ≥ 8.34 μmol/L (n = 152) were considered above the normal concentration. Providing the subjects with a daily combined supplement of 1 mg of folic acid, 0.02 mg vitamin B-12, and 7.2 mg pyridoxal, for 8 weeks, resulted in a reduction in homocysteine concentrations of 27.9%.

Ubbink et al.[47] using a similar combination of these three vitamins observed a 62% reduction in plasma homocysteine concentrations. Additional studies have demonstrated that vitamin B-6 has an important role in the regulation of homocysteine.[43,44] Andersson et al.[158] noted that premenopausal women have considerably lower serum homocysteine concentrations than men or postmenopausal women.[159,160] Nevertheless, inadequate intake of folic acid appears to be the main determinant of homocysteine-related increase in coronary heart disease.[40]

Subjects afflicted with the inborn error, cystathionine β-synthase deficiency, have elevated plasma concentrations of homocysteine.[167] These subjects often have a diminished cystathionine β-synthase activity which responds to high levels of pyridoxine supplementation to reduce the elevated plasma homocysteine concentrations.

Vitamin B-6 Interactions

Vitamin B-6 has been associated with a number of clinical conditions,[75] such as carpal tunnel syndrome.[1,2] Carpal tunnel syndrome is a condition that affects the median nerve at the wrist to cause impairment of nerve function. Some patients with the syndrome have been reported to benefit by pyridoxine supplements[1-7] while other investigators have not observed any benefit.[8,9] The supplements used are quite high, usually 50 to 200 mg of pyridoxine daily for over 12 weeks.[2]

Smoking is associated with low plasma pyridoxal 5′-phosphate concentrations.[193] Plasma pyridoxal 5′-phosphate and pyridoxal concentrations were reported to be lower in smokers than in non-smokers.[194] However, erythrocyte pyridoxal 5′-phosphate and pyridoxal concentrations did not differ between smokers and non-smokers.[194] Pyridoxal 5′-phosphate concentrations have been reported to be depressed in asthmatics.[201,202]

Pyridoxal kinase catalyzes the phosphorylation of pyridoxal, pyridoxine, and pyridoxamine to form pyridoxal 5′-phosphate, pyridoxine 5′-phosphate, and pyridoxamine 5′-phosphate, respectively. Pyridoxal kinase is activated by zinc.[197] Zinc may have a role in the regulation of vitamin B-6 metabolism.[197] The essentiality of riboflavin in the interconversion of the vitamin B-6 forms is also recognized.[256]

Vitamin B-6 Drug Interactions and Antagonists

A number of drugs are known that can impair vitamin B-6 utilization.[68,92,93,97] Included are the antituberculosis drug, isonicotinic acid hydrazide (isoniazid),[203] penicillamine, cycloserine, and hydralazine, and L-dopa.[97] A number of naturally occurring vitamin B-6 antagonists also exist including agaritine (mushrooms), linatine (flax seed meal), canaline (jack bean), canavanine (jack bean), gyromitrin (mushrooms), and mimosine (mimosa). At low levels of vitamin B-6 in the diet, epsilon-pyridoxyllysine demonstrated antivitamin B-6 activity.[26] A number of other vitamin antagonists have been reported to occur naturally in the diet.[27-31]

Use of Oral Contraceptive Agents

The use of low dose oral contraceptives do not appear to have any long-term effects on vitamin B-6 requirements or status.[101,103,185,189] Masse et al.[190] conducted a detailed study on the effect of oral contraceptives on the vitamin B-6 status in 23 young women. Assessment of vitamin B-6 status was based on measurement of pyridoxal and pyridoxal 5'-phosphate concentrations in the plasma and erythrocytes. As a functional test, erythrocyte aspartate aminotransferase (EAST) activity coefficients were measured. Although the metabolism of vitamin B-6 was altered with the use of the oral contraceptive agent, the study provided little evidence of an increased requirement for vitamin B-6.

Alkaline Phosphatase

Diseases and conditions that are associated with elevated plasma alkaline phosphatase activity can reduce pyridoxal 5'-phosphate concentrations.[75] Such may occur with certain bone or hepatic disorders.[75] Plasma alkaline phosphatase activity may increase with age.[75] Conversely, patients with hypophosphatasia have markedly increased circulating pyridoxal 5'-phosphate levels.[76]

Protein Intake and Vitamin B-6 Requirements

The requirement for vitamin B-6 is related to the level of protein intake.[77,82,86,196,207-209,215] The relationship of the level of dietary protein to vitamin B-6 requirements of men has been summarized by Linkswiler[82] and in women by Hansen et al.[207] and Donald.[209] The results of numerous studies indicate that vitamin B-6 requirement for men consuming diets containing 100 to 150 g of protein daily is between 1.5 and 2.0 mg per day. The study conducted in 1994 by Pannemans et al.[187] indicated an age-dependent difference in the protein intake-related vitamin B-6 requirements. Elderly subjects appeared to require less vitamin B-6 at a higher protein intake when compared with young adults. From a detailed study conducted on subjects maintained in a metabolic unit, it was found that the vitamin B-6 requirements of elderly women and elderly men were approximately 1.90 and 1.96 mg/day, respectively.[208] In a study on the vitamin B-6 requirement of young women, Huang et al.[210] found a requirement of 1.94 mg/day of vitamin B-6 (or 0.019 mg vitamin B-6/gram of protein ingested).

Vitamin B-6 and Immune Function

Vitamin B-6 has an important role in the modulation of the immune response and infection.[49,50,56,70] Immune function is particularly impaired in the elderly by vitamin B-6 deficiency and with HIV infection.[51,52,54-56] Mitogenic response of elderly subjects to T- and B-cell mitogens and interleukin-2 formation was affected by a decrease in vitamin B-6 status.[52] Vitamin B-6 deficiency induced in healthy adults (*n* = 8) significantly decreased the percentage and total number of lymphocytes, mitogenic responses of peripheral blood lymphocytes to T- and B-cell mitogens, and interleukin-2 production.[53] Vitamin B-6 supplements corrected these impairments.

Vitamin B-6 and Alcohol

Alcohol has a systemic effect on the maintenance of blood pyridoxal 5'-phosphate concentrations.[147,148,181] Biochemical evidence of a vitamin B-6 deficiency has been noted in 20–30% of alcoholic patients. Clinical signs of a vitamin B-6 deficiency is often observed in alcoholic patients in the form of convulsions, peripheral neuropathy and sideroblastic anemia.[181]

Toxicity

Several reviews have considered the safety of vitamin B-6.[57-61] Since little vitamin B-6 is stored in the body, an excess intake of the vitamin is excreted unaltered or as its metabolite, 4-pyridoxic acid. Consequently, excess intakes of vitamin B-6 are usually removed readily from the body without any evidence of toxicity. Data have indicated that vitamin B-6 doses of less than 500 mg/day were safe over a period of as long as 6 years.[57-59] Doses above 500 mg/day are commonly associated with neuropathy that is usually reversible upon cessation of supplementation.[58-67] In review of the data, toxic effects can apparently occur with prolonged intakes of between 300 and 500 mg/day. Intakes of no more than 200 mg/day of pyridoxine are recommended without medical advice.[67-69]

Summary

Plasma pyridoxal 5'-phosphate (PLP) concentrations can serve as a sensitive indicator of vitamin B-6 status and can provide information as to the body stores of the vitamin. However, pyridoxal 5'-phosphate levels can be influenced by several non-nutritive factors, including physical exercise, pregnancy, and level of plasma alkaline phosphatase activity. As a functional measure of vitamin B-6 status, the xanthurenic acid excretion following a tryptophan load remains a sensitive test. The determinations of erythrocyte transaminase activities and activity coefficients for aspartate aminotransferase (EAST) or alanine aminotransferase (EALT) are sensitive measures of vitamin B-6 status. The erythrocyte transaminase activities are generally considered to be a long-term indicator of vitamin B-6 status and of dietary intake of the vitamin. Urinary excretion of 4-pyridoxic acid provides short-term information on vitamin B-6 status. The excretion of 4-pyridoxic acid correlates well with the dietary intake of vitamin B-6. Urinary excretion of vitamin B-6 provides information comparable to the urinary 4-pyridoxic acid measurements. However, 4-pyridoxic acid is easily determined with the use of HPLC.

References

1. Ellis, J. M., Folkers, K., Levy, M., Shizukuishi, S., Lewandowiski, J., Nishu, S., Schubert, H. A., and Ulrich, R., Response of vitamin B-6 deficiency and the carpal tunnel syndrome to pyridoxine, *Proc. Natl. Acad. Sci.*, 79, 7494, 1982.
2. Ellis, J. M. and Folkers, K., Clinical aspects of treatment of carpal tunnel syndrome with vitamin B-6, *Ann. N.Y. Acad. Sci.*, 585, 302, 1990.
3. Ellis, J. M., Treatment of carpal tunnel syndrome with vitamin B-6, *Southern Med. J.*, 80, 882, 1987.
4. Kasdan, M. L. and James, C., Carpal tunnel syndrome and vitamin B-6, *Plastic Reconstructive Surg.*, 79, 456, 1987.
5. Salked, R. M. and Stotz, R., Vitamin B-6 deficiency: An etiological factor of the carpal tunnel syndrome, in *Vitamin B-6: Its Role in Health and Disease*, Reynolds, R. D. and Leklem, J. E., Eds., Alan R. Liss, Inc. New York, 1985, 463.
6. Guzman, F. J. L., Gonzalez-Buitrago, J. M., de Arriba, F., Mateos, F., Moyano, J. C., and Lopez-Alburquerque, T., Carpal tunnel syndrome and vitamin B-6, *Klin. Wochenschr.*, 67, 38, 1989.
7. Fuhr, J. E., Farrow, A., Nelson, H. S., Jr., Vitamin B-6 levels in patients with carpal tunnel syndrome, *Arch. Surg.*, 124, 1329, 1989.
8. Amadio, P. C., Carpal tunnel syndrome, pyridoxine, and the work place, *J. Hand Surg.*, 12A, 875, 1987.
9. Scheyer, R. D. and Haas, D. C., Pyridoxine in carpal tunnel syndrome, *Lancet*, 2, 42, 1985.
10. Sauberlich, H. E., Bioavailability of vitamins, *Prog. Food Nutr. Sci.*, 9, 1, 1985.
11. Sauberlich, H. E., Vitamins – How much is for keeps, *Nutrition Today*, January/February, 20, 1987.
12. Reynolds, R. D., Bioavailability of vitamin B-6 from plant foods, *Am. J. Clin. Nutr.*, 48, 863, 1988.
13. Gregory, J. F., III, Bioavailability of vitamin B-6 from plant foods, *Am. J. Clin. Nutr.*, 49, 717, 1989.
14. Tarr, J. B., Tamura, T., and Stokstad, E. L. R., Availability of vitamin B-6 and pantothenate in an average American diet, *Am. J. Clin. Nutr.*, 34, 1328, 1981.
15. Gregory, J. F., III, The bioavailability of vitamin B-6: recent findings, *Ann. N.Y. Acad. Sci.*, 585, 86, 1990.
16. Anonymous, Role of glycosylated vitamin B-6 in human nutrition, *Nutr. Rev.*, 48, 251, 1990.
17. Gregory, J. F., III, Trumbo, P. R., Bailey, L. B., Toth, J. P., Baumgartner, T. G., and Cerda, J. J., Bioavailability of pyridoxine-5′-β-D-glucoside determined in humans by stable-isotopic methods, *J. Nutr.*, 121, 177, 1991.
18. Hansen, C. M., Leklem, J. E., and Miller, L. T., Vitamin B-6 status indicators decrease in women consuming a diet high in pyridoxine glucoside, *J. Nutr.*, 126, 2512, 1996.
19. Nakano, H., McMahon, L. G., and Gregory, J. F., III, Pyridoxine-5′-β-D-glucoside exhibits incomplete bioavailability as a source of vitamin B-6 and partially inhibits the utilization of co-ingested pyridoxine in humans, *J. Nutr.*, 127, 1508, 1997.
20. Gregory, J. F., III and Ink, S. F., Identification and quantification of pyridoxine-β-glucoside as a major form of vitamin B-6 in plant-derived foods, *J. Agric. Food Chem.*, 35, 76, 1987.
21. Kant, A. K. and Block, G., Dietary vitamin B-6 intake and food sources in the U.S. population: NHANES-II, 1976-1980, *Am. J. Clin. Nutr.*, 52, 707, 1990.
22. Dong, M. H., McGown, E. L., Schwenneker, B. W., and Sauberlich, H. E., Thiamin, riboflavin, and vitamin B-6 contents of selected foods as served, *J. Am. Diet. Assoc.*, 76, 156, 1980.
23. Sauberlich, H. E., Vitamin B-6, vitamin B-12, and folate, in *Meat and Health*, Volume 6, Person, A. M. and Dutson, T. R., Eds., Elsevier Applied Sciences, New York, 1990, 461.
24. Ferroli, C. E. and Trumbo, P. R., Bioavailability of vitamin B-6 in young and older men, *Am. J. Clin. Nutr.*, 60, 68, 1994.
25. Lumeng, L., Lui, A., and Li, T. K., Plasma content of B-6 vitamers and its relationship to hepatic vitamin B-6 metabolism, *Clin. Invest.*, 66, 688, 1980.

26. Gregory, J. F., III, Effects of epsilon-pyridoxyllysine bound to dietary protein on the vitamin B-6 status of rats, *J. Nutr.*, 110, 995, 1980.

27. Rechcigl, M., Jr. Ed., *Handbook of Naturally Occurring Food Toxicants*, CRC Press, Boca Raton, FL, 1983.

28. *Toxicants Occurring Naturally in Foods*, 2nd edition, National Academy of Sciences, Washington D.C., 1973.

29. Brin, M., Vitamin B-6: Chemistry, absorption, metabolism, catabolism, and toxicity, in *Human Vitamin B-6 Requirements*, National Academy of Sciences, Washington D.C., 1979, 1.

30. Bauernfeind, J. C. and Miller, O. N., Vitamin B-6: Nutritional and pharmaceutical usage, stability, bioavailability, antagonists, and safety, in *Human Vitamin B-6 Requirements*, National Academy of Sciences, Washington D.C., 1978, 78.

31. Klosterman, H. J., Vitamin B-6 antagonists of natural origin, *J. Agric. Food Chem.*, 22, 13, 1978.

32. Rinehart, J. F. and Greenberg, L. D., Arterioscleratic lesions in pyridoxine deficient monkeys, *Am. J. Pathol.*, 25, 481, 1949.

33. McCully, K. S., Vascular pathology of homocysteinemia: implications for the pathogenesis of arteriosclerosis, *Am. J. Pathol.*, 56, 111, 1969.

34. Vermaak, W. J. H., Barnard, H. C., Potgieter, G. M., and du Theron, H., Vitamin B-6 and coronary artery disease: epidemiological observations and case studies, *Atherosclerosis*, 63, 235, 1987.

35. Labadarios, D., Brink, P. A., Weich, H. F. H., Visser, L., Louw, M. E. J., Shephard, G. S., and van Stuijvenberg, M. E., Plasma vitamin A, E, C, and B-6 levels in myocardial infarctions, *S. Afr. Med. J.*, 71, 561, 1987.

36. Vermaak, W. J. H., Barnard, H. C., van Dalen, E. M. S. P., and Potgieter, G. M., Vitamin B-6 adaptive response during myocardial infraction, in *Clinical and Physiological Applications of Vitamin B-6*, Alan R. Liss, Inc., New York, 1988, 219.

37. Serfontein, W. J. and Ubbink, J. B., Vitamin B-6 and myocardial infraction, in *Clinical and Physiological Applications of Vitamin B-6*, Alan R. Liss, Inc., New York, 1988, 201.

38. Schrijver, J. and Kok, F. J., Vitamin B-6 status after heart attack, in *Clinical and Physiological Applications of Vitamin B-6*, Alan R. Liss, Inc., New York, 1988, 225.

39. Shultz, T. D., Roth, W. J., and Howie, B. J., Vitamin B-6 to protein-bound homocysteine interrelationship as a possible risk factor for coronary heart disease among Seventh-Day Adventist men, in *Clinical and Physiological Application of Vitamin B-6*, Alan R. Liss, Inc., New York, 1988, 177.

40. Selhub, J., Jacques, P. F., Boston, A. G., D'Agostino, R. B., Wilson, P. W. F., Belavger, A. J., O'Leary, D. H., Wolfe, P. A., Schaefer, E. J., and Rosenberg, I. H., Association between homocysteine concentrations and extracranial carotid-artery stenosis, *N. Engl. J. Med.*, 332, 286, 1995.

41. Selhub, J., Jacques, P. F., Wilson, P. W., Rush, D., and Rosenberg, I. H., Vitamin status and intake as primary determinants of homocysteinemia in elderly populations, *JAMA*, 270, 2693, 1993.

42. Joosten, E., van den Berg, A., Riezler, R., Naurath, H. J., Lindenbaum, J., Stabler, S. P., and Allen, R. H., Metabolic evidence that deficiencies of vitamin B-12 (cobalamin), folate, and vitamin B-6 occur commonly in elderly people, *Am. J. Clin. Nutr.*, 58, 468, 1993.

43. Brattson, L., Israelsson, B., Norrving, B. et al., Impaired homocysteine metabolism in early-onset cerebral and peripheral occlusive arterial disease: effects of pyridoxine and folic treatment, *Atherosclerosis*, 81, 51, 1990.

44. Ubbink, J. B., Vermaak, W. J., van de Merwe, A., and Becker, P. J., Vitamin B-12, vitamin B-6, and folate nutritional status in men with hyperhomocysteinemia, *Am. J. Clin. Nutr.*, 57, 47, 1993.

45. Ueland, P. M., Refsum, H., and Brattstrom, L., Plasma homocysteine and cardiovascular disease, in *Atherosclerotic Cardiovascular Disease, Hemostasis, and Endothelial Function*, Francis, R. B., Jr., Eds., Marcel Dekker, New York, 1992, 183.

46. Kang, S. –S., Wong. P. W., and Malinow, M. R., Hyperhomocyst(e)inemia as a risk factor for occlusive vascular disease, *Annu. Rev. Nutr.*, 12, 279, 1992.

47. Stampfer, M. J., Malinow, M. R., Willett, W. C. et al., A prospective study of plasma homocyst(e)ine and risk of myocardial infraction in U.S. physicians, *JAMA*, 268, 877, 1992.

48. Woodside, J. V., Yarnell, J. W. G., McMaster, D., Young, I. S., Harmon, D. L., McCrum, E., Patterson, C. C., Gey, K. F., Whitehead, A. S., and Evans, A., Effect of B-group vitamins and antioxidant vitamins on hyperhomocysteinemia: a double-blind, randomized, factorial-design, controlled trial, *Am. J. Clin. Nutr.*, 67, 858, 1998.

49. Chandra, R. K. and Puri, S., Vitamin B-6 modulation of immune response and infection, in *Current Topics in Nutrition and Disease*, Volume 13, Reynolds, R. D. and Leklem, J. E., Eds., Alan R. Liss, Inc., New York, 1985, 163.

50. Stinnett, J. D., *Nutrition and the Immune Response*, CRC Press, Boca Raton, FL, 1983, 127.

51. Meydani, S. N., Hayek, M., and Coleman, L., Influence of vitamin E and B-6 on immune response, *N. Y. Acad. Sci.*, 669, 125, 1992.

52. Meydani, S. N., Ribaya-Mercado, J. D., Russell, R. M., Sahyoun, N., Morrow, F. D., and Gerrhoff, S. N., The effect of vitamin B-6 on the immune response of healthy elderly, *Ann. N.Y. Acad. Sci.*, 587, 303, 1990.

53. Meydani, S. N., Ribaya-Mercado, J. D., Russell, R. M., Sahyoun, N., Morrow, F. D., and Gershoff, S. N., Vitamin B-6 deficiency impairs interleukin 2 production and lymphocyte proliferation in elderly adults, *Am. J. Clin. Nutr.*, 53, 1275, 1991.

54. Talbott, M. C., Miller, L. T., and Kerkvliet, N. I., Pyridoxine supplementation: effect on lymphocyte responses in elderly persons, *Am. J. Clin. Nutr.*, 46, 659, 1987.

55. Baum, M. K., Shor-Posner, G., Bonvehi, P., Cassetti, I., Lu, E., Mantero-Atienza, E., Beach, R. S., and Sauberlich, H. E., Influence of HIV infection on vitamin status and requirements, *Ann. N.Y. Acad. Sci.*, 669, 165, 1992.

56. Anonymous, Vitamin B-6 and immune function in the elderly and HIV-seropositive subjects, *Nutr. Revs.*, 50, 145, 1992.

57. Bendick, A., Safety issues regarding the use of vitamin supplements, *Ann. N.Y. Acad. Sci.*, 669, 300, 1992.

58. Cohen, M. and Bendich, A., Safety of pyridoxine — a review of human and animal studies, *Toxicol. Lett.*, 34, 129, 1986.

59. Bendich, A. and Cohen, M., Vitamin B-6 safety issues, *Ann. N.Y. Acad. Sci.*, 585, 321, 1990.

60. Sauberlich, H. E., Relationship of vitamin B-6, vitamin B-12, and folate to neurological and neuropsychiatric disorders, in *Micronutrients in Health and in Disease Prevention*, Bendich, A. and Butterworth, C. E., Jr., Eds., Marcel Dekker, New York, 1991, 187.

61. Hathcock, J. N., Safety of vitamins and mineral supplements, in *Micronutrients in Health and in Disease Prevention*, Bendich, A. and Butterworth, C. E. Jr., Eds., Marcel Dekker, New York, 1991, 439.

62. Dalton, K. and Dalton, M. J. T., Characteristics of pyridoxine overdose neuropathy syndrome, *Acta Neurol. Scan.*, 76, 8, 1987.

63. Podell, R. N., Nutritional supplementation with megadoses of vitamin B-6, *Postgrad. Med.*, 77, 113, 1985.

64. Schaumburg, H., Kaplan, J., Windebank, A., Vick, N., Rasmus, S., Pleasure, D., and Brown, M. J., Sensory neuropathy from pyridoxine abuse, A new megavitamin syndrome, *N. Engl. J. Med.*, 309, 445, 1983.

65. Berger, A. and Schaumburg, H. H., More on neuropathy from pyridoxine abuse, *N. Engl. J. Med.*, 311, 986, 1984.

66. Parry, G. J. and Bredesen, D. E., Sensory neuropathy with low-dose pyridoxine, *Neurology*, 35, 1466, 1985.

67. Bassler, K. –H., Use and abuse of high dosages of vitamin B-6, in *Elevated Dosages of Vitamins: Benefits and Hazards*, Walter, P., Brubacher, G., and Stahelin, H., Eds., Hans Huber Publication, Lewiston, 1989, 120.

68. Lemonine, A. and Le Devehat, C., Clinical conditions requiring elevated dosages of vitamins, in *Elevated Dosages of Vitamins: Benefits and Hazards*, Walter, P., Brubacher, G., and Stahelin, H., Eds., Hans Huber Publications, Lewiston, 1989, 129.

69. Butterworth, C. E., Jr., Vitamin safety: a current appraisal 1994 update, *VNIS: Vitamin Nutrition Information Services*, 5, 1, 1994.

70. Chandra, R. K. and Sudhakaran, L., Regulation of immune responses by vitamin B-6, *Ann. N.Y. Acad. Sci.*, 585, 404, 1990.

71. Robinson, K., Mayer, E. L., Miller, D. P., Green, R. et al., Hyperhomocysteinemia and low pyridoxal phosphate: common and independent reversible risk factors for coronary artery disease, *Circulation*, 92, 2825, 1995.

72. Smolin, L. A., Crenshaw, T. D., Kurtycz, D., and Benevenga, N. J., Homocyst(e)ine accumulation in pigs fed diets deficient in vitamin B-6: relationship to atherosclerosis, *J. Nutr.*, 113, 2122, 1983.

73. Smolin, L. A. and Benevenga, N. J., Accumulation of homocyst(e)ine in vitamin B-6 deficiency: a model for the study of cystathionine β-synthase deficiency, *J. Nutr.*, 112, 1264, 1982.

74. Dudman, N. P. B., Guo, X. –W., Gordon, R. B., Dawson, P. A., and Wilchen, D. E. L., Human homocysteine catabolism: three major pathways and their relevance to development of arterial occlusive disease, *J. Nutr.*, 126, 1295S, 1996.

75. Merrill, A. H. and Henderson, J. M., Diseases associated with defects in vitamin B-6 metabolism or utilization, *Annu. Rev. Nutr.*, 7, 137, 1987.

76. Whyte, M. P., Mahuren, J. D., Vrabel, L. A., and Coburn, S. P., Markedly increased circulatng pyridoxal 5′-phosphate levels in hypophosphatasia, *J. Clin. Invest.*, 76, 752, 1985.

77. Sauberlich, H. E., Vitamin B-6 status assessment: past and present, in *Methods in Vitamin B-6 Nutrition, Analysis and Status Assessment*, Leklem, J. E. and Reynolds, R. D., Eds., Plenum Press, New York, 1981, 203.

78. Lepkovsky, S., Roboz, E., and Hargen-Smith, A. J., Xanthurenic acid and its role in the tryptophan metabolism of pyridoxine-deficient rats, *J. Biol. Chem.*, 149, 195, 1943.

79. Greenberg, L. D., Bohr, D. F., McGrath, H., and Rinehart, J. F., Xanthurenic acid excretion in the human subjects on pyridoxine-deficient diet, *Arch. Biochem.*, 21, 237, 1949.

80. Brown, R. R., The tryptophan load test as an index of vitamin B-6 nutrition, in *Methods in Vitamin B-6 Nutrition, Analysis and Status Assessment*, Leklem, J. E. and Reynolds, R. D., Eds., Plenum Press, New York, 1981, 321.

81. Leklem, J. E., Rose, D. P., and Brown, R. R., Effects of oral contraceptives on urinary metabolites excretion after administration of L-tyrptophan or L-kynurenine sulfate, *Metabolism*, 22, 1499, 1973.

82. Linkswiler, H. M., Vitamin B-6 requirements of men, in *Human Vitamin B-6 Requirements*, National Academy of Science, Washington D.C., 1978, 279.

83. Vitamin B-6: Its role in health and disease, *Current Topics in Nutrition and Disease*, Volume 13, Reynolds, R. D. and Leklem, J. E., Eds., Alan R. Liss, Inc., New York, 1985, 510.

84. *Methods in Vitamin B-6 Nutrition, Analysis and Status Assessment*, Leklem, J. E. and Reynolds, R. D., Eds., Plenum Press, New York, 1981, 401.

85. Dakshinamurti, K., Ed., Vitamin B-6, *Ann. N. Y. Acad. Sci.*, 585, 567, 1990.

86. Canham, J. E., Baker, E. M., Harding, R. S., Sauberlich, H. E., and Plough, I. C., Dietary protein – its relationship to vitamin B-6 requirements and function, *Ann. N.Y. Acad. Sci.*, 166, 16, 1969.

87. Sauberlich, H. E., Canham, J. E., Baker, E. M., Raica, N., Jr., and Herman, Y. F., Human vitamin B-6 nutrition, *J. Sci. Ind. Res.*, 29, 528, 1970.

88. Sauberlich, H. E., Canham, J. E., Baker, E. M., Raica, N., Jr., and Herman, Y. F., Biochemical assessment of the nutritional status of vitamin B-6 in the human, *Am. J. Clin. Nutr.*, 25, 629, 1972.

89. Linkswiler, H., Biochemical and physiological changes in vitamin B-6 deficiency, *Am. J. Clin. Nutr.*, 20, 547, 1967.

90. Linkswiler, H., Methionine metabolite excretion as affected by a vitamin B-6 deficiency, in *Methods in Vitamin B-6 Nutrition, Analysis and Status Assessment*, Leklem, J. E. and Reynolds, R. D., Eds., Plenum Press, New York, 1980, 373.

91. Sturman, J. A., Vitamin B-6 and sulfur amino acid metabolism, in *Methods in Vitamin B-6 Nutrition, Analysis and Status Assessment*, Leklem, J. E. and Reynolds, R. D., Eds., Plenum Press, New York, 1980, 341.

92. Sauberlich, H. E., Vitamin B-6 group: Active compounds and antagonists, in *The Vitamins*, Volume II, Sebrell, W. H. Jr. and Harris, R. S., Eds., Academic Press, New York, 1968, 33.

93. Sauberlich, H. E., Vitamin B-6, in *The Vitamins*, Volume VII, Gyorgy, P. and Pearson, W. N., Eds., Academic Press, New York, 1967, 169.

94. Sauberlich, H. E., Vitamin B-6 group: biochemical systems and biochemical detection of deficiency, in *The Vitamins*, Volume II, Sebrell, W. H. Jr. and Harris, R. S., Eds., Academic Press, New York, 1968, 44.

95. Bitsch, R., Vitamin B-6, *Int. J. Vit. Nutr. Res.*, 63, 278, 1993.
96. Kretsch, M. J., Sauberlich, H. E., Skala, J. H., and Johnson, H. L., Vitamin B-6 requirement and status assessment: young women fed a depletion diet followed by a plant- or animal-protein diet with graded amounts of vitamin B-6, *Am. J. Clin. Nutr.*, 61, 1091, 1995.
97. Bhagavan, H. N., Interactions between vitamin B-6 and drugs, in *Vitamin B-6: Its Role in Health and Disease*, Reynolds, R. D. and Leklem, J. E., Eds., Alan, R. Liss, Inc., New York, 1985, 401.
98. Gregory J. F., III and Kirk, J. R., Determinations of urinary 4-pyridoxic acid using high performance liquid chromatography, *Am. J. Clin. Nutr.*, 32, 879, 1979.
99. Schultz, T. D. and Leklem, J. E., Urinary 4-pyridoxic acid, urinary vitamin B-6 and plasma pyridoxal phosphate as measures of vitamin B-6 status and dietary intake in adults, in *Methods in Vitamin B-6 Nutrition: Analysis and Status Assessment*, Leklem, J. E. and Reynolds, R. D., Eds., Plenum Press, New York, 1981, 297.
100. Leklem, J. E., Brown, R. R. Rose, D. P., and Linkswiler, H. M., Vitamin B-6 requirements of women using oral contraceptives, *Am. J. Clin. Nutr.*, 28, 535, 1977.
101. Leklem, J. E., Brown, R. R., Rose, D. P., Linkswiler, H. M., and Arend, R. A., Metabolism tryptophan and niacin in oral contraceptive users receiving controlled intakes of vitamin B-6, *Am. J. Clin. Nutr.*, 28, 146, 1975.
102. Rose, D. P., Leklem, J. E., Brown, R. R., and Linkswiler, H. M., Effect or oral contraceptives and vitamin B-6 deficiency on carbohydrate metabolism, *Am. J. Clin. Nutr.*, 28, 872, 1975.
103. Sauberlich, H. E., Human requirements for vitamin B-6, *Vit. Horm.*, 22, 807, 1964.
104. Baker, E. M., Canham, J. E., Nunes, W. T., Sauberlich, H. E., and McDowell, M. E., Vitamin B-6 requirement for adult men, *Am. J. Clin. Nutr.*, 15, 59, 1964.
105. Kelsay, J., Baysal, A., and Linkswiler, H., Effect of vitamin B-6 depletion on the pyridoxal, pyridoxamine and pyridoxine content of the blood and urine of men, *J. Nutr.*, 94, 490, 1968.
106. Donald, E. A., McBean, L. D., Simpson, M. H. W., Sun, M. F., and Aly, H. E., Vitamin B-6 requirement of young adult women, *Am. J. Clin. Nutr.*, 24, 1028, 1971.
107. Storvick, C. A. and Peters, J. M., Methods for the determination of vitamin B-6 in biological materials, *Vit. Horm.*, 22, 833, 1964.
108. Haskell, B. E. and Snell, E. E., Microbiological determination of the vitamin B-6 group, *Methods in Enzymology*, Volume 18A, McCormick, D. B. and Wright, L. L., Eds., Academic Press, New York, 1970, 512.
109. Van den Berg, H., Schruers, W. H. P., and Joosten, G. P. A., Evaluation of the vitamin status in pregnancy, *Int. J. Vit. Nutr. Res.*, 48, 12, 1978.
110. Barnard, H. C., de Kok, J. J., Vermaak, W. J. H., and Potgieter, G. M., A new perspective in the assessment of vitamin B-6 nutritional status during pregnancy in humans, *J. Nutr.*, 117, 1303, 1987.
111. van der Vange, N., van den Berg, H., Kloosterboer, H. J., and Haspels, A. A., Effects of seven low-dose combine contraceptives on vitamin B-6 status, *Contraception*, 40, 377, 1989.
112. Sauberlich, H. E., Dowdy, R. P., and Skala, J. H., *Laboratory Tests for the Assessment of Nutritional Status*, CRC Press, Boca Raton, FL, 1974.
113. Baysal, A., Johnson, B. A., and Linkswiler, H., Vitamin B-6 depletion in man: blood vitamin B-6, plasma pyridoxal-phosphate, serum cholesterol, serum transaminases and urinary vitamin B-6 and 4-pyridoxic acid, *J. Nutr.*, 89, 19, 1966.
114. Cinnamon, A. D. and Beaton, J. R., Biochemical assessment of vitamin B-6 status in man, *Am. J. Clin. Nutr.*, 23, 696, 1970.
115. Cheney, M., Sabry, Z. I., and Beaton, G. H., Erythrocyte glutamic-pyruvic transaminase activity in man, *Am. J. Clin. Nutr.*, 16, 337, 1965.
116. Raica, N. Jr. and Sauberlich, H. E., Blood cell transaminase activity in human vitamin B-6 deficiency, *Am. J. Clin. Nutr.*, 15, 67, 1964.
117. Skala, J. H., Gretz, D., and Waring, P. P., An automated continuous-flow procedure for simultaneous measurement of erythrocyte alanine and aspartate aminotransferase activities, *Nutr. Res.*, 7, 731, 1987.
118. Skala, J. H., Waring, P. P., Lyons, M. F., Rusnak, M. G., and Alleto, J. S., Methodology for determination of blood aminotransferases, in *Methods in Vitamin B-6 Nutrition: Analysis and Status Assessment*, Leklem, J. E. and Reynolds, R. D., Eds., Plenum Press, New York, 1981, 171.

119. Sloger, M. S. and Reynolds, R. D., Pyridoxal 5'-phosphate in whole blood plasma and blood cells of postpartum nonlactating and lactating rats and their pups, *J. Nutr.*, 111, 823, 1981.

120. Giusti, G., Ruggiero, G., and Cacciatores, L., A comparative study of some spectrophotometric and colorimetric procedures for the determination of serum glutamic-oxaloacetic and glutamic-pyruvic transaminase in hepatic diseases, *Enzymol. Biol. Clin.*, 10, 17, 1969.

121. Reitman, S. and Frankel, S., A colorimetric method for the determination of serum glutamic oxalacetic and glutamic-pyruvic transaminases, *Am. J. Clin. Pathol.*, 28, 56, 1957.

122. Karmen, A., A note on the spectophotometric assay of glutamic oxaloacetic transaminase in human blood serum, *Clin. Invest.*, 34, 131, 1955.

123. Wroblewski, F. and La Due, J. S., Serum glutamic pyruvic transaminase in cardiac and hepatic disease, *Proc. Soc. Exp. Biol. Med.*, 91, 569, 1956.

124. Snell, E. E., Vitamin B-6 analysis: some historical aspects, in *Methods in Vitamin B-6 Nutrition: Analysis and Status Assessment*, Leklem, J. E. and Reynolds, R. D., Eds., Plenum Press, New York, 1981, 1.

125. Sauberlich, H. E., Kretsch, M. J., Johnson, H. L., and Nelson, R. A., Animal products as a source of vitamins, in *Animal Products in Human Nutrition*, Beitz, D. C. and Hansen, R. G., Eds., Academic Press, New York, 1982, 340.

126. Meister, A., On the transamination of enzymes, *Ann. N.Y. Acad. Sci.*, 585, 13, 1990.

127. Coburn, S. P. and Mahuren, J. D., A versatile cation-exchange procedure for measuring the seven major forms of vitamin B-6 in biological samples, *Anal. Biochem.*, 129, 310, 1983.

128. Leklem, J. E., Vitamin B-6, in *Modern Nutrition in Health and Disease*, Shils, M. E., Olson, J. A., and Shike, M., Eds., Lea & Febiger, Philadelphia, 1994, 383.

129. Lumeng, L., Li, T. –K., Lui, A., and Roudebush, R. L., The interorgan transport and metabolism of vitamin B-6, in *Vitamin B-6: Its Role in Health and Disease*, Reynolds, R. D., and Leklem, J. E., Eds., Alan R. Liss, Inc., New York, 1985, 35.

130. Sauberlich, H. E., Interaction of vitamin B-6 with other nutrients, in *Vitamin B-6: Its Role in Health and Disease*, Reynolds, R. D., and Leklem, J. E., Eds., Alan R. Liss, Inc., New York, 1985, 193.

131. Gyorgy, P., Vitamin B-2 and the pellagra-like dermatitis in rats, *Nature*, 133, 498, 1934.

132. Gyorgy, P., Vitamin B-2 complex. I. Differentiation of lactoflavin and "rat antipellagra" factors, *Biochem. J.*, 29, 741, 1935.

133. Gyorgy, P., Developments leading to the metabolic role of vitamin B-6, *Am. J. Clin. Nutr.*, 24, 1250, 1971.

134. Coursin, D. B., Vitamin B-6 metabolism in infants and children, *Vitam. Horm.*, 22, 755, 1964.

135. Harris, J. W. and Horrigan, D. C., Pyridoxine-responsive anemia: prototype and variations on the theme, *Vitam. Horm.*, 22, 721, 1964.

136. Kretsch, M. J., Sauberlich, H. E., and Newbrun, E., Electroencephalographic changes and periodontal status during short-term vitamin B-6 depletion of young, nonpregnant women, *Am. J. Clin. Nutr.*, 53, 1266, 1991.

137. Gyorgy, P. and Eckhart, R. E., Vitamin B-6 and skin lesions in rats, *Nature*, 144, 512, 1939.

138. Harris, S. A. and Folkers, K., Synthetic vitamin B-6, *Science*, 89, 347, 1939.

139. Haskell, B. E., Analysis of vitamin B-6, in *Human Vitamin B-6 Requirements*, National Academy of Sciences, Washington D.C., 1978, 61.

140. Lumeng, L. and Li, T. –K., Pyridox (al, amine) 5'-phosphate hydrolase from rat liver, in *Method in Enzymology*, Volume 62D, McCormick, D. B., and Wright, L. D., Eds., Academic Press, New York, 1979, 568.

141. Hamefelt, A., A simplified method for determination of pyridoxal phosphate in biological samples, *Upsala J. Med. Sci.*, 91, 105, 1986.

142. Camp, V. M., Chipponi, J., and Faraj, B. A., Radioenzymatic assay for direct measurement of plasma pyridoxal 5'-phosphate, *Clin. Chem.*, 29, 642, 1983.

143. Chabner, B. and Livingston, D., A simple enzymatic assay for pyridoxal phosphate, *Anal. Biochem.*, 34, 413, 1970.

144. Haskell, B. F. and Snell, E. E., An improved apotryptophanase assay for pyridoxal phosphate, *Anal. Biochem.*, 45, 567, 1972.

145. Shane, B., Vitamin B-6 and blood, in *Human Vitamin B-6 Requirements*, National Academy of Sciences, Washington D.C., 1978, 111.
146. Lumeng, L., Lui, A., and Li, T. K., Microassay of pyridoxal phosphate using tyrosine apodecarboxylase, in *Methods in Vitamin B-6 Nutrition*, Leklem, J. E. and Reynolds, R. D., Eds., Plenum Press, New York, 1981, 57.
147. Lui, A., Lumeng, L., and Li, T. –K., The measurement of plasma vitamin B-6 compounds: comparisons of a cation-exchange HPLC method and the L-tyrosine apodecarboxylase assay, *Am. J. Clin. Nutr.*, 41 1236, 1985.
148. Li, T. –K. and Lumeng, L., Vitamin B-6 metabolism in alcholism and alcoholic liver disease, in *Vitamin B-6: Its Role in Health and Disease*, Reynolds, R. D. and Leklem, J. E., Eds., Alan R. Liss, Inc., New York, 1985, 257.
149. Araki, A. and Sako, Y., Determination of free and total homocysteine in human plasma by high-performance liquid chromatography with fluorescence detection, *J. Chromatogr.*, 422, 43, 1987.
150. Smolin, L. A. and Schneider, J. A., Measurement of total plasma cysteamine using high-performance liquid chromatography with electrochemical detection, *Anal. Biochem.*, 168, 374, 1988.
151. Malinow, M. R., Kang, S. S., Taylor, L. M. et al., Prevalence of hyperhomocyst(e)inemia in patients with peripheral arterial occlusive disease, *Circulation*, 79, 1180, 1989.
152. Pancharuniti, N., Lewis, C. A., Sauberlich, H. E., Perkins, L. L., Go, R. C. P., Alvarez, J. O., Macaluso, M., Acton, R. T., Copeland, R. B., Cousins, A. L., Gore, T. B., Cornwell, P. E., and Roseman, J. M., Plasma homocyst(e)ine, folate, and vitamin B-12 concentrations and risk for early-onset coronary artery disease, *Am. J. Clin. Nutr.*, 59, 940, 1994.
153. Olszewski, A. J. and Szostak, W. B., Homocysteine content of plasma proteins in ischemic heart disease, *Atherosclerosis*, 69, 109, 1988.
154. Malloy, M. H., Rassin, D. K., and Gaull, G. E., Plasma cyst(e)ine in homocyst(e)inemia, *Am. J. Clin. Nutr.*, 34, 2619, 1981.
155. Stabler, S. P., Marcell, P. D., Podell, E. R. et al., Elevation of total homocysteine in the serum of patients with cobalamin or folate deficiency detected by capillary gas chromatography-mass spectrometry, *J. Clin. Invest.*, 81, 466, 1988.
156. Jacobsen, D. W., Gatautis, V. J., Green, R., Robinson, K., Savon, S. R., Secic, M. J. J., Otto, J. M., and Taylor, L. M. Jr., Rapid HPLC determination of total homocysteine and other thiols in serum and plasma: sex differences and correlation with cobalamine and folate levels in healthy subjects, *Clin. Chem.*, 40, 873, 1994.
157. Refsum, H., Ueland, P. M., and Svrdal, A. M., Fully automated fluorescence assay for determining total homocysteine in plasma, *Clin. Chem.*, 35, 1921, 1989.
158. Andersson, A., Brattstrom, L., Israelsson, B., Isaksson, A., Hamfelt, A., and Hultberg, B., Plasma homocysteine before and after methionine loading with regard to age, gender, and menopausal status, *Eur. J. Clin. Invest.*, 22, 79, 1992.
159. Boers, G. H., Smals, A. G., and Trijbels, F. J., Unique efficiency of methionine metabolism in premenopausal women may protect against vascular disease in the reproductive years, *J. Clin. Invest.*, 72, 1971, 1983.
160. Wilcken, D. E. L. and Gupta, V. J., Cysteine-homocysteine mixed disulfide: differing plasma concentrations in normal men and women, *Clin. Sci.*, 57, 211, 1979.
161. Kredich, N. M., Kendall, H. E., and Spence, F. J. Jr., A sensitive radiochemical enzyme assay for S-adenosyl-L-homocysteine and L-homocysteine, *Anal. Biochem.*, 116, 503, 1981.
162. Miller, J. W., Rebaya-Mercado, J. D., Russell, R. M., Shepard, D. C., Morrow, F. D., Cochary, E. F., Sadowski, J. A., Gershoff, S. N., and Selub, J., Effect of vitamin B-6 deficiency on fasting plasma homocysteine concentrations, *Am. J. Clin. Nutr.*, 55, 1154, 1992.
163. Ubbink, J. B., Vermaak, W. J. –H., and Bissbort, S., Rapid high-performance liquid chromatographic assay for total homocysteine levels in human serum, *J. Chromatogr.*, 565, 441, 1991.
164. Ubbink, J. B., Serfontein, W. J., and de Villiers, L. S., Stability of pyridoxal-5-phosphate semicarbazone: application in plasma vitamin B-6 analyses and population surveys of vitamin B-6 nutritional status, *J. Chromatogr.*, 342, 277, 1985.

165. Cornwell, P. E., Morgan, S. L, and Vaughn, W. H., Modification of a high-performance liquid chromatographic method for assay of homocysteine in human plasma, *J. Chromatogr.*, 617, 136, 1993.

166. Hoes, M. J. A. J. M., Kreutzer, E. K. J., and Sijben, N., Xanthurenic acid excretion in urine after oral intake of 5 grams of L-tryptohan by healthy volunteers: standardization of the reference values, *J. Clin. Chem. Clin. Biochem.*, 19, 259, 1981.

167. Kang, S.–S., Wong, P. W. K., and Malinow, M. R., Hyperhomocyst(e)inemia as a risk factor for occlusive vascular disease, *Ann. Rev. Nutr.*, 12, 279, 1992.

168. Graham, I. M., Daly, L. E., Refsum, H. M., Robinson, K., Brattstrom, L. E., Ueland, P. M. et al., Plasma homocysteine as a risk factor for vascular disease, The European Concerted Action Project, *JAMA*, 277, 1775, 1997.

169. Shimizu, S., Ohshiro, T., Yamada, H., Totani, M., and Murachi, T., Specific enzymatic assay method for homocysteine and its application to the screening of neonatal homocystinuria, *Biotechnol. Appl. Biochem.*, 8, 153, 1986.

170. Refsum, H., Helland, S., and Ueland, P. M., Radioenzymic determination of homocysteine in plasma and urine, *Clin. Chem.*, 31, 624, 1985.

171. Sauberlich, H. E., Newer laboratory methods for assessing nutriture of selected B-complex vitamins, *Annu. Rev. Nutr.*, 4, 377, 1984.

172. Chauhan, M. S. and Dakshinamurti, K., Fluorometric assay of B-6 vitamers in biological materials, *Clin. Chim. Acta*, 109, 159, 1981.

173. Dakshinamurti, K. and Chauhan, M. S., Chemical analysis of pyridoxine vitamers, in *Methods in Vitamin B-6 Nutrition: Analysis and Status Assessment*, Leklem, J. E. and Reynolds, R. D., Eds., Plenum Press, New York, 1981, 99.

174. Miller, L. T. and Edwards, M., Microbiological assay of vitamin B-6 in blood and urine, in *Methods in Vitamin B-6 Nutrition: Analysis and Status Assessment*, Leklem, J. E. and Reynolds, R. D., Eds., Plenum Press, New York, 1981, 45.

175. Shin-Buehring, Y., Rasshofer, R., and Endres, W., A new enzymatic method for pyridoxal-5-phosphate determination, *J. Inher. Metab. Dis.*, 4, 123, 1981.

176. Shin, Y. S., Rasshofer, R., Friedrich, B., and Endres, W., Pyridoxal-5′-phosphate determination by a sensitive micromethod in human blood, urine and tissues; its relation to cystathioninuria in neurblastoma and biliary atresia, *Clin. Chim. Acta*, 127, 77, 1983.

177. Leinert, J., Simon, I., and Hotzel, D., Evaluation of methods to determine the vitamin B-6 status of humans. 1. αEGOT: methods and validation, *Int. J. Vit. Nutr. Res.*, 51, 145, 1981.

178. Leinert, J., Simon, I., and Hotzel, D., Methods and their evaluation in the determination of vitamin B-6 status in man, 2. αEGOT: reliability of the parameter, *Int. J. Vit. Nutr. Res.*, 52, 24, 1982.

179. Babson, A. L., Arndt, E. G., and Sharkey, L. J., A revised colorimetric glutamic oxalacetic transaminase, *Clin. Chim. Acta.*, 26, 419, 1969.

180. Carey, R. N., Westgard, J. O., and Dial, M. D., Evaluation of analytic methods which measure the activity of aspartate amino-transferase: results of testing AST methods, in *Quality Control in Laboratory Medicine*, Henry, J. B. and Giegel, J. L., Eds., Masson Publication, New York, 1977, 149.

181. Bonjour, J. P., Vitamins and alcoholism, III. Vitamin B-6, *Int. J. Vit. Nutr. Res.*, 50, 215, 1980.

182. Coburn, S. P., Location and turnover of vitamin B-6 pools and vitamin B-6 requirements of humans, *Ann. N.Y. Acad. Sci.*, 585, 76, 1990.

183. Tillotson, J. A., Sauberlich, H. E., Baker, E. M., and Canham, J. E., Use of carbon-14 labeled vitamins in human nutrition studies: Pyridoxine, *Proceedings of the Seventh International Congress of Nutrition*, 5, 554, 1966.

184. Bosse, T. R. and Donald, E. A., The vitamin B-6 requirement in oral contraceptive users, I. Assessment by pyridoxal level and transferase activity in erythrocytes, *Am. J. Clin. Nutr.*, 32 1015, 1979.

185. Leklem, J. E., Linkswiler, H. M., Brown, R. R., Rose, D. P., and Anand, C. R., Metabolism of methionine in oral contraceptive users and control women receiving controlled intakes of vitamin B-6, *Am. J. Clin. Nutr.*, 30, 1122, 1977.

186. Lui, A., Lumeng, L., Aronoff, G. R., and Li, T. –K., Relationship between body store of vitamin B-6 and plasma pyridoxal-P clearance: Metabolic balance studies in humans, *J. Lab. Clin. Med.*, 106, 491, 1985.

187. Pannemans, D. L. E., van den Berg, H., and Westerterp, K. R., The influence of protein intake on vitamin B-6 metabolism differs in young and elderly humans, *J. Nutr.*, 124, 1207, 1994.

188. Ink, S. L. and Henderson, L. M., Vitamin B-6 metabolism, *Annu. Rev. Nutr.*, 4, 455, 1984.

189. Miller, L. T., Do oral contraceptive agents affect nutrient requirements? Vitamin B-6, *J. Nutr.*, 116, 1344, 1986.

190. Masse, P. G., van den Berg, H., Duguay, C., Beaulieu, G., and Simard, J. M., Early effect of a low dose (30 μg) ethinyl estradiol-containing Triphasil® on vitamin B-6 status, A follow-up study on six menstrual cycles, *Int. J. Vit. Nutr. Res.*, 66, 46, 1996.

191. Kang,-Yoon, S. A., Kirksey, A., Giacoia, G. P., and West, K. D., Vitamin B-6 adequacy in neonatal nutrition: associations with preterm delivery, type of feeding, and vitamin B-6 supplementation, *Am. J. Clin. Nutr.*, 62, 932, 1995.

192. Sax, S. M. and Moore, J. J., Determination of glutamic oxalacetic transaminase activity by coupling of oxalacetate with diazonium salts, *Clin. Chem.*, 13, 175, 1967.

193. Serfontein, W. J., Ubbink, J. B., de Villiers, L. S., and Becker, P. J., Depressed plasma pyridoxal-5'-phosphate levels in tobacco smoking men, *Athersclerosis*, 59, 341, 1986.

194. Vermaak, W. J. H., Ubbink, J. B., Barnard, H. C., Potgieter, G. M., van Jaasveld, H., and Groenewald, A. J., Vitamin B-6 nutrition status and cigarette smoking, *Am. J. Clin. Nutr.*, 51, 1058, 1990.

195. Hattori, M., Kotake, Y., and Kotake, Y., Studies on the urinary excretion of xanthurenic acid in diabetes, *Acta Vitaminol. Enzymol.*, 6, 221, 1984.

196. Anonymous, Dietary protein and vitamin B-6 requirements, *Nutr. Revs.*, 45, 23, 1987.

197. Anonymous, Zinc and the regulation of vitamin B-6 metabolism, *Nutr. Rev.*, 48, 255, 1990.

198. Leklem, J. E., Vitamin B-6: a status report, *J. Nutr.*, 120, 1503, 1990.

199. Leklem, J. E., Vitamin B-6 metabolism and function in humans, in *Clinical and Physiological Applications of Vitamin B-6*, Leklem, J. E and Reynolds, R. D., Eds., Alan R. Liss, Inc., New York, 1988, 3.

200. Canham, J. E., Nunes, W. T., and Eberlin, E. W., Electroencephalographic and central nervous system manifestations of B-6 deficiency and induced B-6 dependency in normal human adults, *Proceedings of the Sixth International Congress of Nutrition*, Edinburgh, August 1963, E. L. S. Livingstone, London, 1964, 537.

201. Reynolds, R. D. and Natta, C. L., Depressed plasma pyridoxal phosphate concentrations in adult asthmatics, *Am. J. Clin. Nutr.*, 41, 684, 1985.

202. Delport, R., Ubbink, J. B., Serfontein, W. J., Becker, P. J., and Walters, L., Vitamin B-6 nutritional status in asthma: the effect of theophylline therapy on plasma pyridoxal-5'-phosphate and pyridoxal levels, *Int. J. Vit. Nutr. Res.*, 58, 67, 1987.

203. Pellock, J. M., Howell, J., Kending, E. L. Jr., and Baker, H., Pyridoxine deficiency in children treated with isoniozid, *Chest*, 87, 658, 1985.

204. Lowik, M. R. H., van den Berg, H., Westenbrink, S., Wedel, M., Schrijver, J., and Ockhuizen, T., Dose-response relationship regarding vitamin B-6 in elderly people: a nationwide nutritional survey (Dutch Nutritional Surveillance System), *Am. J. Clin. Nutr.*, 50, 391, 1989.

205. Schuster, K., Bailey, L. B., Cerda, J. J., and Gregory, J. F. III., Urinary 4-pyridoxic acid excretion in 24-hour versus random urine samples as a measurement of vitamin B-6 status in humans, *Am. J. Clin. Nutr.*, 39, 466, 1984.

206. Hansen, C. M., Leklem, J. E., and Miller, L. T., Changes in vitamin B-6 status indicators of women fed a constant protein diet with varying levels of vitamin B-6, *Am. J. Clin. Nutr.*, 66, 1379, 1997.

207. Hansen, C. M., Leklem, J. E., and Miller, L. T., Vitamin B-6 status of women with a constant intake of vitamin B-6 changes with three levels of dietary protein, *J. Nutr.*, 126, 1891, 1996.

208. Ribaya-Mercado, J. D., Russell, R. M., Sahyoun, N., Morrow, F. D., and Gershoff, S. N., Vitamin B-6 requirements of elderly men and women, *J. Nutr.*, 121, 1062, 1991.

209. Donald, E. A., Vitamin B-6 requirements of young women, in *Human Vitamin B-6 Requirements*, National Academy of Science, Washington D.C., 1978, 226.

210. Huang, Y. –C., Chen, W., Evans, M. A., Mitchell, M. E., and Schultz, T. D., Vitamin B-6 requirement and status assessment of young women fed a high-protein diet with various levels of vitamin B-6, *Am. J. Clin. Nutr.*, 67, 208, 1998.

211. Kant, A. K., Moser-Veillon, P. B., and Reynolds, R. D., Effect of age on changes in plasma, erythrocyte, and urinary B-6 vitamers after an oral vitamin B-6 load, *Am. J. Clin. Nutr.*, 48, 1284, 1988.

212. Woodring, M. J. and Storvick, C. A., Effect of pyridoxine supplementation on glutamic-pyruvic transaminase and *in vitro* stimulation in erythrocytes of normal women, *Am. J. Clin. Nutr.*, 23, 1385, 1970.

213. Sampson, D. A. and O'Connor, D. K., Analysis of vitamin B-6 vitamers and pyridoxic acid in plasma, tissues and urine using high-performance liquid chromatography, *Nutr. Res.*, 9, 259, 1989.

214. Kamp, J. L., Westrick, J. A., and Smolen, A., B-6 vitamer concentrations in mouse plasma, erythrocyte and tissues, *Nutr. Res.*, 15, 415, 1995.

215. Miller, L. T., Leklem, J. E., and Shultz, T. D., The effect of dietary protein on the metabolism of vitamin B-6 in humans, *J. Nutr.*, 115, 1663, 1985.

216. Reddy, S. K., Reynolds, M. S., and Price, J. M., The determination of 4-pyridoxic acid in human urine, *J. Biol. Chem.*, 233, 691, 1985.

217. Ubbink, J. B., Bissort, S., van den Berg, I., de Villiers, L., and Becker, P. J., Genetic polymorphism of glutamate-pyruvate transaminase (alanine aminotransferase): influence on erythrocyte activity as a marker of vitamin B-6 nutritional status, *Am. J. Clin. Nutr.*, 50, 1420, 1989.

218. Raiten, D. J., Reynolds, R. D., Andon, M. B., Robbin, S. T., and Fletcher, A. B., Vitamin B-6 metabolism in premature infants, *Am. J. Clin. Nutr.*, 53, 78, 1991.

219. Heiskanen, K., Siimes, M. A., Perheentupa, J., and Salmenpera, L., Reference ranges for erythrocyte pyridoxal 5'-phosphate concentration and the erythrocyte aspartate transaminase stimulation test in lactating mothers and their infants, *Am. J. Clin. Nutr.*, 59, 1297, 1994.

220. Heiskanen, K., Kallio, M., Salmenpera, L., Siimes, M. A., Ruokonen, I., and Perheentupa, J., Vitamin B-6 status during childhood: tracking from 2 months to 11 years of age, *J. Nutr.*, 125, 2985, 1995.

221. Schuste, K., Bailey, L. B., and Mahan, C. S., Vitamin B-6 status of low-income adolescent and adult pregnant women and the condition of their infants at birth, *Am. J. Clin. Nutr.*, 34, 1731, 1981.

222. Borschel, M. W., Kirksey, A., and Hannemann, R. E., Effects of vitamin B-6 intake on nutriture and growth of young infants, *Am. J. Clin. Nutr.*, 43, 7, 1986.

223. Vuilleumier, J. P., Keller, H. E., and Keck, E., Clinical chemical methods for the routine assessment of the vitamin status in human populations, part III: The apoenzyme stimulation tests for vitamin B-1, B-2, and B-6 adapted to the Cobas-Bio Analyzer, *Int. J. Vit. Nutr. Res.*, 60, 126, 1990.

224. Lemoine, A., Le Devehat, C., Codaccioni, J. L., Monger, A., Bermond, P., and Salkeld, R. M., Vitamins B-1, B-2, B-6 and C status in hospital inpatients, *Am. J. Clin. Nutr.*, 33, 2595, 1980.

225. Manore, M. M., Vaughan, L. A., Carroll, S. S., and Leklem, J. E., Plasma pyridoxal 5'-phosphate concentration and dietary vitamin B-6 intake in free-living, low-income elderly people, *Am. J. Clin. Nutr.*, 50, 339, 1989.

226. Lee, C. M. and Leklem, J. E., Differences in vitamin B-6 status indicator responses between young and middle-aged women fed constant diets with two levels of vitamin B-6, *Am. J. Clin. Nutr.*, 42, 226, 1985.

227. Bapurao, S., Raman, L., and Tulpule, P. G., Biochemical assessment of vitamin B-6 nutritional status in pregnant women with orolingual manifestations, *Am. J. Clin. Nutr.*, 36, 581, 1982.

228. Tolonen, M., Schrijver, J., Westermarck, T., Halme, M., Tuominen, S. E. J., Frilander, A., Keinonen, M., and Sarna, S., Vitamin B-6 status of Finnish elderly: comparison with Dutch younger adults and elderly, The effect of supplementation, *Int. J. Vit. Nutr. Res.*, 58, 73, 1988.

229. McCullough, A. L., Kirksey, A., Wachs, T. D., McCabe, G. P., Bassily, N. S., Bishry, Z., Galal, O. M., Harrison, G. G., and Jerome, N. W., Vitamin B-6 status of Egyptian mothers: relation to infant behavior and maternal-infant interactions, *Am. J. Clin. Nutr.*, 51, 1067, 1990.

230. Changbumrung, S., Schelp, F. P., Hongtong, K., Buavatana, T., Supawan, V., and Migasena, P., Pyridoxine status in preschool children in Northeast Thailand: a community survey, *Am. J. Clin. Nutr.*, 41, 770, 1985.

231. Trumbo, P. R. and Wang, J. W., Vitamin B-6 status indices are lower in pregnant than in nonpregnant women but urinary excretion of 4-pyridoxic acid does not differ, *J. Nutr.*, 123, 2137, 1993.

232. Vermaak, W. J. H., Ubbink, J. B., Banard, H. C., Potgieter, G. M., van Jaarsveld, H., and Groenewald, A. J., Vitamin B-6 nutrition status and cigarette smoking, *Am. J. Clin. Nutr.*, 51, 1058, 1990.

233. Giraud, D. W., Martin, H. D., and Driskell, J. A., Erythrocyte and plasma B-6 vitamer concentrations of long-term tobacco smokers, chewers, and nonusers, *Am. J. Clin. Nutr.*, 62, 104, 1995.

234. Driskell, J. A., McChrisley, B., Reynolds, L. K., and Moak, S. W., Plasma pyridoxal 5'-phosphate concentrations in obese and nonobese black women residing near Petersburg, VA, *Am. J. Clin. Nutr.*, 50, 37, 1989.

235. Driskell, J. A. and Moak, S. W., Plasma pyridoxal phosphate concentrations and coenzyme stimulation of erythrocyte alanine aminotransferase activities of white and black adolescent girls, *Am. J. Clin. Nutr.*, 43, 599, 1986.

236. Andon, M. B. and Reynolds, R. D., A comparison of plasma pyridoxal 5'-phospahte concentrations in capillary (finger prick) and venous blood, *Am. J. Clin. Nutr.*, 45, 1461, 1987.

237. Rose, C. S., Gyorgy, P., Butler, M., Andres, R., Brin, M., and Spiegel, H., Age differences in vitamin B-6 status of 617 men, *Am. J. Clin. Nutr.*, 29, 847, 1976.

238. Coburn, S. P., Mahuren, J. D., Schaltenbrand, W. E., Weber, J., and Conley, R. E., Comparison of pyridoxal 5'-phosphate (PLP) determinations in plasma by cation-exchange HPLC and a kit based on tyrosine decarboxylase, *Clin. Chem.*, 42, No. 6, S301, 1996 (Abstract).

239. Ubbink, J. B., Serfontein, W. J., and de Villiers, L. S., Analytical recovery of protein-bound pyridoxal-5'-phosphate in plasma analysis, *J. Chromatogr. Med. Appl.*, 375, 399, 1986.

240. Hess, D. and Viulleumier, J. P., Assay of pyridoxal-5'-phosphate, pyridoxal and pyridoxic acid in biological material, *Int. J. Vit. Nutr. Res.*, 59, 338, 1989.

241. Smith, G. P., Samson, D., Peters, T. J., A fluorimetric method for the measurement of pyridoxal and pyridoxal phosphate in human plasma and leucocytes, and its application to patients with sideroblastic marrow, *J. Clin. Pathol.*, 36, 701, 1983.

242. McCrisley, B., Thye, F. W., McNair, H. M., and Driskell, J. A., Plasma B-6 vitamer and 4-pyridoic acid concentrations of men fed controlled diets, *J. Chromatogr. Biomed. Appl.*, 428, 35, 1988.

243. Schrijver, J., Speek, A. J., and van den Berg, H., Pyridoxal 5'-phosphate (PLP) in whole blood by HPLC, in *Nutritional Assessment – A Manual for Population Studies*, Fidaza, F., Ed., Hans Huber Publication, Bern, 1990.

244. Sauberlich, H. E., Goad, W., Herman, Y. F., Milan, F., and Jamison, P., Biochemical assessment of the nutritional status of the Eskimos of Wainwright, Alaska, *Am. J. Clin. Nutr.*, 25, 437, 1972.

245. Driskell, J. A. and Moak, S. W., Plasma pyridoxal phosphate concentrations and coenzyme stimulation of erythrocyte alanine aminotransferase activities of white and black adolescent girls, *Am. J. Clin. Nutr.*, 43, 599, 1986.

246. Smith, J. L., Wickiser, A. A., Korth, L. L., Grandjean, A. C., and Schaefer, A. E., Nutritional status of an institutionalized age population, *Am. Coll. Nutr.*, 3, 13, 1984.

247. Fries, M. E., Chrisley, B. M., and Driskell, J. A., Vitamin B-6 status of a group of preschool children, *Am. J. Clin. Nutr.*, 34, 2706, 1981.

248. Driskell, J. A., Clark, A. J., Bazzarre, T. L., Chopin, L. F., McCoy, H., Kenney, M. A., and Moak, S. W., Vitamin B-6 status of southern adolescent girls, *J. Am. Diet. Assoc.*, 85, 46, 1985.

249. Driskell, J. A., Clark, A. J., and Moak, S. W., Longitudinal assessment of vitamin B-6 status in Southern adolescent girls, *J. Am. Diet. Assoc.*, 87, 307, 1987.

250. Crozier, P. G., Cordain, L., and Sampson, D. A., Exercise-induced changes in plasma vitamin B-6 concentrations do not vary with exercise intensity, *Am. J. Clin. Nutr.*, 60, 552, 1994.

251. Schrijver, J., Speek, A. J., and Schreurs, W. H. P., Semi-automatic fluorometric determination of pyridoxal-5'-phosphate (vitamin B-6) in whole blood by high-performance liquid chromatography, *Int. J. Vit. Res.*, 51, 216, 1981.

252. Gregory, J. F. III, Methods for determination of vitamin B-6 in foods and other biological materials: a critical review, *J. Food Comp. Anal.*, 1, 105, 1988.

253. Bayoumi, R. A. and Rosalki, S. B., Evaluation of methods of coenzyme activation of erythrocyte enzyme for detection of deficiency of vitamin B-1, B-2, and B-6, *Clin. Chem.*, 22, 3, 1976.

254. Rosalki, S. B., Detection of vitamin B deficiency by red cell enzyme activation tests, in *Quality Control in Laboratory Medicine*, Henry, J. B. and Giegel, J. L., Eds., Masson Publishing, New York, 1977, 121.

255. Kok, F. J., Schrijver, J., Hofman, A., Witterman, J. C. M., Kruyesson, D. A. C. M., Remme, W. J., and Valkenburg, H. A., Low vitamin B-6 status in patients with acute myocardial infarction, *Am. J. Cardiol.*, 63, 513, 1989.

256. Madigan, S. M., Tracey, F., McNulty, H., Eaton-Evans, J., Coulter, J., McCartney, H., and Strain, J. J., Riboflavin and vitamin B-6 intakes and status and biochemical response to riboflavin supplementation in free-living elderly people, *Am. J. Clin. Nutr.*, 68, 389, 1998.

257. Kimura, M., Kanehira, K., and Yokoi, K., Highly sensitive and simple liquid chromatographic determination in plasma of B-6 vitamers, especially pyridoxal 5'-phosphate, *J. Chromatogr.*, A722, 296, 1996.

258. Gregory, J. F. III, Nutritional properties and significance of vitamin glycosides, *Annu. Rev. Nutr.*, 18, 277, 1998.

259. Euronut SENEC study, Nutritional status: blood vitamins A, E, B-6, B-12, folic acid and carotene, *Eur. J. Clin. Nutr.*, 45, 63, 1991.

Folate (Folic Acid, Pteroylmonoglutamic Acid, Folacin)

Converting metric units to International System (SI) units:

Folic Acid:
molecular weight: 441.41

ng/mL × 2.266 = nmol/L

nmol/L × 0.441 = ng/mL

5-Formyltetrahydrofolic acid (folinic acid, leucovorin, CF, citrovorum factor)
molecular weight: 473.45

ng/mL × 2.112 = nmol/L

nmol/L × 0.473 = ng/mL

5-Methyltetrahydrofolic acid
molecular weight: 459.46

ng/mL × 2.179 = nmol/L

nmol/L × 0.459 = ng/mL

Tetrahydrofolic acid
molecular weight: 445.44

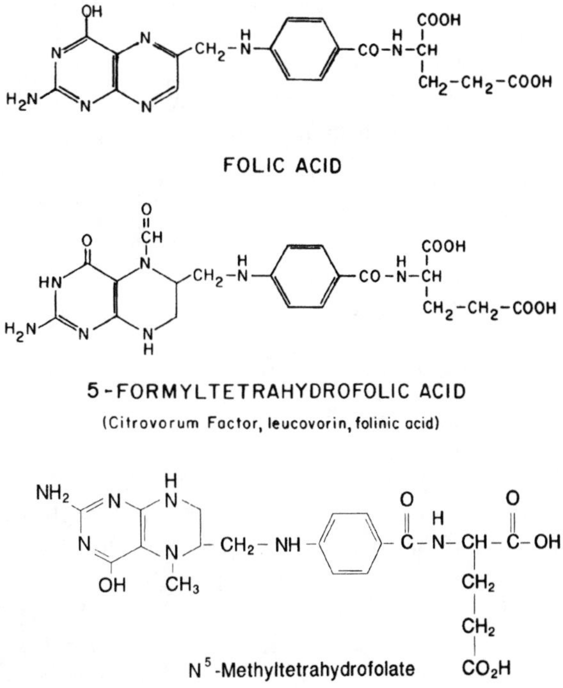

FOLIC ACID

5-FORMYLTETRAHYDROFOLIC ACID

(Citrovorum Factor, leucovorin, folinic acid)

N^5-Methyltetrahydrofolate

FIGURE 18

Structure of folic acid, N^5-methyltetrahydrofolate, and 5-formyltetrahydrofolic acid.

Introduction

Folate is used as the generic descriptor for folic acid and related compounds exhibiting qualitatively the biological activity of folic acid. 5-Formyltetrahydrofolic acid is the most stable of the tetrahydrofolic acid cofactors. Folic acid is the commercially available synthetic form of folate. Only small amounts of folic acid occur in nature. Quantities of 5-formyltetrahydrofolic acid (Leucovorin) are produced for use as a rescue agent in conjunction with the use of antifolate therapy.[47]

The History of Folate

The history of folate was confused by the fact that anemias due to a deficiency of folate or of vitamin B-12 have the common morphological features of megaloblastic erythropoiesis. In 1926, Addisonian pernicious anemia was recognized as a condition associated with diet. However, the subsequent efforts of Lucy Wills, working in India in 1931, demonstrated that another factor, now known as folate, was associated with the megaloblastic anemia of pregnant women.[37-39] The dietary factor became known as the Wills factor which was found to be identical to an unknown substance essential for chicks, monkeys, and a number of microorganisms, such as *Lactobacillus casei*, now *L. rhamnosus*. Subsequently, Mitchell et al.[40] in 1941 isolated a compound from spinach that was active for *Streptococus faecalis* (now called *Enterococcus hirae*) and was given the name folic acid. In 1946, Angier et al.[41,42] reported on the structure and synthesis of folic acid. The discovery of 5-formyltetrahydrofolic acid (citrovorum factor, Lecovorin)[43-46] revealed the importance of reduced folates and the function of folates in single-carbon transport. Early animal studies demonstrated the essentiality of both vitamin B-12 and folic acid in the ability of homocysteine to replace methionine in the diet.[109]

Leucovorin is used to reverse the (a) toxicity of methotrexate (leucovorin rescue), (b) and to potentiate the cytotoxic effects of 5-fluorouracil in the treatment of childhood leukemia.[47]

The synthetic folic acid, pteroylmonoglutamic acid, consists of a pteridine nucleus, p-aminobenzoic acid, and glutamic acid. Folic acid is readily converted in the body to the active tetrahydrofolic acid. Folates are unstable to light.

Food Sources of Folate

Folate contents of foods have been difficult to obtain. Over 150 forms of folate are known to exist in foods. Measurement of the folate content in foods requires special treatment of samples in order to obtain the total folate content.[55,56,147,148] Consequently, folate contents utilized in food composition tables commonly have underestimated values. However, the assessment of the adequacy of dietary intake of folate requires not only the knowledge of the nutrient content of the foods ingested, but also the extent to which the folate present in the diet is available for absorption and utilization.[48,50,51,53,54,67,147] The bioavailability of folate is poor for many foods.[49-52,67] Moreover, because of lability, as much as 50 to 95% of the folate present in foods may be lost during home preparation and food processing.

Recognizing the inadequacies of data available, Subar et al.[57] summarized the folate content of commonly consumed foods. The following is the folate content of common food items found in the U.S. diet.[57]

Folate Content of Some Common Food Items in the U.S. Diet[57]

Items Prepared for Consumption	Folate Content (μg/100g)
Liver	428
Eggs	43
Orange juice	41
Fortified cereals	991
Cooked cereals	15
Pizza	16
Veal	16
Milk (2% fat)	5
Corn	43
Broccoli	65
Cauliflower	53
Turnip greens or mustard greens	54
Green peas	46
Green beans	28
Tomatoes	10
Bananas	19
Beef steaks	8
Hamburgers	21
Hot dogs	30
Pork chops	55
Cheese, cheddar	18
Fried fish	4–15
Spinach	128
Pinto or navy beans (cooked)	100
Strawberries	17
Sweet potatoes	17

Dietary data collected during Second National Health and Nutrition Examination Survey (NHANES-II), indicated that the United States adults had a mean daily intake of folate of 242 μg for men and 207 μg for women.[57] Similar folate intakes were observed during the Third National Health and Nutrition Examination Survey (NHANES-III). Daily folate intake was 270 μg for males aged 50 to 59 years, and 207 μg for females aged 50 to 59 years.

Folate Metabolism and Functions

Folate Metabolism

The biochemistry, functions, and metabolism of folate has been reviewed in detail by Krumdieck[73] and others.[30,61-65,67,138,249]

The major forms of folate in foods occur as polyglutamates. In order for these folates to be utilized by the human requires the hydrolysis of the polyglutamate folates to the monoglutamate forms.[3,62,63,67] The intraluminal polyglutamate hydrolysis is catalyzed by the intestinal brush border enzyme pteroylpolyglutamate hydrolase.[191] The enzyme cleaves the polyglutamyl chain one residue at a time. As a result the bioavailability of food folates is commonly less than that of folic acid.[48,50,55,56,67,71] Alcohol as well as some factors in foods may impair the utilization of folate.[4,61] Crohn's disease, tropical sprue, celiac disease, and other malabsorption syndromes adversely affect the absorption of folate. The normal body stores of 5 to 10 mg of folate is considered adequate to prevent a folate deficiency for about 50 days in the normal adult male.[6,65]

Serum Folate

The major form of folate in serum is 5-methyltetrahydrofolate and is the principal methyl donor for the formation of methionine from homocysteine.[62-65] This reaction requires the participation of the vitamin B-12 requiring enzyme, methionine synthase. In a vitamin B-12 deficiency, homocysteine is not remethylated and accumulates in the blood while folate accumulates as 5-methyltetrahydrofolate.[30,62]

Folate Functions

Folate participates in numerous metabolic functions.[62,63,65] The functions include (a) methylation of deoxyuridylate to thymidylate in DNA synthesis, (b) catabalism of histidine, (c) interconversion of serine and glycine, (d) formate formation and utilization, (e) methylation of uracil residues in transfer RNA, (f) methione formation from homocysteine, and (g) choline synthesis. The folate polyglutamates serve as functional coenzymes in the body tissues.[62-65] The coenzymes participate primarily in one-carbon transfers such as in pyrimidine and purine biosynthesis, formate metabolism, and amino acid interconversions (e.g., homocysteine to methionine formation, serine and glycine interconversions, histidine degradation to glutamic acid).

Megaloblastic anemia is an outcome of prolonged folate deficiency. The deficiency is associated with hypersegmentation of peripheral blood neutrophils.[7,65] Excretion of increased amounts of forminoglutamic acid occurs with prolonged folate deficiency (i.e., after 7 weeks of deficiency).

Folate and Vitamin B-12 Interaction

Deficiency of vitamin B-12 may also result in an identical megaloblastic anemia since both folate and vitamin B-12 are required for the synthesis of thymidylate in the formation of DNA.[64,65] However, folate deficiency occurs considerably more frequently than vitamin B-12 deficiency.[7] In a vitamin B-12 deficiency a patient is subjected to the "methylfolate trap" condition whereby the folate is metabolically unavailable for thymidylate formation and DNA synthesis.[7,30] Consequently, folate accumulates as 5-methyltetrahydrofolate, which is metabolically inactive in the absence of vitamin B-12.

Occurrence of Folate Deficiency

General

An inadequate folate nutritional status is relatively common as a result of low dietary intakes, pregnancy, excessive alcohol consumption, medications, and other influences.[57,61,93,94,247,250] Nutrition surveys often indicate that the folate intake of segments of the U.S. population is less than adequate.[57,93] Consequently, measurements to assess folate status are often performed in clinical laboratories.

Plasma folate concentrations fall rather rapidly when subjects are maintained on a folate deficient diet.[50,175] Red blood cell concentrations of folate fall considerably slower, reflecting the red cell life span of 120 days. Folate incorporated into the red cells at their formation is retained nearly entirely throughout their lifespan.[29,50]

When the rate of red cell synthesis increases as during rapid growth of infants, pregnancy, and adolescents, the folate requirement to support the growth is increased.[247] During these periods, a higher risk of folate deficiency may be observed.[5,8,9,13,14,16,89,93,98,100,140,179,180] Adolescent females are commonly observed to have a folate status less than adequate, based on serum and red cell folate concentrations.[93,181,209,247]

Pregnancy and Folate Status

TABLE 26

Effect of Folic Acid Supplements on Plasma and Erythrocyte Folacin Concentrations During Pregnancy (Mean Values)

Measurement	Non-Pregnant	Trimester of Pregnancy		
		1	2	3
Plasma folate (nmol/L)				
No folate supplement ($n = 101$)	13–45	13.8	10.2	10.2
Folate supplemented 200 µg/day with folic acid ($n = 105$)		15.0	15.9	14.3
Erythrocyte folate (nmol/L)				
No folate supplement ($n = 101$)	374	356	315	267
Folate supplemented 200 µg/day with folic acid ($n = 105$)		374	431	424

Adapted from *Laboratory Indices of Nutritional Status in Pregnancy.*[8]

Folate deficiency in pregnancy is one of the most frequently occurring nutritional diseases.[8,9,89,93,98,201,247] During pregnancy and lactation, folate deficiency may result in megaloblastic anemia.[5,100] Folate supplementation during pregnancy can prevent the development of a folate deficiency.[8,9,13,14,89,98] Erythrocyte and serum folate measurements have proven to be a useful biochemical test for evaluating folate nutritional status in pregnancy.[8,9,16,65,89,100,204-208]

Catabolism of folate during the second and third trimester of pregnancy has been reported to increase, and then returned to baseline postpartum.[174] This increased rate of folate catabolism would produce an extra need of 200 to 300 µg/day of dietary folate. In a small study, a decrease in folate status in the pregnant women during the third trimester was of predictive value of the newborn weight.[173]

Elderly Population

Folate deficiency occurs commonly in the elderly.[199,211] Folate status of population groups has been the subject of several reviews.[100-184] The folate nutritional status of elderly population was reviewed earlier by Grinblat[183] and more recently by Bailey[98,247] and by Sauberlich.[100]

Readers are referred to these sources for extensive information on the folate status of various population groups including elderly, adults, adolescents, pregnant women, and infants. In the United States, the National Health and Nutrition Examination Surveys (NHANES) have provided extensive information regarding the incidence of folate deficiency in various population groups.[93,98,100] In the Health and Nutrition Examination Survey (HANES I), 6% of the elderly had low serum folate levels (< 6.7 nmol/L; < 3.0 ng/mL).[185] Age alone does not appear to cause a decrease in the ability to absorb folate polyglutamates.[202]

A similar incidence of low plasma folate concentrations in elderly persons was noted by Hanger et al.[186] in Christchurch, New Zealand. A prevalence of 1% were with low serum folate levels and 3.3% were with low red cell folate levels. Serum vitamin B-12 concentrations were low in 7.3% of the elderly subjects. The lower limits of the reference ranges used were 43 nmol/L serum folate; 297 nmol/L red cell folate; and 114 pmol/L for serum vitamin B-12.

In a Canadian study by Basu et al.[187] on 156 elderly free-living subjects (65 to 77 y), 9 to 14% of the subjects were found to have low plasma folate levels. Garry, et al.[188] examined the folate nutritional status of 270 health elderly in New Mexico. They observed that 8% had low plasma folate concentrations (< 3.0 ng/mL) and only 3% had red blood cell folate concentrations of less than 140 ng/ml. The investigators concluded that folate deficiency was not a major medical problem of this population.

Information on Folate Status From Nutrition Surveys

Folate data from the Second National Health and Nutrition Examination Survey (NHANES-II) conducted during the period of 1976 through 1980 were summarized by Senti and Pilch.[93,98,100,137,138,189] Because of some methodological problems, the conclusions should be accepted with caution.[223] Nevertheless, percentage of individuals with low serum folate, low red cell folate, and with both low serum and red cell folate values were lowest in children aged 6 months to 9 years (2, 2, and 2%, respectively); males aged 10 to 19 years (3, 5, 2%, respectively; and female aged 45 to 74 years [9, 4, and 2%, respectively]).[100] Females aged 20 to 44 years appeared to be the age group at greatest risk for developing folate deficiency (low serum folate, 15%; low red cell folate, 13%). The distribution was based on serum folate values of <30 ng/mL or red cell folate values of <140 ng/mL, values considered deficient. Because of serious methodological problems folate data collected during the Third National Health and Nutrition Examination Survey (NHANES-III, 1988–1994) were unreliable for evaluating the folate nutriture of the U.S. population.[223]

Folate Nutritional Status

General

Folate nutritional status has gained increased importance with the apparent participation of the vitamin in (a) occurrence of neural tube defects,[19,29,60,221] (b) risk of cardiovascular disease,[20,30,84-86,95,192,233,234,250] (c) incidence of certain cancers,[21,31,32,90,96,178,201] and (d) neurological conditions.[66,97] Low folate nutritional status has been shown to be associated with an increased risk of coronary heart disease.[228,229,246,250,255]

Signs and Symptoms of a Folate Deficiency State

Folate deficiency results in megaloblastic anemia which is identical to that caused by a deficiency of vitamin B-12.[1,2,7-9,62,64,92,190] Folate deficiency is seldom associated with the neurologic abnormalities that occur frequently with vitamin B-12 deficiency.[97] Depapillation of the tongue may result with severe folate deficiency. Folate deficiency may also result in alterations in intestinal function resulting from abnormalities in the rapid turnover of the cells of the intestinal villi. Other clinical manifestations of a folate deficiency include fatigue, weak, tired, irritability, anorexia, diarrhea, forgetfulness, and sore tongue.[6,7,10,65,247]

Folate Deficiency and Tropical Sprue

Tropical sprue syndrome is characterized by diarrhea, anorexia, weight loss, and malabsorption.[1] The disease responds to treatment with folic acid and antimicrobial therapy. Tropical sprue occurs in a number of areas of the world including Central America, Puerto Rico, India, Philippines, and other parts of Southeast Asia. Malabsorption of folate is common in patients with tropical sprue. Although the mechanism of the malabsorption is not fully understood, patients may absorb monogtutamates (e.g., folic acid) normally, but fail to absorb polyglutamates, the predominant form in foods.[2]

Folate and Neural Tube Defects

The recognition that folic acid supplementation in preconception and early pregnancy reduced the prevalence of neural tube defects has placed an increased importance to folate nutritional status.[17,18,81-83,183,201,221] These findings were initially reported by Smithells et al.[218] and by Lawerence et al.[219] and later by Milunsky et al.[23] and the MRC Vitamin Study Research Group.[25] Extensive literature exists regarding the level of folic acid supplementation required for an optimum benefit.[22-28,222] Many of these studies have been summarized by Wald,[19] Scott et al.,[29,60] Roe,[217] and Butterworth and Bendich.[59]

Factors Influencing Folate Status

Cigarette Smoking

Several investigators have reported that subjects who smoke cigarettes have a lower concentration of folate in their plasma and red blood cells than that of nonsmokers.[93,98,101-103] Plasma folate concentrations of the smokers rose to the concentrations of the nonsmokers when provided with a daily folate intake of 1.49 µmol (658 µg).[103] Similar observations were reported by Witter et al.[101]

Folate Levels in Smoking and Non-Smoking Non-Pregnant Adult Women

	Nonsmoker	Smoker	P
Serum folate			
ng/mL	7.0 ± 5.6	4.7 ± 2.4	.009
RBC folate			
ng/mL	160 ± 70	110 ± 42	.001

From Reference 101.

Use of Oral Contraceptive Agents and Folate Status

Earlier investigations indicated that the concentration of folate in blood serum was low in women who were users of oral contraceptive agents.[107,108] Other studies found no difference in serum folate concentrations between users and nonusers of oral contraceptive agents.[30,61,77,93,98,100,107,108,137]

In 1982, Grace et al.[76] studied the folate status in 170 girls, aged 12 to 19 years. Serum folate concentrations of < 5 ng/mL were found in 37% of the users of oral contraceptive agents and 21% of the nonusers. Whole-blood folate concentrations of <150 ng/mL were found in 15% of the oral contraceptive users and in 15% of the nonusers.

Recently, Green et al.[78] studied the influence of the use of currently available oral contraceptive agents on the folate status in 129 adolescent females. The use of oral contraceptive agents was found not to be associated with lower serum or red blood cell folate concentrations or with higher serum homocysteine concentrations. Serum vitamin B-12 concentrations were lower among oral contraceptive users than nonusers.

Nutrient Interaction of Folate and Zinc

In 1984, Mukherjee et al.[34] and Milne et al.[35] reported on a possible adverse effect of folic acid supplements on zinc status in the human. These studies and the subsequent numerous investigations on the subject were extensively evaluated by Tamura.[33,87] The human intestinal musosol brush border folate conjugase is a zinc-dependent enzyme.[33,36] Tamura[33] concluded from his review that if there "is any adverse effect of folic acid supplementation on zinc nutriture or on pregnancy outcome it must be extremely subtle." Kauwell et al.[88] also observed no adverse effects of folic acid supplementation on zinc status. Conversely, zinc intake did not impair folate utilization.

Genetic Defects Involving Folate[97,119,120]

Fragile X-Syndrome

This inherited disorder is second only to Down's syndrome among the genetic causes of mental retardation.[97,117] The fragile X-syndrome affects approximately one male in 2,610 and one female in 4,221.[97,117] Some reports indicate that early treatment of patients with high levels of folate may be of some benefit.[117]

5,10-Methylenetetrahydrofolate Reductase Deficiency

This enzyme catalyzes the formation of the methyl donor, 5-methyltetrahydrofolate, which is the main form of folate in plasma and tissues. Therefore, patients with this enzyme deficiency have reduced concentrations of folate in erythrocytes, plasma, and spinal cord.[121-123]

In addition, the patients may have elevated concentrations of homocysteine in their blood and urine, along with reduced plasma concentrations of methionine.[121-124] To prevent the neurological deterioration that occurs in children with this disorder, requires prompt therapy with N^5-formyletetrahydrofolate (leucovorin).[125,126] In some cases additional supplements of vitamin B-6, vitamin B-12, methionine, and betaine are necessary to prevent the neurological changes.[126]

Evaluation of Folate Nutritional Status

TABLE 27
Correlations Between Biochemical and Dietary Measurements of Folate in Adult Men

Parameter	No. of Subjects	r	p
Serum folate vs. dietary folate	526	0.23	0.00001
Erythrocyte folate vs. dietary folate	526	0.20	0.00001
Erythrocyte folate vs. serum folate	283	0.65	0.00001
Whole blood folate vs. serum folate	283	0.65	0.00001

From Kretsch, Sauberlich, and Skala, Letterman Army Institute Report No. 192; December, 1984.[216]

A number of procedures have been employed to provide information concerning the nutritional status of folacin in the individual subjects. Some of these procedures have proven suitable for nutrition surveys. The procedures include the following:

Plasma folacin concentrations
Red blood cell folacin concentrations
Plasma homocysteine concentrations
Neutrophil hypersegmentation
DU suppression test
Formiminoglutamic acid excretion
Urinary excretion of folacin

Use of Serum/Plasma and Erythrocyte Folate Concentrations

For evaluating folate nutritional status, the measurement of serum or plasma folate concentrations is most commonly performed. However, plasma folate concentrations are probably a relatively poor indicator of the degree of folate deficiency.[7,11,12,65] Low plasma concentrations of folate may reflect recent low dietary intake while providing little information about the tissue reserves of the vitamin.[7,50] Consequently, low plasma folate concentrations are not necessarily associated with megaloblastic anemia.[7,11,12] Nevertheless, erythrocyte folate concentrations correlated with serum folate concentrations ($r = 0.65$).[216] A very similar correlation was observed by Kirke et al. ($r = 0.71$).[215]

The erythrocyte folate concentration has come to be considered a more accurate and less variable quantitative index than plasma folate as to the severity of folacin deficiency.[7,10,12,65] However, erythrocyte folate measurements do not distinguish between megaloblastic anemia due to vitamin B-12 deficiency and that due to a folate deficiency.[64,239] With a vitamin

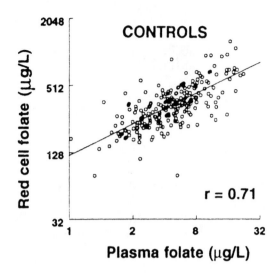

FIGURE 19
Correlations between red cell folate and plasma folate concentrations (*n* = 247).[115] (With permission.)

B-12 deficiency, folate concentrations in the plasma may be elevated while low concentrations may be observed in the erythrocytes.[7,10,15] Low folate concentrations for both plasma and erythrocytes provide strong evidence of a folate deficiency.

A folate depletion and repletion study was conducted in adult nonpregnant women maintained on a metabolic unit.[50] Omission of folate from the diet produced a prompt fall in the plasma folate concentrations. After 28 days of deficiency, plasma folate concentrations had fallen an average of 60%. By the end of this depletion period, the erythrocyte folate concentrations had fallen approximately 15%. For instance, plasma folate concentrations in Group A subjects had fallen to 8.2 nmol/L (3.6 ng/mL). At this state, abnormal changes were observed in neutrophil hypersegmentation and in lymphocyte deoxyuridine suppression.[50]

In another study, the effects of folic acid supplementation was investigated.[213] Women who were receiving 209 µg/day of food folates were supplemented with an additional 400 µg/day of folic acid for 3 months. Their erythrocyte folate concentrations increased from an initial mean of 351 µg/L to a mean of 492 µg/L at the end of 3-month period.

Laboratory cutoff guides for folate status should correspond to folate levels at which the earliest biochemical, physiological, behavioral, functional, or morphological changes appear.[65,247] In this respect, Jagerstad and Pietrzik[236] found red blood cell folate concentrations of <250 nmol/L to be associated with hypersegmentation of >3.6 lobes. This represents an inadequate folate status. Consequently, plasma folate concentrations of <7.0 nmol/L and red blood cells folate concentrations of <300 nmol/L have been considered indicative of folate deficiency.

Leucocytes also contain relatively high levels of folate. Leucocytes from normal subjects have been reported to contain 60 to 123 ng of folate/ml of packed cells with a mean value of 92 ng/ml.[237] Values as high as 262 to 1,028 ng/ml cells have also been reported. The leucocyte folate levels correlated well with red cell folate values but less so with serum folate values.[237,238] The procedure did not distinguish between patients with pernicious anemia and those deficient in folate.[237] Hence, considering the technical difficulties involved, the method provides no apparent advantage over the measurement of folate in serum and red blood cells.

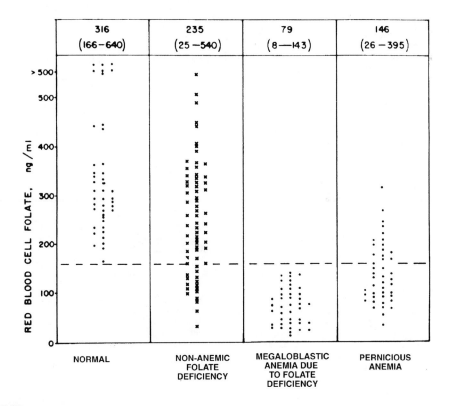

FIGURE 20
The mean, range, and distribution of red blood cell folate levels of healthy control subjects, nonanemic patients with subnormal serum folate levels, patients with megaloblastic anemia due to folate deficiency, and patients with pernicious anemia. (From Hoffrand, Newcombe, and Mollin.[12] With permission from BMJ Publishing Group.)

Guidelines Used to Evaluate Blood Folate Data

Based on the results of controlled human folate deficiency studies and on the treatment of folate deficient patients, guidelines have been developed and used in evaluating plasma and erythrocyte folate data.[6,9,50,69,111,140]

The following guidelines have frequently been used for the interpretation of plasma and red blood cell folate concentrations.[9]

| | Less than Acceptable (at risk)* | | |
Measurement	Deficient (High Risk) nmol/L	Low (Medium Risk) nmol/L	Acceptable (Low Risk) nmol/L
Plasma folate (all ages)	< 6.8 (< 3.0)	6.8 – 13.4 (3.0 – 5.9)	≥ 13.4 (≥ 6.0)
Red blood cell folate (all ages)	< 317 (< 140)	317 – 354 (140 – 159)	≥ 356 (≥ 160)

* ( ) = ng/mL

The following guidelines have also been used for the interpretation of serum or plasma and red blood cell folate concentrations (Tables 28 to 32).

TABLE 28

World Health Organization Guidelines

Nutrient	Normal Range	Probable Deficiency	Normal	Probable Deficiency
Serum B-12, pg/ml	150–1000	< 100	110–738 pmol/L	< 74 pmol/L
Serum folate, ng/ml	6–20	< 3	13.4–44.5 nmol/L	< 6.7 nmol/L
Red cell folate, ng/ml	150–700	< 100	334–1558 nmol/L	223 nmol/L

WHO Technical Report Series No. 503 (1972).[220]

TABLE 29

Pan American Health Organization Guidelines for Serum Folate Concentrations

	Serum Folate Concentrations	
Category (All Ages)	ng/ml	nmol/L
Deficient	< 3.0	< 6.4
Low	3.0–4.9	6.4–10.9
Acceptable or high	> 5.0	> 11.1

G. Arroyave, *Metabolic Adaptation and Nutrition*, p. 98, Pan American Health Organization Scientific Publication No. 222, 1971.

TABLE 30

Guidelines for Evaluating Folate Data from the National Health and Nutrition Examination Survey III

	ng/mL	nmol/L
Erythrocyte folate		
Deficient	<140	<312
Low	<150	<334
Normal	150–600	150–1336
Plasma folate		
Deficient	<2.0	<4.5
Low	2.0–4.0	4.5–9.0
Normal	4.0–18.0	9.0–4.0

NHANES III.[189,223]

TABLE 31

Guidelines for the Diagnosis of Folate Deficiency

		ng/mL	nmol/L
Lindenbaum and Allen[65,91]			
Serum folate*	Deficient	2.1	4.7
Serum folate*	Low	4.0	8.9
Erythrocyte folate**	Deficient	<150	334

* Measured by radioassay.

** Measured by *L. rhamnosus* microbiological assay.

TABLE 32

Plasma Concentrations of Homocysteine, Vitamin B-12, Folate, and Pyridoxal-5'-phosphate in Normal Men and Women

Measurement in Plasma	Subjects		
	Men (n = 380)	Women (n = 204)	All (n = 584)
Folate (nmol/L)	8.55 ± 5.19	9.75 ± 6.58	8.97 ± 5.74
Vitamin B-12 (pmol/L)	238 ± 102	236 ± 116	237 ± 107
Pyridoxal-5'-phosphate (nmol/L)	42 ± 38	41 ± 51	42 ± 43
Homocysteine (μmol/L)	9.7 ± 4.9	7.6 ± 4.1	9.0 ± 4.7

Adapted from Lussier-Cacan et al.[214]

Determination of Plasma and Erythrocyte of Folate Concentrations

Radioassay Procedures

Earlier commercial radioassay kits for measuring folate concentrations in plasma and serum had difficulties that resulted in questionable or erroneous values.[139,150,151,223,240] With subsequent modifications, the commercial radioassay kits provide serum folate concentrations that are generally comparable to *L. casei* (*L. rhamnosus*) microbiological assay.[65,96,115,137,139] Many of the kits are designed to measure simultaneously serum concentrations of both folate and vitamin B-12 which is convenient for diagnostic needs (e.g., Magic Vitamin B-12/Folate Radioassay, Chiron Diagnostics Corp., Norwood, MA; Quantaphase B-12/Folate Radioassay, Bio-Rad Diagnostic Group, Hercules, CA; B-12/Folate Simul-TRAC, ICN Pharmaceuticals, Costa Mesa, CA; DiaSorin, Stillwater, MN).

The radioassay procedures have the advantage of avoiding interference from the presence of antibiotics in the serum samples. However, the procedures involve the use of radioisotopes and the need for a gamma isotope counter. The variability in results with radioassays between laboratories is perplexing.[153-155,223,224]

Improved standardized methods and diagnostic kits for serum and red cell folate measurements are essential. Suitable reference materials need to be used.[223,224,244] Gunter and Twite[241] have used lyophilize serum and lyophilized human blood as quality control materials for serum and erythrocyte folate analyses by radioassay. The materials were stable over a two-year period.

O'Broin et al.[243] have used finger-stick blood samples to determine folate concentrations. They used the mean cell hemoglobin concentration to interconverts red cell and hemoglobin folate data.

The radioassay kits were designed for the measurement of folate in serum. Their applications to the measurement of folate in red cells are not adequately established. The folate present in erythrocytes is complex when compared to the folates present in serum, which leads to uncertainties in the reliability, accuracy, and precision of the kits.[150,155,240] Until well validated, the use of radioassay kits for the measurement of erythrocyte folate concentrations cannot be recommended. The microbiological assay has been long established as a satisfactory method to measure folate in erythrocyte.[50,55,65,99,139,148,150,223,240]

Microbiological Assays for Folate

Microbiological procedures have been used since 1941 for the measurement of folate.[43,44,156] The assay medium developed by Teply and Elvehjem in 1945[157] continues to be used with only slight modification. *Lactobacillus rhamnosus* (ATCC 7469), formerly called *L. casei*, is commonly used as the assay organism for it responds to the widest spectrum of folates.[148,158] The microbiological assay for folates in serum, plasma, and whole blood has been detailed in a number of sources.[55,65,99,138,150,159-161,200,240] The microbiological assay remains the only practical method for measurement of the folate content of foods.[159]

Formerly, investigators without experience in performing microbiological assays considered the folate assay difficult to establish and time consuming. However, with the use of cryoprotected *L. rhamnosus (L. casei)* cultures[162,163] and the introduction of the 96-well plate and computer assisted microplate reader, the assay is easier to perform, less time consuming, and more reproducible.[159,164-166,169] Full details are provided in the publication of Molloy and Scott.[168]

The stability of folate in long-term storage of plasma or whole blood samples (at –70°C) may be enhanced with the presence of a reducing agent (e.g., ascorbic acid).[137,138,167,168,170,244] Kirke et al.[215] found over a 6-year storage period that the plasma folate of 14 samples deteriorated by $19.2 \pm 6.4\%$. There was no deterioration in erythrocyte folate concentrations when stored diluted with 1% ascorbic acid. The samples were stored at –20°C. However, in unpublished studies, we found that erythrocyte samples without added ascorbic acid and held at –70°C for several years were without significant loss of folate as measured by *L. rhamnosus (L. casei)* assay.[99,200]

Gunter et al.[244] conducted an interlaboratory comparison study to assess differences among methods. The results underscored the urgent need for developing and validating reference methods for plasma and whole-blood folate measurements. Gunter et al.[244] stabilized serum samples with the addition of 1 mg of ascorbic acid per mL of serum and held frozen at –70°C. Whole-blood samples were diluted 10-fold and held frozen at –70°C. Thus, 0.5 mL of whole blood was diluted with 4.5 mL of 10 g/L ascorbic acid diluent. Heparin or EDTA may be used as the anticoagulant.[245]

The folates are present in the red blood cells as polyglutamyl forms and must be hydrolyzed to the monoglutamates before they can be measured by microbiological assay or radioassay. Most of the folate in whole blood is located in the red blood cells. The hydrolysis can be easily accomplished by lysing the whole blood and allowing the plasma cojugase present to hydrolyze the polyglutamates.

Folate Status and Homocysteine Metabolism

Plasma Homocysteine and Folate Status

Homocysteine concentrations in plasma can serve as a marker for nutritional inadequacies for folate, vitamin B-6, and vitamin B-12.[171,172,199,201] Concentrations of plasma homocysteine are almost always elevated in deficiencies of folate or vitamin B-12.[242] The prevalence of high plasma homocysteine increases with age with an inverse association with plasma folate concentrations.[30,172,208,212]

The studies of Joosten et al.[199] suggest that the prevalence of tissue deficiencies of folate, vitamin B-12 and vitamin B-6 as demonstrated by elevated serum homocysteine concentrations is substantially higher than that estimated by measuring the serum concentrations of folate, vitamin B-12, and vitamin B-6.

Jacob et al.[175-177] conducted a moderate folate depletion study with eight postmenopausal women maintained in a metabolic unit. The subjects were fed a diet that provided only

56 µg/day of folate. After 41 days on the low folate diet, their plasma folate concentrations had fallen from an initial concentration of 9.8 µmol/L to 9.3 µmol/L. Plasma homocysteine concentrations rose during this period from an initial concentration of 9.8 µmol/L to 12.5 µmol/L. Lymphocyte DNA hypomethylation occurred, which was reversed with 286 to 516 µg/day of folate repletion. The elevated plasma homocysteine concentration did not decrease with an intake of 286 µg/day of folate, but did with a folate daily intake of 516 µg.

McCully made the initial report linking plasma homocysteine concentrations with arteriosclerotic vascular disease.[95,203] Hyperhomocysteinema is caused primarily by inherited enzyme deficiencies or nutritional deficiencies. Less frequently the hyperhomocysteinemia is drug-induced due to the use of antagonists of folate, vitamin B-6, or vitamin B-12. As an example, methotrexate because of its antifolate effect may produce an increase in fasting plasma homocysteine concentrations.[58]

The enzyme deficiencies associated with the cause of hyperhomocysteinemia are cystathionine β-synthase, methionine synthase, and methylenetetrahydrofolate reductase. Nutritional deficiencies of folate, vitamin B-12, or vitamin B-6 may induce hyperhomocysteinemia. Folate deficiency appears to be the most common cause of elevated plasma homocysteine concentrations. Vitamin B-12 (cobalamin) deficiency and vitamin B-6 deficiency have been considered in separate chapters. The clinical implications of hyperhomocysteinemia have been described in detail in the excellent reviews of Green and Jacobsen,[30] Lindenbaum and Allen,[65] and Kang et al.[230-232]

In the absence of deficiencies of vitamin B-12 and vitamin B-6, plasma concentrations of homocysteine can serve as a form of functional test of folate status.[233,234] Patients with an established folate deficiency megaloblastic anemia have a high correlation with their plasma homocysteine concentrations.[91] For the interpretation of the folate status, it is essential that a vitamin B-12 deficiency is not simultaneously present. Savage et al.[91] reported that 96% of the patients with a proven vitamin B-12 deficiency had elevated serum homocysteine concentrations.

Lindenbaum, Allen, and Savage[91] found in another study with alcoholic patients that in half of their patients with megaloblastic changes, the serum folate concentration was above 4.7 nmol/L (2.1 ng/mL). The investigators indicated that if the cutoff point for folate deficiency was raised to 8.9 nmol/L (4.0 ng/mL), excellent sensitivity would be achieved, but with a very low specificity.[91] They reported that the sensitivity of the erythrocyte folate concentrations as measured by *Lactobacillus rhamnosus* assay and the serum homocysteine concentration were both good. Homocysteine is stable in frozen plasma or serum samples.[234]

Figure 21 presents a relationship of plasma homocysteine concentrations to plasma folate concentrations in 209 adult males.[212] Plasma folate concentrations at the lower range considered to be normal in the United States (> 6.8 nmol/L)[100,137,138,189] were inadequate to prevent elevations in plasma homocysteine concentrations. The World Health Organization considered plasma folate concentrations above 13.6 nmol/L (6.0 ng/mL) as acceptable.[200] The NHANES-II considered plasma folate concentrations of less than 6.8 nmol/L (3.0 ng/mL) low.[189] In the NHANES-II project, the plasma folate concentration as measured by microbiological assay was 12.2 nmol/L for adult males and 13.4 nmol/L for adult females. These results would suggest that in order to prevent elevations in plasma homocysteine concentrations, the low lower acceptable plasma folate concentration is approximately 15 nmol/L (6.6 ng/mL).

Considerable variation exists between investigators regarding normal plasma homocysteine concentrations and those concentrations that relate to a risk of coronary vascular disease. Bouskey et al.[84] summarized the reports of 27 studies on the subject. Several guidelines have been used to evaluate plasma homocysteine data (Tables 33–36).

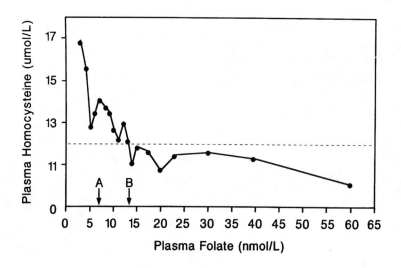

FIGURE 21

Relationship of plasma homocysteine concentrations to plasma folate concentrations in 209 adult males. (A) Indicates lower limit of normal plasma folate as used by NHANES-II (6.8 nmol/L); (B) Indicates lower limit of normal plasma folate as used by WHO (13.6 nmol/L). Homocysteine concentrations above the dotted line are considered elevated.[212] (With permission.)

TABLE 33

Guidelines for Evaluating Plasma Homocysteine Data

Study	Plasma Homocysteine Concentrations (μmol/L)	References
Framingham Heart Study		Selhub et al.[192,253]
Normal or low level	≤ 9.1	
Elevated (risk) level	≥ 14.4	
United States Physician Study		Stampfer et al.[171,254]
Elevated (risk) level	> 15.8	
International Study of Elderly		Joosten et al.[199]
Elevated (risk) level	> 13.9	

TABLE 34

Tentative Guidelines For Evaluating Hyperhomocysteinemia

	Plasma Homocysteine Concentrations (μmol/L)	
Risk Level	Malino,[86] Kang[236]	Jacobsen[225]
Normal/Low	<15	<12
Moderate	16–30	12–25
Intermediate	31–100	26–50
Severe	>100	>50

Mild (15 to 25 μmol/L) and intermediate (26 to 50 μmol/L) hyperhomocysteinemia is frequently seen in patients with cardiovascular disease such as stroke, coronary artery disease, and peripheral vascular disease.[255] The upper limit of normal plasma homocysteine has been suggested to be <12 μmol/L.[225] Other studies indicate that a plasma homocysteine concentration of less than 10 μmol/L would be desirable (see accompanying tables). For example, Wilcken et al.[226] found normal adults to have a plasma homocysteine concentration of 4.2 ± 0.8 μmol/L. Coronary artery patients with a plasma homocysteine concentration of

TABLE 35
Relationship of Age on Plasma Homocysteine Concentrations*
(Hordaland Norway Homocysteine Study)

Age (years)	Plasma Homocysteine Concentrations	
	Men	Women
40–42	10.8 µmol/L (*n* = 5918)	9.1 µmol/L (*n* = 6348)
65–67	12.3 µmol/L (*n* = 1386)	11.0 µmol/L (*n* = 1932)

* Mean values.
From Nygard et al.[251,252]
Subjects characterized by high folate intakes, nonsmoking status, and moderate coffee consumption had lower plasma homocysteine concentrations of approximately 2–4 µmol/L.[252]

TABLE 36
Summary of Criteria used to Evaluate Folate Status in the Absence of
Vitamin B-12 Deficiency[93]

Criterion	Range
Megaloblastic Anemia	
Plasma folate concentration:	
Deficiency (high risk)	< 6.7 nmol/L (< 3.0 ng/mL)
Marginal (moderate risk)	6.7–13.4 nmol/L (3–5 ng/mL)
Acceptable (low risk)	> 13.4 nmol/L (> 6.0 ng/mL)
Erythrocyte folate concentration:	
Deficiency (high risk)	< 312 nmol/L cells (< 140 ng/mL)
Marginal (moderate risk)	312–356 nmol/L cells (140–160 ng/mL)
Acceptable (low risk)	> 356 nmol/L cells (> 160 ng/mL)
dU Suppression test	Acceptable: < 10%
Neutrophil hypersegmentation	Acceptable: lobe average of < 3.6
FIGLU excretion	Deficient: elevated after histidine load
Plasma homocysteine concentration	Undesirable: > 12 µmol/L

FIGLU = formiminoglutamic acid.

< 9 µmol/L had after 4 years a mortality of 3.8% compared to 24.7% in the patients with a plasma homocysteine concentration of 15 µmol/L or higher.[227]

Black subjects maintain a relatively lower homocysteine concentration than non-black subjects suggesting a more efficient metabolism of homocysteine by blacks.[75] The South African black population has a lower prevalence of coronary heart disease than the white population.[75]

Plasma Homocysteine Concentrations in Blacks Compared to Adult Whites

	Black Men (*n* = 52)	White Men (*n* = 195)
Plasma homocysteine concentrations (µmol/L)	9.7 ± 3.3	13.4 ± 4.7

From Reference 75.

In some subjects with low normal concentrations of serum folate (e.g., 4.7 to 8.9 nmol/L; 2.1 to 4.0 ng/mL) and with low normal serum concentrations of vitamin B-12 (e.g., 141 to 162 pmol/L; 191 to 220 pg/mL) had elevated concentrations of serum homocysteine.[230-232]

Recently, a kit has become commercially available for measuring total plasma homocysteine.[248] The measurement utilizes electrochemical detection and requires 200 µL of sample. The kit (system) is available form Bioanalytical Systems, Inc., West Lafayette, IN.

Hypersegmentation of Neutrophils

The earliest hematological sign of folate deficiency is an increase in the hypersegmentation of the nuclei of the neutrophilic polymorphonuclear leucocytes.[6,7,10,12,50,65,111,116] With the onset of megaloblastic anemia the neutrophils, instead of having a normal average lobe number of approximately 3.2, will be observed to have an increase in the percentage of cells with five or more nuclear lobes.[7]

Hypersegmentation has been considered to exist when more than 5% of the neutrophils have five or more lobes.[7] A lobe average greater than 3.5 has also been considered hypersegmentation.[7,134] Hypersegmented neutrophils may be estimated according to the procedure of Herbert.[6]

Following the changes in the neutrophils, the next hematologic alteration that may be noted in folacin deficiency is a gradual appearance of macroovalocytosis, with gradual increase in the mean corpuscular volume.[7,111]

Megaloblastic bone marrow changes also occur with dietary folate deprivation.[7,111] Usually the severity of the bone marrow changes will relate directly with the degree of anemia present. However, the morphological changes in the peripheral blood usually occur before the appearance of an overtly megaloblastic bone marrow.[6,10]

It should be noted that the histological findings indicated above are identical for the megaloblastic anemias caused by either a deficiency in folic acid or vitamin B-12. Hence morphological changes alone cannot be used to distinguish between these two vitamin deficiencies. However, the presence of neutrophil hypersegmentation can be highly specific for the diagnosis of a vitamin B-12 or a folacin deficiency. Further laboratory measurements can readily establish which deficiency, if not both, is present.

In a folacin depletion and repletion investigation with young women, neutrophil hypersegmentation observations were performed. Although neutrophil hypersegmentation determinations can be easily performed, in this study they did not provide a reliable early indicator of folate status.[50]

Another report indicated that plasma folate concentrations of less than 9.1 nmol/L (<4.0 ng/mL), and red blood folate concentrations less than 567 nmol/L (<250 ng/mL) corresponded with an increasing neutrophil lobe average >3.5.[113,114]

Deoxyuridine Suppression Test (dUST)

The deoxyuridine suppression test (dUST) has been used to evaluate the functional status of certain folate-dependent and cobalamin-dependent enzyme reactions in short-term cultures of living cells.[130-141] The test measures the effect of deoxyuridine in suppressing the uptake of tritrated labeled thymidine into DNA, which is abnormal in a folate or vitamin B-12 deficiency.[135-136] When folate and vitamin B-12 are deficient, the degree of suppression is less pronounced because of impaired *de novo* synthesis of thymidylate and greater utilization of the salvage pathway.[130,135] The deoxyuridine suppression test can reflect nutritional folate or vitamin B-12 deficiencies in lymphocytes formed earlier and surviving into the early phases of repletion.[133,134,149]

The original procedure was based on the use of cultured bone marrow cells and was subsequently modified.[127-131] However, for ease of performing dUST, a procedure was developed that used small volumes of whole blood rather than suspensions of bone marrow or

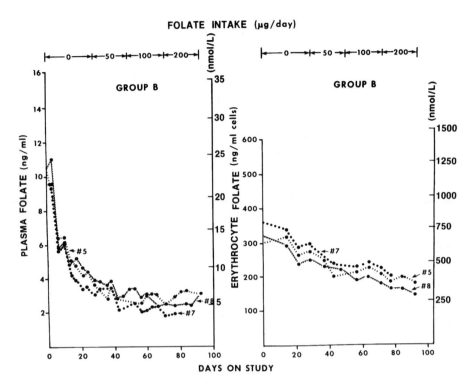

FIGURE 22

Effect of folate intake on the folate concentrations in plasma and erythrocytes in young women. Folate supplements were provided in natural forms from food items.[50] (With permission.)

isolated lymphocytes.[132-136] The lymphocyte deoxyuridine suppression test[132] was studied during a folate depletion and repletion study with nonpregnant women maintained on a metabolic unit.[50]

The greatest suppression was noted at the end of the folate depletion when the plasma and erythrocyte folate concentrations were the lowest. The dUST values returned to normal at the end of the folate repletion. Variability existed among the volunteer subjects, which may have been a reflection of differences between individuals in folate status. Tamura et al.[35] evaluated the deoxyuridine suppression test using whole blood samples from 245 women. They observed that the dUST values had a significant negative correlation with plasma and erythrocyte folate concentrations. However, it was concluded that comparable information could probably be obtained more expeditiously and with lower expense through erythrocyte folate assays. To distinguish between the two vitamins, the effect of *in vitro* added folate or vitamin B-12 in the test is observed.

Formiminoglutamic Acid Excretion (FIGLU Test)

Several indirect tests for evaluating folate status are based on the increased urinary excretion of formiminoglutamic acid (FIGLU) and of its immediate precursor, urocanic acid, that occurs in the deficient subjects.[111,144,145] These compounds arise from histidine metabolism which is normally converted to glutamic acid through the participation of formiminotransferase and tetrahydrofolic acid. In folate deficiency, the conversion is inhibited and the amounts of FIGLU and urocanic acid in the urine are increased.[146] The excretion of these compounds can be greatly increased in the deficient subject by administering an oral load of 2 to 25 g of L-histidine.[146]

The excretion of FIGLU or of FIGLU-plus-urocanic acid has been used as an index of folate deficiency, particularly in research studies. For nutrition surveys, the procedure is impractical. Unfortunately, the FIGLU and urocanate excretion test is not entirely specific. Patients with pernicious anemia often have a positive test[111] and, hence, the test does not distinguish between the anemia of vitamin B-12 deficiency and the anemia of folate deficiency. Similarly, abnormal amounts of FIGLU and urocanic acid may be excreted by subjects suffering from liver damage, protein malnutrition, and congenital formiminotransferase deficiency. A number of methods are available for measuring FIGLU, but the procedure of Tabor and Wyngarden has been commonly used.[143] In our experience as well as others, subjects complained of nausea and stomach distress after ingestion of the histidine.[50,142] Moreover, the FIGLU test lacks the sensitivity and specificity desired. Although the FIGLU test represent a form of functional test, it has been replaced by more convenient and practical procedures and is now seldom used.

Urinary Excretion of Folate

Folate normally is effectively reabsorbed by the proximal renal tubule, with little loss of intact folate.[62,68] In a folate depletion and repletion study with nonpregnant women, the urinary excretion of folate fell promptly with the omission of the vitamin from the diet (Figure 23).[50] However, even after 28 days of folate deficiency, measurable amounts of folate were present in the urine (i.e., 10 to 15 nmol [24 hr]).[50] *Lactobacillus casei (L. rhamnosus)* folate assay was used to measure the folate available in untreated urine samples. With intakes of folate up to 300 µg/day, only a slight increase in the urinary excretion of folate occurred. In another study, subjects fed diets providing 200, 300, or 400 µg/day of folate had a mean daily excretion of folate of 3.8 ± 0.93, 5.5 ± 0.25, and 21.2 ± 12 nmol, respectively.[210] Normal subjects on an average diet have been reported to excrete daily only 11.3 to 90.6 nmol (5–40 µg) of free folate.[69-72]

Urinary excretion of folate has been reported to continue even with advanced folate depletion with the presence of megaloblastic anemia. Thus, the measurement of urinary concentrations of folate has limited, if any, usefulness as an indicator of folate nutritional status. Folate catabolites, such a p-aminobenzoylaglutamate, have been studied as a possible indicator of folate requirements and metabolism.[110]

Gregory et al.[79] have studied the 24-hr urinary excretion of folate following a single oral dose of isotopically labeled folate ($[^2H_4]$ folate). The results suggested that the excretion of the isotopically labeled folate may serve as a functional indicator of folate nutritional status.

Folate Safety and Toxicity

Folate supplementation has been of concern because of the potential ability of folate supplements to mask the anemia that normally develops in vitamin B-12 deficiency. Folate can induce a hematological response in vitamin B-12 deficient patients, but fails to prevent the

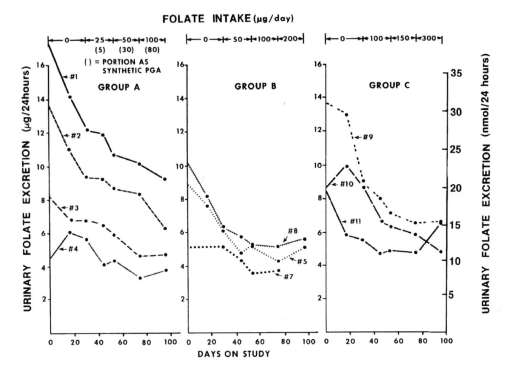

FIGURE 23

Effect of folate intake on the urinary excretion of microbiologically available folate using the *L. rhamnosus* assay.[50] (With permission.)

irreversable neurological manifestations of a vitamin B-12 deficiency.[64] This view is based on a small number of confirmed cases.

Clinical experience indicates that the cases in which vitamin B-12 deficiency is masked by folic acid are extremely rare.[74] No evidence exists that daily supplements of 0.4 mg of folic acid increased the risk of masking a vitamin B-12 deficiency. Intakes of 1.0 mg/day are not likely to mask a vitamin B-12 deficiency. Wald et al.[25] found in a study with 1,817 women that a folic acid supplement of 4.0 mg per day was without adverse effect. In a study with young women, a daily supplement of 10 mg of folic acid for 6 months was without any observed adverse effects.[80] With the more common use of plasma vitamin B-12 measurements, overlooking a case of folate masking has become less likely.

Large supplements of folic acid can reverse the effectiveness of anticonvulsant medications (e.g., phenytoin [Dilatin], phenobarbital, and pyrimidone).[74,89,105] However, the interference of folic acid supplementation is variable. A variety of other folic acid antagonists exist that are used to treat diverse illnessess.[90] Some of the more common folate antagonists are methotrexate, pyrimethamine (Daraprin), trimethoprim, sulfasalazine, trimetrexate, and piritrexim.[47,74,90,104]

Summary

Deficiency of folate results in megaloblastic anemia which cannot be distinguished from that caused by a deficiency of vitamin B-12. Consequently, plasma or serum vitamin B-12 measurements should be performed in conjunction with folate nutritional assessments.

Folate nutritional status is usually evaluated through the measurement of folate concentrations in serum and erythrocytes. Microbiological assays or radioassays are used for the measurements. Plasma folate concentrations above 13.4 nmol/L (6.0 ng/mL) are considered acceptable while values less than 6.7 nmol/L (3.0 ng/mL) are considered deficient. Erythrocyte concentrations above 256 nmol/L (160 ng/mL) are considered acceptable while values less than 312 nmol/L (140 ng/mL) are considered deficient. The erythrocyte folate concentrations have been regarded as a more accurate and less variable quantitative index than serum folate as to the severity of a folate deficiency in an individual subject. Folate plays important roles in the prevention of megaloblastic anemia of pregnancy, in cancer prevention, coronary heart disease, stroke, and of neural tube defects.

References

1. Banwell, J. G., Malabsorption syndromes, in *Tropical and Geographic Medicine*, Warren, K. S. and Mahmoud, A. A. F., Eds., McGraw-Hill, New York, 1984, 14.
2. Corcino, J. J., Reisenauer, A. M., and Halsted, C. H., Jejunal perfusion of simple and conjugated folates in tropical sprue, *J. Clin. Invest.*, 58, 298, 1976.
3. Halsted, C. H., Reisenauer, A. M. Romero, J. J. et al., Jejunal perfusion of simple and conjugated folates in celiac sprue, *J. Clin. Invest.*, 59, 933, 1977.
4. Krumdieck, C. L., Newman, A. J., and Butterworth, C. E., A naturally occurring inhibitor of folic acid conjugase (pteroylpolyglutamate hydrolase) in beans and other pulses, *Am. J. Clin. Nutr.*, 26, 460, 1973.
5. Metz, J., Folate deficiency conditioned by lactation, *Am. J. Clin. Nutr.*, 23, 843, 1970.
6. Herbert, V., Experimental nutritional folate deficiency in man, *Trans. Assoc. Am. Physicians*, 75, 307, 1962.
7. Herbert, V. and Das, K. C., Anemias due to nuclear maturation defects (megaloblastic anemias), in *Medicine for the Practicing Physician*, 3rd edition, Hurst, J. W., Ed., Butterworth-Heinemann, Boston, 1992, 851.
8. Sauberlich, H. E., Vitamin indices, in *Laboratory Indices of Nutritional Status in Pregnancy*, National Academy of Sciences, Washington D.C., 1978, 109.
9. Sauberlich, H. E., Detection of folic acid deficiency in populations, Food and Nutrition Board, Folic acid: Biochemistry and physiology in relation to the human nutrition requirement, National Academy of Sciences, Washington D.C., 1977, 213.
10. Herbert, V., Folic acid, *Annu. Rev. Med.*, 16, 359, 1965.
11. Blakley, R. L., The biochemistry of folic acid and related pteridimes, in *Frontiers of Biology*, Volume 13, Neuburger, A. and Tatum, E. L., Eds., North-Holland Publishing Co., Amsterdam, The Netherlands, 1969, 570.
12. Hoffbrand, A. V., Newcombe, B. F. A., and Molin, D. L., Method of assay of red cell folate activity and the value of the assay as a test for folate deficiency, *J. Clin. Pathol.*, 19, 17, 1966.
13. Metz, J., Festenstein, H., and Welch, P., Effect of folic acid and vitamin B-12 supplementation on tests of folate and vitamin B-12 nutrition in pregnancy, *Am. J. Clin. Nutr.*, 16, 472, 1965.
14. Iyengar, L., Folic acid requirements of Indian pregnant women, *Am. J. Obstet. Gynecol.*, 111, 13, 1971.
15. Nixon, P. F. and Bertino, J. R., Interrelationships of vitamin B-12 and folate in man, *Am. J. Med.*, 48, 555, 1970.
16. Rothman, D., Folic acid in pregnancy, *Am. J. Obstet. Gynecol.*, 108, 149, 1970.
17. Hibbard, E. D. and Smithells, R. W., Folic acid metabolism and human embryopathy, *Lancet* I, 1254, 1965.
18. Smithells, R. W., Seller, M. J., Harris, R., Fielding, D. W., Schorah, C. J., Nevin, N. C., Sheppard, S., Read, A. P., Walker, S., and Wild, J., Further experience of vitamin supplementation for prevention of neural tube defect recurrences, *Lancet* I, 1027, 1983.

19. Wald, N., Folic acid and the prevention of neural tube defects, *Ann. N.Y. Acad. Sci.*, 678, 112, 1993.
20. Anonymous, Homocysteine, folic acid, and the prevention of vascular disease, *Nutr. Rev.*, 47, 247, 1989.
21. Butterworth, C. E., Hatch, K. D., Macaluso, M., Cole, P., Sauberlich, H. E., Soong, S.–J., Borst, M., and Backer, V. V., Folate deficiency and cervical dysplasia, *JAMA*, 267, 528, 1992.
22. Mulinare, J. J., Cordero, F., Erickson, J. D., and Berry, R. J., Periconceptional use of multivitamins and the occurrence of neural tube defects, *JAMA*, 260, 3141, 1988.
23. Milunskey, A., Jick, H., Jick, S. S., Bruell, C. L., MacLaughin, D. S., Rothman, K. J., and Willett, W., Multivitamin/folic acid supplementation in early pregnancy reduces the prevalence of neural tube defects, *JAMA*, 262, 2847, 1989.
24. Schorah, C. J. and Smithells, R. W., A possible role for preconceptional multivitamin supplementation in the prevention of the recurrence of neural tube defects, in *Micronutrients in Health and Disease Prevention*, Bendich, A. and Butterworth, C. E., Eds., Marcel Dekker, New York, 1991, 263.
25. Wald, N., Sneddon, J., Densem, J., Frost, C., and Stone, R., Medical Research Council Vitamin Study Research Group, Prevention of neural tube defects: Results of the Medical Research Council Vitamin Study, *Lancet*, 338, 131, 1992.
26. Mulinare, J., Epidemiologic associations of multivitamin supplementation and occurrence of neural tube defects, *Ann. N.Y. Acad. Sci.*, 678, 130, 1993.
27. Mills, J. L. and Raymond, E., Effects of recent research on recommendations for preconceptional folate supplement use, *Ann. N.Y. Acad. Sci.*, 137, 1993.
28. Bower, C., Stanley, F. J., and Nicol, D. J., Maternal folate status and the risk for neural tube defects, *Ann. N.Y. Acad. Sci.*, 678, 146, 1993.
29. Scott, J. M., Weir, D. G., and Kirke, P. N., Folate and neural tube defects, in *Folate in Health and Disease*, Bailey, L. B., Ed., Marcel Dekker, New York, 1995, 329.
30. Green, R. and Jacobson, D. W., Clinical implications of hyperhomocysteinemia, in *Folate in Health and Disease*, Bailey, L. B., Ed., Marcel Dekker, New York, 1995, 75.
31. Mason, J. B. Folate status: effects on carcinogenesis, in *Folate in Health and Disease*, Bailey, L. B., Ed., Marcel Dekker, New York, 1995, 361.
32. Priest, D. G. and Bunni, M. A., Folates and folate antagonists in cancer chemotherapy, in *Folate in Health and Disease*, Bailey, L. B., Ed., Marcel Dekker, New York, 1995, 379.
33. Tamura, T., Nutrient interaction of folate and zinc, in *Folate in Health and Disease*, Bailey, L. B., Ed., Marcel Dekker, New York, 1995, 287.
34. Mukherjee, M. D., Sandstead, H. H., Ratnaparkhi, M. V., Johnson, L. K., Milne, D. B., and Stelling, H. P., Maternal zinc, iron, folic acid, and protein nutriture and outcome of human pregnancy, *Am. J. Clin. Nutr.*, 40, 496, 1984.
35. Milne, D. B., Canfield, W. K., Mahalko, J. R., and Sandstead, H. H., Effect of oral folic acid supplements on zinc, copper, and iron absorption and excretion, *Am. J. Clin. Nutr.*, 39, 535, 1984.
36. Chandler, C. J., Wang, T. T. Y., and Halsted, C. H., Pterolypolyglutamate hydrolase from human jejunal brush borders, purification and characterization, *J. Biol. Chem.*, 261, 928, 1986.
37. Wills, L., Nature of the haemopoietic factor in marmite, *Lancet*, 1, 1283, 1933.
38. Wills, L., Treatment of "pernicious anemia of pregnancy" and "tropical anemia" with special reference to yeast extract as a curative agent, *Br. Med. J.*, 1, 1059, 1931.
39. Wills, L. and Evans, P. D. F., Tropical macrocytic anaemia: its relation to pernicious anemia, *Lancet*, 2, 416, 1938.
40. Mitchell, H. K., Snell, E. E., and Williams, R. J., Concentration of "folic acid," *J. Am. Chem. Soc.*, 63, 2284, 1941.
41. Angier, R. B., Boothe, J. H., Hutchings, B. L., Mowat, J. H., Semb, J., Stokstad, E. L. R. et al., The structure and synthesis of the liver *L. casei* factor, *Science*, 103, 667, 1946.
42. Angier, R. B., Boothe, J. H., Hutchings, B. L., Mowat, J. H., Semb, J., Stokstad, E. L. R., SubbaRow, Y., Waller, C. W., Caswlich, D. B., Fahrenbach, M. J., Hultquist, M. E., Kuh, E., Northey, E. H., Seeger, D. R., Sickles, J. P., and Smith, J. M., Synthesis of a compound identical with *L. casei* factor isolate from liver, *Science*, 102, 227, 1945.
43. Stokstad, E. L. R., Historical perspective on key advances in the biochemistry and physiology of folates, in *Folic Acid Metabolism in Health and Disease*, Picciano, M. F., Stokstad, E. L. R., and Gregory, J. F. III, Eds., Wiley-Liss, New York, 1990, 1.

44. Welch, A. D., Folic acid: Discovery and the exciting first decade, *Perspect. Biol. Med.*, 27, 64, 1983.
45. Stokstad, E. L. R. and Jukes, T. H., Sulfanamides and folic acid antagonists: A historical review, *J. Nutr.*, 117, 1335, 1987.
46. Sauberlich, H. E. and Baumann, C. A., A factor required for the growth of *Leuconostoc citrovorum*, *J. Biol. Chem.*, 176, 165, 1948.
47. Sauberlich, H. E., Antagonists of folate – Their biochemical and clinical importance, *Nutrition*, 18, 214, 1994.
48. Sauberlich, H. E., Bioavailability of vitamins, *Prog. Food & Nutr. Sci.*, 9, 1, 1985.
49. Anonymous, How do foods affect folate bioavailability, *Nutr. Rev.*, 48, 326, 1990.
50. Sauberlich, H. E., Kretsch, M. J., Skala, J. H., Johnson, H. L., and Taylor, P. C., Folate requirement and metabolism in nonpregnant women, *Am. J. Clin. Nutr.*, 46, 1016, 1987.
51. Sauberlich, H. E., Vitamin: how much for keeps, *Nutr. Today*, Jan.-Feb., 20, 1987.
52. Tamura, T. Biovailability of folic acid in fortified food, *Am. J. Clin. Nutr.*, 66, 1299, 1997.
53. Gregory, J. F. III., Bhandari, S. D., Bailey, L. B., Toth, J. P., Baumgartner, T. G., and Cerda, J. J., Relative bioavailability of deuterium-labeled monoglutamyl tetrahydrofolates and folic acid in human subjects, *Am. J. Clin. Nutr.*, 55, 1147, 1992.
54. Pfeiffer, C. M., Rogers, L. M., Bailey, L. B., and Gregory, J. F. III., Absorption of folate from fortified cereal-grain products and of supplemental folate consumed with or without food determined by using a dual-label stable-isotope protocol, *Am. J. Clin. Nutr.*, 66, 1388, 1997.
55. Tamura, T., Mizuno, Y., Johnston, K. E., and Jacob, R. A., Food folate assay with protease, α-amylase, and folate conjugase treatments, *J. Agr. Food Chemistry*, 45, 135, 1997.
56. Martin, J. I., Landen, W. O. Jr., Saliman, A. G. M., and Eitenmiller, R. R., Application of a tri-enzyme extraction for total folate determination in foods, *J. Assoc. Off. Anal. Chem.*, 73, 805, 1990.
57. Subar, A. F., Block, G., and James, L. D., Folate intake and food sources in the US population, *Am. J. Clin. Nutr.*, 50, 508, 1989.
58. Refsum, H., Helland, S., and Ueland, P. M., Fasting plasma homocysteine as a sensitive parameter of antifolate effect: A study of psoriasis patients receiving low-dose methotrexate treatment, *Clin. Pharmacol. Ther.*, 46, 510, 1989.
59. Butterworth C. E. and Bendich, A., Folic acid and the prevention of birth defects, *Annu. Rev. Nutr.*, 16, 73, 1996.
60. Scott, J. M., Kirke, P. N., and Weir, D. G., The role of nutrition in neural tube defects, *Annu. Rev. Nutr.*, 10, 277, 1990.
61. Halsted, C. H., Alcohol and folate interaction: clinical implications, in *Folate in Health and Disease*, Bailey, L. B., Ed., Marcel Dekker, New York, 1995, 313.
62. Shane, B., Folate chemistry and metabolism, in *Folate in Health and Disease*, Bailey, L. B., Ed., Marcel Dekker, New York, 1995, 1.
63. Wagner, C., Biochemical role of folate in cellular metabolism, in *Folate in Health and Disease*, Bailey, L. B., Ed., Marcel Dekker, New York, 1995, 23.
64. Savage, D. G. and Lindenbaum, J., Folate-cobalamin interactions, in *Folate in Health and Disease*, Bailey, L. B., Ed., Marcel Dekker, New York, 1995, 237.
65. Lindenbaum, J. and Allen, R. H., Clinical spectrum and diagnosis of folate deficiency, in *Folate in Health and Disease*, Bailey, L. B., Ed., Marcel Dekker, New York, 1995, 43.
66. Bottiglieri, T., Crellin, R. F., and Reynolds, E. H., Folates and neuropsychiatry, in *Folate in Health and Disease*, Bailey, L. B., Ed., Marcel Dekker, New York, 1995, 435.
67. Gregory, J. F. III, The bioavailability of folates, in *Folate in Health and Disease*, Bailey, L. B., Ed., Marcel Dekker, New York, 1995, 195.
68. Selhub, J., Emmanouel, D., Stavopoulos, T., and Arnold, R., Renal folate absorption and the kidney folate binding protein, *Am. J. Physiol.*, 252, F75, 1987.
69. Herbert, V., Nutritional requirements of vitamin B-12 and folic acid, *Am. J. Clin. Nutr.*, 21, 743, 1968.
70. Retief, F. P., Urinary folate excretion after ingestion of pteroylmonoglutamic acid and food folate, *Am. J. Clin. Nutr.*, 22, 352, 1969.
71. Tamura, T. and Stokstad, E. L. R., The availability of food folate in man, *Br. J. Haematol.*, 25, 513, 1973.

72. Cooperman, J. M., Pesci-Bourel, A., and Lubby, A. L., Urinary excretion of folic acid in man, *Clin. Chem.*, 16, 375, 1970.
73. Krumdieck, C. L., Folic acid, in *Present Knowledge in Nutrition*, 6th edition, Brown, M. L., Ed., International Life Sciences Institute, Nutrition Foundation, Washington D.C., 1994, 179.
74. Butterworth, C. E. Jr. and Tamura, T., Folic acid safety and toxicity: a brief review, *Am. J. Clin. Nutr.*, 50, 353, 1989.
75. Ubbink, J. B., Delport, R., and Vermaak, W. J. H., Plasma homocysteine concentrations in population with a low coronary heart disease prevalence, *J. Nutr.*, 126, 1254S, 1996.
76. Grace, E., Emans, S. J., and Drum, D. E., Hematologic abnormalities in adolescents who take oral contraceptive pills, *J. Pediatr.*, 101, 771, 1982.
77. Webb, J. L., Nutritional effects of oral contraceptive use: a review, *J. Reprod. Med.*, 25, 150, 1980.
78. Green, T. J., Houghton, L. A., Donovan, U., Gibson, R. S., and O'Connor, D. L., Oral contraceptives did not effect biochemical folate indexes and homocysteine concentrations in adolescent females, *J. Am. Diet. Assoc.*, 98, 49, 1998.
79. Gregory, J. F. III, Willamson, J., Bailey, L. B., and Toth, J. P., Urinary excretion of [^{2}H$_4$] folate by nonpregnant women following a single oral dose of [^{2}H$_4$] folic acid is a functional index of folate nutritional status, *J. Nutr.*, 128, 1907, 1998.
80. Butterworth, C. E. Jr., Hatch, K. D., Soong, S.–J., Cole, P., Tamura, T., Sauberlich, H. E., Borst, M., Macaluso, M., and Baker, V., Oral folic acid supplementation for cervical dysplasia: a clinical intervention trial, *Am. J. Obset. Gyneol.*, 166, 803, 1992.
81. Czeizel, A. E. and Dudes, I., Prevention of the first occurrence of neural tube defects by periconceptional vitamin supplementation, *N. Engl. J. Med.*, 327, 1832, 1992.
82. Werler, M. M., Shapiro, S., and Mitchell, A. A., Periconceptional folic acid exposure and risk of occurrent neural tube defects, *J. Am. Med. Assoc.*, 269, 1257, 1993.
83. Zimmermann, M. B. and Shane, B., Supplemental folic acid, *Am. J. Clin. Nutr.*, 58, 127, 1993.
84. Boushey, C. J., Beresford, S. A., Omenn, G. S., and Motulsky, A. G., A quantitative assessment of plasma homocysteine as a risk factor for vascular disease: probable benefits of increasing folic acid intakes, *JAMA*, 274, 1049, 1995.
85. den Heijer, M. D., Koster, T., Blom, H. J., Bos, G. M. J., Briet, E., Reitsma, P. H., Vandenbroucke, J. P., and Rosndaal, F. R., Hyperhomocysteinemia as a risk factor for deep-vein thrombosis, *N. Eng. J. Med.*, 334, 759, 1996.
86. Malinow, M. R., Plasma homocyst(e)ine: a risk factor for arterial occlusive diseases, *J. Nutr.*, 126, 1238S, 1996.
87. Tamura, T., Goldenberg, R. L., Freeberg, L. E., Cliver, S. P., Cutter, G. R., and Hoffman, H. J., Maternal serum folate and zinc concentrations and their relationships to pregnancy outcome, *Am. J. Clin. Nutr.*, 56, 365, 1992.
88. Kauwell, G. P., Bailey, L. B., Gregory, J. F. III, Bowling, D. W., and Cousins, R. J., Zinc status is not adversely affected by folic acid supplementation and zinc intake does not impair folate utilization in human subjects, *J. Nutr.*, 125, 66, 1995.
89. Bailey, L. B., Folate requirements and dietary recommendations, in *Folate in Health and Disease*, Bailey, L. B., Ed., Marcel Dekker, New York, 1995, 123.
90. Morgan, S. L. and Baggott, J. E., Folate antagonists in nonneoplastic disease: proposed mechanisms of efficacy and toxicity, in *Folate in Health and Disease*, Bailey, L. B., Ed., Marcel Dekker, New York, 1995, 405.
91. Savage, D. G., Lindenbaum, J., Stabler, S. P., and Allen, R. H., Serum methymalonic acid and total homocysteine for diagnosing cobalamine and folate deficiencies, *Am. J. Med.*, 96, 239, 1994.
92. Herbert, V., Making sense of laboratory test of folate status; Folate requirements to sustain normality, *Am. J. Clin. Nutr.*, 26, 199, 1997.
93. Sauberlich, H. E., Evaluation of folate nutrition in population groups, in Evaluation of Folic Acid Metabolism in Health and Disease, Picciano, M. F., Ed., Wiley-Liss, New York, 1990, 211.
94. Roe, D. A., Drug effects on nutrient absorption, transport, and metabolism, *Drug-Nutrient Interact.*, 4, 117, 1985.
95. McCully, K. S., Micronutrients, homocysteine metabolism, and atherosclerosis, in *Micronutrients in Health and in Disease Prevention*, Bendich, A. and Butterworth, C. E. Jr., Eds., Marcel Dekker, New York, 1991, 69.

96. Butterworth, C. E. Jr., Folate deficiency and cancer, in *Micronutrients in Health and Disease Prevention*, Bendich, A. and Butterworth, C. E., Jr. Eds., Marcel Dekker, New York, 1991, 165.

97. Sauberlich, H. E., Relationship of vitamin B-6, vitamin B-12, and folate to neurological and neuropsychiatric disorders, in *Micronutrients in Health and Disease Prevention*, Bendich, A. and Butterworth, C. E. Jr., Eds., Marcel Dekker, New York, 1991, 187.

98. Bailey, L. B., Folate nutrition in adolescents and adults, in *Folic Acid Metabolism in Health and Disease*, Picciano, M. F., Stokstad, E. L. R. and Gregory, J. F. III, Eds., Wiley-Liss, New York, 1990, 253.

99. Tamura, T., Microbiological assay of folate, in *Folic Acid Metabolism in Health and Disease*, Picciano, M. E., Stokstad, E. L. R., and Gregory, J. F. III, Eds., Wiley-Liss, New York, 1990, 121.

100. Sauberlich, H. E., Folate status of U.S. population groups, in *Folate in Health and Disease*, Bailey, L. B., Ed., Marcel Dekker, New York, 1995, 171.

101. Witter, F. R., Blake, D. A., and Baumgardner, R. et al., Folate, carotene, and smoking, *Am. J. Obstet. Gynecol.*, 144, 857, 1982.

102. Heimburger, D. C., Localized deficiencies of folic acid in aerodigestive tissues, *Ann. N.Y. Acad. Sci.*, 669, 87, 1992.

103. Piyathilake, C. J., Macalusa, M., Hine, R. J., Richards, E. W., and Krumdieck, C. L., Local and systemic effects of cigarette smoking on folate and vitamin B-12, *Am. J. Clin. Nutr.*, 60, 559, 1994.

104. Lambie, D. G. and Johnson, R. H., Drugs and folate metabolism, *Drugs*, 30, 145, 1985.

105. Dansky, L. V., Andermann, E., Rosenblatt, D., Sherwin, A. L., and Andermann, F., Anticonvulsants, folate levels, and pregnancy outcome: a prospective study, *Annu. Neurol.*, 21, 176, 1987.

106. Ortega, R. M., Lopez-Sobaler, A. M., Gonzalez-Gross, M. M., Redondo, R. M., Marzanna, I., Zamora, M. J., and Andres, P., Influence of smoking on folate intake and blood folate concentrations in a group of elderly Spanish men, *J. Am. Coll. Nutr.*, 13, 68, 1994.

107. Shojania, A. M., Oral contraceptive: effects on folate and vitamin B-12 metabolism, *CMA J.*, 126, 244, 1982.

108. Hettiarahchy, N. S., Srikantha, S. S., and Coreo, S. M. X., The effect of oral contraceptive therapy and of pregnancy on serum folate levels of rural Sri Lankan women, *Br. J. Nutr.*, 50, 495, 1983.

109. Sauberlich, H. E., Methionine, homocystine, choline, folic acid and vitamin B-12 in the nutrition of the mouse, *J. Nutr.*, 68, 141, 1959.

110. McParlin, J., Courtney, G., McNulty, H., Weir, D., and Scott, J., The quantitative analysis of endogenous folate catabolites in human urine, *Anal. Biochem.*, 206, 256, 1992.

111. Herbert, V., Biochemical and hematologic lesions of folic acid deficiency, *Am. J. Clin. Nutr.*, 20, 562, 1967.

112. Lindenbaum, J. and Nath, B. J., Megaloblastic anaemia and neutrophil hypersegmentation, *Br. J. Haematol.*, 44, 511, 1980.

113. Pietrzik, K., Concept of borderline vitamin deficiencies, in *Nutritional Status Assessment of Individuals and Population Groups*, Fidaza, F., Ed., Proceedings of a workshop of the Group of European Nutritionists held at Garada Lake, Italy, Institute of Nutrition and Food Science Perugia, 1984, 43.

114. Hages, M. and Pietrzick, K., Evaluation of the folacin status in children with consideration of the cobalamin and iron status, *Int. J. Vit. Nutr. Res.*, 55, 59, 1985.

115. Sage, R. E., Evaluation of a commercial radioassay for the simultaneous estimation of vitamin B-12 and folate, with subsequent derivation of the normal reference range, *J. Clin. Pathol.*, 37, 1327, 1984.

116. Kitay, D. Z., Hogan, W. J., Eberle, B., and Mynt, T., Neutrophil hypersegmentation and folic acid deficiency, *Am. J. Obset. Gynec.*, 104, 1163, 1969.

117. Simensen, R. J. and Rogers, R. C., Fragile -X syndrome, *Am. Family Phys.*, 39, 185, 1989.

118. Erbe, R. W. and Wang, J.–C. C., Folate metabolism in humans, *Am. J. Med. Genetics*, 17, 277, 1984.

119. Chanarin, I., The folates, in *Vitamins in Medicine*, 4th edition, Volume 1, Barker, B. M. and Bender, D. A., Eds., Heinemann Medical, Ltd., London, 1980, 247.

120. Davis, R. E., Clinical chemistry of folic acid, *Adv. Clin. Chem.*, 25, 233, 1986.

121. Clayton, P. T., Smith, I., Harding, B., Hyland, K., Leonard, J. V., Leeming, R. J., Subacute combined degeneration of the spinal cord, dementia and parkinsonism due to an inborn error of folate metabolism, *J. Neurol. Neurosurg. Psychiat.*, 49, 920, 1986.

122. Rowe, P. B., Inherited disorders of folate metabolism, in *The Metabolic Basis of Inherited Disease*, Stanbury, J. R., Wyngaarden, J. B., Fredrickson, D. C., Goldstein, J. L., and Brown, M. S., Eds., McGraw-Hill, New York, 1983, 498.

123. Hyland, K., Smith, I., Bottiglieri, T., Perry, T., Wendel, U., Clayton, P. T., and Leonard, J. V., Demyelination and decreased S-adenosylmethionine in 5,10-methylene tetrahydrofolate reductase deficiency, *Neurology*, 38, 459, 1988.

124. Kang, S.–S., Wong, P. W. K., Zhou, J., Sora, J., Lessick, M., Ruggie, N., and Greevich, G., Thermolabile methylenetetrahydrofolate reductase in patients with coronary artery disease, *Metabolism*, 37, 611, 1988.

125. Harpey, J. P., LeMoal, G., Zittoun, J., Follow-up in a child with 5,10-methylenetetrahydrofolate reductase deficiency, *J. Pediatr.*, 103, 1007, 1983.

126. Wendel, U. and Bremer, H. J., Betaine in the treatment of homocystinuria due to 5,10-methylenetetrahydrofolate reductase deficiency, *Eur. J. Pediatr.*, 142, 147, 1984.

127. Killmann, S.–A., Effect of deoxyuridine on incorporation of tritiated thymidine: difference between normablasts and megaloblasts, *Acta Med. Scand.*, 175, 483, 1964.

128. Petty, A. C. and Burman, J. F., New micro method for deoxyuridine suppression test, *J. Clin. Pathol.*, 39, 1155, 1986.

129. Metz, J., Kelly, A., Swett, V. C., Waxman, S., and Herbert, V., Deranged DNA synthesis by bone marrow from vitamin B-12 deficient humans, *Br. J. Haematol.*, 14, 575, 1968.

130. Metz, J., The deoxyuridine suppression test, *CRC Crit. Rev. Clin. Lab. Sci.*, 20, 205, 1984.

131. Das, K. C. and Hoffbrand, A. V., Lymphocyte transformation in megaloblastic anaemia: morphology and DNA synthesis, *Br. J. Haematol.*, 19, 459, 1970.

132. Das, K. C., Manusselis, C., and Herbert, V., Simplifying lymphocyte culture and the deoxyuridine suppression test by using whole blood (0.1 mL) instead of separated lymphocytes, *Clin. Chem.*, 26, 72, 1980.

133. Das, K. C. and Herbert, V., The lymphocyte as a marker of part nutritional status: persistence of abnormal lymphocyte deoxyuridine (dU) suppression test and chromosomes in patients with past deficiency of folate and vitamin B-12, *Br. J. Haematol.*, 38, 219, 1978.

134. Das, K. C., Herbert, V., Colman, N., and Longo, D. C., Unmasking covert folate deficiency in iron-deficient subjects with neutrophil hypersegmentation: dU suppression test on lymphocytes and bone marrow, *Br. J. Haematol.*, 39, 357, 1978.

135. Tamura, T., Soong, S.–J., Sauberlich, H. E., Hatch, K. D., Cole, P., and Butterworth, C. E. Jr., Evaluation of the deoxyuridine suppression test by using whole blood samples from folic acid-supplemented subjects, *Am. J. Clin. Nutr.*, 51, 80, 1990.

136. Das, K. C. and Herbert, V., *In vitro* DNA synthesis by megaloblastic bone marrow: Effect of folates and cobalamins on thymidine incorporation and *de novo* thymidylate synthesis, *Am. J. Hematol.*, 31, 11, 1989.

137. Assessment of the folate nutritional status of the U.S. population based on data collected in the second national health and nutrition survey, 1976–1980, Senti, F. R. and Pilch, S. M., Eds., Federation of American Societies for Experimental Biology, Bethesda, MD, 1984.

138. Anderson, S. A. and Talbot, J. M., A review of folate intake, methodology, and status, Life Sciences Federation of American Societies for Experimental Biology, Bethesda, MD, 1981.

139. Colman, N., Laboratory assessment of folate status, *Clin. Lab. Med.*, 1, 775, 1981.

140. Food and Nutrition Board, National Research Council, *Folic Acid: Biochemistry and Physiology in Relation to the Human Nutrition Requirements*, National Academy of Sciences, Washington D.C., 1977.

141. Wichramasinghe, S. N. and Saundrs, J., Correlations between the deoxyuridine-suppressed value and some conventional haematological parameters in patients with folate or vitamin B-12 deficiency, *Scand. J. Haematol.*, 16, 121, 1976.

142. Armstrong, P., Rae, P. W. H., Gray, W. M., and Spence, A. A., Nitrous oxide and formiminoglutamic acid: excretion in surgical patients and anaesthetists, *Br. J. Anaesthesia*, 66, 163, 1991.

143. Tabor, H. and Wyngarden, L., A method for the determination of formiminoglutamic acid in urine, *J. Clin. Invest.*, 37, 824, 1958.
144. Today's tests: histidine loading (FIGlu excretion) test, *Br. Med. J.*, 1, 100, 1969.
145. Zalusky, R. and Herbert, V., Urinary formiminoglutamic acid a test of folic acid deficiency, *Lancet*, 2, 108, 1962.
146. Chanarin, I., Studies on urinary formiminoglutamic acid excretion, *Proc. R. Soc. Med.*, 57, 384, 1964.
147. Ball, G. F. M., Folate, in *Bioavailability and Analysis of Vitamins in Foods*, Chapman & Hall, New York, 1998, 439.
148. Ball, G. F. M., *Water-Soluble Vitamin Assays in Human Nutrition*, Chapman & Hall, New York, 1994.
149. Wickramasinghe, S. N. and Saunders, J. E., Results of three years' experience with the deoxyuridine suppression test, *Acta Haemat.*, 58, 193, 1977.
150. McGown, E. L., Lewis, C. M., Dong, M. H., and Sauberlich, H. E., Results with commercial radioassay kits compared with microbiological assay of folate in serum and whole-blood, *Clin. Chem.*, 24, 2186, 1978.
151. Dawson, D. W., Fish, D. I., Frew, I. D. O., Roome, T., and Tilston, I., Laboratory diagnosis of megaloblastic anemia: current methods assessed by external quality assurance trials, *J. Clin. Pathol.*, 40, 393, 1987.
152. Gilois, C. R. and Dunbar, D. R., Measurement of low serum and red cell folate levels: a comparison of analytical methods, *Med. Lab. Sci.*, 44, 33, 1987.
153. Brown, R. D., Uhr, E., Watman, R., Hughs, W., and Arnold, B., The impact of the QAP survey on the performance of red cell folate assays, *Pathology*, 23, 365, 1991.
154. Shane, B., Tamura, T., and Stokstad, E. L. R., Folate assay: a comparison of radioassay and microbiological methods, *Clin. Chim Acta*, 100, 13, 1980.
155. Brown, R. D., Jun, R., Hughes, W., Watman, R., Arnold, B., and Kronenberg, H., Red cell folate assays: some answers to current problems with radioassay variability, *Pathology*, 22, 82, 1990.
156. Stokstad, E. L. R., Isolation of a nucleotide essential for the growth of *Lactobacillus casei*, *J. Biol. Chem.*, 139, 475, 1941.
157. Teply, L. J. and Evehjem, C. A., The titrimetric determination of "*Lactobacillus casei factor*" and "folic acid", *J. Biol. Chem.*, 157, 303, 1945.
158. Krumdieck, C. L., Tamura, T., and Eto, I., Synthesis and analysis of the pteroylpolyglutamates, *Vitam. Horm.*, 40, 45, 1983.
159. Tamura, T., Determination of food folate, *Nutr. Biochem.*, 9, 285, 1998.
160. Cooperman, J. M., Microbiological assay of folic acid activity in serum and whole blood, *Methods Enzymol.*, Part B, 18, 629, 1971.
161. Bird, O. D. and McGlohon, V. M., Differential assays of folic acid in animal tissues, in *Analytical Microbiological*, Volume 2, Kavanagh, F., Ed., Academic Press, New York, 1972, 409.
162. Grossowicz, N., Waxman, S., and Schreiber, C., Cryoprotected *Lactobacillus casei*: An approach to standardization of microbiological assay of folic acid in serum, *Clin. Chem.*, 27, 745, 1981.
163. Wilson, S. D. and Horne, D. W., Use of glycerol-cryoprotected *Lactobacillus casei* for microbiological assay of folic acid, *Clin. Chem.*, 28, 1198, 1982.
164. Newman, E. M. and Tsai, J. F., Microbiological analysis of 5-formyltetrahydrofolic acid and other folates using an automatic 96-well plate reader, *Anal. Biochem.*, 154, 509, 1986.
165. Horne, D. W. and Patterson, D., *Lactobacillus casei* microbiological assay of folic acid derivatives in 96-well microtiter plates, *Clin. Chem.*, 34, 2357, 1988.
166. Horne, D. W., Microbiological assays of folate in 96-well microtiter plates, *Methods Enzymol.*, 281, 38, 1997.
167. Wilson, S. D. and Horne, D. W., Evaluation of ascorbic acid in protecting labile folic acid derivatives, *Proc. Natl. Acad. Sci.*, 80, 6500, 1983.
168. Molloy, A. M. and Scott, J. M., Microbiological assay for serum, plasma, and red cell folate using cryopreserved, microtiter plate method, *Methods Enzymol.*, 281, 43, 1997.
169. O'Broin, S. and Kelleher, B., Microbiological assay on microtitire plates of folate in serum and red cells, *J. Clin. Pathol.*, 45, 344, 1992.

170. Gilois, C. R., Stone, J., Lai, A. P., and Wierzbicki, A. S., Effect of haemolysate preparation on measurement of red cell folate by a radioisotopic method, *J. Clin. Pathol.*, 43, 160, 1990.

171. Stampfer, M. J. and Willett, W. C., Homocysteine and marginal vitamin deficiency, The importance of adequate vitamin intake, *JAMA*, 270, 2726, 1993.

172. Selhub, J., Jacques, P. F., Wilson, P. W. F., Rush, D., and Rosenberg, I. H., Vitamin status and intake as primary determinants of homocysteinemia in an elderly population, *JAMA*, 270, 2693, 1993.

173. Frelut, M. L., de Courcy, G. P., Christides, J.–P., Blot, P., and Navarro, J., Relationship between maternal folate status and fetal hypotrophy in a population with a good socio-economical level, *Int. J. Vit. Nutr. Res.*, 65, 267, 1995.

174. McParthin, J., Halligan, A., Scott, J. M., Darling, M., and Weir, D. G., Accelerated folate breakdown in pregnancy, *Lancet*, 341, 148, 1993.

175. Jacob, R. A., Gretz, D. M., Taylor, P. C., James, S. J., Pogribony, I. P., Miller, B. J., Henning, S. M., and Swendseid, M. E., Moderate folate depletion increases plasma homocysteine and decreases lymphocyte DNA methylation in postmenopausal women, *J. Nutr.*, 128, 1204, 1998.

176. Jacob, R. A., Pianalto, F. S., Henning, S. H., Zhang, J. Z., and Swendseid, M. E., *In vivo* methylation capacity is not impaired in healthy men during short-term dietary folate and methyl group restriction, *J. Nutr.*, 125, 1495, 1995.

177. Jacob, R. A., Wu, M. M., Henning, S. M., and Swendseid, M. E., Homocysteine increases as folate decreases in plasma of healthy men during short-term dietary folate and methyl group restriction, *J. Nutr.*, 124, 1072, 1994.

178. Glynn, S. A. and Abanes, D., Folate and cancer: a review of the literature, *Nutr. Cancer*, 22, 101, 1994.

179. Picciano, M. F., Folate nutrition in infancy, in *Folic Acid Metabolism in Health and Disease*, Picciano, M. F., Stokstad, E. L. R., and Gregory, J. F. III, Eds., Wiley-Liss, New York, 1990, 237.

180. Picciano, M. F., Folate nutrition in lactation, in *Folate in Health and Disease*, Bailey, L. B., Ed., Marcel Dekker, New York, 1995, 153.

181. Clark, A. J., Mossholder, S., and Gates, R., Folacin status in adolescent females, *Am. J. Clin. Nutr.*, 46, 302, 1987.

182. Grinblat, J., Folate status in the aged, *Clinics in Geriatric Med.*, 1, 711, 1985.

183. Picciano, M. F., Green, T., and O'Connor, D. L., The folate status of women and health, *Nutr. Today*, 29, 20, 1994.

184. Shojania, A. M., Folic acid and vitamin B-12 deficiency in pregnancy and in the neonatal period, *Clinics in Perinatology*, 11, 433, 1984.

185. Lowenstein, F. W., Nutritional status of the elderly in the United States of America, 1971–1974, *J. Am. Coll. Nutr.*, 1, 165, 1982.

186. Hanger, H. C., Sainsbury, R., Gilchrist, N. L., Beard, M. E. J., and Duncan, J. M., A community study of vitamin B-12 and folate levels in the elderly, *J. Am. Geriatr. Soc.*, 39, 1155, 1991.

187. Basu, T. K., Donald, E. A., Hargreaves, J. A., Thompson, G. W., Overton, T. R., Chao, E., and Petersons, D., Vitamin B-12 and folate status of a selected group of free-living older persons, *J. Nutr. for the Elderly*, 11, 5, 1992.

188. Garry, P. J., Goodwin, J. S., and Hunt, W. C., Folate and vitamin B-12 status in a healthy elderly population, *J. Am. Geriatr. Soc.*, 32, 719, 1984.

189. Senti, F. R. and Pilch, S. M., Analysis of folate data from the Second National Health and Nutrition Examination Survey (NHANES II), *J. Nutr.*, 115, 1398, 1985.

190. Shane, B. and Stokstad, E. L. R., Vitamin B-12 – folate interrelationship, *Annu. Rev. Nutr.*, 5, 115, 1985.

191. Halsted, C. H., Intestinal absorption of dietary folates, in *Folic Acid Metabolism in Health and Disease*, Picciano, M. F., Stokstad, E. L. R. and Gregory, J. F. III, Eds., Wiley-Liss, New York, 1990, 23.

192. Selhub, J., Jacques, P. F., Boston A. G., D'Agostino, R. B., Wilson, P. W. F., Belanger, A. J., O'Leary, D. H., Wolf, P. A., Schaefer, E. J., and Rosenberg, I. H., Association between plasma homocysteine concentrations and extracranial carotid-artery stenosis, *N. Engl. J. Med.*, 332, 286, 1995.

193. Elwood, P. L., Shinton, N. K., Wilson, C. L. et al., Hemoglobin, vitamin B-12, and folate levels in the elderly, *Br. J. Haematol.*, 21, 557, 1971.
194. Bailey, L. B., Wagner, P. A., Jernigan, J. A. et al., Folacin and iron status of an elderly population, *Fed. Proc.*, 41, 951, 1982 (Abstract).
195. Vir, S. C. and Love, A. H. G., Nutritional status of institutionalized and noninstitutionalized aged in Belfast, Northern Ireland, *Am. J. Clin. Nutr.*, 32, 1934, 1979.
196. Evans, D. M. D., Pathy, M. S., Saneskin, N. G., Anemia in geriatric patients, *Gerontol. Clin.*, 10, 228, 1968.
197. Varadi, S. and Elwis, A., Folic acid deficiency in the elderly, *Br. Med. J.*, 2, 410, 1966.
198. Carney, M. W. P., Charg, T. K. N., and Launly, M. et al., Red cell folate concentrations in psychiatric patients, *J. Affective Disord.*, 19, 207, 1990.
199. Joosten, E., van den Berg, A., Riezler, R., Naurath, H. J., Lindenbaum, J., Stabler, S. P., and Allen, R. H., Metabolic evidence that deficiencies of vitamin B-12 (cobalamin), folate, and vitamin B-6 occur commonly in elderly people, *Am. J. Clin. Nutr.*, 58, 468, 1993.
200. Tamura, T., Freeberg, L. E., and Cornwell, P. E., Inhibition by EDTA of growth of *Lactobacillus casei* in the folate microbiological assay and its reversal by added manganese or iron, *Clin. Chem.*, 36, 1993, 1990 (Abstract).
201. Butterworth, C. E. Jr., Folate status, women's health, pregnancy outcome, and cancer, *Am. Coll. Nutr.*, 12, 438, 1993.
202. Russell, R. M., Implications of gastric atrophy for vitamin and mineral nutriture, in *Nutrition and Aging*, Hutchinson, M. L. and Murro, H. N., Eds., Academic Press, New York, 1986, 59.
203. McCully, K. S., Vascular pathology of homocysteinemia: implications for the pathogenesis of arteriosclerosis, *Am. J. Pathol.*, 56, 111, 1969.
204. Tamura, T., Goldenberg, R. L., Johnston, K. E., Cliver, S. P., Hoffman, H. J., Serum concentrations of zinc, folate, vitamin A and E, and proteins, and their relationships to pregnancy outcome, *Acta Obstet. Gynecol. Scand.*, 76, 63, 1997.
205. Worthington-White, D. A., Behnke, M., and Gross, S., Premature infants require additional folate and vitamin B-12 to reduce the severity of the anemia of prematurity, *Am. J. Clin. Nutr.*, 60, 930, 1994.
206. Goldenberg, R. L., Tamura, T., Cliver, S. P., Cutter, G. R., Hoffman, H. J., and Copper, R. L., Serum folate and fetal growth retardation: A matter of compliance, *Obestet. Gynecol.*, 79, 719, 1992.
207. Scholl, T. O., Hediger, M. L., Schall, J. I., Khoo, C. –S., and Fischer, R. L., Dietary and serum folate: their influence on the outcome of pregnancy, *Am. J. Clin. Nutr.*, 63, 520, 1996.
208. Caudill, M. A., Cruz, A. C., Gregory, J. F. III, Hutson, A. D., and Bailey, L. B., Folate status response to controlled folate intake in pregnant women, *J. Nutr.*, 127, 2363, 1997.
209. Tsui, J. C. and Nordstrom, J. W., Folate status of adolescents: effects of folic acid supplementation, *J. Am. Diet. Assoc.*, 90, 1551, 1990.
210. O'Keefe, C. A., Bailey, L. B., Thomas, E. A., Hofler, S. A., Davis, B. A., Cerda, J. J., and Gregory, J. F. III, Controlled dietary folate affects folate status in nonpregnant women, *J. Nutr.*, 125, 2717, 1995.
211. Blundell, E. L., Matthews, J. H., Allen, S. M., Middelton, A. M., Morris, J. E., and Wickramasinge, S. N., Importance of low serum vitamin B-12 and red cell folate concentrations in elderly hospital patients, *J. Clin. Pathol.*, 38, 1179, 1985.
212. Lewis, C. A., Pancharuniti, N., and Sauberlich, H. E., Plasma folate adequacy as determined by homocysteine level, *Ann. N.Y. Acad. Sci.*, 669, 360, 1992.
213. Cuskelly, G. J., McNulty, H., and Scott, J. M., Effect of increasing dietary folate on red-cell folate: implications for prevention of neural tube defects, *Lancet*, 347, 657, 1996.
214. Lussier-Cacan, S., Xhignesse, M., Piolot, A., Selhub, J., Davignon, J., and Genest, J. Jr., Plasma total homocysteine in healthy subjects: sex-specific relation with biological traits, *Am. J. Clin. Nutr.*, 64, 587, 1996.
215. Kirke, P. N., Molloy, A. M., Daly, L. E., Burke, H., Weir, D. G., and Scott, J. M., Maternal plasma folate and vitamin B-12 are independent risk factors for neural tube defects, *Quarterly J. Med.*, 86, 703, 1993.

216. Kretsch, M. J., Sauberlich, H. E., and Skala, J. H., Nutritional status assessment of Marines before and after the installation of the "Multi-Restaurant" food service system at the Twenty-nine Palms Marine Corps Base, CA, Letterman Army Institute Report No. 192, December, 1984.

217. Roe, D. A., Evaluation of publicly available scientific evidence regarding certain nutrient-disease relationships. 1. Folic acid and neural tube defects, Life Sciences Research Office, Federation of American Societies for Experimental Biology, Bethesda, MD, December, 1991.

218. Smithells, R. W., Sheppard, S., Schorah, C. J., Seller, M. J., Nevin, N. C., Harris, R., Read, A. P., and Fielding, D. W., Apparent prevention of neural tube defects by periconceptional vitamin supplementation, *Arch. Dis. Child.*, 56, 911, 1981.

219. Laurence, K. M., James, N., Miller, M. H., Tennant, G. B., and Campbell, H., Double-blind randomized controlled trial of folate treatment before conception to prevent recurrence of neural-tube defects, *Br. Med. J.*, 282, 1509, 1981.

220. WHO Report, Nutritional anemias: Report of a WHO Group of Experts, Geneva, Switzerland, October 11–15, 1971, WHO technical report series no. 503, Geneva, Switzerland, 1972.

221. Centers for Disease Control, Recommendations for use of folic acid to reduce the number of cases of spina bifida and other neural tube defects, Atlanta, *MNWR (Morbidity and Mortality Weekly Report)*, 41, 1, 1992.

222. Rush, D., Periconceptional folate and neural tube defect, *Am. J. Clin. Nutr.*, 59, 511S, 1994.

223. Raiten, D. J. and Fisher, K. D., Assessment of folate methodology used in the third National Health and Nutrition Examination Survey (NHANES-III, 1988-1994), *J. Nutr.*, 125, 1371S, 1995.

224. van den Berg, H., Finglas, P. M., and Bates, C., FLAIR intercomparisons on serum and red cell folate, *Int. J. Vit. Nutr. Res.*, 64, 288, 1994.

225. Jacobsen, D., Determinants of hyperhomocysteinemia: a matter of nature or nurture, *Am. J. Clin. Nutr.*, 64, 641, 1996.

226. Wilcken, D. E. L., Dudman, N. P. B., Tyrrell, P. A., and Robertson, M. R., Folic acid lowers elevated plasma homocysteine in chronic renal insufficiency: possible implications for prevention of vascular disease, *Metabolism*, 37, 697, 1988.

227. Nygard, O., Nordrehaug, J. E., Refsum, H., Ueland, P. M., Farstad, M., and Vollset, S. E., Plasma homocysteine levels and mortality in patients with coronary artery disease, *N. Engl. J. Med.*, 337, 230, 1997.

228. Morrison, H. I., Schaubel, D., Desmeules, M., and Wigle, D. T., Serum folate and risk of fatal coronary heart disease, *JAMA*, 275, 1893, 1996.

229. Pancharuniti, N., Lewis, C. A., Sauberlich, H. E., Perkins, L. L., Go, R. C. P., Alvarez, J. O., Macaluso, M., Acton, R. T., Copeland, R. B., Cousins, A. L., Gore, T. B., Cornwell, P. E., and Roseman, J. M., Plasma homocyst(e)ine, folate, and vitamin B-12 concentrations and risk for early-onset coronary heart disease, *Am. J. Clin. Nutr.*, 59, 940, 1994.

230. Kang, S. S., Wong, P. W. K., and Malinow, M. R., Hyperhomocyst(e)inemia as a risk factor for occlusive vascular disease, *Annu. Rev. Nutr.*, 12, 279, 1992.

231. Kang, S. S., Wong, P. W. K., and Norusis, M., Homocysteinemia due to folate deficiency, *Metabolism*, 36, 458, 1987.

232. Kang, S.-S., Treatment of hyperhomocyst(e)inemia: physiological basis, *J. Nutr.*, 126, 1273S, 1996.

233. Ueland, P. M. and Refsum, H., Plasma homocysteine, a risk factor for vascular disease: plasma levels in health, disease, and drug therapy, *L. Clin. Med.*, 114, 473, 1989.

234. Ueland, P. M., Refsum, H., Stabler, S. P., Malinow, M. R., Anderson, A., and Allen, R. H., Total homocysteine in plasma or serum: methods and clinical applications, *Clin. Chem.*, 39, 1764, 1993.

235. Allen, R. H., Stabler, S. P., Savage, D. G., and Lindenbaum, J., Metabolic abnormalities in cobalamin (vitamin B-12) and folate deficiencies, *FASEB J.*, 7, 1344, 1993.

236. Jagerstad, M. and Pietrzik, K., Folate, *Internat. J. Vit. Nutr. Res.*, 63, 285, 1993.

237. Hoffbrand, A. F. and Newcombe, B. F. A., Leucocyte folate in vitamin B-12 and folate deficiency and in leukemia, *Br. J. Haematol*, 13, 954, 1967.

238. Vilter, R. W., Will, J. J., Wright, T., and Rullman, D., Interrelationships of vitamin B-12, folic acid and ascorbic acid in the megaloblastic anemias, *Am. J. Clin. Nutr.*, 12, 130, 1963.

239. Hoffbrand, A. V., Newcombe, B. F. A., and Mollin, D. L., Method of assay of red cell folate activity and the value of the assay as a test for folate deficiency, *J. Clin. Pathol.*, 19, 17, 1966.
240. Sauberlich, H. E., Newer laboratory methods for assessing nutriture of selected B-complex vitamins, *Annu. Rev. Nutr.*, 4, 377, 1984.
241. Gunter, E. W. and Twite, D. B., Improved materials for long-term quality-control assessment of erythrocyte folate analysis, *Clin. Chem.*, 36, 2139, 1990.
242. Stabler, S. P., Marcell, P. D., Podell, E. R., Allen, R. H., Savage, D. G., and Lindenbaum, J., Elevation of total homocysteine in the serum of patients with cobalamin or folate deficiency detected by capillary gas chromatography-mass spectrometry, *J. Clin. Invest.*, 81, 466, 1988.
243. O'Broin, S. D., Kelleher, B. P., Davoren, A., and Gunter, E. W., Field-study screening of blood folate concentrations: specimen stability and finger-stick sampling, *Am. J. Clin. Nutr.*, 66, 1398, 1997.
244. Gunter, E. W., Bowman, B. A., Caudill, S. P., Twite, D. B., Adams, M. J., and Sampson, E. J., Results of an international round robin for serum and whole-blood folate, *Clin. Chem.*, 42, 1689, 1996.
245. O'Broin, S. D., Temperley, I. J., and Scott, J. M., Erythrocyte, plasma, and serum folate: specimen stability before micorbiological assay, *Clin. Chem.*, 26, 522, 1980.
246. Jacobsen, D. W., Serum and erythrocyte folates: a matter of life and premature death, *Clin. Chem.*, 42, 1579, 1996.
247. Bailey, L. B., Folate status assessment, *J. Nutr.*, 120, 1508, 1990.
248. Solomon, B. P. and Dude, C. T., Homocysteine determination in plasma, *Current Separations*, 17, 1, 1998.
249. Chanarin, I., The folates, in *Vitamins in Medicine*, Volume 1, Barker, B. M. and Bender, D. A., Eds., William Heinemann Medical Books, London, 1980, 247.
250. Mayer, E. L., Jacobsen, D. W., and Robinson, K., Homocysteine and coronary atherosclerosis, *J. Am. Coll. Cardiol.*, 27, 517, 1996.
251. Nygard, O., Vollset, S. E., Refsum, H., Stensvold, I., Tverdal, A., Nordrehaug, J. E., Ueland, P. M., and Kvale, G., Total plasma homocysteine and cardiovascular risk profile, *JAMA*, 274, 1526, 1995.
252. Nygard, O., Refsum, H., Ueland, P. M., and Vollset, S. E., Major lifestyle determinants of plasma total homocysteine distribution: the Hordaland Homocysteine Study, *Am. J. Clin. Nutr.*, 67, 263, 1998.
253. Selhub, J., Jacques, P. F., Bostom, A. G., D'Agonstino, R. B., Wilson, P. W. F., Belanger, A. J., O'Leary, D. H., Wolf, P. A., Rush, D., Schaefer, E. J., and Rosenberg, I. H., Relationship between plasma homocysteine, vitamin status and extracranial carotid-artery stenosis in the Framingham Study population, *J. Nutr.*, 126, 1258S, 1996.
254. Stampfer, M. J., Malinow, M. R., Willet, W. C., Newcomer, L. M., Upson, B., Ullmann, D., Tishler, P. V., and Hennekens, C. H., A prospective study of plasma homocyst(e)ine and risk of myocardial infarction in US physicians, *J. Am. Med. Assoc.*, 268, 877, 1992.
255. Brattstrom, L., Vitamins as homocysteine-lowering agents, *J. Nutr.*, 126, 1276S, 1996.

Vitamin B-12 (Cyanocobalamin, Corrinoids)

Converting metric units to International System (SI) units:

pg/mL × 0.7378 = pmol/L

pmol/L × 1.3554 = pg/mL

molecular weight: 1355.4 (cyanocobalamin)

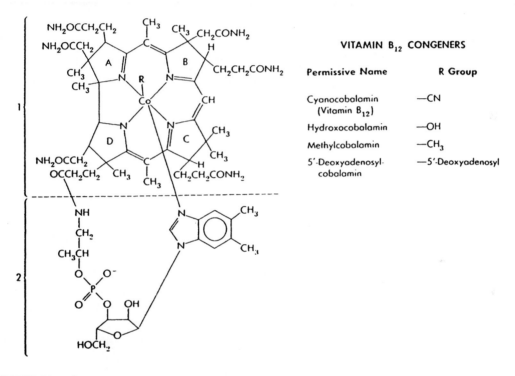

VITAMIN B_{12} CONGENERS	
Permissive Name	**R Group**
Cyanocobalamin (Vitamin B_{12})	—CN
Hydroxocobalamin	—OH
Methylcobalamin	—CH_3
5′-Deoxyadenosyl-cobalamin	—5′-Deoxyadenosyl

FIGURE 24
Structure of vitamin B-12.

Vitamin B-12 and cobalamin are used as a generic descriptor for all corrinoids that can be converted to 5′-deoxyadenosylcobalamin or methylcobalamin. Cyanocobalamin is the commercially available form of vitamin B-12. This form is stable and readily converted in the body to metabolically active vitamin B-12.

History of Vitamin B-12

The history of vitamin B-12 has been both interesting and perplexing. In 1922, an anemia was described that was considered to be associated with a digestive disorder. This condition

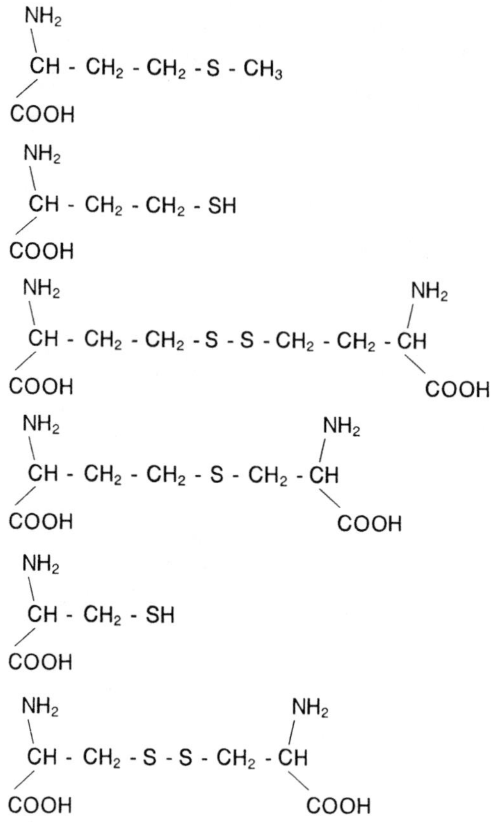

$$\begin{array}{l} NH_2 \\ | \\ CH - CH_2 - CH_2 - S - CH_3 \\ / \\ COOH \end{array} \qquad \text{methionine}$$

$$\begin{array}{l} NH_2 \\ | \\ CH - CH_2 - CH_2 - SH \\ / \\ COOH \end{array} \qquad \text{homocysteine}$$

$$\begin{array}{l} NH_2 \qquad\qquad\qquad\qquad NH_2 \\ | \qquad\qquad\qquad\qquad\quad | \\ CH - CH_2 - CH_2 - S - S - CH_2 - CH_2 - CH \\ / \qquad\qquad\qquad\qquad\qquad\qquad\quad \backslash \\ COOH \qquad\qquad\qquad\qquad\qquad\qquad COOH \end{array} \qquad \text{homocystine}$$

$$\begin{array}{l} NH_2 \qquad\qquad\qquad NH_2 \\ | \qquad\qquad\qquad\quad | \\ CH - CH_2 - CH_2 - S - CH_2 - CH \\ / \qquad\qquad\qquad\qquad\qquad \backslash \\ COOH \qquad\qquad\qquad\qquad COOH \end{array} \qquad \text{cystathionine}$$

$$\begin{array}{l} NH_2 \\ | \\ CH - CH_2 - SH \\ / \\ COOH \end{array} \qquad \text{cysteine}$$

$$\begin{array}{l} NH_2 \qquad\qquad\qquad NH_2 \\ | \qquad\qquad\qquad\quad | \\ CH - CH_2 - S - S - CH_2 - CH \\ / \qquad\qquad\qquad\qquad\quad \backslash \\ COOH \qquad\qquad\qquad\qquad COOH \end{array} \qquad \text{cystine}$$

FIGURE 25
Structures of methionine metabolites.

became known as Addisonian pernicious anemia.[214] In 1926, Minot and Murphy established that a dietary factor was associated with this megloblastic anemia.[215] Subsequently, Castle and Ham stated that, "The nutritional defect in such patients is apparently caused by the failure of a reaction which occurs in the normal individual between a substance in the food (extrinsic factor) and a substance in the normal gastric secretion (intrinsic factor)."[214,216] In 1944, a red crystalline substance was isolated by Rickes et al.[217] and termed vitamin B-12. It was soon found that only microgram quantities of the vitamin were required to produce a positive hematologic response in pernicious anemia patients.

Function of Vitamin B-12 (Cobalamin)

Vitamin B-12 serves as the cofactor for two enzymatic reactions:[42,90,91,95,97] (1) L-methylmalonyl-CoA mutase, an adenosylcobalamin-dependent enzyme, converts L-methylmalonyl-CoA to succinyl-CoA. In a vitamin B-12 deficiency, L-methylmalonyl-CoA accumulates resulting in its cleavage by a specific hydrolase to methylmalonic acid. This reaction is essential for the metabolism of odd-chain length fatty acids. (2) The methylation of homocysteine by methionine synthase requires the availability of a methyl group from N_5-methyl-tetrahydrofolate and methylcobalamin as a coenzyme (Figure 26). Impairment

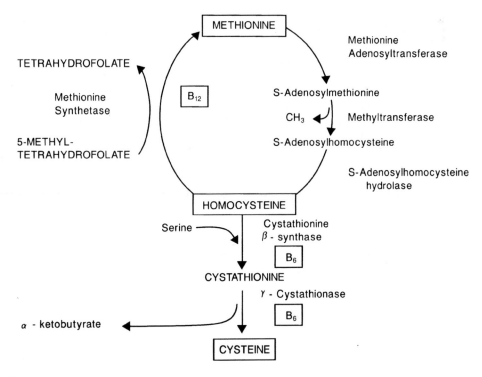

FIGURE 26
Participation of vitamin B-12, folate, and vitamin B-6 in the metabolism of methionine and homocysteine.[90] (With permission.)

of this reaction affects DNA synthesis that may lead to macrocytic megaloblastic anemia. In a vitamin B-12 deficiency, homocysteine concentrations rise in the serum.

The majority of the vitamin B-12 is stored in the liver where it is present as 5'-deoxyadenosylcobalamin (65 to 75%), hydroxycobalamin (20–30%), and methylcobalamin (1–5%).[192] The predominant form in plasma is methylcobalamin (135–425 pmol/L).

Sources of Vitamin B-12

Microorganisms are the source of all vitamin B-12 in nature. Hence, all plants and plant food are devoid of vitamin B-12 unless contaminated by microorganisms. Consequently, animal products serve as the virtual sole source of vitamin B-12 in the food supply:[192] meats contributed 69%, dairy items 21%, and eggs 8.5%. Cereals, fortified with vitamin B-12, provide only a small amount of the vitamin (1.6%). Vitamin B-12 is quite stable to heat and to the usual cooking practices.

Vitamin B-12 Deficiency

Vitamin B-12 deficiency develops slowly over a period of time. The deficiency may be reflected in fatigue or generalized weakness, indigestion, glossitis, stomatitis, pallor, diarrhea, or depression.[89] Unexplained neuropsychiatric signs or symptoms may be associated with a vitamin B-12 deficiency.[90,91,197] The most common cause is the result of malabsorption of the vitamin due to a lack of gastric production of intinsic factor; namely, pernicious anemia. An increased risk of vitamin B-12 deficiency may result from ileal disease or resection, gastrectomy, tropical sprue, gluten enteropathy, or pancreatic insufficiency.

Vitamin B-12 (cobalamin) deficiency results in a megaloblastic anemia which is identical to the megaloblastic anemia that results from a folacin deficiency.[198] Megaloblastic anemia is characterized by the presence in the blood of large, immature, and dysfunctional red and white blood cells.[202] In addition, a vitamin B-12 deficiency may result in neurologic symptoms even in the absence of anemia.[50,200,201] Vitamin B-12 deficiency, metabolism, requirement, and assessments have been the topic of numerous reviews.[90,91,155,189,199]

Occurrence of Vitamin B-12 Deficiency

In the Elderly

Many investigators have reported an increased prevalence of low serum vitamin B-12 concentrations in the elderly.[31,32,42,47-56,88,89,206,222] As documented by elevated plasma concentrations of methylmalonic acid, up to 15% of the elderly population had a vitamin B-12 deficiency.[42] A detailed study was conducted as to prevalence of vitamin B-12 deficiency in the 548 surviving members of the original Framingham Study.[31] Low serum vitamin B-12 concentrations (< 258 pmol/L) were found in 40.5% of the subjects. For 29 of these subjects, serum concentrations of under 148 pmol/L were found. Elevated serum methylmalonic acid and elevated serum total homocysteine concentrations confirmed, in a functional manner, the presence of vitamin B-12 deficiency in this elderly group.

From survey data, it has been estimated that 2 to 5 million Americans over 60 years have subnormal serum vitamin B-12 concentrations.[40] Vitamin B-12 deficiency in the elderly population has been documented by the presence of elevated serum methylmalonic acid levels and by the total homocysteine information.[42] Stabler et al.[42] found that 60 to 66% of the elderly subjects with elevated serum total homocysteine concentrations also had elevated serum methylmalonic acid concentrations. These subjects may be completely free of hematologic abnormalities.

Other Countries

Information is limited as to the occurrence of vitamin B-12 deficiency in developing countries.[37,38] World Health Organization reports indicate that the prevalence of vitamin B-12 deficiency was low. New information indicates that vitamin B-12 deficiency may be more prevalent than had been realized.

Sweden and United Kingdom

In Sweden and the United Kingdom, vitamin B-12 deficiency as a result of impaired absorption due to a lack of intrinsic factor (pernicious anemia) occurs in nearly 1% of the individuals over the age of 60 years.[87]

Rural Mexico

A study was conducted on rural Mexican children, adults and lactating women on their vitamin B-12 status.[33,74] Based on plasma vitamin B-12 concentrations, 19% to 41% of the subjects had deficient vitamin B-12 levels. The vitamin B-12 deficiency was probably caused by malabsorption of vitamin B-12. This was supported by the finding of a high prevalence of low holotransabalamin II concentrations in the groups studied.[33] The radio-assay for vitamin B-12 used purified hog intrinsic factor and thereby only biological active vitamin B-12 was measured.[74]

Zimbabwe

In Zimbabwe, vitamin B-12 deficiency is the primary cause of megaloblastic anemia.[39] In a study of 144 consecutive patients with megalablastic anemia, 86% were diagnosed with vitamin B-12 deficiency. Neurological dysfunction (70%) and elevated serum concentrations of methylmalonic acid and homocysteine (98%) were found in the majority of the patients.

Guatemala

In a study of a rural Guatemalan village, 38% of the elderly population of ≥ 60 years of age were found to have vitamin B-12 deficiency.[41] Of the elderly men and women, 18% were classified as at risk of anemia.

Vegetarian/Vegan

Vegetarian diets have long been recognized to be deficient in vitamin B-12.[6-8] A strict vegetarian diet (vegan) is devoid of vitamin B-12 since plants do not produce vitamin B-12. Only contamination with vitamin B-12 synthesizing bacteria can provide their vitamin B-12 needs.[6] Fermented foods and seaweed (algae) have been considered a source of vitamin B-12.[11,12] However, most of the apparent vitamin B-12 in these sources are analogues of the true vitamin B-12.[6] In one study, plasma vitamin B-12 concentrations of vegans were reported as 193 (mean) pmol/L, compared to 311 (mean) pmol/L for omnivorous controls.[12] Occasionally cases of vitamin B-12 deficiency with anemia or neurological abnormalities are observed.[6,9,10] Infants born of vegetarian mothers, may suffer from a vitamin B-12 deficiency.[61,62] Vitamin B-12 therapy corrected the condition. Vitamin B-12 deficiency may occur in non-vegetarians due to poor food choices.[14]

Nitrous Oxide and Vitamin B-12

Nitrous oxide gas has been widely used as an anesthetic.[1-5] Studies have suggested that nitrous oxide oxidizes vitamin B-12 and thereby interferes with the function of vitamin B-12.[3,91] Patients who received nitrous oxide during surgery were found to have had megaloblastic bone-marrow aspirates and abnormal dU suppression tests.[3] In another study,[1] twelve patients anesthetized with nitrous oxide had postoperative increased plasma levels of homocysteine and folate, indicating vitamin B-12 inactivation. The patients returned to normal within several days.

In a study of 21 dentists who regularly used nitrous oxide in their surgeries, serum vitamin B-12 and folate concentrations were within normal limits.[2] However, three of the dentists were found to have abnormal deoxyuridine tests and abnormal white blood cells when bone marrow aspirates were examined. In another study, Koblin et al.[5] studied the exposure of 23 surgical patients to nitrous oxide. Using urinary excretion of formiminoglutamic acid (FIGLU) as markers of vitamin B-12 deficiency, nitrous oxide exposure produced only a transient increase in FIGLU excretion. Without a histidine load, the FIGLU test is a comparatively insensitive marker for vitamin B-12 deficiency.

Laboratory Methods for Assessment of Vitamin B-12 Status

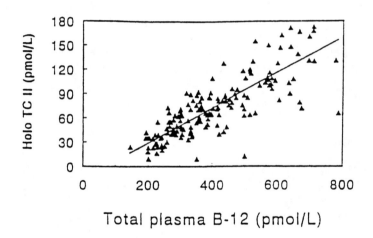

Total plasma B-12 (pmol/L)

FIGURE 27
Correlation between total vitamin B-12 and holotranscobalamin II in children (n = 167).[223] (With permission.)

Vitamin B-12 (Cobalamin) Assays

Serum concentrations of vitamin B-12 provide information as to the vitamin B-12 nutritional status. Low body stores of vitamin B-12 are associated with low serum levels of the vitamin. Vitamin B-12 measurements may be performed by either microbiological assays or by radioassay techniques.[208,210] The availability of suitable quality controls remains a problem.

Vitamin B-12 Radioassay Procedures

Some of the early vitamin B-12 radioassay procedures failed to detect certain patients with pernicious anemia.[72-75,93,96,208,209,218] Subsequent modifications in the commercial radioassay kits appear to have eliminated this problem[72-75,93,96,186] (e.g., Chiron Diagnostic Corp.,

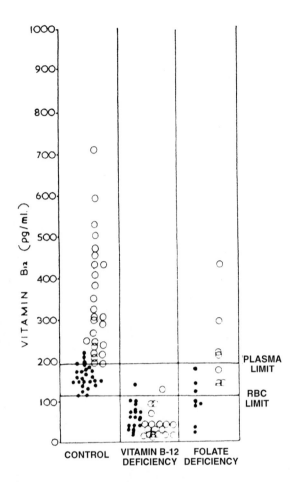

FIGURE 28

Plasma and erythrocyte vitamin B-12 concentrations in normal subjects and in patients with vitamin B-12 deficiency or folacin deficiency (From Omer et al.[191] With permission.)

Norwood, MA; ICN Pharmaceuticals (Diagnostics), Irvine, CA; BioRad Lab., Hercules, CA; DiaSorin, Stillwater, MN). Commercial assay kits are also available that allow for the simultaneous measurement in serum of both vitamin B-12 and folacin (e.g., Chiron Diagnostics Corp., Norwood, MA; BioRad, Hercules, CA; ICN Pharmaceuticals, Irvine, CA). With the ready availability of the commercial kits, the radioassay for vitamin B-12 has proven simple, reliable, and convenient. However, since the kits use ^{57}Co for the vitamin B-12 assay, the availability of a gamma counter is required and radioactive handling procedures applied. Serum or plasma (EDTA) samples may be used. Heparinized samples cannot be used because of interference of heparin in the vitamin B-12 assay. Quality controls are available from the kit manufacturer.

Plasma vitamin B-12 concentrations were measured by radioassay in 380 healthy men and in 204 healthy women.[98] The commercial radioassay kit of Chiron Diagnostic Corp. Norwood, MA, was used to measure the vitamin B-12 levels. The plasma vitamin B-12 concentration was found to be 238 ± 102 pmol/L in the men and 236 ± 116 pmol/L in the women.

A negative vitamin B-12 balance has been defined as a serum vitamin B-12 concentration of <222 pmol/L (<300 pg/mL).[106]

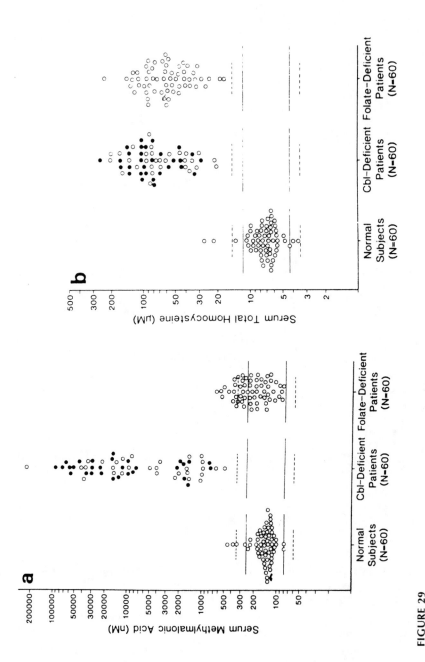

FIGURE 29

(a) Serum concentrations of methylmalonic acid in normal subjects and in vitamin B-12 or folate deficient patients.[128,132] (b) Serum concentrations of total homocysteine in normal subjects and in vitamin B-12 or folate deficient patients.[128,132] (With permission.)

Microbiological Assays for Vitamin B-12

Before the introduction of commercial radioassay kits for measuring vitamin B-12 concentrations in plasma, microbiological assays were used with the vitamin B-12-dependent *Euglena gracilis,*[154] *Escherichia coli,*[162] or *Lactobacillus leichmannii.*[156,170] With the current nomenclature, *Lactobacillus leichmannii* is now known as *Lactobacillus delbrueckii subsp. lactis* (ATCC 4797). Another strain of *L. delbruckii* used for vitamin B-12 assay is available as ATCC 7830. Microbiological assays have also been used for the measurement of vitamin B-12 in erythrocytes and whole blood.[179,191] However, measurements of vitamin B-12 in whole blood or in erythrocytes have no advantage over serum or plasma vitamin B-12 measurements. Just as for the vitamin B-12 radioassay procedures, heparinized plasma sample should not be used in the microbiological vitamin B-12 assays. For those familiar with microbiological assays, the microbial procedures have served well. However, the traditional vitamin B-12 microbiological assay was time-consuming, cumbersome, used test tubes, and required a relatively large sample volume. Moreover, microbial contamination needed to be avoided. In addition, the presence of antibiotics in the subjects serum may cause inhibition in the assay resulting in falsely low values.[157]

Subsequently these disadvantages have been overcome with the use of collistin sulfate resistant strain of *Lactobacillus leichmannii* (ATCC 43787; NCIB 12519).[158,161] The procedure was simplified by introducing the use of 96-well microtitre plates and the plates are read with an automatic plate reader in conjunction with a computerized data reduction program.[158] The vitamin B-12 assay medium has been available from Difco Laboratories, Detroit, MI. The inoculating culture is preserved as aliquots by cryopreservations.[159] Antibiotic interference in samples can be essentially eliminated by enzyme inactivation.[160] The microbiological assay provides an alternative to the use of a radioisotope procedure and the need for a gamma counter.

A number of studies have compared the vitamin B-12 microbiological assay with commercially available radioisotope dilution assay kits.[146,163-169] In general, the results obtained with the commercial radioassay kits agree closely with the microbiological assay results. In some instance, the radioassay values for serum vitamin B-12 were somewhat higher than those obtained with the microbiological assay.[164,168]

Serum Methylmalonic Acid Measurement

Serum methylmalonic acid concentrations are elevated with a deficiency of vitamin B-12, but not by a folate deficiency.[100,154] The lack of adenosylcobalamin blocks the conversion of methylmalonate-CoA to succinyl-CoA. Urinary excretion of methylmalonic acid also increases with vitamin B-12 deficiency. Serum levels of cystathionine are also increased in most subjects with a vitamin B-12 or folate deficiency.[63,92]

Urinary and serum methylmalonic acid levels are often used to screen individuals and populations for cobalamin (vitamin B-12) deficiency.[31,32,42-47,57-61,63-71] An increase in methylmalonic acid concentrations in serum or plasma appears to be an early if not the first indicator of a vitamin B-12 deficiency.[66,68,98] Measurement of serum methylmalonic acid have been useful in identifying subjects with a vitamin B-12 deficiency, even with a subclinical deficiency.[70,100]

Early methods for the measurement of methylmalonic acid in urine and serum lacked sensitivity and specificity. This has been overcome with the development of highly sensitive and specific methods utilizing gas chromatography-mass spectrometry techniques.[58-60,63,69]

Methylmalonic acid and homocysteine are stable in serum and urine for several years when stored at $-70°C$. Plasma total homocysteine levels have been reported to be elevated in over 90% of subjects with clinical vitamin B-12 deficiency or with folate deficiency.[63] Elevation in plasma methylmalonic acid is slightly more sensitive than the increase in total homocysteine in vitamin B-12 deficiency.[63] For diagnostic purpose, folate therapy does not correct an elevated methylmalonic acid nor an elevated total homocysteine in vitamin B-12 deficient subjects.[99] Methylmalonic acid concentrations in plasma are elevated in nearly all subjects with neurologic or hematologic abnormalities due to vitamin B-12 deficiency.[42] The elevated methylmalonic acid concentrations fall with cobalamin therapy.[50,60,63,97]

Elderly men and women were reported to have serum methylmalonic acid concentrations of 208 ± 162 nmol/L. Serum vitamin B-12 concentrations less than 221 pmol/ L (300 pg/mL) were considered vitamin B-12 deficient.[106,107] Out of 100 elderly men and women, 18 subjects had serum vitamin B-12 concentrations of less than 221 pmol/L.[100] Sixteen of the subjects had serum methylmalonic acid concentrations above 271 nmol/L. Methylmalonic acid concentrations above this indicate an inadequate vitamin B-12 status.

Based on the studies of Lindenbaum et al.,[31] the commonly used serum cutoffs for diagnosing vitamin B-12 deficiency are too low. They suggest the use of a cutoff of 258 pmol/L (350 pg/mL) of serum vitamin B-12.

Methylmalonic acid measurements of serum or urine are a more sensitive indicator of vitamin B-12 status than serum levels of the vitamin. Serum methylmalonic acid concentrations of <638 nmol/L were considered acceptable. A serum vitamin B-12 concentration of >250 pmol/L (350 pg/mL) was associated with this serum concentration of methylmalonic acid.[31]

Plasma/Serum Total Homocysteine (t Hcy)

Elevated plasma homocysteine concentrations have been considered an independent risk factor for vascular disease.[97-105, 108-118,122-135,219] Elevated fasting serum concentrations of homocysteine may be caused by a deficiency of folate, vitamin B-12, or vitamin B-6 and less frequent due to inborn errors of metabolism or to renal insufficiency.[6,43,44,61,68,70,71,97-105,141,153,204,211,212,219]

Fasting plasma total homocysteine concentration were measured in a group of healthy men ($n = 380$) and women ($n = 204$).[98] The men had plasma total homocysteine concentrations of 9.7 ± 4.9 μmol/L while women had a lower concentration of 7.4 ± 4.1 μmol/L.

Brattstrom et al.[204] found total plasma homocysteine concentrations of 11.5 ± 0.9 μmol/L ($n = 21$) in normal controls while the concentration of homocysteine of asymptomatic vitamin B-12-deficient subjects was 23.8 ± 3.8 μmol/L ($n = 20$). Vitamin B-12 administration reduced the concentration to 12.2 ± 1.5 μmol/L.

Total plasma homocysteine concentrations can be readily measured by HPLC with fluorescent [103,118-120] or electrochemical [133-137] detection. Homocysteine has also been measured in plasma with an enzymatic procedure.[138,139,211] Using the enzymatic procedure, serum total homocysteine concentration in 18 healthy adults was found to be 9.1 ± 1.5 μmol/L (range: 6.9 to 12.1 μmol/L).[211]

In the author's experience, the fluorescent method of Cornwell et al.[119] and the electrochemical method of Malinow et al.[134] have been equally reliable. Capillary gas chromatography mass spectrometry has also been used as a highly sensitive and specific method for the measurement of serum homocysteine concentrations.[70,100,128,132,140] Homocysteine in plasma is very stable. Samples have been stored at –20°C or –70°C for several years without loss in homocysteine.[103,121]

It should be remembered that total plasma homocysteine concentrations cannot determine whether a subject is deficient in vitamin B-12 or folacin or both.[154] Both deficiencies will cause marked increases in plasma total homocysteine. Excessive intakes of protein and methionine may increase plasma homocysteine concentrations by enhancing the synthesis of homocysteine.[129]

Selhub et al.[127] observed from the Framingham Heart Study that the risk of carotid-artery stenosis was elevated at plasma levels of homocysteine between 11.4 and 14.3 μmol/L. This would indicate that plasma homocysteine levels above 11.4 μmol/L are undesirable, and for a margin of safety, a lower concentration of homocysteine could be considered desirable. Thompson in a recent unpublished study found a plasma homocysteine concentration of 8.3 ± 1.3 μmol/L in 169 young women.[46] The procedure of Cornwell et al.[119] with fluorometric detection was used.

Kang et al. have classified hyperhomocyst(e)inemia as follows:[101,129,219]

State	Plasma Total Homocysteine (μmol/L)
Normal	5–12
Marginal	12–16
Moderate	16–30
Intermediate	31–100
Severe	> 100

Malinow et al.[133] reported on the effect of age and peripheral arterial occlusive disease on plasma homocysteine concentrations as follows:

	Plasma Homocysteine (μmol/L)		
	Control		
Subjects	< 60 yr	> 60 yr	PAOD*
Women	8.58 ± 2.82	9.04 ± 2.16	17.04 ± 8.26
Men	11.18 ± 3.58	10.74 ± 2.16	15.44 ± 5.76

* Peripheral arterial occlusive disease.

Holotranscobalamin II

Plasma concentrations of holotranscobalamin II can provide an early and sensitive measurement of negative vitamin B-12 balance.[6,34-36,76,81] Vitamin B-12 is rapidly depleted from holotranscobalamin II when vitamin B-12 status is low.[35,36]

Herbert[6] found in his patient population that a serum holotranscobalamin II level below 29.6 pmol/L (40 pg/mL) was associated with an inadequate vitamin B-12 consumption or a clinical problem of the stomach, pancreas, or ileum.

Holotranscobalamin II concentrations of <30 pmol/L were considered vitamin B-12 deficient. According to Herbert et al.,[6,35,36] holotranscobalamin II concentrations of <15 pmol/L would indicate that no vitamin B-12 is being absorbed. Borderline low holotranscobalamin II was considered to range from 29.6 to 44.4 pmol/L (40 to 60 pg/mL).[6] Hence, a serum holotranscobalamin II level of >45.0 pmol/L (>60 pg/mL) was considered normal.[6,83,86] Fernandes-Costa et al.[85] found holotranscobalamin II levels were higher in healthy women than that of healthy men.

Several methods have been used to quantitate holotranscobalamin II in serum, but most are modifications of the procedure of Herzlich and Herbert.[34-36,76,79-81] Various investigators have utilized holotranscobalamin II measurements in studies on pregnancy,[82] lactation,[83] race,[84] and sex.[85] Plasma vitamin B-12 and plasma holotranscobalamin II are both measured in the same assay by the use of Microparticle Enzyme Intrinsic Factor Assay (IMX B-12 assay; Abbott Laboratories, Abbott Park, IL).[33,34]

The procedure as described by Allen et al.[33] consists of mixing one mL of plasma with microfine glass particles, which bind the apotranscobalamin II and holotranscobalamin II. The supernate contains the vitamin B-12 bound to transcobalamin I and III (haptocorrins). Plasma holotranscobalamin II was calculated as total plasma vitamin B-12, minus the vitamin B-12 bound to transcobalamin I and III. The vitamin B-12 present was measured with the Abbott Laboratories IMX B-12 Assay.

Deoxyuridine Suppression Tests

The deoxyuridine suppression test can serve as a functional test for vitamin B-12 deficiency.[178] The deoxyuridine suppression test as described by Das et al.[6,171,174] uses whole blood specimens rather than bone marrow cells.[6,172] The deoxyuridine suppression test can assist in the diagnosis of a vitamin B-12 or folate deficiency.[176,187,188] Herbert[173] states that early in vitamin B-12 deficiency, the suppression test becomes abnormal before either plasma homocysteine concentrations or methylmalonic acid concentrations increase.

The deoxyuridine suppression test has been used in a number of investigations.[54,55,175-178,180] The test is somewhat slow and tedious to perform. When compared to other procedures available for the assessment of vitamin B-12 and folacin status, the deoxyuridine suppression test is not practical or reliable for widespread use.[176,188]

Hypersegmented Neutrophil Estimates

The use of granulocyte hypersegmentation counts in the evaluation of vitamin B-12 or folate status has been described by Herbert.[181,182,184] Blood smears have been considered hypersegmented if the mean lobe count was greater than 3.5 or if 6-lobed neutrophils were present.[183,193] Although the procedure is simple to perform, the procedure does not distinguish between a vitamin B-12 deficiency or that of a folacin deficiency.[177,185,186]

Vitamin B-12 (Cobalamin) Absorption Tests

The Schilling test measures vitamin B-12 absorption and not the state of stores of the vitamin.[6,144,148,193] However, the tests can help delineate the cause of the malabsorption.[6,143,148] Thus the test can provide information as to whether the malabsorption is due to a lack of intrinsic factor or to a lack of gastric acid production or enzymic secretion.[147,153,196] A modified Schilling test is used for this purpose whereby an animal protein-bound vitamin B-12 is used instead of crystalline vitamin B-12.[142-153,189,203] Unfortunately, the dual-isotope Schilling test kit (Dacopac-Amersham) used in a number of studies is no longer commercially available.[142,150,151]

Factors Influencing Vitamin B-12 Status

Pernicious anemia is found in all ethnic groups and is relatively frequent in young black women.[153] Ethnic differences appear to exist regarding normal vitamin B-12 concentrations. Reports from Africa have demonstrated that blacks have higher serum vitamin B-12 concentrations than whites.[22-26]

In the United States, blacks also had significantly higher serum vitamin B-12 concentrations than whites.[21,26] Latin-Americans living in the United States had vitamin B-12 concentrations that were intermediate between those of whites and blacks.[21] No sex differences were observed (median of 362 pmol/L) for men and 380 pmol/L for women). Similarly in a military nutrition survey, no significant differences in serum vitamin B-12 levels were observed between male and female military personnel.[27]

In normal elderly subjects, vitamin B-12 absorption from the gut does not decline with age.[88] However, for many, the ability to absorb vitamin B-12 efficiently may decrease with age because the capacity of the stomach to secrete hydrochloric acid may be reduced in many of the elderly.[88,89] Vitamin B-12 deficiency is rare among alcoholics although some may have low serum vitamin B-12 concentrations.[28,29] Cigarette smokers may have depressed concentrations in the plasma and buccal mucosa.[30] Subjects with HIV-1 infection frequently have low serum vitamin B-12 concentrations.[17-20,36,77,78] The deficiency in vitamin B-12 was associated with a deterioration in cognitive performance.[78] Serum homocysteine may be elevated by renal disease without the presence of vitamin B-12 or folate deficiency.[6] In AIDS patients, however, serum homocysteine levels may remain low despite the presence of folate or vitamin B-12 deficiency.[13] Numerous other investigations have reported an impaired vitamin B-12 status in human immunodeficiency virus type 1 (HIV-1) infection.[15-20]

Omeparazole is an inhibitor of gastric acid and used for the treatment of gastroesophageal reflux disease. In a controlled study, omeprazole therapy actually decreased cynocobalamin absorption in a dose-dependent manner.[205]

Interpretation of Vitamin B-12 and Folate Assessment Results

Depending upon the test used in the diagnosis of vitamin B-12 or of folate deficiency, false-positive or false-negative results may occur. Hence, when feasible, the use of more than one diagnostic test should be encouraged. It should be remembered that in subjects with megaloblastic anemia, a low plasma vitamin B-12 concentration does not indicate a vitamin B-12 deficiency unless either the plasma folate concentrations are normal or malabsorption of vitamin B-12 has been demonstrated. Likewise, a low plasma or erythrocyte folate concentration would not confirm a diagnosis of megaloblastic anemia due to folate deficiency unless the plasma vitamin B-12 concentration is normal or it has been demonstrated that the absorption of vitamin B-12 is normal.

Measurements of both serum vitamin B-12 and holotranscobalamin II would provide the most useful information for the assessment of vitamin B-12 status. Holotranscobalamin II measurement provide an early sensitive detection of negative vitamin B-12 balance.

Toxicity

Vitamin B-12 has a very low order of toxicity. The administration of oral doses of 1000 µg of cobalamin per day produced no adverse effects.[221]

Summary

Because of the interaction of vitamin B-12 with folate metabolism, the nutritional status of both vitamins need to be assessed simultaneously.[94,198] Folate deficiency and vitamin B-12 deficiency both produce an identical megaloblastic anemia.

Serum methylmalonic acid and total homocysteine levels are elevated in most subjects with a vitamin B-12 deficiency. Most subjects with a folacin deficiency will not have elevated serum levels of methylmalonic acid but will have elevated serum levels of total homocysteine.[70] Thus the two measurements can be useful in diagnosing subjects with a folate deficiency and a vitamin B-12 deficiency and in distinguishing between these two deficiencies.[68,70]

Vitamin B-12 evaluations may be assisted by neutrophil hypersegmentation measurements, deoxyuridine suppression tests, or formiminoglutamic acid excretion levels. These procedures are not entirely specific to a vitamin B-12 deficiency and, therefore, have received limited utilization.

A negative vitamin B-12 balance has been considered to exist when serum vitamin B-12 concentration are less than 222 pmol/L (<300 pg/mL).[106] With further studies, serum holotranscobalamin II measurements may become the commonly used procedure for the sensitive and early detection of vitamin B-12 deficiency. Currently, for practical reasons, the measurement of serum concentrations of vitamin B-12 is the procedure of choice for the assessment of vitamin B-12 status (Tables 37 to 39).

TABLE 37

Guidelines for the Interpretation of Serum Vitamin B-12 Concentrations

World Health Organization[213] (all age groups)	Deficient	Low	Acceptable
pmol/L	< 110	110–147	≥ 147
pg/mL	< 150	150–200	≥ 201
Lindenbaum et al.[31]*			
pmol/L	—	—	≥ 258
pg/mL	—	—	≥ 350

* *Am. J. Clin. Nutr.* 60:2, 1994.

TABLE 38

Tentative Guides for Vitamin B-12 Assessment

		References
Serum Vitamin B-12		
Deficient:	<258 pmol/L (350 pg/mL)	31
	<222 pmol/L (<300 pg/mL)	106
Serum Methylmalonic Acid		
Acceptable:	< 376 nmol/L	31, 70, 39
Serum Holotranscobalamin II		
Borderline:	29–44 pmol/L (40–60 pg/mL)	6
Normal:	> 45 pmol/L (> 60 pg/mL)	83, 86
Urinary Methylmalonic Acid		
Vitamin B-12 deficient:	> 5.0 µg methylmalonic	
Acid excretion/mg creatinine	(> 20 µg/mL urine)	57, 60, 63

TABLE 39

Vitamin B-12 Guidelines Used in a Study
with Older Dutch Stubjects[222]

Plasma Vitamin B-12	
Mild vitamin B-12 deficiency	<260 pmol/L
Acceptable vitamin B-12 concentration	≥260 pmol
Elevated vitamin B-12 concentrations	>750 pmol/L
Plasma Methylmalonic Acid	
Elevated concentration	>0.32 μmol/L
Acceptable concentration	≤0.32 μmol/L

References

1. Ermens, A. A. A., Refsum, H., Ruprect, J., Spijkers, L. J. M., Guttormsen, A. B., Lindemans, J., Ueland, Per M., and Abels, J., Monitoring cobalamin inactivation during nitrons oxide anesthesia by determination of homocysteine and folate in plasma and urine, *Clin. Pharmacol. Ther.*, 49, 385, 1991.

2. Sweeney, B., Bingham, R. M., Amos, R. J., Petty, A. C., and Cole, P. V., Toxicity of bone marrow in dentists exposed to nitrous oxide, *Br. Med. J.*, 291, 567, 1985.

3. Amess, J. A. L., Burman, J. F., Rees, G. M., Nancikievill, D. G., and Mollin, D. C., Megaloblastic haemopoiesis in patients receiving nitrous oxide, *Lancet*, 339, 1978.

4. Schilling, R. F., Is nitrous oxide a dangerous anesthetic for vitamin B-12-deficient subjects, *JAMA*, 255, 1605, 1986.

5. Koblin, D. D., Tomerson, B. W., Waldman, F. M., Lampe, G. H., Wauk, L. Z., and Eger, E. I. Jr., Effect of nitrous oxide on folate and vitamin B-12 metabolism in patients, *Anesth. Analg.*, 71, 610, 1990.

6. Herbert, V., Staging vitamin B-12 (cobalamin) status in vegetarians, *Am. J. Clin. Nutr.*, 59, 1213S, 1994.

7. Anonymous, Inadequate vegan diets at weaning, *Nutr. Revs.*, 48, 323, 1990.

8. Bar-Sella, P., Rakover, Y., and Ratner, D., Vitamin B-12 and folate levels in long-term vegans, *Isr. J. Med. Sci.*, 26, 309, 1990.

9. Close, G. C., Rastoafarianism and the vegan syndrome, *Brt. Med. J.*, 286, 473, 1983.

10. Stollhoff, K. and Schulte, F. J., Vitamin B-12 and brain development, *Eur. J. Pediatr.*, 146, 205, 1987.

11. Dagnelie, P. C., van Staveren, W. A., and van den Berg, H., Vitamin B-12 from algae appears not to be bioavailable, *Am. J. Clin. Nutr.*, 53, 695, 1991.

12. Rauma, A. –L., Torronen, R., Hanninen, O., and Mykkanen, H., Vitamin B-12 status of long-term adherents of a strict uncooked vegan diet ("Living Food Diet") is compromised, *J. Nutr.*, 125, 2511, 1995.

13. Jacobsen, D. W., Green, R., Herbert, V., Longworth, D. L., and Rehm, S., Decreased serum glutathione with normal cysteine and homocysteine levels in patients with AIDS, *Clin. Res.*, 38, 556A (Abst.), 1990.

14. Narayanan, M. N., Dawson, D. W., and Lewis, M. J., Dietary deficiency of vitamin B-12 is associated with low serum cobalamin levels in non-vegetarians, *Eur. J. Haematol.*, 47, 115, 1991.

15. Boudes, P., Zittoun, J., and Sobel, A., Folate, vitamin B-12, and HIV-infection, *Lancet*, 335, 1401, 1990.

16. Israel, D. S. and Plaisance, K. I., Neutropenia in patients infected with human immunodeficiency virus, *Clin. Pharmacol.*, 10, 268, 1991.

17. Beach, R. S., Morgan, R., Wilke, F., Mantero-Atienza, E., Blaney, N., Shor-Posner, G., Lu, Y., Eisdorfer, C., and Baum, M. K., Plasma vitamin B-12 level as a potential cofactor in studies of human immunodeficiency virus type 1-related cognitive changes, *Arch. Neurol.*, 49, 501, 1992.

18. Ehrenpreis, E. D., Carlson, S. J., Boorstein, H. C., and Craig, R. M., Malabsorption and deficiency of vitamin B012 in HIV-infected patients with chronic diarrhea, *Digest. Disease Sci.*, 39, 2159, 1994.

19. Tang, A. M., Graham, N. M. H., Chandra, R. K., and Saah, A. J., Low serum vitamin B-12 concentrations are associated with faster human immunodeficiency virus type 1 (HIV-1) disease progression, *J. Nutr.*, 127, 345, 1997.

20. Kieburtz, K. D., Giang, D. W., Schiffer, R. B., and Vakil, N., Abnormal vitamin B-12 metabolism in human immunodeficiency virus infection, Association with neurological dysfunction, *Arch. Neurol.*, 48, 312, 1991.

21. Saxena, S. and Carmel, R., Racial differences in vitamin B-12 levels in the United States, *Am. J. Clin. Pathol.*, 88, 95, 1987.

22. Brandt, V., Kerrick, J. E., and Metz, J., The distribution of serum vitamin B-12 concentrations in some population groups in South Africa, *S. Afr. J. Med. Sci.*, 28, 125, 1963.

23. Davies, D. G. and Newson, J., Some haematological and biochemical characteristics of pastoral tribes in Kenya, *East Afr. Med. J.*, 52, 666, 1975.

24. Fernandes-Costa, F. and Metz, J., A comparison of serum transcobalamin levels in white and black subjects, *Am. J. Clin. Nutr.*, 35, 83, 1982.

25. Fleming, A. F., Ogunfunmilade, Y. A., and Carmel, R., Serum vitamin B-12 levels and vitamin B-12 binding proteins of serum and saliva of healthy Nigerians and Europeans, *Am. J. Clin. Nutr.*, 31, 1732, 1978.

26. Kwee, H. G., Bowman, H. S., and Wells, L. W., A racial difference in serum vitamin B-12 levels, *J. Nucl. Med.*, 26, 790, 1985.

27. Kretsch, M. J., Sauberlich, H. E., and Skala, J. H., Nutritional status assessment of marines before and after the installation of the "multi-restaurant" food service system at the Twenty-Nine Palms Marine Corps Base, California, Letterman Army Institute of Research, Presidio of San Francisco, CA, Institute Report No. 192, December 1984.

28. Lindenbaum, J., Folate and vitamin B-12 deficiencies in alcoholism, *Seminars in Heamatol.*, 17, 119, 1980.

29. Gimsing, P., Melgaard, B., Anderson, K., Vilstrup, H., and Hippe, E., Vitamin B-12 and folate function in chronic alcoholic men with peripherol neuropathy and encephalopathy, *J. Nutr.*, 119, 416, 1989.

30. Piyathilake, C. J., Macaluso, M., Hine, R. J., Richards, E. W., and Krumdieck, C. L., Local and systemic effects of cigarette smoking on folate and vitamin B-12, *Am. J. Clin. Nutr.*, 60, 559, 1994.

31. Lindenbaum, J., Rosenberg, I. H., Wilson, P. W. F., Stabler, S. P., and Allen, R. H., Prevalence of cobalamin deficiency in the Framingham Elderly population, *Am. J. Clin. Nutr.*, 60, 2, 1994.

32. Allen, L. H. and Castesline, J., Vitamin B-12 deficiency in elderly individuals: diagnosis and requirements, *Am. J. Clin. Nutr.*, 60, 12, 1994.

33. Allen, L. H., Rosado, J. L., Castesline, J. E., Martinez, H., Lopez, P., Munoz, E., and Black, A. K., Vitamin B-12 deficiency and malabsorption are highly prevalent in rural Mexican communities, *Am. J. Clin. Nutr.*, 62, 1013, 1995.

34. Vu, T., Amin, J., Ramos, M., Flener, V., Vanyo, L., and Tisman, G., Measurement of B-12 on transcobalamin II (holo TCII) using microfilm glass: significance of evaluating B-12 absorption following chemotherapy, *Am. J. Hematol.*, 42, 202, 1993.

35. Herbert, V., Fong, W., Jacobson, J., Stapler, T., Castellar, L., and Tsougranis, M., Less than 20 pg B-12 on transcobalamin II (TC II)/ml serum predicts inability to absorb B-12 from food in AIDS patients, *Clin. Res.*, 37, 853A (Abst.), 1989.

36. Herbert, V., Fong, W., Gulle, V., and Stapler, T., Low holotranscobalamin II is the earliest serum marker for subnormal vitamin B-12 (cobalamin) absorption in patients with AIDS, *Am. J. Hematol.*, 34, 132, 1990.

37. Chanarin, I., O'Shea, A. M., Malkowska, V., and Rinsler, M. G., Megaloblastic anemia in a vegetarian Hindu community, *Lancet*, 1168, 1985.

38. World Health Organization, Publications of the World Health Organization 1973–1977 and 1978–1982, Geneva, Switzerland.

39. Savage, D., Gangaidzo, I., Lindenbaum, J., Kiire, C., Mukvbi, J. M., Moyo, A., Gwanzura, C., Mudenge, B., Bennie, A., Sitima, J., Stabler, S. P., and Allen, R. H., Vitamin B-12 deficiency is the primary cause of megaloblastic anemia in Zimbabwe, *Brit. J. Haematol*, 86, 844, 1994.
40. Carmel, R., Cobalamin, the stomach, and aging, *Am. J. Clin. Nutr.*, 66, 750, 1997.
41. King, J. E., Mazariegos, M., Valdez, C., Castaneda, C., and Solomons, N. W., Nutritional status indicators and their interactions in rural, Guatemalan elderly: a study in San Pedro Ayampuc, *Am. J. Clin. Nutr.*, 66, 795, 1997.
42. Stabler, S. P., Lindenbaum, J., and Allen, R. H., Vitamin B-12 deficiency in the elderly: current dilemas, *Am. J. Clin. Nutr.*, 66, 741, 1997.
43. Joosten, E., Lesaffre, R., and Reizler, R., Are different reference intervals for methylmalonic acid and total homocysteine necessary in elderly people, *Eur. J. Haematol.*, 57, 222, 1996.
44. Rasmussen, K., Moller, J., Lyngbak, M., Pedersen, A. M. H., and Dybkjer, L. Age-and gender-specific reference intervals for total homocysteine and methylmalonic acid in plasma before and after vitamin supplementation, *Clin. Chem.*, 42, 630, 1996.
45. Cox, E. and White, A. M., Methylmalonic acid excretion: an index of vitamin B-12 deficiency, *Clin. Chim. Acta*, 18, 197, 1962.
46. Thomson, S. W., Homocysteine, copper, folic acid, and cervical dysplasia risk, University of Alabama at Birmingham, Personal communication.
47. Norman, E. J. and Morrison, J. A., Screening elderly populations for cobalamin (vitamin B-12) deficiency using the urinary MMA assay by gas chromatography/mass spectrometry, *Am. J. Med.*, 94, 589, 1993.
48. Barber, K. E., Christie, M. L., Thula, R., and Cutfield, R. G., Vitamin B-12 concentrations in the elderly: a regional study, *N. Z. Med. J.*, 102, 406, 1989.
49. Crantz, J. C., Vitamin B-12 deficiency in the elderly, *Clinics in Geriatric Med.*, 1, 701, 1985.
50. Elsborg, L., Lund, V., and Bastrup-Madsen, P., Serum vitamin B12 levels in the aged, *Acta Med. Scand.*, 200, 309, 1976.
51. Basu, T. K., Donald, E. A., Hargreaves, J. A., Thompson, G. W., Overton, T. R., Chao, E., and Peterson, D., Vitamin B-12 and folate status of a selected group of free-living older persons, *J. Nutr. for the Elderly*, 11, 5, 1992.
52. Craig, G. M., Elliot, C., and Hughes, K. R., Masked vitamin B-12 and folate deficiency in the elderly, *Brt. J. Nutr.*, 54, 613, 1985.
53. Garry, P. J., Goodwin, J. S., and Hunt, W. C., Folate and vitamin B-12 status in a healthy elderly population, *J. Am. Geriatr. Soc.*, 32, 719, 1984.
54. Blundell, E. L., Matthews, J. H., Allen, S. M., Middleton, A. M., Morris, J. E., and Wickramasinghe, S. N., Importance of low serum vitamin B-12 and red cell folate concentrations in elderly hospital inpatients, *J. Clin. Pathol.*, 38, 1179, 1985.
55. Matthews, J. H., Clark, D. M., and Abrahamson, G. H., Effect of therapy with vitamin B-12 and folic acid on elderly patients with low concentrations of serum vitamin B-12 or erythrocyte folate but normal blood counts, *Acta Haematol.*, 79, 84, 1988.
56. Logan, R. F., Elwis, A., Forrest, M. J., and Lawernce, A. C. K., Mechanisms of vitamin B-12 deficiency in elderly inpatients, *Age and Aging*, 18, 4, 1989.
57. Rasmussen, K. and Nathan, E., The clinical evaluation of cobalamin deficiency by determination of methylmalonic acid in serum or urine is not invalidated by the presence of heterozygous methylmalonic-acidaemia, *J. Clin. Chem. Clin. Biochem.*, 28, 419, 1990.
58. Rasmussen, K., Solid-phase sample extraction for rapid determination of methylmalonic acid in serum and urine by a stable-isotope-dilution method, *Clin. Chem.*, 35, 260, 1989.
59. Stabler, S. P., Marcell, P. D., Podell, E. R., Allen, R. H., and Lindenbaum, J., Assay of methylmalonic acid in the serum of patients with cobalamin deficiency using capillary gas-chromatography-mass spectrometry, *J. Clin. Invest.*, 77, 1606, 1986.
60. Norman, E. J., Gas chromatography mass spectrometry screening of urinary methylmalonic acid: early detection of vitamin B-12 (cobalamin) deficiency to prevent permanent neurologic disability, *GC-MS News*, 12, 120, 1984.
61. Higgenbotton, M. C., Sweetman, L., and Nyhan, W. L., A syndrome of methylmalonic aciduria, homocystinuria, megalablastic anemia and neurologic abnormalities in a vitamin B-12-deficient breast-fed infant of a strict vegetarian, *N. Engl. J Med.*, 299, 317, 1978.

62. Specker, B. L., Miller, D., Norman, E. J., Greene, H., and Hayes, K. C., Increased urinary methylmalonic acid excretion in breast-fed infants of vegetarian mothers and identification of an acceptable dietary source of vitamin B-12, *Am. J. Clin. Nutr.*, 47, 89, 1988.
63. Matchar, D. B., Feussner, J. R., Millington, D. S., Wilkinson, R. H. Jr., Watson, D. J., and Gale, D., Isotope-dilution assay for urinary methylmalonic acid in the diagnosis of vitamin B-12 deficiency, *Annu. Int. Med.*, 106, 707, 1987.
64. Norman, E. J., Matelo, O. J., and Denton, M. D., Cobalamin (vitamin B12) deficiency detection by urinary methylmalonic acid quantitation, *Blood*, 59, 1128, 1982.
65. Norman, E. J. and Morrison, J. A., Screening elderly populations for cobalamin (vitamin B-12) deficiency using the urinary methylmalonic acid assay by gas chromatography mass spectrometry, *Am. J. Med.*, 94, 589, 1993.
66. Rasmussen, K., Moelby, L., and Jensen, M. K., Studies on methylmalonic acid in humans, II, Relationship between concentrations in serum and urinary excretion, and the correlation between serum cobalamin and accumulation of methylmalonic acid, *Clin. Chem.*, 35, 2277, 1989.
67. Moelby, L., Rasmussen, K., Jensen, M. K., Thomsen, L. H., and Nielsen, G., Serum methylmalonic acid before and after oral L-isoleucine loading in cobalamin-deficiency patients, *Scand. J. Clin. Lab. Invest.*, 52, 255, 1992.
68. Savage, D. G., Lindenbaum, J., Stabler, S. P., and Allen, R. H., Sensitivity of serum methylmalonic acid and total homocysteine determinations for diagnosing cobalamin and folate deficiencies, *Am. J. Med.*, 96, 239, 1994.
69. Marcell, P. D., Stabler, S. P., and Allen, R. H., Quantitation of methylmalonic acid and other dicarboxylic acids in normal serum and urine using capillary gas chromatography-mass spectrometry, *Annu. Biochem.*, 150, 58, 1985.
70. Allen, R. H., Stabler, S. P., Savage, D. G., and Lindenbaum, J., Diagnosis of cobalamin deficiency I. Usefulness of serum methylmalonic acid and total homocysteine concentrations, *Am. J. Hematol.*, 34, 90, 1990.
71. Lindenbaum, J., Savage, D. G., Stabler, S. P., and Allen, R. H., Diagnosis of cobalamin deficiency: II. Relative sensitivities of serum cobalamin, methylmalonic acid, and total homocysteine concentrations, *Am. J. Hematol*, 34, 99, 1990.
72. Shilling, R. F., Fairbanks, V. F., Miller, R., Schmitt, K., and Smith, M. J., "Improved" vitamin B-12 assays: a report on two commercial kits, *Clin. Chem.*, 29, 582, 1983.
73. Kubasik, N. P., Ricotta, M., and Sine, H. E., Commercially-supplied binders for plasma cobalamin (vitamin B-12) analysis – "purified" intrinsic factor, "cobinamide" blocked R-protein binder, and non-purified intrinsic factor-R-protein binder – compared to microbiological assay, *Clin. Chem.*, 26, 598, 1980.
74. Black, A. K., Allen, L. H., Pelto, G. H., de Mata, M. P., and Chavez, A., Iron, vitamin B-12 and folate status in Mexico: Associated factors in men and women and during pregnancy and lactation, *J. Nutr.*, 124, 1179, 1994.
75. Kolhouse, J. F., Kondo, H., Allen, N. C., Podell, E., and Allen, R. H., Cobalamin analogues are present in human plasma and can mask cobalamin deficiency because current radioisotope dilution assays are not specific for the cobalamins, *N. Engl. J. Med.*, 299, 785, 1978.
76. Herzlich, B. and Herbert, V., Depletion of serum holotranscobalamin II. An early sign of negative vitamin B-12 balance, *Lab. Invest.*, 58, 332, 1988.
77. Rule, S. A. J., Hooku, M., Castello, C., Luck, W., and Hoffbrand, A. V., Serum vitamin B-12 and transcobalamin levels in early HIV disease, *Am. J. Hematol.*, 47, 167, 1994.
78. Baum, M. K., Shor-Posner, G., Bonveki, P., Cassetti, I., Lu, Y., Mantero-Atienza, E., Beach, R. S., and Sauberlich, H. E., Influence of HIV infection on vitamin status and requirements, *Annu. NY Acad. Sci.*, 669, 165, 1992.
79. Jacob, E., Wong, K.–T., and Herbert, V., A simple method for the separate measurement of transcobalamins I, II, and III: Normal ranges in serum and plasma in men and women, *J. Lab. Clin. Med.*, 89, 1145, 1977.
80. Benhayoun, S., Adjalla, C., Nicolas, J. P., Gueant, J. L., and Lambert, D., Method for the direct specific measurement of vitamin B-12 bound to transcobalamin II in plasma, *Acta Haematol.*, 89, 195, 1993.

81. Wickramasinghe, S. N. and Fida, S., Correlations between holo-transcobalamin II, holo-haptocorrin, and total B-12 in serum samples from healthy subjects and patients, *J. Clin. Pathol.,* 46, 537, 1993.

82. Fernandes-Costa, F. and Metz, J., Levels of transcobalamins I, II, and III during pregnancy and in cord blood, *Am. J. Clin. Nutr.,* 35, 87, 1982.

83. Casterline, J. E., Allen, L. H., and Ruel, M. T., Vitamin B-12 deficiency is very prevalent in lactating Guatemalan women and their infants at three months postpartum, *J. Nutr.,* 127, 1966, 1997.

84. Fernandes-Costa, F. and Metz, J., A comparison of serum transcobalamin levels in White and Black subjects, *Am. J. Clin. Nutr.,* 35, 83, 1992.

85. Fernandes-Costa, F., van Tonder, S., and Metz, J., A sex difference in serum cobalamin and transcobalamin levels, *Am. J. Clin. Nutr.,* 41, 784, 1985.

86. Tisma, G., Vu, J., Amin, G., Brenner, M., Ramos, M., Flener, V., Cordts, V., Bateman, R., Malkin, S., and Browder, T., Measurement of red blood cell-vitamin B-12: a study of correlation between intracellular B-12 content and concentrations of plasma holotranscobalamin II, *Am. J. Hematol.,* 43, 226, 1993.

87. Chanarin, I., The cobalamins (vitamin B-12), in *Vitamins in Medicine,* Volume 1, 4th edition, Barker, B. M. and Bender, D. A., Eds., William Heinemann, London, 1980.

88. Russell, R. M., Implications of gastric atrophy for vitamin and mineral nutriture, in *Nutrition and Aging,* Hutchinson, M. L. and Munro, H. N., Eds., Academic Press, New York, 1986, 59.

89. Goodman, K. I. and Salt, W. B. II., Vitamin B-12 deficiency: important new concepts in recognition, *Postgraduate Med.,* 88, 147, 1990.

90. Sauberlich, H. E., Relationship of vitamin B-6, vitamin B-12, and folate to neurological and neuropsychiatric disorders, in *Micronutrients in Health and in Disease Prevention,* Bendich, A. and Butterworth, C. E. Jr., Eds., Marcel Dekker, New York, 1991, 187.

91. Metz, J., Cobalamin deficiency and the pathogenesis of nervous systems disease, *Annu. Rev. Nutr.,* 12, 59, 1992.

92. Stabler, S. P., Lindenbaum, J., Savage, D. G., and Allen, R. H., Elevation of serum cystathione levels in patients with cobalamin and folate deficiency, *Blood,* 199, 3404, 1993.

93. Matchar, D. B., McCrory, D. C., Millington, D. S., and Feussner, J. R., Performance of the serum cobalamin assay for diagnosis of cobalamin deficiency, *Am. J. Med. Sci.,* 308, 276, 1994.

94. Colman, N., Laboratory assessment of folate status, *Clinics in Lab. Med.,* 1, 775, 1981.

95. Chanarin, I., Megaloblastic anaemia, cobalamin, and folate, *J. Clin. Pathol.,* 40, 978, 1987.

96. Cooper, B. A. and Whitehead, V. M., Evidence that some patients with pernicious anemia are not recognized by radio dilution assay for cobalamin in serum, *N. Eng. J. Med.,* 299, 816, 1978.

97. Brattstrom, L., Lindgren, A., Israelsson, B., Andersson, A., and Hulberg, B., Homocysteine and cysteine: determinants of plasma level in middle-aged and elderly subjects, *J. Int. Med.,* 236, 633, 1994.

98. Lussier-Cacan, S., Xhignese, M., Piolot, A., Selhub, J., Davignon, J., and Genest, J. Jr., Plasma total homocysteine in healthy subjects: sex-specific relation with biological traits, *Am. J. Clin. Nutr.,* 64, 587, 1996.

99. Stabler, S. P., Allen, R. H., Savage, D. G., and Lindenbaum, J., Clinical spectrum and diagnosis of cobalamin deficiency, *Blood,* 76, 871, 1990.

100. Koehler, K. M., Romero, L. J., Stauber, P. M., Pareo-Tubbeh, S. L., Liang, H. C., Baumgartner, R. N., Garry, P. J., Allen, R. H., and Stabler, S. P., Vitamin supplementation and other variables affecting serum homocysteine and methylmalonic acid concentrations in elderly men and women, *J. Am. Coll. Nutr.,* 15, 364, 1996.

101. Kang, S. S., Wong, P. W. K., and Malinow, M. R., Hypercyst(e)inemia as a risk factor for occlusive vascular disease, *Annu. Rev. Nutr.,* 12, 279, 1992.

102. Ueland, P. M., Refsum, H., and Brattstrom, L., Plasma homocysteine and cardiovascular disease, in *Atherosclerotic Cardiovascular Disease, Hemostasis and Endothelial Function,* Francis, R. B. Jr., Ed., Marcel Dekker, New York, 1992, 183.

103. Ueland, P. M., Refsum, H., Stabler, S. P., Malinow, M. R., Anderson, A., and Allen, R. H., Total homocysteine in plasma or serum: methods and clinical applications, *Clin. Chem.,* 39, 1764, 1993.

104. Green, R. and Jacobsen, D. W., Clinical implications of hyperhomocysteinemia, in *Folate in Health and Disease*, Baily, L. B., Ed., Marcel Dekker, New York, 1995, 75.

105. McCully, K. S., Micronutrients, homocysteine metabolism, and atherosclerosis, in Micronutrients in *Health and in Disease Prevention*, Bendich, A. and Butterworth, C. E. Jr., Eds., Marcel Dekker, New York, 1991, 69.

106. Yao, Y., Yao, S. –L., Yao, S. –S., Yao, G., and Lou, W., Prevalence of vitamin B-12 deficiency among geriatric outpatients, *J. Fam. Practice*, 35, 524, 1992.

107. Pennypacker, L. C., Allen, R. H., Kelly, J. P., Matthews, L. M., Grigsby, J., Kaye, K., Lindenbaum, J., and Stabler, S. P., High prevalence of cobalamin deficiency in elderly outpatients, *J. Am. Geriatr. Soc.*, 40, 1197, 1992.

108. Boushey, C. J., Beresford, S. A. A., Omenn, G. S., and Motulsky, A. G., A quantitative assessment of plasma homocysteine as a risk factor for vascular disease, Probable benefits of measuring folic acid intakes, *JAMA*, 274, 1049, 1995.

109. Selhub, J., Jacques, P. F., Wilson, P. W. F., Rush, D., and Ronsenberg, I. H., Vitamin status and intake as primary determinants of homocysteinemia in an elderly population, *JAMA*, 270, 2693, 1993.

110. Joosten, E., van den Berg, A., and Riezler R. et al., Metabolic evidence that deficiencies of vitamin B-12 (cobalamin), folate, and vitamin B-6 occur commonly in elderly people, *Am. J. Clin. Nutr.*, 58, 468, 1993.

111. Nilsson, K., Gustafson, L., Faldt, R.; Andersson, A., and Hultberg, B., Plasma homocysteine in relation to serum cobalamin and blood folate in a psychogeriatric population, *Eur. J. Clin. Invest.*, 24, 600, 1994.

112. Pancharuniti, N., Lewis, C. A., and Sauberlich, H. E. et al., Plasma homocyst(e)ine, folate, and vitamin B-12 concentrations and risk of early-onset coronary artery disease, *Am. J. Clin. Nutr.*, 59, 940, 1994.

113. Hopkins, P. N., Wu, L. L., and Wu, J. et al., Higher plasma homocyst(e)ine and increased susceptibility to adverse effects of low folate in early familial coronary artery disease, *Arterioscler. Thromb. Vasc. Biol.*, 15, 1314, 1995.

114. Dalery, K., Lussier-Cacan, S., Selhub, J., Davignon, J., Latour, Y., and Genest, J. Jr., Homocysteine and coronary artery disease in French Canadian subjects: relation with vitamins B_{12}, B_6, pyridoxal phosphate, and folate, *Am. J. Cardiol.*, 75, 1107, 1995.

115. Robinson, K., Mayer, E. L., and Miller, D. P. et al., Hyperhomocysteinemia and low pyridoxal phosphate, common and independent reversible risk factors for coronary artery disease, *Circulation*, 92, 2825, 1995.

116. Andersson, A., Brattstrom, L., Israelsson, B., Isaksson, A., Hamfelt, A., and Hultberg, B., Plasma homocysteine before and after methionine loading with regard to age, gender, and menopausal status, *Eur. J. Clin. Invest.*, 22, 79, 1992.

117. Ubbink, J. B., Vermaak, W. J. H., van der Merwe, A., and Becker, P. J., Vitamin B-12, vitamin B-6, and folate nutritional status in men with hyperhomocysteinemia, *Am. J. Clin. Nutr.*, 57, 47, 1993.

118. Araki, A. and Sako, Y., Determination of free and total homocysteine in human plasma by high-performance liquid chromatography with fluorescence detection, *J. Chromatogr.*, 422, 43, 1987.

119. Cornwell, P. E., Morgan, S. L., and Vaughn, W. H., Modification of a high-performance liquid chromatographic method for assay of homocysteine in human plasma, *J., Chromatogr.*, 617, 136, 1993.

120. Ubbink, J. B., Vermaak, W. J. H., and Bissbort, S., Rapid high-performance liquid chromatographic assay for total homocysteine levels in human serum, *J. Chromatogr.*, 565, 441, 1991.

121. Israelsson, B., Brattstrom, L., and Refsum, H., Homocysteine in frozen plasma samples, A short cut to establish hyperhomocysteinemia as a risk factor for arteriosclerosis, *Scand. J. Clin. Lab. Invest.*, 53, 465, 1993.

122. Rosenberg, I. H., Homocysteine, vitamins and arterial occlusive disease: an overview, *J. Nutr.*, 126, 1235S, 1996.

123. Malinow, M. R., Plasma homocyst(e)ine: A risk factor for arterial occlusive diseases, *J. Nutr.*, 126, 1238S, 1996.

124. Refsum, H., Nygard, O., Kvale, G., Ueland, P. M., and Vollset, S. E., The Hordaland homocys-teine study: The opposite tails odds ratios reveal different effects of gender and intake of vitamin supplements at high and low plasma total homocysteine concentrations, *J. Nutr.*, 126, 1244S, 1996.
125. Herzlick, B. C., Lichstein, E., Schulhoff, N., Weinstock, M., Pagala, M., Ravindran, K., Namba, T., Nieto, F. J., Stabler, S. P., Allen, R. H., and Malinow, M. R., Relationship among ho-mocyst(e)ine, vitamin B-12 and cardiac disease in the elderly: Association between vitmain B-12 deficiency and decreased left ventricular ejection fraction, *J. Nutr.*, 126, 1249S, 1996.
126. Ubbink, J. B., Delport, R., and Vermaak, W. J. H., Plasma homocysteine concentrations in a population with a low coronary heart disease prevalence, *J. Nutr.*, 126, 1254S, 1996.
127. Selhub, J., Jacques, P. F., Boston, A. G., D'Agostino, R. B., Wilson, P. W. F., Belanger, A. J., O'Leary, D. H., Wolf, P. A., Rush, D., Schaeffer, E. J., and Rosenberg, I. H., Relationship between plasma homocysteine, vitamin status and extracranial carotid-artery stenosis in the Framing-ham study population, *J. Nutr.*, 126, 1258S, 1996.
128. Stabler, S. P., Lindenbaum, J., and Allen, R. H., The use of homocysteine and other metabolites in the specific diagnosis of vitamin B-12 deficiency, *J. Nutr.*, 126, 1266S, 1996.
129. Kang, S. –S., Treatment of hyperhomocyst(e)inemia: physiological basis, *J. Nutr.*, 126, 1273S, 1996.
130. Brattstrom, L., Vitamins as homocysteine-lowering agents, *J. Nutr.*, 126, 1276S, 1996.
131. Dudman, N. P. B., Guo, X. –W., Gordon, R. B., Dawson, P. A., and Wileken, D. E. L., Human homocysteine catabolism: three major pathways and their relevance to development of arterial occlusive disease, *J. Nutr.*, 126, 1295S, 1996.
132. Allen, R. H., Stabler, S. P., Savage, D. G., and Lindenbaum, J., Metabolic abnormalities in cobalamin (vitamin B-12) and folate deficiency, *FASEB J.*, 7, 1344, 1993.
133. Malinow, M. R., Kang, S. S., Taylor, L. M., Wong, P. W. K., and Coull, B. et al., Prevalence of hyperhomocyst(e)inemia in patients with peripherol arterial occlusive disease, *Circulation*, 79, 1180, 1989.
134. Malinow, M. R., Sexton, G., Averbuch, M., Grossman, M., Wilson, D., and Upson, B., Homocyst(e)inemia in daily practice: levels in coronary artery disease, *Coronary Artery Disease*, 1, 215, 1990.
135. Brattstrom, L., Lindgren, A., Israelsson, B., Malinow, M. R., Norrving, B., Upson, B., and Hamfelt, A., Hyperhomocysteinaemia in stroke: prevalence, cause, and relationships to type of stroke and stroke risk factor, *Eur. J. Clin. Invest.*, 22, 214, 1992.
136. Smolin, L. A. and Benevengea, N. G. H., Accumulaion of homocyst(e)ine in vitamin B-6 deficiency: A model for the study of cystathionine-β-synthase deficiency, *J. Nutr.*, 112, 1264, 1982.
137. Smolin, L. A. and Schneider, J. A., Measurement of total plasma cysteamine using high-performance liquid chromatography with electrochemical detection, *Anal. Biochem.*, 168, 374, 1988.
138. Henning, S., McKee, R. W., and Swendseid, M. E., Hepatic content of S'-adenosylmethionine, S-adenosylhomocysteine and glutathione in rats receiving treatments modulating methyl donor availability, *J. Nutr.*, 119, 1478, 1989.
139. Refsum, H., Helland, S., and Ueland, P. M., Radioenzymatic determination of homocysteine in plasma and urine, *Clin. Chem.*, 31, 624, 1985.
140. Stabler, S. P., Marcell, P. D., Podell, E. R., and Allen, R. H., Quantitation of total homocysteine, total cysteine, and methionine in normal serum and urine using capillary gas chromatography-mass spectrometry, *Anal. Biochem.*, 162, 185, 1987.
141. Kang, S. –S., Wong, P. W., and Norusis, M., Homocysteinemia due to folate deficiency, *Metabolism*, 36, 458, 1987.
142. Joosten, E., Pelemans, W., Devos, P., Lesaffre, E., Goossens, W., Criel, A., and Verhaeghe, R., Cobalamin absorption and serum homocysteine and methylmalonic acid in elderly subjects with low serum cobalamin, *Eur. J. Haematol.*, 51, 25, 1993.
143. Narayanan, M. N., Dawson, D. W., and Lewis, M. J., Dietary deficiency of vitamin B-12 is associated with low serum cobalamin levels in non-vegetarians, *Eur. J. Haematol.*, 47, 115, 1991.

144. International Committee for Standardization in Haematology, Recommended method for the measurement of vitamin B-12 absorption, *J. Nuclear Med.*, 22, 1091, 1981.

145. Henze, E., Manner, S., Clausen, M., Malfertheiner, P., Hellwig, D., Ditschuneit, H., Kornhuber, H., and Adam, W. E., The Schilling test cannot be replaced by an absorption test with unlabeled vitamin B-12, *Klin. Wochenschr.*, 66, 332, 1988.

146. Shojania, A. M., Problems in the diagnosis and investigation of megaloblastic anemia, *CMA J.*, 122, 999, 1980.

147. Carlisle, W. R., New uses for an old test: The Schilling test, *J. Med. Assoc. Alabama*, 51, 16, 1982.

148. Schilling, R. F., Vitamin B-12: Assay and absorption, *Lab. Management*, 20, 31, 1982.

149. Rhode, B. M., Arseneau, P., Cooper, B. A., Katz, M., Gilfix, B. M., and MacLean, L. D., Vitamin B-12 deficiency after gastric surgery for obesity, *Am. J. Clin. Nutr.*, 63, 103, 1996.

150. Domsmtad, P. A., Choy, Y. C., Kim, E. E., and Deland, F. H., Reliability of the dual-isotope Schilling test for the diagnosis of pernicious anemia or malabsorption syndrome, *Am. J. Clin. Pathol.*, 75, 723, 1981.

151. Atrah, H. I., and Davison, R. J. L., A survey and critical evaluation of a dual isotope (Dicopac) vitamin B-12 absorption test, *Eur. J. Nucl. Med.*, 15, 57, 1989.

152. Fairbanks, V. F., Wahner, H. W., and Phyliky, R. L., Test for pernicious anemia: the "Schilling test," *Mayo Clin. Proc.*, 58, 541, 1983.

153. Pruthi, R. K. and Tefferi, A., Pernicious anemia revisited, *Mayo Clin. Proc.*, 69, 144, 1994.

154. Savage, D. G. and Lindenbaum, J., Folate-cobalamin interactions, in *Folate in Health and Disease*, Bailey, L. B., Ed., Marcel Dekker, New York, 1995, 237.

155. Anderson, B. B., Investigations into the Euglena method for assay of vitamin B-12 in serum, *J. Clin. Pathol.*, 17, 14, 1964.

156. Spray, G. H., An improved method for the rapid estimation of vitamin B-12 in serum, *Clin. Sci.*, 14, 661, 1955.

157. Lindenbaum, J., Status of laboratory testing in the diagnosis of megaloblastic anemia, *Blood*, 61, 62, 1983.

158. Kelleher, B. P. and O'Broin, S. D., Microbiological assay for vitamin B-12 performed in 96-well microtitre plates, *J. Clin. Pathol.*, 44, 592, 1991.

159. Kelleher, B. P., Scott, J. M., and O'Broin, S. D., Cryo-preservation of *Lactobacillus leichmannii* for vitamin B-12 microbiological assay, *Med. Lab. Sci.*, 47, 90, 1990.

160. Kelleher, B. P., Scott, J. M., and O'Broin, S. D., Use of beta-lactamase to hydrolyse interferring antibiotics in vitmain B-12 microbiological assay using *Lactobacillus leichmanii*, *Clin. Lab. Haematol.*, 12, 87, 1990.

161. Kelleher, B. P., Walshe, K. W., Scott, J. M., and O'Broin, S. D., Microbiological assay for vitamin B-12 with use of a colistin-sulfate-resistant organism, *Clin. Chem.*, 33, 52, 1987.

162. Sourial, N., Use of an improved *E. coli* method for the measurement of cobalamin in serum: comparison with the *E. gracilis* assay results, *J. Clin. Pathol.*, 34, 351, 1981.

163. Copper, B. A., Fehedy, V., and Blanshay, P., Recognition of deficiency of vitamin B-12 using measurements of serum concentration, *J. Lab. Clin. Med.*, 107, 447, 1986.

164. Kumar, S., Ghosh, K., and Das, K. C., Serum vitamin B-12 levels in an Indian population: an evaluation of three assay methods, *Med. Lab. Sci.*, 46, 120, 1989.

165. Sheridan, B. L. and Pearce, L. C., Vitamin B-12 assays compared by use of patients sera with low vitamin B-12 content, *Clin. Chem.*, 31, 734, 1985.

166. Grinblat, J., Marcus, D. L., Hernandez, F., and Freedman, M. L., Folate and vitamin B-12 levels in an urban elderly population with chronic diseases, Assessment of two laboratory folate assays: microbiologic and radioassay, *J. Am. Geriatr. Soc.*, 34, 627, 1986.

167. Gilois, C. R., Beattie, G., and Mills, S. P., Measurement of vitamin B-12 and serum folic acid: a comparison of methods, *Med. Lab. Sci.*, 43, 140, 1986.

168. Mollin, D. L., Hoffbrand, A. V., Ward, P. G., and Lewis, S. M., Interlaboratory comparison of serum vitamin B-12 assay, *J. Clin. Pathol.*, 33, 243, 1980.

169. England, J. M. and Linnell, J. C., Problems with the serum vitamin B-12 assay, *Lancet*, 2, 1072, 1980.

170. Berg, T. M., de Vries, J. A., van Gasteren, C. J. M., Meewwissen, H., Stevens, G. A. W., and Verbon, F. J., Comparative studies on the microbiological vitamin B-12 assay at two laboratories, *Appl. Environ. Microbiol.*, 31, 459, 1976.
171. Das, K. C., Asiz, M. A., Colman, N., Manusselis, C., and Herbert, V., Eliminating false positive and false negative results in lymphocyte diagnostic dU suppression test (Dx dUST) for folate deficiency by recognizing different "normal" individuals have different folate stores, *Blood*, 78 (Suppl 10), 99a, 1991.
172. Herbert, V., Megaloblastic anemias, *Lab. Invest.*, 52, 3, 1984.
173. Herbert, V., Cobalamin deficiency and neuropsychiatric disorders, *N. Engl. J. Med.*, 319, 1733, 1988 (letter).
174. Das, K. C., Manusslis, C., and Herbert, V., Simplifying lymphocyte culture and deoxyuridine suppression test by using whole blood (0.1 mL) instead of separated lymphocytes, *Clin. Chem.*, 26, 72, 1980.
175. Metz, J., The deoxyuridine suppression test, *CRC Crit. Rev. Clin. Lab. Sci.*, 20, 205, 1984.
176. Tamura, T., Soong, S. -J., Sauberlich, H. E., Hatch, K. D., Cole, P., and Butterworth, C. E. Jr., Evaluation of the deoxyuridine suppression test by using whole blood samples from folic acid-supplemented subjects, *Am. J. Clin. Nutr.*, 51, 80, 1990.
177. Sauberlich, H. E., Kretsch, M. J., Skala, J. H., Johnson, H. L., and Taylor, P. C., Folate requirements and metabolism in nonpregnant women, *Am. J. Clin. Nutr.*, 46, 1016, 1987.
178. Herbert, V. and Das, K. C., Anemias due to nuclear maturation defects (megloblastic anemias), in *Medicine for the Practicing Physician*, Hurst, J. W., Ed., Butterworth-Heinemann, Boston, MA, 1992, 851.
179. Santini, R. and Millan, S., Determination of erythrocyte vitamin B-12 activity, *Am. J. Clin. Nutr.*, 29, 791, 1976.
180. Herbert, V. and Das, K. S., Folic acid and vitamin B-12, in *Modern Nutrition in Health and Disease*, 8th edition, Shils, M. E., Olson, J. A., and Shike, M., Eds., Lea & Febiger, Baltimore, MD, 1994, 402.
181. Herbert, V., Don't ignore low serum cobalamin (vitamin B-12) levels, *Arch. Int. Med.*, 148, 1705, 1988.
182. Herbert, V., Memoli, D., McAleer, E., and Colman, N., What is normal, Variation from the individual's norm for granulocyte "lobe average" and holo-transcobalamin II (holo-TC II) diagnosis vitamin B-12 deficiency before variation from the laboratory norm, *Clin. Res.*, 342, 718, 1986 (Abstr.).
183. Lindenbaum, J. and Nash, B. J., Megaloblastic anaemia and neutrophil hypersegmentation, *Br. J. Haematol.*, 44, 511, 1980.
184. Herbert, V., Experimental nutritional folate deficiency in man, *Trans. Assoc. Am. Physician*, 75, 307, 1962.
185. Thompson, W. G., Cassino, C., Babitz, L., Meola, T., Berman, R., Lipkin, M. Jr., and Freedman, M., Hypersegmented neutrophils and vitamin B-12 deficiency, Hypersegmentation in B-12 deficiency, *Acta Haematol.*, 81, 191, 1989.
186. Dawson, D. W., Fish, D. I., Frew, I. D. O., Roome, T., and Tilston, I., Laboratory diagnosis of megaloblastic anaemia: current methods assessed by external quality assurance trials, *J. Clin. Pathol.*, 40, 393, 1987.
187. Wickramasinghe, S. N. and Saunders, J., Correlation between the deoxyuridine-suppressed value and some conventional haematological parameters in patients with folate or vitamin B-12 deficiency, *Scand. J. Haematol.*, 16, 121, 1976.
188. Mathews, J. H. and Wickramasinghe, S. N., The deoxyuridine suppression test performed on phytahaemagglutin-stimulated peripheral blood cells fails to relfect *in vivo* vitamin B-12 of folate deficiency, *Eur. J. Haematol.*, 40, 174, 1988.
189. Goodman, K. I. and Salt, W. B., Vitamin B-12 deficiency: Important new concepts in recognition, *Postgraduate Med.*, 88, 147, 1990.
190. Green, R., Macrocytic anemias, in *Medicine for the Practicing Physician*, 4th edition, Hurst, J. W., Ed., Appleton & Lange, Stamford, CT, 1996, 821.

191. Omer, A., Finlayson, N. D. C., Shearman, D. J. C., Simson, R. R., and Girdwood, R. H., Erythrocyte vitamin B-12 activity in health, polycythemia, and in deficiency of vitamin B-12 and folate, *Blood*, 35, 73, 1970.

192. Sauberlich, H. E., Vitamin B-6, vitamin B-12 and folate, in *Meat and Health, Advances in Meat Research*, Volume 6, Pearson, A. M. and Dutson, T. R., Eds., Elsevier Applied Science, New York, 1990, 461.

193. Ward, P. C. J., Investigation of macrocytic anemia, *Postgrad. Med.*, 65, 203, 1979.

194. Anonymous, Unrecognized cobalamin-responsive neuropsychiatric disorders, *Nutr. Res.*, 47, 208, 1989.

195. Martin, D. C., B-12 and folate deficiency dementia, *Clin. Geri. Med.*, 4, 841, 1988.

196. Brugge, W. R., Goff, J. S., Allen, N. C., Podell, E. R., and Allen, R. H., Development of a dual label Schilling test for pancreatic exocrine function based on the differential absorption of cobalamin bound to intrinsic factor and R-protein, *Gastroenterology*, 78, 937, 1980.

197. Beck, W. S., Cobalamin and the nervous system, *N. Engl. J. Med.*, 318, 1752, 1988.

198. Scott, J. and Weir, D., Folate/vitamin B-12 inter-relationships, *Essays Biochem.*, 28, 63, 1994.

199. Grasbeck, R., Biochemistry and clinical chemistry of vitamin B-12 transport and the related diseases, *Clin. Biochem.*, 17, 99, 1984.

200. Healton, E. B., Savage, D. G., Brust, J. C. M., Garrett, T. J., and Lindenbaum, J., Neurologic aspects of cobalamin deficiency, *Medicine*, 70, 229, 1991.

201. Lindenbaum, J., Healton, E. B., Savage, D. G., Brust, J. C. M., Garrett, T. J., Podell, E. R., Marchell, P. D., Stabler, S. P., and Allen, R. H., Neuropsychiatric disorders caused by cobalamin deficiency in the absence of anemia or macrocystosis, *N. Engl. J. Med.*, 318, 1720, 1988.

202. Allen, R., Megaloblastic anemias, in *Cecil Textbook of Medicine*, 19th edition, Wyngaarden, J. B. et al., Eds., W. B. Saunders, Philadelphia, 1992, 847.

203. Carmel, R., Sinow, R. M., Siegel, M. E., and Samloff, I. M., Food cobalamin malabsorption occurs frequently in patients with unexplained low serum cobalamin levels, *Arch. Interm. Med.*, 148, 1715, 1988.

204. Brattstrom, L., Israelsson, B., Lindgarde, F., and Hultberg, B., Higher total plasma homocysteine in vitamin B-12 deficiency than in heterozygosity for homocysteine due to cystathione β-synthase deficiency, *Metabolism*, 37, 175, 1988.

205. Marcuard, S. P., Albernaz, L., and Khozanie, P. G., Omeprazole therapy causes malabsorption of cyanocobalamin (vitamin B-12), *Annu. Int. Med.*, 120, 211, 1994.

206. Carethers, M., Diagnosing vitamin B-12 deficiency: a common geriatric disorder, *Geriatrics*, 43, 89, 1988.

207. Thompson, W. G., Babitz, L., Cassino, C., Freedman, M., and Lipkin, M., Evaluation of current criteria used to measure vitamin B-12 levels, *Am. J. Med.*, 82, 291, 1987.

208. Lee, D. S. C. and Griffiths, B. W., Human serum vitamin B-12 assay methods – A review, *Clin. Biochem.*, 18, 261, 1985.

209. LeFebvre, R. J., Virji, A. S., and Mertens, B. F., Erroneously low results due to high nonspecific binding encountered with a radioassay kit that measures "true" serum vitamin B-12, *Am. J. Clin. Pathol.*, 74, 209, 1980.

210. O'Sullivan, J. J., Leeming, R. J., Lynch, S. S., and Pollock, A., Radioimmunoassay that measures serum vitamin B-12, *J. Clin. Pathol.*, 45, 328, 1992.

211. Chu, R. C. and Hall, C. A., The total serum homocysteine as an indicator of vitamin B-12 and folate status, *Am. J. Clin. Pathol.*, 90, 446, 1988.

212. Hall, C. A. and Chu, R. C., Serum homocysteine in routine evaluation of potential vitamin B-12 and folate deficiency, *Eur. J. Haematol.*, 45, 143, 1990.

213. *Nutritional Anaemias*, Report of a WHO Scientific Group, World Health Organization Technical Report Series No. 405, World Health Organization, Geneva, Switzerland, 1968.

214. Castle, W. B., A century of curiosity about pernicious anemia, *Trans. Am. Clin. Climatol. Assoc.*, 73, 54, 1961.

215. Minot, G. R. and Murphy, W. P., Treatment of pernicious anemia by a special diet, *J. Am. Med. Assoc.*, 87, 470, 1926.

216. Castle, W. B., Development of knowledge concerning the gastric intrinsic factor and its relation to pernicious anemia, *N. Engl. J. Med.*, 249, 603, 1953.

217. Rickes, E. L., Brink, N. G., Koniuszy, F. R., Wood, T. R., and Folkers, K., Crystalline vitamin B-12, *Science*, 107, 396, 1948.
218. Cohen, K. L. and Donaldson, R. M., Unreliability of radiodilution assays as screening tests for cobalamin (vitamin B-12) deficiency, *JAMA*, 244, 1942, 1980.
219. Pietrzik, K. and Bronstrup, A., Causes and consequences of hyperhomocyst(e)inemia, *Int. J. Vit. Nutr. Res.*, 67, 389, 1997.
220. Mason, J. B. and Miller, J. W., The effects of vitamins B-12, B-6, and folate on blood homocysteine levels, *Ann. N.Y. Acad. Sci.*, 669, 197, 1992.
221. Hathcock, J. N. and Troendle, G. J., Oral cobalamin for treatment of pernicious anemia, *JAMA*, 265, 96, 1991.
222. van Asselt, D. Z. B., de Groot, L. C. P. G. M., van Steveren, W. A., Blom, H. J., Wevers, R. A., Biemond, I., and Hoefnagels, W. H. L., Role of cobalamin intake and atrophic gastritis in mild cobalamin deficiency in older Dutch subjects, *Am. J. Clin. Nutr.*, 68, 328, 1998.
223. Allen, L. H., Rosado, J. L., Casterline, J. E., Martinez, H., Lopez, P., Munoz, E., and Black, A. K., Vitamin B-12 deficiency and malabsorption are highly prevalent in rural Mexican communities, *Am. J. Clin. Nutr.*, 62, 1013, 1995.

Niacin (Nicotinic Acid, Nicotinamide)

Nicotinic acid (3-pyridinecarboxylic acid)
molecular weight: 123.1

Nicotinamide (3-pyridinecarboxamide)
molecular weight: 122.1

N′-methylnicotinamide
molecular weight: 138.1

2-pyridone (N′-methyl-2-pyridone-5-carboxamide)
molecular weight: 153.1

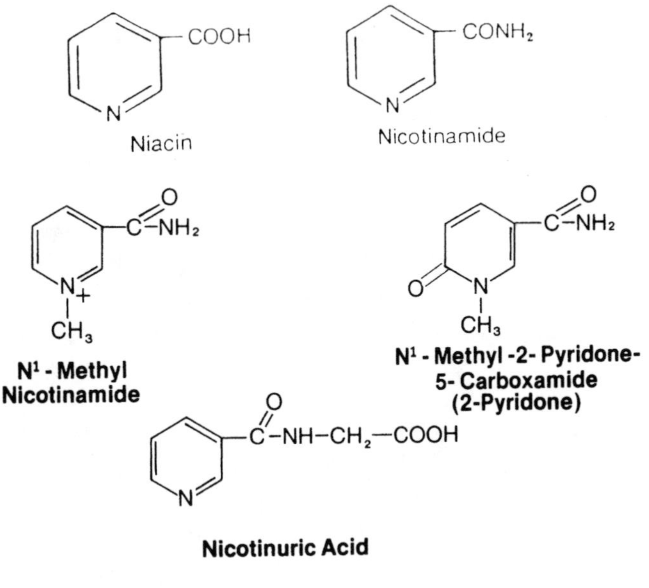

FIGURE 30
Structures of niacin and nicotinamide
and of niacin metabolites.

History of Niacin

Columbus encountered corn and cornmeal in the New World and introduced it into
Europe, where it was slowly accepted. Europeans considered it fit only for animal consumption. Nevertheless, by 1600, corn had been accepted into the diet even as far as China
and the East Indies. In 1735, Don Gaspar Casal, physician to King Philip V of Spain,
described a skin condition which was given the name "mal de la rosa."[8-13] In 1740, a similar

condition was recognized in Italy and given the term "pellagra" (rough skin). With the widespread use of corn (maize), pellagra subsequently spread throughout most of Europe.

The first case of pellagra in the U.S. was described in 1864 in Utica, NY. By 1907, pellagra began to appear with alarming speed in the southern states. In 1917, 170,000 cases of pellagra were reported. In 1930 alone, 7,146 deaths from pellagra were reported.

Pellagra was considered a transmitted disease or one caused by moldy corn, however, Dr. Joseph Goldberger of the U.S. Public Health Service demonstrated that pellagra was a dietary disease. He was proven correct with the isolation of nicotinic acid in 1937 by Conrad A. Elvehjem and co-workers at the University of Wisconsin who demonstrated its ability to cure canine black tongue (analogous to human pellagra).[15] Soon thereafter, Tom D. Spies, at the University of Alabama in Birmingham, used nicotinic acid to dramatically treat four subjects with classical pellagra.[16] It was subsequently found that the human was capable of converting tryptophan to nicotinic acid.[12,14,22-26]

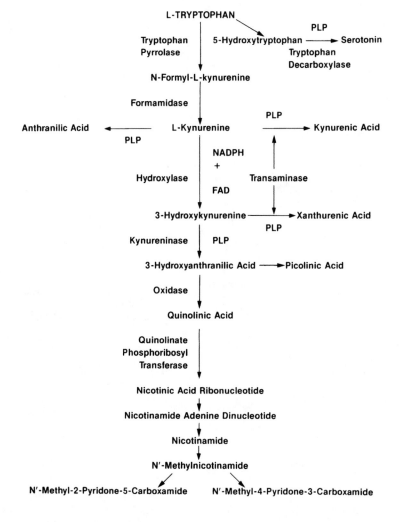

FIGURE 31

Metabolic conversion of tryptophan to nicotinamide in the human. Reactions involving pyridoxal 5'-phosphate are indicated as PLP.

Sources of Niacin

Niacin is used in a generic application to nicotinic acid and nicotinamide. Niacin is very stable in storage, cooking, and baking. Although red meats, fish, and poultry serve as good sources of niacin, most cereals and legumes provide significant amounts. Lesser amounts are found in vegetables and fruits.[12,22] Food sources that are high in tryptophan may also contribute significantly to the niacin needs. On average, 35 μmol of tryptophan (60 mg) can be converted to 1 μmol of niacin (1 mg). Evidence indicates that excess leucine present in the diet such as with the use of millet (jowar), may impair the conversion of tryptophan to niacin.[29,30] While niacin is present in a free form in millet (jowar),[32] biologically unavailable bound forms of niacin are present in wheat, cereal products, and corn.[12,13,33-37] An appreciable amount of biological available niacin is even present in brewed coffee.[38]

Niacin Deficiency (Pellagra)

Niacin deficiency is usually associated with diarrhea, dermatitis, dementia, and finally death.[19] In acute pellagra, the mucous membranes of the gastrointestinal and genitourinary tracts become severely inflamed. The mouth and tongue become very sore, swollen, and reddened. Skin changes are particularly pronounced on the parts of the skin exposed to sunlight.

With the ready availability of nicotinic acid (the widespread niacin fortification of foods and with improved diets) pellagra has been virtually eradicated. Pellagra may still be encountered among the Bantus of South Africa, in parts of Egypt and Brazil, and in areas of India where jowar, a form of millet, serves as the main staple in the diet. Poor niacin nutritional status has been reported in school children in the Transvaal Province of South Africa despite niacin fortification of maize meal.[58] Pellagra has also been observed in alcoholics in Brazil,[59,60] and in Mozambican women.[83] Pellagra is seldom seen in the United States; when it is observed it is generally associated with alcoholism and concurrent poor diet. Occasionally, subjects with Hartnup's disease or Crohn's disease have been observed to have the symptoms of pellagra that are corrected with intramuscular administration of nicotinic acid.[13,18,27,28] A pellagra syndrome has been observed in patients treated with isoniazid.[48]

Functions

Niacin participates in more than 200 reactions that are involved in the metabolism of fatty acids, amino acids, and carbohydrates.[12,20,22] Metabolically, niacin serves as a component of the cosubstrates nicotinamide adenine dinucleotide (NAD) and nicotinamide adenine dinucleotide phosphate (NADP).[23] They function as hydrogen acceptors in oxidative reactions or in the reduced forms the cosubstrates function as hydrogen donors in reductive reactions. Hence, tissues with a high respiration rate, such as the central nervous system, are most extensively affected by a niacin deficiency. The body readily converts nicotinic acid to nicotinamide, but very little NAD or NADP is stored in the body. Hence, under experimental conditions, a niacin deficiency was produced in 50 days in adult humans fed a corn diet containing about 4.7 mg of niacin and 190 mg of tryptophan.[19,21]

Although little niacin is present in plasma, appreciable amounts are present in the erythrocytes and leucocytes as NAD.[61,74,91] The following concentrations of NAD were observed in normal adult humans:[67] erythrocytes, 90 µg/L; serum, 0.5 µg/mL; leucocytes, 70 µg/mL; and whole blood, 30 µg/mL.

Methods for the Assessment of Niacin Status

Niacin can be measured microbiologically, chemically, or enzymatically.[20,22,81] Chemical methods are often used to measure niacin metabolites present in the urine.[22,42] More recent procedures for assessing niacin nutritional status have been summarized in a review.[12]

Microbiological Methods

Tetrahymena pyriformis has been used to assay nicotinic acid.[53] Protozoans responds equally to both nicotinic acid and nicotinamide. The growth density of the protozoan is measured and a standard curve established. The assay range of sensitivity is from 1 to 300 ng/mL. Blood and urine samples were autoclaved prior to assay. Using this procedure, the nicotinic acid activity of blood was found to be 2.7 to 9.6 µg/mL and serum was 0.016 to 0.05 µg/mL.[54]

The microbiological assay for niacin was one of the earliest microbiological assay procedures developed.[55] The assay organism used is *Lactabacillus plantarum* ATCC No. 8014. Assay medium used for the assay is commercially available (Difco Laboratories, Detroit, MI). *L. plantarum* responds essentially equally to nicotinic acid, nicotinamide, and nicotinuric acid. The assay range was 3 to 30 ng/mL. *L. plantarum* has also been used in a radiometric microbiological assay for niacin in biological fluids.[82]

Pediococcus acidilactici ACCT No. 8042 (*Leuconostoc mesenteroides* P-60) has also been used. This organism responds only to nicotinic acid.

In the author's laboratory, a simplified microbiological assay procedure has been employed to measure niacin concentrations in plasma (unpublished data). The procedure uses *L. plantarum* as the assay organism and the assay medium was obtained from Difco Laboratories. The nicotinic acid standard was obtained from the National Institute of Standards and Technology, Gaithersburg, MD. The procedure was an adaptation of the microbiological assay of folic acid employed by Tamura[57] to provide a niacin assay procedure. The procedure utilized 96-well microplates. The bacterial growth was measured with a microplate reader interfaced with a personal computer. The microprocedure minimizes sample requirements and permits a large number of samples to be readily analyzed.

Chemical Methods

Because of low sensitivity and specificity, chemical methods used to analyze foods for niacin have not been satisfactory for measuring niacin in biological specimens.[12,22]

N'-methylnicotinamide

Formerly, niacin metabolites such as N'-methylnicotinamide, were measured by fluorometric procedures based on the reaction of ketones with the metabolite in an alkaline solution to form a fluorescent product.

Ketones react with N'-methylnicotinamide in alkaline solution to form a fluorescent product, which in the presence of acid is converted to a more stable blue fluorescent product which is measured with a photofuorometer. Methyl-ethyl ketone is usually the ketone of choice although acetone has been used.[42-44] This simple procedure was used extensively to measure N'-methylnicotinamide in urine specimen collected during the numerous international nutrition surveys conducted by the International Committee for National Defense of the National Institutes of Health.[42] Improved methods are available for the analysis of N'-methylnicotinamide in urine that are highly sensitive and reproducible.[12,22,45,46] The spectrophotofluorometric procedure of Carpenter and Kodicek has been a reliable method for the measurement of N'-methylnicotinamide in urine.[44] Sensitive fluorometric procedures are also available to measure N'-methylnicotinamide in serum.[47] The procedures are based on the early Huff and Perlzwig method.[43]

High-Performance Liquid Chromatography Procedures (HPLC)

The measurements of the two metabolites, N'-methylnicotinamide and N'-methyl-2-pyridone-5-carboxamide, have been greatly facilitated by the availability of high-performance liquid chromatography (HPLC).[12,39,51,56,61-64,70-72]

The HPLC procedure of Carter is simple, sensitive, specific, and accurate for measuring N'-methyl-2-pyridone-5-carboxamide and N'-methylnicotinamide in urine specimens.[64] After a simple anion-exchange clean-up of the urine sample, the two metabolites are quantitated with the use of HPLC. A simple HPLC method has been described by Kutnink et al.[70] for determining N'-methylnicotinamide in urine samples. Human urine samples can be analyzed directly without need for prior extraction or ion exchange cleanup. The procedure has been exceedingly reliable and rapid.

With the use of a linear ion-pair mobile phase gradient HPLC, McKee et al.[84] were able to separate and quantitate nicotinamide, nicotinic acid, nicotinamide, nicotinuric acid, N'-methylnicotinamide, and N'-methyl-2-pyridone-5-carboxamide in human urine.

Terry and Simon,[72] following separate ion-exchange extractions measured simultaneously N'-methylnicotinamide and N'-methyl-2-pyridone-5-carboxamide. A number of other similar HPLC procedures have been described and applied to urine or plasma samples.[56,71,85]

Measurement of N'-Methyl-4-Pyridone-5-Carboxamide

Shibata and colleagues have reported on HPLC methods for the determination of the urinary concentrations of N'-methy-2-pyridone-5-carboxamide, N'-methyl-4-pyridone-5-carboxamide, and nicotinamide.[88-90] Previously, because of analytical difficulties little information was available on the urinary excretion by the human of N'-methyl-4-pyridone-5-carboxamide. Shibata and Matsu[90] reported that Japanese women excreted 7.1 ± 3.3 µmol/d of N'-methyl-4-pyridone-5-carboxamide. In comparison, 59.8 ± 26.5 μmol/d of N'-methyl-2-pyridone-5-carboxamide and 31.1 ± 12.3 μmol/d of N'-methylnicotinamide were excreted.[90]

Assessment of Niacin Status

Much of the niacin in certain foods such as corn (maize) is in a bound form frequently unavailable to the human (e.g., niacytin).[33-37] Consequently, dietary intake information may be misleading with respect to niacin nutrition. Thus biochemical information has been considered more useful than dietary data for evaluating niacin nutritional status (Tables 40 to 42).[41]

TABLE 40
Guidelines Used For Evaluating Niacin Status

1. ICNND Guide to Interpretation N'-methylnicotinamide Excretion Data[42]

Subjects	Deficient	Low	Acceptable	High
Adults (males and non-pregnant and non-lactating females)				
mg/g creatinine	< 0.5	0.5–1.59	1.6–4.29	> 4.3
mg/6 hr/g creatinine	< 0.2	0.2–0.59	0.6–1.59	> 1.6
Pregnant women[52,80]				
mg/g creatinine				
1st trimester	< 0.5	0.5–1.59	1.6–4.29	> 4.3
2nd trimester	< 0.6	0.6–1.99	2.0–4.99	> 5.0
3rd trimester	< 0.8	0.8–2.49	2.5–6.49	> 6.5

2. Ratio Urinary 2-pyridone/N'-methylnicotinamide[49-51,72]

All age groups: <1.0 at risk of niacin deficiency

3. Urinary 2-pyridone Excretion[65,66]

Niacin Status	mg/g creatinine
Normal	> 4.0
Low	2.0–3.9
Deficient	< 2.0

4. Erythrocyte NAD/Erythrocyte NADP Ratio[74]

Controlled metabolic unit study (n = 7 men)
Ratio < 1.0 indicated at risk of a niacin deficiency

TABLE 41
Effect of Niacin Nutriture on Levels of Niacin Metabolites in Plasma in Young Men

Days on Diet	Niacin Equivalents Consumed/Day	Plasma Niacin Metabolites (μg/DL) (n = 7)		
		2-Pyridone	N'-Methylnicotinamide	Ratio
35	6	1.3 ± 2.3	2.0 ± 0.9	0.65
35	10	3.7 ± 0.9	2.3 ± 0.5	1.61
28	28	16.3 ± 5.9	3.0 ± 2.1	5.43

From References 73, 91.

TABLE 42
Urinary Excretion of Niacin Metabolites by Mozambican Women

Metabolite	Control ($n = 9$)	Without Signs of Pellagra ($n = 9$)	With Pellagra ($n = 10$)
2-pyridone*			
mg/g creatinine	3.87 ± 3.63	1.35 ± 2.53	0.5 ± 0.49
mmol/24-hr urine	557 ± 199	152 ± 104	42 ± 9
N'-methylnicotinamide			
mg/g creatinine	2.40 ± 1.11	1.83 ± 0.52	2.00 ± 0.79
mmol/24-hr urine	273 ± 50	162 ± 17	213 ± 41
2-Pyridone/N'-methylnicotinamide Ratio			
mg/g creatinine	1.61	0.73	0.25
mmol/24-hr urine	1.95	0.90	0.18

* 2-pyridone = N'-methyl-2-pyridone-5-carboxamide.
Data reported by Dillon et al.[83]

Although information on niacin requirements is extensive, biochemical procedures for assessing niacin nutritional status are limited. The amount of nicotinic acid present in serum or urine is small and does not respond appreciably to changes in nicotinic acid intake. However, measurement of metabolites of niacin present in urine and serum have been useful as an indirect marker of niacin status.

Unfortunately, few laboratory procedures are available for assessing niacin nutrition in humans.[11,17,20,39] Most often, products of niacin metabolism excreted in the urine are measured.[17,39] The first clinical signs of a niacin deficiency occurs shortly after the urinary excretion of niacin metabolites has stabilized at low levels.[19] Urinary excretion of niacin metabolites falls to very low levels in pellagra patients. The excretion of N'-methyl-2-pyridone-5-carboxamide (2-pyridone) falls more precipitously than N'-methylnicotinamide.[21,49,76-78] Based on the excretion of these metabolites, niacin-loading tests have been proposed for the evaluation of niacin nutritional status.[76] However, these loading tests have seen little use. Since the body stores little excess niacin, the sum of the urinary excretion of N'-methylnicotinamide and N'-methyl-2-pyridone-5-carboxamide in a 24-hour period can reflect the dietary intake of niacin and tryptophan (Tables 40 and 41).[79]

Although the metabolites of niacin are numerous, the major metabolites excreted into the urine are N'-methyl-nicotinamide, N'-methyl-2-pyridone-5-carboxamide, N'-methyl-4-pyridone-5-carboxamide, and nicotinuric acid (glycine conjugated nicotinic acid).[12,17,20-23] In animal products, niacin is present largely as nicotinamide nucleotides.

The adult human normally excretes 20 to 30% of their niacin intakes as N'-methylnicotinamide and 40 to 60% as the N'-methyl-2-pyridone-5-carboxamide. Only small amounts of intact niacin are excreted in the urine and the level excreted is only slightly influenced by dietary intakes of niacin or typtophan. Consequently, measurements of intact niacin are not useful for assessing niacin status.

When only a random urine specimen is available, such as with field studies, the ratio of 2-pyridone to N'-methylnicotinamide can serve as a screening method for evaluating niacin status.[79,91] The ratio was unaffected by level of creatinine excretion, age, or accuracy of collection period.[79] A ratio of less than 1.0 would be indicative of a niacin deficiency.[79] The ratio correlated well with the occurrence of clinical symptoms of niacin deficiency (Table 42).[83]

With a niacin deficiency, the urinary excretion for 2-pyridone is reduced more profoundly than that of N'-methynicotinamide.[12,49] Some investigators have suggested that low 2-pyridone excretion levels alone can serve to evaluate a niacin nutritional status.[73,91] Relating urinary excretion of niacin metabolites to creatinine excretion has also been used as an indicator of niacin status.[59] Functional tests for the evaluation of niacin nutritional status based on NADP or NAD cosubstrate roles have not been developed.

With the availability of rapid, simple, and reliable HPLC methods to measure 2-pyridone and N'-methylnicotinamide, it is possible to use the ratio of these two metabolites as an index of niacin nutritional status. Formerly, 2-pyridone measurements were avoided because the assay was tedious to perform. As noted above, an advantage of the ratio is that random urine specimens may be used instead of 24-hr urine collection. The 2-pyridone: N'-methylnicotinamide ratio is not influenced by age or creatinine excretion. Terry and Simon[72] reported that for 50 normal adults a ratio of 3.60 ± 1.06 (range 1.76 to 5.9) was observed. A ratio of less than 1.0 was considered indicative of a niacin deficiency. Similar criteria were reported by DeLang and Joubert.[51]

Plasma Metabolites and Niacin Status

In a controlled study performed on 7 young men maintained on varying niacin equivalents, plasma and urine concentrations of 2-pyridone and N'-methylnicotinamide were measured.[73,91] The investigators concluded from their findings that 2-pyridone levels of plasma were a better marker of niacin deficiency than the levels of N'-methylnicotinamide in either plasma or urine.[73,91] The plasma ratios of 2-pyridone: N'-methylnicotinamide also appear informative. If these findings are confirmed and extended, only a blood plasma specimen would be necessary to evaluate the niacin nutritional status of an individual.[91]

Pyridine Nucleotides and Niacin Status

HPLC techniques have been applied in the measurement of nicotinamide, nicotinic acid, and their metabolites in urine and plasma.[12,56,71,72] The pyridine nucleotides and related compounds may also be separated by HPLC.[68] This procedure may have application in that the niacin nutritional status may relate to the ratio of NAD:NADP in the erythrocytes.[17,74] A decrease in the ratio may identify subjects with a poor niacin status.[17] A ratio below 1.0 would be indicative of an individual at risk of developing a niacin deficiency.[74] A micromethod was used to measure the pyridine nucleotides.[75] This approach to the evaluation of niacin status may be worthy of further study.

Children (10 to 13 Years)

Niacin status was determined in 25 children by measuring urinary excretion of N'-methyl-2-pyridone-5-carboxamide (2-pyridone) with the use of a HPLC procedure.[58,64] The niacin metabolite excretion was related to the excretion of creatinine in two hour urine collections. Using this procedure, 28% of the rural black South African children studied were low or deficient in niacin.[58]

Niacin status was classified on the following basis of 2-pyridone excretion.[65,66]

Urinary 2-pyridone Excretion	
> 4 mg/g creatinine	Normal niacin status
2.0 to 3.9 mg/g creatinine	Low
< 2.0 mg/g creatinine	Deficient

Pregnancy

The excretion of N'-methylnicotinamide increases gradually during the second trimester of pregnancy, reaches a plateau during the third trimester, and returns rapidly to normal post-partum (Table 40).[52,80] Comparable information on the urinary excretion of 2-pyridone is needed in order to determine whether the ratio of the two niacin metabolites would provide improved information as to the niacin status.

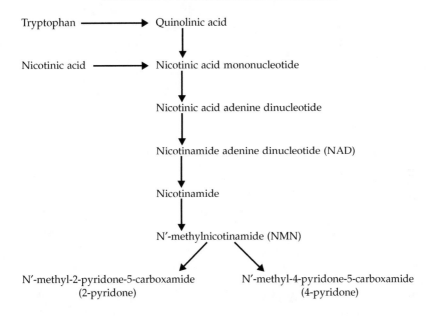

Metabolism of Nicotinic Acid and Nicotinamide

Tryptophan ⟶ Quinolinic acid

Nicotinic acid ⟶ Nicotinic acid mononucleotide

↓

Nicotinic acid adenine dinucleotide

↓

Nicotinamide adenine dinucleotide (NAD)

↓

Nicotinamide

↓

N'-methylnicotinamide (NMN)

↙ ↘

N'-methyl-2-pyridone-5-carboxamide N'-methyl-4-pyridone-5-carboxamide
(2-pyridone) (4-pyridone)

Toxicity (Niacin)

Nicotinic acid is used in large doses to treat hyperlipedemia (Types II–V).[1-7,13] Nicotinic acid, but not nicotinamide, will produce flushing as a consequence of histamine release.[2-4] Most subjects taking niotinic acid at a level of 3 grams per day experience the flushing, with about one-half of the patients developing a tolerance to this side effect.[2-4] Other toxic effects of high doses of nicotinoic acid (usually 3 gram/day) include stomach pain, diarrhea, and nausea.[2-7] Nicontic acid ingestion has been associated also with a number of other adverse effects such as some cardiac arrhythmias, dermatologic problems, hepatotoxicity, and elevated serum levels of uric acid.[2-5] These conditions are usually reversed when the high intakes of niacin are discontinued. Measurements of blood levels of nicotinic acid or its metabolites are not useful in evaluating toxic effects, although obtaining information on the status of plasma enzymes of hepatic origin (e.g., serum transaminases) and other liver function tests is warranted if not essential.[5,7] The majority of the toxic effects of high intakes of niacin are associated with the use of sustained-release niacin rather than with immediate-release niacin preparations.[5]

Summary

The most commonly used procedure to assess niacin nutritional status has been the measurement of the niacin metabolites, N'-methylnicotinamide and N'-methyl-2-pyridone-5-carboxamide (2-pyridone), in the urine. Under normal circumstances, adults excrete 20 to 30% of their nicotinic acid as the N'-methylnicotinamide form and 40 to 60% as the 2-pyridone. Thus, a ratio of 1.3 to 4 exists between 2-pyridone/N'-methylnicotinamide under normal conditions. A ratio value of less than 1.0 is considered to be indicative of a latent niacin deficiency. The excretion of 2-pyridone falls more markedly than that of N'-methylnicotinamide with a niacin deficiency. The advent of HPLC procedures has permitted a sensitive, accurate, specific, and rapid means of measuring both metabolites in both urine and plasma. The measurement of 2-pyridone and N'-methylnicotinamide concentrations in plasma appears to provide a more reliable ratio of the metabolites than comparable measurements on urine. The ratio of NAD:NADP in the erythrocytes holds promise as another means to identify niacin inadequacy in individuals.

References

1. Vavos, J. G., Patel, S. T., Falko, J. M., Newman, H. A. I., and Hill, D. S., Effects of nicotinic acid therapy on plasma lipoproteins and very low density lipoprotein apoprotein C subspecies in hyperlipoproteinemia, *J. Clin. Endocrin. Metab.*, 54, 1210, 1982.
2. Zollner, N., Effects of nicotinic acid, nicotinamide, and pyridylcarbinol in pharmacologic dosages on lipid metabolism in humans, *Int. J. Vit. Nutr. Res.*, 30 (Supplement), 114, 1989.
3. DiPalma, J. R. and Thayer, W. S., Use of niacin as a drug, *Annu. Rev. Nutr.*, 11, 169, 1991.
4. Alhadeff, L., Gualtieu, C. T., and Lipton, M., Toxic effects of water-soluble vitamins, *Nutr. Rev.*, 42, 33, 1984.
5. McKenny, J. M., Proctor, J. D., Harris, S., and Chinchili, V. M., A comparison of the efficacy and toxic effects of sustained- vs. immediate-release niacin in hypercholesterolemic patients, *JAMA*, 271, 672, 1994.
6. The Coronary Drug Project Research Group, Clofibrate and niacin in coronary artery disease, *JAMA*, 231, 360, 1975.
7. Expert panel on detection, evaluation, and treatment of high blood cholesterol in adults, Summary of the Second Report of the National Cholesterol Education Program (NCEP) Expert Panel on Detection, Evaluation, and Treatment of High Blood Cholesterol in Adults (Adult Treatment Panel II), *JAMA*, 269, 3015, 1993.
8. Major, R. H., *Classic Descriptions of Disease*, C. C. Thomas Publications, Springfield, IL, 1932, 575.
9. Carpenter, K. C., *Pellagra*, Academic Press, New York, 1981.
10. McCollum, E. V., *A History of Nutrition*, Houghton Mifflin Company, Boston, 1957.
11. Sebrell, W. H. Jr., History of pellagra, *Fed. Proc.*, 40, 1520, 1981.

12. Sauberlich, H. E., Nutritional aspects of pyridine nucleotides, in *Pyridine Nucleotide Coenzymes: Chemical, Biochemical, and Medical Aspects*, Vol. 2B, Dolphin, D., Paulson, R., and Avramovic, O., Eds., John Wiley & Sons, Inc., New York, 1987.
13. Darby, W. J., McNutt, K. W., and Todhunter, E. N., Niacin, *Nutr. Revs.*, 33, 289, 1975.
14. Krehl, W. A., Discovery of the effect of tryptophan on niacin deficiency, *Fed. Proc.*, 40, 1527, 1981.
15. Elvehjem, C. A., Madden, R. J., Strong, F. M., and Woolley, D. W., Relation of nicotinic acid and nicotinic acid amide to canine black tongue, *Am. Chem. Soc.*, 59, 1767, 1937.
16. Spies, T. D., Cooper, C., and Blankenhorn, M. A., The use of nicotinic acid in treatment of pellagra, *JAMA*, 110, 622, 1938.
17. Swendseid, M. E. and Jacob, R. A., Niacin, in *Modern Nutrition in Health and Disease*, 8th edition, Shils, M. E., Olson, J. A., and Shike, M., Eds., Lea & Febiger, Philadelphia, 1994, 376.
18. Pollack, S., Enat, R., Haim, S., Zinder, O., and Barzilai, D., Pellagra as the presenting manifestation of Crohn's disease, *Gastraenterology*, 85, 948, 1982.
19. Goldsmith, G. A., Vitamin B-complex, *Progress in Food and Nutrition Sciences*, Vol. 1, 559, 1975.
20. Bender, D. A., Niacin, in *Vitamin in Medicine*, Volume 1, 4th edition, William Heinemann Medical Books, London, 1980, 315.
21. Goldsmith, G. A., Sarett, H. P., Register, U. D., and Gibben, J., Studies of niacin requirement in man. I. Experimental pellagra in subjects on corn diets low in niacin and tryptophan, *J. Clin. Invest.*, 31, 533, 1952.
22. Hankes, L. V., Nicotinic acid and nicotinamide, in *Handbook of Vitamins*, Machlin, L. J., Ed., Marcel Dekker, Inc., New York, 1984, 329.
23. Henderson, L. M., Niacin, *Annu. Rev. Nutr.*, 3, 289, 1983.
24. Patterson, J. I., Brown, R. R., Linkswiler, H., and Harper, A. E., Excretion of tryptophan-niacin metabolites by young men: effects of tryptophan, leucine, and vitamin B_6 intakes, *Am. J. Clin. Nutr.*, 33, 2157, 1980.
25. Horwitt, M. K., Harvey, C. C., Rothwell, W. S., Cutler, J. L., and Hafferon, D., Tryptophan-niacin relationship in man, *J. Nutr.*, 60, 1, 1956.
26. Goldsmith, G. A., Miller, O. N., and Unglaub, W. G., Efficiency of tryptophan as a niacin precursor in man, *J. Nutr.*, 73, 172, 1961.
27. Halvorsen, K. and Halvorsen, S., Harnup disease, *Pediatrics*, 31, 29, 1963.
28. Moran, J. R. and Green, H. L., The B vitamins and vitamin C in human nutrition, II. Conditional B vitamins and vitamin C, *Am. J. Dis. Childr.*, 133, 308, 1979.
29. Bender, D. A., Effects of a dietary excess of leucine on the metabolism of tryptophan in the rat: a mechanism for the pellagragenic action of leucine, *Brit. J. Nutr.*, 50, 25, 1983.
30. Gopalan, C. and Srikantia, S. G., Leucine and pellagra, *Lancet*, 1, 954, 1960.
31. Horwitt, M. K., Harper, A. E., and Henderson, L. M., Niacin-tryptophan relationship for evaluating niacin equivalents, *Am. J. Clin. Nutr.*, 34, 423, 1981.
32. Belavady, B. and Gopalan, C., Availability of nicotinic acid in jowar *(Sorgum vulgare)*, *Indian J. Biochem.*, 3, 44, 1966.
33. Mason, J. B., Gibson, N., and Kodicek, E., The chemical nature of the bound nicotinic acid of wheat bran: studies of nicotinic acid-containing macromolecules, *Brit. J. Nutr.*, 30, 297, 1973.
34. Ghosh, H. P., Sarkar, P. K., and Guha, B. C., Distribution of the bound form of nicotinic acid in natural materials, *J. Nutr.*, 79, 451, 1963.
35. Kodicek, E. and Wilson, P. W., The isolation of niacytin, the bound form of nicotinic acid, *Biochem. J.*, 76, 27P, 1960.
36. Kodicek, E., Some problems connected with the availability of niacin in cereals, *Bibl. Nutr. Diet*, 23, 86, 1976.
37. Carter, E. G., and Carpenter, K. J., The bioavailability for humans of bound niacin from wheat bran, *Am. J. Clin. Nutr.*, 36, 855, 1982.
38. Smith, R. F., Niacin content of coffee, *Nature*, 197, 1321, 1963.
39. Sauberlich, H. E., Assessment of vitamin B_1, vitamin B_2, niacin, and pantothenic acid, in *Nutritional Status Assessment of the Individual*, Livingston, G. E., Ed., Food and Nutrition Press, Trumbull, 1989, 295.

40. Sauberlich, H. E., Skala, J. H., and Dowdy, R. P., *Laboratory Tests for the Assessment of Nutritional Status*, CRC Press, Inc., Boca Raton, FL, 1974.

41. Pearson, W. N., Assessment of nutritional status: biochemical methods, in *Nutrition*, Volume III, Beaton, G. H. and McHenry, E. W., Eds., Academic Press, New York, 1966, 265.

42. *Manual for Nutrition Surveys*, 2nd edition, Interdepartmental Committee on Nutritional Defense, National Institutes of Health, Bethesda, MD, 1963.

43. Huff, J. W. and Perlzweig, W. A., The fluorescent condensation product of N'-methylnicotinamide and acetone, II. A sensitive method for the determination of N'-methylnicotinamide in urine, *J. Biol. Chem.*, 167, 157, 1947.

44. Carpenter, K. J. and Kodicek, E., The fluorometric estimation of N'-methylnicotinamide and its differentiation from coenzyme I, *Biochem. J.*, 46, 421, 1950.

45. Price, J. M., Brown, R. R., and Yess, N., Testing the functional capacity of the tryptophan-niacin pathway in man by analysis of urinary metabolites, *Adv. Metab. Disease*, 2, 159, 1965.

46. Vivian, V. M., Reynolds, M. S., and Price, J. M., Use of ion exchange resins for the determination of N'-methylnicotinamide, *Anal. Biochem.*, 10, 274, 1965.

47. Clark, B. R., Halpern, R. M., and Smith, R. A., A fluormetric method for quantitation in the picomole range of N'-methylnicotinamide and nicotinamide in serum, *Anal. Biochem.*, 68, 54, 1975.

48. Bender, D. A. and Russel-Jones, R., Isoniazid-induced pellagra despite vitamin B_6 supplementation, *Lancet*, 2, 1125, 1979.

49. Vivian, V. M., Chalouyska, M. M., and Reynolds, M. S., Some aspects of tryptophan metabolism in human subjects, I. Nitrogen balances, blood pyridine nucleotides and urinary excretion of N'-methylnicotinamide and N'-methyl-2-pyridone-5-carboxamide on a low-niacin diet, *J. Nutr.*, 66, 587, 1958.

50. DuPessis, J. P., An evaluation of biochemical criteria for use in nutrition surveys, Council for Scientific and Industrial Research Report No. 261, National Nutrition Research Institute, Pretoria, 1967.

51. DeLang, D. J. and Joubert, C. P., Assessment of nicotinic acid status of population groups, *Am. J. Clin. Nutr.*, 15, 169, 1964.

52. Darby, W. J., McGanity, W. J., and Martin, M. P. et al., The Vanderbilt Cooperative study of maternal and infant nutrition, IV. Dietary, laboratory and physical findings in 2,129 delivered pregnancies, *J. Nutr.*, 51, 565, 1953.

53. Baker, H. and Frank, O., Eds., Nicotinic acid, in *Clinical Vitaminology: Methods*, and *Interpretation*, Interscience Publication, New York, 1968.

54. Baker, H., Frank, O., Pasher, I., Hunter, S. H., and Sobotka, H., Nicotinic acid assay in blood and urine, *Clin. Chem.*, 6, 572, 1960.

55. Snell, E. E. and Wright, L. D., A microbiological assay for the determination of nicotinic acid, *J. Biol. Chem.*, 139, 675, 1941.

56. Sauberlich, H. E., Newer laboratory methods for assessing nutriture of selected B-complex vitamins, *Annu. Rev. Nutr.*, 4, 377, 1984.

57. Tamura, T., Microbiological assay of folates, in *Folic Acid Metabolism in Health and Disease*, Picciano, M. F., Stokstad, E. L. R. and Gregory, J. F. III., Eds., Wiley-Liss, New York, 1990, 121.

58. Soldenhoff, M. and van der Westhuyzen, J., Niacin status of schoolchildren in Transvaal Province, South Africa, *Int. J. Vit. Nutr. Res.*, 58, 208, 1988.

59. Vannucchi, H., Mellow de Oliveira, J. A., and Dutra de Oliveira, J. E., Tryptophan metabolism in alcoholic pellagra patients: measurements of urinary metabolites and histochemical studies of related muscle enzymes, *Am. J. Clin. Nutr.*, 35, 1368, 1982.

60. Vannucchi, H. and Moreno, F. S., Interaction of niacin and zinc metabolism in patients with alcoholic pellagra, *Am. J. Clin. Nutr.*, 50, 364, 1989.

61. Joubert, C. P. and de Lange, J., A modification of the method for the determination of N'-methyl-2-pyridone-carboxylamide in human urine and its application in the evaluation of nicotinic acid status, *Proc. Nutr. Soc. South Africa*, 3, 60, 1962.

62. Walters, C. J., Brown, R. R., Kaihara, M., and Price, J. M., The excretion of N'-methyl-2-pyridone-5-carboxamide by man following ingestion of several known or potential precursors, *J. Biol. Chem.*, 217, 489, 1955.

63. Price, J. M., The determination of N′-methyl-2-pyridone-5-carboxamide in human urine, *J. Biol. Chem.*, 211, 117, 1954.

64. Carter, E. G. A., Quantitation of urinary niacin metabolites by reversed-phase liquid chromatography, *Am. J. Clin. Nutr.*, 36, 926, 1982.

65. Louw, M. E. J., DuPlessis, J. P., and Laubscher, N. F., A biochemical evaluation of the nutrition status of rural and urban pedimales, *S. Afri. Med. J.*, 46, 1139, 1972.

66. Nel, A., DuPlessis, J. P., and Fellingham, S. A., Biochemical evaluation, *S. Afr. Med. J.*, 45, 1315, 1971.

67. Ijichi, H., Ichiyamo, A., and Hayaishi, O., Studies on the biosynthesis of nicotinamide adenine dinucleotide, *J. Biol. Chem.*, 241, 3701, 1966.

68. Benofsky, C., Preparation of alpha-NADP+, *Methods Enzymology*, 66, 23, 1980.

69. Clark, B. R., Fluorometric quantitation of picomole amounts of 1-methylnicotinamide and nicotinamide in serum, *Methods Enzymology*, 66, 5, 1980.

70. Kutnink, M. A., Vannucchi, H., and Sauberlich, H. E., A simple high performance liquid chromatography procedure for the determination of N′-methylnicotinamide in urine, *J. Liq. Chromtogr.*, 7, 969, 1984.

71. Sandhu, J. S. and Fraser, D. R., Measurement of niacin metabolites in urine by high pressure liquid chromatography; a simple, sensitive assay of niacin nutritional status, *Int. J. Vit. Nutr. Res.*, 51, 139, 1981.

72. Terry, R. C. and Simon, M., Determination of niacin metabolites 1-methyl-5-carboxylamide-2-pyridine and N-1-methylnicotinamide in urine by high-performance liquid chromatography, *J. Chromatogr.*, 232, 261, 1982.

73. Jacob, R. A., McKee, R. W., McKee, C. S., Fu-Liu, C. S., and Swendseid, M. E., Plasma markers of human niacin status, *Fed. Proc.*, 46, 1159, 1987.

74. Fu, C. S., Swendseid, M. E., Jacob, R. A., and McKee, R. W., Biochemical markers for assessment of niacin status in young men: levels of erythrocyte niacin coenzymes and plasma tryptophan, *J. Nutr.*, 119, 1949, 1989.

75. Nisselbaum, J. S. and Green, S., A simple ultramicromethod for determination of pyridine nucleotides in tissues, *Anal. Biochem.*, 27, 212, 1969.

76. Unglaub, W. G. and Goldsmith, G. A., Evaluation of vitamin adequacy: urinary excretion test, in *Methods for Evaluation of Nutritional Adequacy and Status*, Spector, H., Peterson, M. S., and Friedemann, T. E., Eds., National Academy of Sciences, National Research Council, Washington D.C., 1954, 69.

77. Goldsmith, G. A., Rosenthal, H. L., and Unglaub, W. G., Niacin requirement on "corn" and "wheat" diets low in tryptophan, *Fed. Proc.*, 12, 415, 1953.

78. Rosenthal, H. L., Goldsmith, G. A., and Sarett, H. P., Excretion of N′-methylnicotinamide in urine of human subjects, *Proc. Soc. Exp. Biol. Med.*, 82, 208, 1953.

79. Prinsloo, J. G., DuPlessis, J. P., Kruger, H., DeLange, D. J., and DeVilliers, L. S., Protein nutrition status in childhood pellagra. Evaluation of nicotinic acid status and creatinine excretion, *Am. J. Clin. Nutr.*, 21, 98, 1968.

80. Sauberlich, H. E., Vitamin indices, in *Laboratory Indices of Nutritional Status in Pregnancy*, Pitkin, R. M., Ed., Food and Nutrition Board, National Research Council, National Academy of Sciences, Washington D.C., 1978, 109.

81. Ball, G. F. M., *Water-soluble Vitamin Assays in Human Nutrition*, Chapman & Hall, New York, 1994.

82. Kertcher, J. A., Guilarte, T. R., Chen, M. F., Rider, A. A., and Medntyre, P. A., A radiometric microbiological assay for the biologically active forms of niacin, *J. Nucl. Med.*, 20, 419, 1979.

83. Dillion, J. C., Malfait, P., Demaux, G., and Foldi-Hope, C., Les metabolites urinaires de la niacine au cours de la pellagre, *Annu. Nutr. Metab.*, 36, 181, 1992.

84. McKee, R. W., Kang-Lee, Y. AE., Panqus, M., and Swenseid, M. E., Determination of nicotinamide, and metabolic products in urine by high-performance liquid chromatography, *J. Chromatg.*, 230, 309, 1982.

85. DeVries, J. X., Gunthert, W., and Ding, R., Determination of nicotinamide in human plasma and urine by ion-pair reversed-phase high-performance liquid chromatography, *J. Chromatgr.*, 221, 161, 1980.

86. Hengen, N., Seiberth, V., and Hengen, M., High-performance liquid-chromatographic determination of free nicotinic acid and its metabolite, nicotinuric acid, in plasma and urine, *Clin. Chem.*, 24, 1740, 1978.

87. Hengen, N. and de Vries, J. X., Nicotinic acid and nicotinamide, in *Modern Chromatographic Analyses of the Vitamin*, de Leeheer, A. P., Lambert, W. E., and de Ruyter, M. G. M., Eds., Marcel Dekker, Inc., New York, 1985, 342.

88. Shibata, K., Kawada, T., and Iwai, K., Microdetermination of N'-methyl-2-pyridone-5-carboxamide, a major metabolite of nicotinic acid and nicotinamide, in urine by high-performance liquid chromatography, *J. Chromatogr.*, 417, 173, 1987.

89. Shibata, K., Kawada, T., and Iwai, K., Simultaneous micro-determination of nicotinamide and its major metabolites, N'-methyl-2-pyridone-5-carboxamide and N'-methyl-4-pyridone-3-carboxamide, by high-performance liquid chromatography, *J. Chromatogr.*, 424, 23, 1988.

90. Shibata, K. and Matsuo, H., Correlation between niacin equivalent intake and urinary excretion of its metabolites, and N'-methyl-4-pyridone-3-carboxamide, in humans consuming a self-selected food, *Am. J. Clin. Nutr.*, 50, 114, 1989.

91. Jacob, R. A., Swendseid, M. E., McKee, R. W., Fu, C. S., and Clemens, R. A., Biochemical markers for assessment of niacin status in young men: urinary and blood levels of niacin metabolites, *J. Nutr.*, 119, 591, 1989.

Pantothenic Acid

Converting metric units to International System (SI) units:

$\mu g/mL \times 4.56 = \mu mol/L$

molecular weight: 219.23

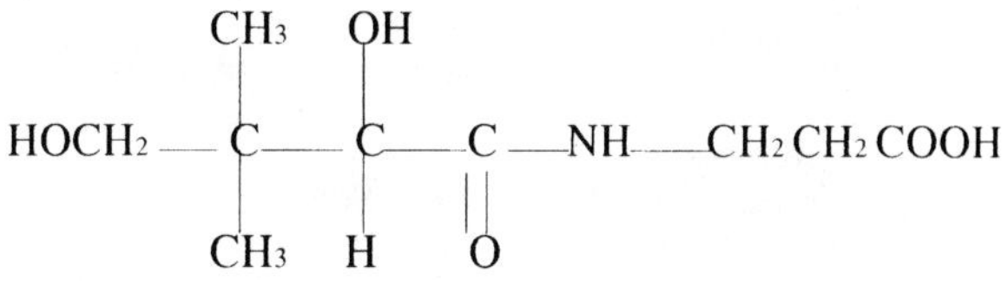

$$HOCH_2 - \underset{\underset{CH_3}{|}}{\overset{\overset{CH_3}{|}}{C}} - \underset{\underset{H}{|}}{\overset{\overset{OH}{|}}{C}} - \underset{\underset{O}{||}}{C} - NH - CH_2 CH_2 COOH$$

FIGURE 32
Structure of pantothenic acid.

General

Pantothenic acid is present in varying amounts in virtually all plant and animal foods.[13,45,46,50] Good sources of the vitamin are legumes, oat cereal, and meats, particularly liver. Milk, vegetables, and fruits contain lesser amounts. The average American diet provides approximately 4 to 7 mg/day of pantothenic acid. Pantothenic acid is a component of two coenzymes; namely, coenzyme A and acyl carrier protein.[1,14,15] The majority of the pantothenic acid in food is present as a component of coenzyme A.[45,46]

During digestion, pantothenic acid is released from coenzyme A. The absorbed pantothenic acid is taken up by the body cells for phosphorylation and resynthesis of coenzyme A.[1,8,9,14,15] The limited information available indicates that 40 to 60% of the pantothenic acid present in the average American diet is bioavailable.[6,7] Because pantothenic acid contains a peptide linkage, it may be destroyed by heat at either in alkaline or acid pH. Losses in pantothenic acid occur during food processing.[10] Losses of over 50% may occur in canned vegetables and processed meat.[7,10,11] Processed and refined grains lost up to 74% of the pantothenic acid that was present in the whole grain product.[7] For example, the refining of flour resulted in a loss of 54 to 58% in pantothenic acid. Thus, a diet without whole grain and containing certain processed meats could be low in pantothenic acid.[5,23,45]

Pantothenic Acid Deficiency

Experimental studies have demonstrated the need for pantothenic acid in the human.[12,13,17] Human pantothenic acid deficiency is rare, but its occurrence is associated with fatigue and depression.[4] A condition referred to as the "burning feet" syndrome was reported among prisoners of war in the Far East[20] and in malnourished subjects in India and Surinam.

Pantothenic acid preparations were effective in treating the condition; other vitamin B-complex vitamins were ineffective. In a few other instances, such as in Surinam, the burning feet syndrome described has been associated with a multiple B-complex vitamin deficiency state that included a deficiency of pantothenic acid. Chronic malnourished patients and poorly nourished alcoholic patients have been observed with low blood and urine levels of pantothenic acid.

In controlled studies, volunteer subjects placed on a pantothenic acid deficient diet and supplemented with the pantothenic acid antagonist, omega methyl pantothenic acid, developed a deficiency syndrome.[7,12,19,33] Symptoms of the syndrome included malaise, fatigue, insomnia, vomiting, abdominal distress, burning cramps, and parasthesis of the hands and feet. However, the study did not provide for the development of suitable measurements to assess a pantothenic acid deficiency (Tables 43 to 46).

TABLE 43
Pantothenic Acid Content of Blood and Urine of Adolescents

	Pantothenic Acid Content		
Parameter	**Females** (*n* = 32)	**Males** (*n* = 25)	**All** (*n* = 57)
Dietary intake (mg/day)	4.1 ± 1.2	6.3 ± 2.1	5.1 ± 1.9
Whole blood (ng/ml)	344 ± 113	412 ± 1.03	374 ± 113
Whole blood (μmol/L)	1.57 ± 0.52	1.88 ± 0.47	1.17 ± 0.52
Erythrocytes (ng/ml)	301 ± 93	376 ± 104	334 ± 104
Urine (mg/g creatinine)	4.5 ± 1.9	3.3 ± 1.3	4.0 ± 1.8

Eissenstat et al.[23]
Analysis performed by RIA.[41]

TABLE 44
Urinary Excretion of Pantothenic Acid (PA)

	Period of Study			
	I (7 days)	**II–IV** (21 days)	**V–VII** (21 days)	**VII–X** (21 days)
Group A (*n* = 6)				
PA intake (mg/day)	7	0	0	0
Urinary PA excretion (mg/day)	3.05 ± 0.2	1.86 ± 0.4	1.07 ± 0.5	0.79 ± 0.2
Group B (*n* = 4)				
PA intake (mg/day)	7	10	10	10
Urinary PA excretion (mg/day)	3.95 ± 0.2	4.42 ± 1.1	5.47 ± 0.6	5.84 ± 1.3

Subjects on a pantothenic acid-free experimental diet.
From Reference 13.

Results from rabbit studies indicate that wound healing is enhanced with pantothenic acid supplements.[35,36] The requirement for pantothenic acid appears to be related to energy intake.

Functions

Pantothenic acid, as the functional form of coenzyme A, has a central role in fatty acid, carbohydrate, and amino acid metabolism, in the acetylation of some drugs, and in acetyl

TABLE 45

Urinary Excretion of Pantothenic Acid by Subjects on Known Intakes of the Vitamin

Subjects	Pantothenic Acid (mg) Intake (per day)	Urinary Excretion (per day)	References
8 college women	2.8**	3.2	Fox et al.[19,24]
	7.8**	4.5	
	12.8**	5.6	
6 men	0	0.78	Fox et al.[25]
4 men	10	5.53	
11 girls; 7–9 years	4.49**	2.85	Pace et al.[18]
12 girls; 7–9 years	5.00**	1.71	
12 girls; 7–9 years	2.79**	1.31	
Students	12.4**	6.2	Koyangi et al.[26]
8 men	12.0**	7.4	Cohenour and Calloway[27]
5 non-pregnant girls	3.3**	2.5	Cohenour and Calloway[27]
14 girls, postpartum	4.1**	3.5	Cohenour and Calloway[27]
26 lactating women	8.9	4.7	Song et al.[22]

** Double enzyme system used to determine total pantothenic acid intake (e.g., alkaline phosphatase and chicken liver enzyme).[28-30,55]

TABLE 46

Comparison of Microbiological Assay with the Radioimmunoassay for the Measurement of Pantothenic Acid

Subjects (*n*)	Pantothenic Dietary Intakes (mg/day)	Pantothenic Acid Assay Microbiological Assay	Radioimmunoassay
Whole Blood (ng/ml)			
Non-Institutionalized (*n* = 45)	11.1 ± 1.7	527 ± 28	537 ± 27
Institutionalized (*n* = 22)	10.1 ± 1.4	558 ± 27	615 ± 47
Urinary Excretion (mg/g creatinine)			
Non-Institutionalized (*n* = 63)	10.3 ± 1.4	6.4 ± 1.2	8.0 ± 0.9
Institutionalized (*n* = 24)	10.3 ± 1.4	7.1 ± 1.0	8.8 ± 1.0

Data from Srinivasan et al.[21]

group transfers in the biosynthesis of porphyrins and steroids.[1,14-16] Propionate metabolism in man requires pantothenic acid and biotin in its conversion to methylmalonic acid.[32] Pantothenic acid is the prosthetic group on acyl carrier protein which is concerned with the synthesis of fatty acids. More than 70 enzymes are known to require coenzyme A or acyl carrier protein.

Methods for the Determination of Pantothenic Acid

Microbiological Assay

The microbiological assay provides for a sensitive measurement of pantothenic acid. The assay range is from 0.02 μg/mL. The assay for pantothenic acid was among the earliest microbiological assay to be developed and remains the most practical means to measure the vitamin in biological materials.[53,54]

Pantothenic acid can be measured in whole blood, plasma, and urine by microbiological assay using *Lactobacillus plantarum* (ATCC 8014).[6,28-30,39,40,42,47,51] Although other microorganism have been used, including the yeast *Saccharomyces uvarum*, *L. plantarum* has been the most suitable[28,30,51] and can be used with 96-well titration plates. Whole blood samples require an enzyme treatment to convert the coenzyme A to free pantothenic acid.[6,28,44,51] The microorganisms do not respond to coenzyme A.

Radioimmunoassay and ELISA

The radioimmunoassay for pantothenic acid provides an alternative method for measuring the vitamin in blood and other tissues.[41,46,51] The assay correlates well with the microbiological assay.[21,41] (Table 46) The procedure is sensitive and specific, but requires the preparation of suitable antibodies and the use of radiolabeled pantothenic acid.

A sensitive enzyme-linked immunosorbent assay (ELISA) for measuring pantothenic acid in foods has been reported.[51,52] The assay has not however been applied to blood or urine samples but such an application appears feasible.

Gas Chromatography

Several gas chromatographic methods have been described for measuring pantothenic acid in foodstuffs.[34,51] The methods compared favorable with the microbiological assay procedure for determining pantothenic acid. The yeast *Saccharomyces uvarum* 4228 was used as the test organism in the microbiological assay. However, the gas chromatographic methods were not applied to plasma or whole blood measurements of pantothenic acid. Gas chromatography has been used for the measurement of pantothenic acid in urine. Quantitative measurements of the vitamin in the range of 0.5 to 1000 μg/mL urine were possible.[36,37]

Functional Assessment

Although erythrocytes contain high concentrations of coenzyme A, no practical functional assessment of procedure based upon a coenzyme A-dependent enzyme present in erythrocytes has been developed. Attempts have been made to develop a functional test based on acetylation of sulfanilamide by erythrocytes.[49] In our experience such tests were not promising for application to the human and attempts were discontinued.

Assessment of Pantothenic Acid Status

Without evidence that pantothenic acid deficiency is of common occurrence, little interest has existed in developing tests for assessing pantothenic acid deficiency. Nutritional status of pantothenic acid has been assessed primarily by indirect approaches that include (a) assessing dietary intakes of the vitamin and by (b) the determination of blood and urinary pantothenic acid levels (Tables 43 to 46).

Blood Measurements

Serum contains free pantothenic acid, but is devoid of coenzyme A. Erythrocytes contain considerably more pantothenic acid, primarily as coenzyme A. Studies reported before

1975 on the pantothenic acid concentrations in whole blood may be considered unreliable and erroneously high because of inadequacies in the pantothenic acid liberation techniques used.[13,44] Hence it has been suggested that whole blood total pantothenic acid concentrations of <4.6 µmol/L (1.0 mg/L) may be normal and should not be considered indicative of a deficiency.[44] Hansen et al.,[23,44] using optimized analytical conditions, reported the normal range of whole blood pantothenic acid was 1.57 to 2.66 µmol/L (344 to 583 µg/L). These blood concentrations of pantothenic acid are considerably lower than those reported earlier by Frey et al.[13]

To avoid hemolysis problems that may give rise to falsely high free pantothenic acid values in plasma, measurement of total blood pantothenic acid would be more reliable and would be recommended.[28] Plasma pantothenic acid concentrations are not a reliable indicator of pantothenic acid intakes.[23] The concentrations respond little to changes in pantothenic acid intakes.

The knowledge on the catabolism of pantothenic acid in the human is incomplete, although it is recognized that some of the vitamin is metabolized to carbon dioxide. It has been suggested also that the intestinal flora may contribute to the pantothenic acid needs of the human. Certainly additional human studies are required to ascertain fully the usefulness of blood pantothenic acid concentrations in evaluating the nutritional status of this vitamin in the human.

Urine Measurement

Urinary excretion of pantothenic acid may provide a more reliable indicator of pantothenic acid status than blood pantothenic acid levels. Nearly all of the pantothenic acid in urine is in a free state and does not require the enzymatic treatment required for whole blood and erythrocyte pantothenate measurements.[22,44] Since urinary excretion of pantothenic acid is closely related to the dietary intake of the vitamin, urinary excretion has served as an indicator of pantothenic acid status (Table 45).[6,13,23,48] Urinary excretion of pantothenic acid can range widely between individuals, but an excretion of <1 mg/day of the vitamin is generally considered abnormally low. The following figure illustrates the relationship between pantothenic acid intake and urinary pantothenate excretion.[6] Other studies relating pantothenic acid intake to urinary excretion of pantothenate are summarized in Table 46.[55]

Pantothenic Acid Status in Population Groups

Adolescent Population

Despite the widespread occurrence of pantothenic acid in most foods, a large percentage of the adolescent population, because of food choices, have low intakes of the vitamin that fall below the 4 mg/day, the safe and adequate intake suggested by the Food and Nutrition Board.[16,23] In studies with preadolescent children and adolescents, dietary intakes of pantothenic acid were highly correlated with urinary excretion of the vitamin.[18,23] Levels of pantothenic acid in erythrocytes also correlated well with dietary intakes of pantothenic acid and its urinary excretion. Pantothenic acid content of whole blood was 344 ± 114 ng/mL for females ($n = 32$) and 412 ± 103 ng/mL for males ($n = 25$).[23] The pantothenic acid analyses were performed by radioimmunoassay.[41] Results of the radioimmunoassay correlated well with those obtained by *Lactobacillus plantarum* microbiological assay.[21,41]

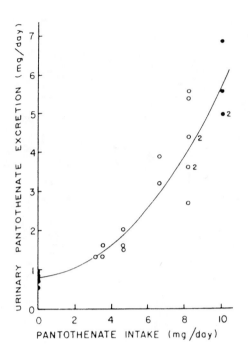

FIGURE 33

Relationship between urinary pantothenic acid excretion and pantothenic acid intake.[6,13] (With permission.)

Pregnancy and Lactation

Similarly, pantothenic acid intakes by pregnant and lactating women may often be considered low. Blood levels of pantothenic acid were reported lower in pregnant and lactating women than that of non-pregnant women.[43]

Toxicity

No cases of pantothenic acid toxicity have been reported in the human. The toxicity of pantothenic acid is extremely low since humans have tolerated intakes of 10 gr/day without adverse effects.[1,2] In clinical studies, this level of intake of pantothenic acid has been consumed for weeks without any toxic effects. Vitamin preparations commonly provide oral intakes of 5 to 10 mg per day. The related panthenol likewise is safe at high levels of intake.[3]

Summary

Relatively limited interest has existed concerning the role of pantotheinc acid in human nutrition. Consequently, the techniques to study human pantothenic acid nutriture are inadequate. Several methods are available to measure pantothenic acid in whole blood, erythrocytes, plasma, and urine, but the methods must be conducted with care. Urine pantothenic acid measurements are perhaps the easiest to conduct and interpret. The urinary excretion of pantothenic acid is closely related to its dietary intake. In contrast, the relationship of blood pantothenic acid concentrations to the nutritional status of the vitamin in the human remains unclear.[13] Functional precedures are not available for the nutritional assessment of pantothenic acid. Urinary excretion of pantothenic acid by an adult of less than 1 mg/day is considered indicative of a poor pantothenate nutritional status.

References

1. Plesofsky-Vig, N. Pantothenic acid and coenzyme A, in *Modern Nutrition in Health and Disease*, 8th edition, Shils, M. E., Olson, J. A., and Shike, M., Eds., Lea & Febiger, Philadelphia, 1994, 395.
2. Miller, D. R. and Hayes, K. C., Vitamin excess and toxicity, in *Nutritional Toxicology*, Vol. 1, Hathcock, J. N., Ed., Academic Press, New York, 1982, 81.
3. Komar, V. I., The use of pantothenic acid preparations in treating patients with viral hepatitis A, *Ter. Arkh.*, 63, 58, 1991.
4. Wagner, A. F. and Folkers, K., *Vitamins and Coenzymes*, John Wiley & Sons, New York, 1964.
5. Sauberlich, H. E., Bioavailability of vitamins, *Prog. Food Nutr. Sci.*, 9, 1, 1985.
6. Tarr, J. B., Tamura, T., and Stokstad, E. L. R., Availability of vitamin B_6 and pantothenate in an average American diet in man, *Am. J. Clin. Nutr.*, 34, 1328, 1981.
7. Schroeder, H. A., Losses of vitamins and trace elements resulting from processing and preservation of foods, *Am. J. Clin. Nutr.*, 24, 562, 1971.
8. Sugarman, B. and Munro, H. N., ^{14}C-Pantothenate accumulation by isolated adipocytes from adult rats of different ages, *J. Nutr.*, 110, 2297, 1980.
9. Abiko, Y., Metabolism of CoA, in *Metabolic Pathways*, Greenberg, D. M., Ed., Academic Press, New York, 1975, 7, 1.
10. Latymer, E. A. and Coates, M. E., The availability to the chick of pantothenic acid in foods, *Br. J. Nutr.*, 1982, 47, 131.
11. Fennema, O., Effect of processing on nutrition value of foods: freezing, in *Handbook of Nutritive Value of Processed Food, Food for Human Use*, Rechcigl, N. Jr. Ed., CRC Press, Boca Raton, FL, 1982, I, 31.
12. Hodges, R. E., Bean, W. B., Ohlson, M. A., and Bleiler, R. E., Factors affecting human antibody responses. V. Combined deficiencies of pantothenic acid and pyridoxine, *Am. J. Clin. Nutr.*, 11, 187, 1962.
13. Fry, P. C., Fox, H. M., and Tao, H. G., Metabolic response to a pantothenic acid deficient diet in humans, *J. Nutr. Sci. Vitaminol.*, 22, 339, 1976.
14. Plesofsky, N. and Brambl, R., Pantothenic acid and coenzyme A in cellular modification of proteins, *Annu. Rev. Nutr.*, 8, 461, 1988.
15. Combs, G. F. Jr., *The Vitamins*, Academic Press, Inc., New York, 1992, 345.
16. *Recommended Dietary Allowances*, 10th edition., Food and Nutrition Board, National Academy Press, Washington D.C., 1989, 169.
17. Hodges, R. E., Bean, W. B., Ohlson, M. A., and Bleiler, B., Human pantothenic acid deficiency produced by omega-methylpantothenic acid, *J. Clin. Invest.*, 38, 1421, 1959.
18. Pace, J. K., Stier, L. B., Taylor, D. D., and Goodman, P. S., Metabolic patterns in preadolescent children. V. Intake and urinary excretion of pantothenic acid and of folic acid, *J. Nutr.*, 74, 345, 1961.
19. Fox, H. M. and Linkswiler, H., Pantothenic acid excretion on three levels of intake, *J. Nutr.*, 75, 451, 1961.
20. Glusman, M., Syndrome of "burning feet" (nutritional melalgia) as manifestations of nutritional deficiency, *Am. J. Med.*, 3, 211, 1947.

21. Srinivasan, V. N., Christensen, N., Wyse, B. W., and Hansen, R. G., Pantothenic acid nutritional status in the elderly — institutionalized and non-institutionalized, *Am. J. Clin. Nutr.*, 34, 1736, 1981.

22. Song, W. O., Chan, G. M., Wyse, B. W., and Hansen, R. G., Effect of pantothenic acid status on the content of the vitamin in human milk, *Am. J. Clin. Nutr.*, 40, 317, 1984.

23. Eissenstat, B. R., Wyse, B. W., and Hansen, R. G., Pantothenic acid status of adolescents, Am. *J. Clin. Nutr.*, 44, 931, 1986.

24. Fox, H. M., Linkswiler, H., and Geschwender, D., Effect of altering the pantothenic acid intakes on the urinary excretion of this vitamin, *Fed. Proc.*, 18, 2068, 1968.

25. Fox, H. M., Lee, S., and Chen, C. S. L., Response to alterations in pantothenic acid content of the diet, *Fed. Proc.*, Abstract, 23, 1964.

26. Koyanagi, T., Harcyama, S., Kiruchi, R., Takanohoshi, R., Oikawa, K., and Akazawa, N., Effect of administration of thiamin, riboflavin, ascorbic acid, and vitamin A to students on their pantothenic acid contents in serum and urine, *Tohoku J. Exp. Med.*, 98, 357, 1969.

27. Cohenour, S. H. and Calloway, D. H., Blood, urine, and dietary pantothenic acid levels of pregnant teenagers, *Am. J. Clin. Nutr.*, 25, 512, 1972.

28. Hatano, M., Microbiological assay of pantothenic acid in blood and urine, *J. Vitaminol.*, 8, 134, 1962.

29. Ishiguro, K., Kobayashi, S., and Kaneta, S., Pantothenic acid content of human blood, *Tohoku J. Exp. Med.*, 74, 65, 1961.

30. Bird, O. D. and Thompson, R. Q., Pantothenic acid, in *The Vitamins*, Volume VII, 2nd edition, Gyorgy, P. and Pearson, W. N., Eds., Academic Press, New York, 1967, 209.

31. Knott, R. P., Toxicity of pantothene, PSEBM, 95, 340, 1957.

32. McCormick, D. B., Biotin, *Nutr. Rev.*, 33, 97, 1975.

33. Lubin, R., Daum, K. A., and Bean, W. B., Studies on pantothenic acid metabolism, *Am. J. Clin. Nutr.*, 4, 420, 1956.

34. Davidek, J., Velisek, J., Cerna, J., and Davidek, T., Gas chromatographic determination of panothenic acid, *J. Micronutr. Analysis*, 1, 39, 1985.

35. Grenier, J. F., Aprahamian, M., Genot, C., and Dentinger, A., Pantothenic acid (vitamin B_5) efficiency on wound healing, *Acta Vitaminol. Enzymol.*, 4, 81, 1982.

36. Aprahamian, M., Dentinger, A., Stock-Damge, C., Kouassi, J.–C., and Grenier, J. F., Effects of supplemental pantothenic acid on would healing: experimental study in rabbit, *Am. J. Clin. Nutr.*, 41, 578, 1985.

37. Schulze zur Viesel, E., Hesse, C., and Holtzel, D., Gaschromatographische Bestimmung von Pantothensourer in Urin, *Z. Klin. Chem. Klin. Biochem.*, 12, 498, 1974.

38. Novelli, G. D., Methods for determination of coenzyme A, in *Methods of Biochemical Analysis*, Vol. II, Glick, D., Ed., Interscience Publishers, New York, 1955, 194.

39. Pennington, D., Snell, E. E., and Williams, R. J., An assay method for pantothenic acid, *J. Biol. Chem.*, 135, 213, 1940.

40. Pantothenic acid, in *Methods of Vitamin Assay*, The Association of Vitamin Chemists, Inc., Eds., (Freed, M., Chairman, Methods Committee), 3rd edition, New York, Interscience Publishers., 1966, 197.

41. Wyse, B. W., Wittwer, C., and Hansen, R. G., Radio-immunoassay for pantothenic acid in blood and other tissues, *Clin. Chem.*, 25, 108, 1979.

42. Baker, H., Frank, O., Pasher, I., Dinnerstein, A., and Sobotka, H., An assay for pantothenic acid in biological fluids, *Clin. Chem.*, 6, 36, 1960.

43. Song, W. O., Wyse, B. W., and Hansen, R. G., Pantothenic acid status of pregnant and lactating women, *J. Am. Diet. Assoc.*, 85, 192, 1985.

44. Wittwer, C. T., Schweitzer, C., Pearson, J., Song, W. O., Windham, C. T., Wyse, B. W., and Hansen, R. G., Enzymes for liberation of pantothenic acid in blood: use of plasma pantetheinase, *Am. J. Clin. Nutr.*, 50, 1072, 1989.

45. Walsh, J. H., Wyse, B. W., and Hansen, R. G., Pantothenic acid content of 75 processed and cooked foods, *J. Am. Diet. Assoc.*, 78, 140, 1981.

46. Walsh, J. H., Wyse, B. W., and Hansen, R. G., A comparison of microbiological and radioimmunoassay methods for the determination of pantothenic acid in foods, *J. Food Biochem.*, 3, 175, 1980.
47. Difco Supplementary Literature, Difco Laboratories, Detroit, 1972, 447.
48. Sauberlich, H. E., Assessment of vitamin B_1, vitamin B_2, niacin, and pantothenate acid, in *Nutritional Status Assessment of the Individual*, Livingston, G. F., Ed., Food and Nutrition Press, Trumbull, 1989, 295.
49. Ellestad, J. J., Nelson, R. A., Adson, M. A. et al., Pantothenic acid and coenzyme A activity in blood and colonic mucosa from patients with chronic ulcerative colitis, *Fed. Proc.*, 29, 820, 1970. (Abstract)
50. United States Department of Agriculture, Human Nutrition Information Service, Composition of Foods, U. S. Government Printing Office, Washington D.C., Agriculture Handbooks 8–1 to 8–16, 1976.
51. Ball, G. F. M., *Water-soluble Vitamin Assays in Human Nutrition*, Chapman & Hall, New York, 1994.
52. Finglas, P. M., Faulks, R. M., Morris, H. C., Scott, K. J., and Morgan, M. R. A., The development of an enzyme-linked immunosorbent assay (ELISA) for the analysis of pantothenic acid and analogues. II. Determination of pantothenic acid in foods, *J. Micronutr. Anal.*, 4, 47, 1988.
53. Snell, E. E. and Wright, L. D., A microbiological method for determination of nicotinic acid, *J. Biol. Chem.*, 139, 675, 1941.
54. Skeggs, H. R. and Wright, L. D., The use of *Lactobacillus arabinosus* in the microbiological determination of pantothenic acid, *J. Biol. Chem.*, 156, 21, 1944.
55. Sauberlich, H. E., Dowdy, R. P., and Skala, J. H., *Laboratory Tests for the Assessment of Nutritional Status*, CRC Press, Boca Raton, FL, 1974, 89.

Biotin

Converting metric units to International System (SI) units:

pg/mL × 4.098 = pmol/L

pmol/L × 0.244 = pg/mL

molecular weight: 244.31

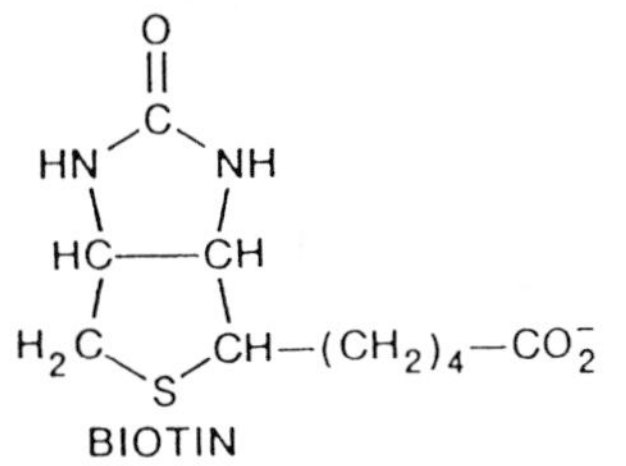

FIGURE 34
Structure of biotin.

BIOTIN

Introduction

The early history on biotin has been summarized in a number of reviews.[3-5,16-20,28,41,49] Biotin occurs widely in foods, but usually at very low concentrations. Egg yolk, kidney, liver, and dairy products are good sources of biotin while fruits, most vegetables, bread products and meats are poor sources of the vitamin.[2] Much of the biotin in foods is in a protein bound form. Proteolylic enzymes release the bound biotin as biocytin.[1-5,20] Biocytin requires the action of the enzyme biotinadase (EC 3.5.1.1.2) to release the biotin to a free state.[1-5,20] Intestinal flora of the human is capable of synthesizing biotin.[18,20,72] The extent and significance of this enteral source of biotin is uncertain.[18,20,42] However, prolonged use of certain antibiotics may result in reduced biotin status.[18,42]

Biotin Deficiency

A dietary deficiency is rarely observed. The consumption of large quantities of raw whole eggs or raw egg white has resulted in a biotin deficiency.[1,6,15,23,41] The avidin present in the egg white binds the biotin present in the diet to render it unavailable to the human.[6,18,23,41,42] Symptoms of a biotin deficiency included nausea, anorexia, vomiting, pallor, glossitis, depression, and a dry, scaly dermititis.[20,23,39,41]

Early total parenteral nutrition preparations were devoid of biotin. Prolonged use of such preparations resulted in a biotin deficiency.[21,22,26,47,54,55] Biotin supplements promptly corrected the condition. Biotin supplements may have beneficial effects in treating seborrheic dermatitis of infancy on Leiner's disease.[18,20,42]

185

Chronic hemodialysis may produce a biotin deficiency due to loss of free biotin in the dialysate.[24] Biotin replacement therapy corrected the deficiency. A biotin deficiency may be induced also with the use of certain anticonvulsant drugs such as primidone, phenytoin, phenobarbital, and carbamazapine.[20,25,45]

The biotin-dependent multiple carboxylase deficiency syndrome occurs in infants and children in between 1 in 17,500 and 1 in 340,000 births.[20,27-29,80] Biotin nutritional status in children and adults was normal in vegetarians (vegans), lactovegetarians, and in those consuming mixed diets.[8] The plasma and urine concentrations were determined with use of ^{125}I-avidin assay.[53]

Biochemical and clinical manifestation of a biotin deficiency have been described in children suffering from protein-energy malnutrition.[56] The malnourished children had plasma biotin concentration lower than those of normal children. The plasma and urinary biotin concentrations were determined with use of an isotope dilution assay. A further study indicated that measurements of activities of the carboxylases were better indicators of biotin status than plasma biotin concentration.[57]

With the use of the avidin competition assay developed by the investigators, the values reported appear to be unusually high. Biotin concentrations in plasma were found to be 1.4 ± 0.6 nmol/L for marasmus subjects ($n = 10$); 3.6 ± 0.09 nmol/L for kwashiorhkor subjects ($n = 4$); and 4.0 ± 0.3 nmol/L for normal subjects ($n = 14$).[57]

Recently, Mock et al.[76,81] have provided evidence that the biotin status decreases during pregnancy. Biotin nutritional status was assessed longitudinally in 13 pregnant women by measurement of excretion 3-hydroxyisovaleric acid and by determination of urinary excretion of biotin concentrations; 12 non-pregnant women served as controls. The excretion of 3-hydroxyvaleric acid increased during pregnancy. Serum concentrations and urinary excretions of biotin decreased during the later stages of pregnancy.

Function of Biotin

Carboxylases

At least nine biotin-dependent enzymes are known, representing one transcarboxylase, two decarboxylases, and six carboxylases.[1-5,42] Carboxylases for acetyl-CoA (EC 6.4.1.2), β-methylcrotonyl-CoA (EC 6.4.1.4), propionyl-CoA (EC 6.4.1.3), and pyruvate (EC 6.4.1.1) are found in human tissues.[1-5,20,30,41,42,70,73,80] Thus, all biotin-containing enzymes in the human are concerned with the transfer of a carbonyl group.

Pyruvate carboxylase catalyzes the formation of oxaloacetic acid from pyruvate.

Propionyl-CoA carboxylase catalyzes the carboxylation of propionyl-CoA to methylmalonyl-CoA, thus participates in the catabolism of propionic acid, isoleucine, valine, methionine, and threonine, and in the oxidation of odd-numbered fatty acids.

3-Methylcrotonyl-CoA carboxylase participates in the formation of 3-methylglutaconyl-CoA from 3-methylcrotonyl-CoA and thus participates in the catabolism of leucine.

Acetyl-CoA carboxylase catalyzes the formation of malonyl-CoA which is used in fatty acid synthesis and fatty acid chain elongation.

Patients with genetic defects in the activities of these enzymes have been reported.[20,27,29,41,66,80] In some patients the organic aciduria associated with the defects responds to treatment with high levels of biotin.[20,31,66,67,74] The activities of carboxylases have been measured with the use of the assay of Burri et. al.[58]

Holocarboxylase Synthetase

Holocarboxylase synthetase is essential for the transfer of biotin to the apocarboxylase for their activation. This involves the formation of biotinylated lysine (biocytin).[5,20,31] Patients with abnormal holocarboxylase synthetase are recognized and may respond to treatment with high doses of biotin (e.g., 10 mg/day).[20,31,46,70,79]

Biotinidase Deficiency

Genetic defect resulting in reduced biotinidase activity (EC 3.5.1.12) have been reported.[1-5,20, 32-35,38,42,69] This defect prevents the liberation of biotin from biotin-containing compounds in the circulation and leads to the excretion of biocytin in the urine.[1,20,34,68] The condition has been referred to as late-onset multiple carboxylase deficiency. Patients with this deficiency often have low serum concentrations of biotin.[38] To overcome this defect requires treatment with pharmacologic doses of biotin.[20,36]

For the most part, the lack of the biotinidase enzyme negates the usefulness of much of the biotin found in foods. However, some biotin is present in food in the free state. This amount of free biotin may provide partial protection for biotinidase-deficient patients so that their symptoms may be mild.[37,38] Various procedures are available to measure biotinidase activity in serum.[38,39,59,60-67] Wolf and Secor McVoy[39,59] have described a sensitive radioassay for serum biotinidase activity that is based on the liberation of [^{14}C-carboxyl]-p-aminobenzoate from N-biotinyl [^{14}C-carboxyl]-p-aminobenzoate.

Biotin Determination

Determination of biotin in blood and other test materials requires that the bound biotin must be released by papain digestion or by sulfuric acid hydrolysis.[13] However, nearly all of the biotin in plasma is present in a free form. In addition to microbiological assays, gas chromatographic, avidin binding assays, colorimeteric, polarographic and isotope dilution methods have been proposed for the measurement of biotin.[13,18,42,43,69,71,75,77,78]

The use of these different methods has resulted in a wide range of biotin concentrations in blood and urine that have been difficult to interpret or report. Nevertheless, with a given procedure and control populations, reduced levels of biotin in blood or urine have been reported for elderly, alcoholics, pregnant and lactating women, epileptics, and children with seborrheic dermatitis and Leiner's disease.[2,18,42-45,76]

The flagellate *Ochromonas danica* has been used successfully as the test organism to measure biotin concentrations in blood, urine, and other biological tissues.[48] With healthy human adults (n = 600), the following biotin concentrations were observed: blood, 215 to 750 pg/ml (mean = 485); serum, 200 to 700 pg/ml (mean = 400); and urine, 6 to 50 µg/24-hr collection (mean = 29). Also using the *O. danica* assay, no indications of a biotin deficiency were observed in surveys of elderly persons,[50] school children,[51] or mothers and newborns at parturition.[52]

The microbiological assay, using *Lactobacillus plantarium* (ATCC 8014; formerly *L. arabinosus*) as the assay organism, is commonly used to measure biotin.[9,10,13,78] The organism responds to free biotin and to biotin sulfoxide.[9,64] In a comparison study, the competitive protein binding assay[13,76,78] correlated well with the microbiological assay (*L. plantarum*) for the determination of biotin in plasma (r = 0.926) and urine (r = 0.934).[13] The less often used *L. rhamnosus* formerly called *Lactobacillus casei* (ATCC 7469) responds also to bound biotin.[9]

The assay is sensitive with a standard curve ranging from 0 to 0.1 ng/mL of biotin used.[9,11] Biotin was stable in plasma and urine samples stored at −18°C for one year.[13]

Biotin Assessment

Urine

Various studies have investigated the urinary excretion of biotin as an index of biotin nutritional status.[6-8,13,14,18,63,76] Studies using HPLC in conjunction with an avidin-binding assay have demonstrated that in addition to biotin, numerous biotin metabolites were excreted in human urine.[6,7,63,76-78] Consequently, microbiological assays on urine may overestimate the concentration of biotin;[63] however, the avidin-binding assay also measures biotin analogues in addition to biotin. To overcome these difficulties requires the use of HPLC to separate biotin from these other avidin-binding substances in urine.[6-8,64,76-78] Biotin analogues identified in human urine include bisnorbiotin, biotin-dl-sulfoxide, and bisnorbiotin methyl ketone (Table 47).[7,63,64]

Serum and Plasma

Literature values for plasma and whole blood biotin concentrations are variable and show no agreement. Values reported before 1975 are therefore difficult to interpret and may be unreliable.[18] Thus, earlier studies reported normal concentrations of biotin in plasma ranged from 1.4 to 3.0 nmol/L (195–722 ng/L).[20] A patient with a human biotin deficiency had a plasma biotin concentration of 0.64 nmol/L (156 ng/L).[20] Plasma biotin concentration of <1.02 nmol/L was considered to indicate biotin deficiency. Bartlett et al.[75] reported that normal biotin concentrations in serum ranged from 200 to 500 ng/L. The discrepancies between the earlier analytical results and those of recent reports may relate to the degree of specificity of the methods employed.

Most of the biotin in human serum is in a free form.[65] Human serum contains biotin as well as several biotin metabolites including biotin sulfoxide and bisnorbiotin.[14,64,76-78] A number of these substances can be measured with avidin-binding assays.[64,76-78] The concentration of these compounds in the serum of 15 fasting adults was found as follows:[14]

Compound*	Concentration (pmol/L)	% of total
Biotin	230 ± 16	58
Bisnorbiotin	163 ± 8	41
Biotin sulfoxide	7 ± 2	2

* Biotin and the analogues were separated by HPLC followed by detection with a sequential solid-phase avidin-binding assay.[78]

Experimental Biotin Deficiency in the Human

Experimentally, a marginal biotin deficiency was induced in the normal adults.[6] During the study, various indicators of biotin status were examined. The urinary excretion of both

TABLE 47

Some Literature Reports on Biotin Concentrations of Biological Specimens

Analysis	Concentrations	References
The following results were obtained with an avidin-binding assay.[63]		
Normal Adults		
Serum biotin (*n* = 15)	244 ± 61 pmol/L	64
Serum bisnorbiotin (*n* = 15)	189 ± 135 pmol/L	64
Urine bisnorbiotin (*n* = 10)	17.4 ± 4.2 nmol/L	63
Urine biotin (*n* = 10)	26.7 ± 8.8 nmol/L	63
Normal Adults (*n* = 6)		
Urine biotin	35 ± 14 nmol/24 hr	7
Urine bisnorbiotin	68 ± 48 nmol/24 hr	7
Urine biotin sulfone	5 ± 5 nmol/24 hr	7
Normal Adults (*n* = 15)		
Serum biotin	230 ± 16 pmol/L	14
Serum bisnorbiotin	163 ± 8 pmol/L	14
Normal Adults		
Serum biotin (*n* = 15)	244 ± 61 pmol/L	6
Serum bisnorbiotin	189 ± 135 pmol/L	6
Urine biotin (*n* = 10)	41 ± 18 nmol/24 hr	6
Urine bisnorbiotin	26 ± 10 nmol/24 hr	6
The following results were obtained with Ochromonas danica *assay.*[48] *The reported values are considerably higher than those obtained by avidin-binding assay, indicating differences in specifity.*		
Blood biotin (*n* = 600)	485 (215–750) pg/mL	48
Serum biotin (*n* = 600)	400 (200–700) pg/mL	48
Urine biotin (*n* = 600)	29 (6–50) µg/24–hr	48
Plasma biotin determined by L. plantarum *microbiological assay.*		
Normal Adults (*n* = 112)		
Plasma biotin	1.63 ± 0.49 nmol/L	45
Patients on long-term therapy with anticonvulsants (*n* = 404)		
Plasma biotin	0.90 ± 0.29 nmol/L	45
Radiometric – microbiological assay used.[71]		
Normal Adults		
Men (*n* = 15)		
Plasma biotin	260 ± 91 pg/mL	71
Women (*n* = 23)		
Plasma biotin	228 ± 94 pg/mL	71

biotin and bisnorbiotin decreased significantly during the 3-week depletion period; however, serum concentrations of biotin did not decrease significantly.[6,64] A trend of decreasing plasma biotin concentrations was observed which may have become significant with a longer biotin deficiency period.

The experimental biotin deficiency resulted in a significant increase in the urinary excretion of 3-hydroxyisovaleric acid.[6] Within 10 days on the biotin deficient diet, a marked

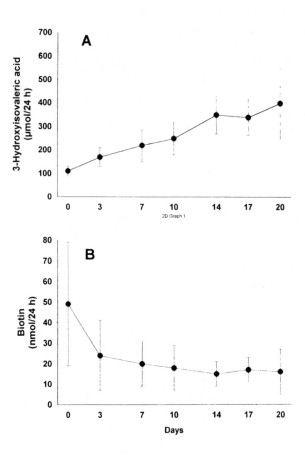

FIGURE 35
Urinary excretion of 3-hydroxyisovaleric acid and biotin in 10 subjects fed a biotin-deficient diet for 20 days.[6]
(With permission.)

increase had occurred in the urinary excretion of the acid. This may reflect a decreased activity of the biotin-dependent methylcrotonyl-CoA carboxylase. The investigators suggest that these preliminary studies indicate that the urinary excretion of 3-hydroxyisovaleric acid could serve as an indicator of biotin status.[6]

From the study it was concluded that a decrease in the urinary excretion of biotin and an increase in the urinary excretion of 3-hydroxyisovaleric acid are early sensitive indicators of biotin deficiency and that the serum concentrations of biotin is not.[6] Additional investigations are necessary to establish the validity of these observations and to develop less technical analytical procedures.

Toxicity

Although there are no reports of biotin toxicity, it is probably very low. No adverse effects were observed in infants who received biotin injections of 10 mg per day for 6 months.[12] Excess biotin is excreted rapidly into the urine.[13]

Summary

The occurrence of a biotin deficiency in the general population appears exceedingly rare. Biotin deficiency when observed is usually in association with genetic defects, drug interactions, prolonged total parenteral nutrition, or unusual diet habits. Procedures to evaluate a biotin status are limited although some new approaches may provide a more reliable means. Plasma concentrations of biotin are probably not a sensitive or early indicator of a biotin status.[6,76,78] Measurement of urinary excretion levels of biotin and of 3-hydroxyisovaleric acid appear to be the most useful procedures currently available to assess biotin status. Valid guidelines and reference standards need to be established for the interpretation of the values obtained. Less technically demanding procedures are also required to permit their general practical use.

References

1. Dakshinamurti, K., Biotin, in *Modern Nutrition in Health and Disease*, 8th edition, Shils, M. E., Olson, J. A., and Shike, M., Eds., Lea & Febiger, Philadelphia, 1994, 426.
2. Combs, G. F. Jr., *The Vitamins*, Academic Press, Inc., New York, 1992, 329.
3. Dakshinamurti, K. and Bhangvan, H. N., Ed., Biotin, *Ann. N.Y. Acad. Sci.*, 447, 441, 1985.
4. Dakshinamurti, K. and Chauhan, J., Biotin, *Vit. Horm.*, 45, 337, 1989.
5. Dakshinamurti, K. and Chauhan, J., Regulation of biotin enzymes, *Annu. Rev Nutr.*, 8, 211, 1988.
6. Mock, N. I., Malik, M. I., Stumbo, P. J., Bishop, W. P., and Mock, D. M., Increased urinary excretion of 3-hydroxyisovaleric acid and decreased urinary excretion of biotin are sensitive early indicators of decreased biotin status in experimental biotin deficiency, *Am. J. Clin. Nutr.*, 65, 951, 1997.
7. Zempleni, J., McCormick, D. B., and Mock, D. M., Identification of biotin sulfone, bisnorbiotin methyl ketone, and tetranorbiotin-/-sulfoxide in human urine, *Am. J. Clin. Nutr.*, 65, 508, 1997.
8. Lombard, K. A. and Mock, D. M., Biotin nutritional status of vegans, lactoovovegetarians, and nonvegetarians, *Am. J. Clin. Nutr.*, 50, 486, 1989.
9. *Methods of Vitamin Assay*, Freed, M., Ed., Interscience Publishers, New York, 1966, 245.
10. Wright, L. D. and Skeggs, H. R., Determination of biotin with *Lactobacillus arabinosus*, *Proc. Soc. Exp. Biol. Med.*, 56, 95, 1944.
11. *Difco Manual*, Dehydrated culture media and reagents for microbiology, 10th edition, Difco Laboratories, Detroit, MI, 1984, 1076.
12. Miller, D. R. and Hayes, K. C., Vitamin excess and toxicity, in *Nutritional Toxicology*, Volume I, Hathcock, J. N., Ed., Academic Press, New York, 1982, 81.
13. Bitsch, R., Salz, L., and Hotzel, D., Studies on bioavailability of oral biotin doses for humans, *Int. J. Vit. Nutr. Res.*, 59, 65, 1989.
14. Mock, N. and Mock, D., Biotin represents about half of total identified avidin-binding substances in human serum, *FASEB J.*, 8, A447, 1994.
15. Baugh, C. M., Malone, J. H., and Butterworth, C. E. Jr., Human biotin deficiency: a case history of biotin deficiency induced by raw egg consumption in cirrhotic patient, *Am. J. Clin. Nutr.*, 21, 173, 1968.
16. Gyorgy, P. and Langer, B. W. Jr., Biotin XI, Deficiency effects in and requirements of man, in *The Vitamins*, Volume II, 2nd edition, Academic Press, New York, 1968, 347.
17. Mistry, S. P., Biotin, in *Vitamins in Medicine*, Volume I, 4th edition, Barker, B. M. and Bender, D. A., Eds., William Heinemann Medical Books, London, 1980, 381.
18. Bojour, J. P., Biotin in man's nutrition and therapy – a review, *Int. J. Vit. Nutr. Res.*, 47, 107, 1977.

19. McCormick, D. B., Biotin, *Nutr. Rev.*, 33, 97, 1975.
20. Sweetman, L. and Nyhan, W. L., Inheritable biotin-treatable disorders and associated phenomena, *Annu. Rev. Nutr.*, 6, 317, 1986.
21. Mock, D. M., Baswell, D. C., Baker, H., Holman, R. T., and Sweetman, L., Biotin deficiency complicating parenteral alimentation, *J. Pediatrics*, 106, 762, 1988.
22. McClain, C. J., Baker, H., and Onstad, G. R., Biotin deficiency in an adult during home parenteral nutrition, *JAMA*, 247, 3116, 1982.
23. Syndenstricher, V. P., Singal, S. A., Briggs, A. P., DeVaughn, N. M., and Isbell, H., Observation on the "egg-white injury" in man, *JAMA*, 118, 1199, 1942.
24. Yatzidis, H., Koutsicos, D., Alaveras, A. G., Papastephanides, C., and Frangos-Plemenos, M., Biotin for neurologic disorders of uremia, *N. Engl. J. Med.*, 305, 764, 1981.
25. Krauser, K. H., Berlit, P., and Bonjur, J. P., Impaired biotin status in anticonvulsant therapy, *Annu. Neurol.*, 12, 485, 1982.
26. Mock, D. M., deLorimer, A. A., Liebman, W. M., Sweetmen, L., and Baker, H., Biotin deficiency: an unusual complication of parenteral alimentation, *N. Engl. J. Med.*, 304, 820, 1981.
27. Wolf, B. and Feldman, G. L., The biotin-dependent carboxylase deficiency, *Am. J. Hum. Genet.*, 34, 699, 1982.
28. Mock, D. M., Biotin, in *Present Knowledge In Nutrition*, Ziegler, E. E., and Filer, L. J. Jr., Eds., International Life Sciences Institutes, Nutrition Foundation, Washington D.C., 1996, 220.
29. Roth, K. S., Yang, W., Allan, L., Saunders, M., Grand, R. A., and Dakshinamurti, K., Prenatal administration of biotin in biotin responsive multiple carboxylase deficiency, *Pediatr. Res.*, 16, 126, 1982.
30. Sauberlich, H. E., Interactions of thiamin, riboflavin, and other vitamins, *Ann. N.Y. Acad. Sci.*, 355, 80, 1980.
31. Roth, K. S., Yang, W., Foreman, J. W., Rothman, R., and Segal, S., Holocarboxylase synthetase deficiency: a biotin-responsive organic acidemia, *J. Pediatr.*, 96, 845, 1980.
32. Wolf, B., Grier, R. E., Allen, R. J., Goodman, S. I., and Kien, C. L., Biotinidase deficiency: the enzymatic defect in late-onset multiple carboxylase deficiency, *Clin. Chim. Acta*, 131, 273, 1983.
33. Wolf, B., Grier, R. E., Parker, W. D., Goodman, S. I., and Allen, R. J., Deficient biotinidase activity in late-onset multiple carboxylase deficiency, *N. Engl. J. Med.*, 308, 161, 1983.
34. Wolf, B., Grier, R. E., Secor Mcvoy, J. R., and Heard, G. S., Biotinidase deficiency: a novel vitamin recycling defect, *J. Inherit. Metab. Dis.*, 8 (Suppl. 1), 53, 1985.
35. Wolf, B., Heard, G. S., Jefferson, L. G., Proud, V. K., Nance, W. E., and Weissbecker, K. A., Clinical findings in four children with biotinidase deficiency detected through a statewide neonatal screening program, *N. Engl. J. Med.*, 313, 16, 1985.
36. Dionisi-Vici, C., Bachmann, C., Graziana, M. C., and Sabetta, G., Case report: laryngeal stridor as a leading symptom in a biotinidase-deficient patient, *J. Inherit. Metab. Dis.*, 11, 312, 1988.
37. Wolf, B., Heard, G. S., Secor McVoy, J. R., and Raetz, H. M., Biotinidase deficiency: the possible role of biotinidase in the processing of dietary protein-bound biotin, *J. Int. Metab. Dis.*, 7 (Suppl. 2), 121, 1984.
38. Wolf, B., Heard, G. S., Secor McVoy, J. R., and Grier, R. E., Biotinidase deficiency, *Ann. N.Y. Acad. Sci.*, 447, 252, 1985.
39. Wolf, B., Biotinidase deficiency, *Laboratory Management*, October, 31, 1987.
40. Bates, H. M., Biotinidase deficiency: screening and treatment, *Laboratory Management*, April, 15, 1987.
41. Roth, K. S., Biotin in clinical medicine – a review, *Am. J. Clin. Nutr.*, 34, 1967, 1981.
42. Bonjour, J.-P., Biotin in human nutrition, *Ann. N.Y. Acad. Sci.*, 447, 97, 1985.
43. Bojour, J. P., Biotin, in *Handbook of Vitamins*, Machlin, L. J., Ed., Marcel Dekker, New York, 1984, 403.
44. Bojour, J. P., Vitamins and alcoholism. VIII. Biotin, *Int. J. Vit. Nutr. Res.*, 50, 439, 1980.
45. Krause, K.-H., Bonjour, J. P., Berlit, P., and Kochen, W., Biotin status of epileptics, *Ann. N.Y. Acad. Sci.*, 447, 297, 1985.
46. Sweetman, L., Two forms of biotin-responsive multiple carboxylase deficiency, *J. Inherit. Metab. Dis.*, 4, 53, 1981.

47. McClain, C. J., Biotin deficiency complicating parenteral alimentation, *J. Am. Med. Assoc.*, 250, 1028, 1983.
48. Baker, H., Assessment of biotin status: clinical implications, *Ann. N.Y. Acad. Sci.*, 447, 129, 1985.
49. Murthy, P. N. A. and Mistry, S. P., Biotin, *Prog. Fed. Nutr. Sci.*, 2, 405, 1977.
50. Baker, H., Frank, O., Thind, I. S., Jaslow, S. P., and Louria, D. B., Vitamin profiles in elderly person living at home or in nursing homes versus profile in healthy young subjects, *J. Am. Geriatrics Soc.*, 27, 444, 1979.
51. Baker, H., Frank, O., Feingold, S., Christakis, G., and Ziffer, H., Vitamins, total cholesterol and triglycerides in 642 New York City school children, *Am J. Clin. Nutr.*, 20, 850, 1967.
52. Baker, H., Frank, O., Thomson, A. D., Langer, A., Munves, E. D., DeAngelis, B., and Kaminetzky, H., Vitamin profile of 174 mothers and newborns at parturition, *Am. J. Clin. Nutr.*, 28, 56, 1975.
53. Mock, D. M. and DuBois, D. B., A sequential, soild-phase assay for biotin in physiologic fluids that correlates with expected biotin status, *Anal. Biochem.*, 153, 272, 1986.
54. Mock, D. M., Johnson, B. B., and Holman, R. T., Effects of biotin deficiency on serum fatty acid composition: evidence for abnormalities in humans, *J. Nutr.*, 188, 342, 1988.
55. Innis, S. M. and Allardyce, D. B., Possible biotin deficiency in adults receiving long-term total parenteral nutrition, *Am. J. Clin. Nutr.*, 37, 185, 1983.
56. Velazquez, A., Martin-del-Compo, C., Baez, A., Zamudio, S., Quiterio, M., Aguilar, J. L., Perez-Ortiz, B., Sanchez-Ardines, M., Guzman-Hernandez, J., and Casanueva, E., Biotin deficiency in protein-energy malnutrition, *Eur. J. Clin. Nutr.*, 43, 169, 1988.
57. Velazquez, A., Teran, M., Baez, A., Gutievez, J., and Rodriguez, R., Biotin supplementation affects lymphocyte carboxylases and plasma biotin in severe protein-energy malnutrition, *Am. J. Clin. Nutr.*, 61, 385, 1995.
58. Burri, B. J., Sweetman, L., and Nyhan, W. L., Heterogeneity of holocarboxylase synthetase in patients with biotin-responsive multiple carboxylase deficiency, *Am. J. Hum. Genet.*, 37, 326, 1985.
59. Wolf, B. and Secor McVoy, J. R., A sensitive radioassay for biotinidase activity: deficient activity in tissues of serum biotinidase-deficient individuals, *Clin. Chim. Acta*, 135, 275, 1984.
60. Thuy, L. E., Ziebinska, B., Sweetman, L., and Nyhan, W. L., Determination of biotinidase activity in human plasma using [^{14}C] biocytin as substrate, *Ann. N.Y. Acad. Sci.*, 447, 434, 1985.
61. Ebrahim, H. and Dakshinamurti, K., A fluorometric assay for biotinidase, *Anal. Biochem.*, 154, 282, 1986.
62. Wastell, H., Dale, G., and Barlett, K., A sensitive fluorimetric rate assay for biotinidase using a new derivative of biotin, biotinyl-6-aminoquinoline, *Anal. Biochem.*, 140, 69, 1984.
63. Mock, D. M., Lankford, G. L., and Cazin, J. Jr., Biotin and biotin analogs in humam urine: biotin accounts for only half of the total, *J. Nutr.*, 123, 1844, 1993.
64. Mock, D. M., Lankford, G. L., and Mock, N. I., Biotin accounts for only half of the total avidin-binding substances in human serum, *J. Nutr.*, 125, 941, 1995.
65. Mock, D. M. and Malik, M. I., Distribution of biotin in human plasma: most of the biotin is not bound to protein, *Am. J. Clin. Nutr.*, 56, 427, 1992.
66. Thoene, J., Baker, H., Yoshino, M., and Sweetman, L., Biotin-responsive carboxylase deficiency associated with subnormal plasma and urinary excretion, *N. Engl. J. Med.*, 304, 817, 1981.
67. Blom, W., van den Berge, G. B., Huijmas, J. G. M., Przyrembel, H., Fernandes, J., Scholte, H. R., and Sanders-Woudstra, J. A. R., Neurologic action of megadoses of vitamins, *Bibliotheca Nutr. Diet.*, 38, 120, 1986.
68. Bonjour, J. P., Bausch, J., Suormala, T., and Baumgartner, E. R., Detection of biocytin in urine of children with congential biotinidase deficiency, *Int. J. Vit. Res.*, 54, 223, 1984.
69. Dakshinamurti, K., Landman, A. D., Ramamurti, L., Constable, R. J., Isotope dilution assay for biotin, *Anal. Biochem.*, 61, 225, 1974.
70. Bartlett, K., Ghneim, H. K., Stirk, H.-J., and Wastell, H., Enzyme studies in biotin-responsive disorders, *J. Int. Metab. Dis.*, 8 (Suppl. 1), 46, 1985.
71. Guilarte, T. R., Radiometric-microbiological assay of biotin in human plasma, *Ann. N. Y. Acad. Sci.*, 447, 398, 1985.
72. Bitsch, R., Toth-Dersi, A., and Hoetzel, D., Biotin deficiency and biotin supply, *Ann. N. Y. Acad. Sci.*, 447, 133, 1985.

73. Gravel, R. A. and Robinson, B. H., Biotin-dependent carboxylase deficiencies (Propionyl CoA and pyruvate carboxylases), *Ann. N.Y. Acad. Sci.*, 447, 225, 1985.

74. Swick, H. M. and Kien, C. L., Biotin deficiency without organic aciduria, *Ann. N.Y. Acad. Sci.*, 447, 430, 1985.

75. Dakshinamurti, K. and Allan, L., Isotope dilution assay for biotin: use of ^{3}H biotin, *Methods Enzymol.*, 62, 284, 1979.

76. Mock, D. M., Stadler, D. D., Stratton, S. L., and Mock, N. I., Biotin status assessed longitudinally in pregnant women, *J. Nutr.*, 127, 710, 1997.

77. Mock, D. M. and Heird, G. M., Urinary biotin analogs are biotin metabolites, *Am. J. Physiol. Endocrinol. Metab.*, 272, 83, 1997.

78. Mock, D. M., Determinations of biotin in biological fluids, in *Vitamins and Coenzymes*, Parts 1 and 2, Volume 279, Section V, (A volume of *Methods in Enzymology*), McCormick, D. B., Suttie, J. W. and Wagner, C., Eds., Academic Press, San Diego, CA, 1997.

79. Sweetman, L., Burri, B. J., and Nyhan, W. L., Biotin holocarboxylase synthetase deficiency, *Ann. N.Y. Acad. Sci.*, 447, 288, 1985.

80. Baumgartner, E. R. and Suormala, T., Multiple carbocylase deficiency: inherited and acquired disorders of biotin metabolism, *Int. J. Vit. Nutr. Res.*, 67, 377, 1997.

81. Mock, D. M., Biotin status: Which are valid indicators and how do we know? *J. Nutr.*, 129, 4985, 1999.

Retinol (Vitamin A)

Converting metric units to International System (SI) units:

Retinol

$\mu g/mL \times 3.49 = \mu mol/L$

$\mu mol/L \times 0.287 = \mu g/mL$

molecular weight: 286.5

β-Carotene

$\mu g/mL \times 1.86 = \mu mol/L$

$\mu mol/L \times 0.537 = \mu g/mL$

molecular weight: 536.9

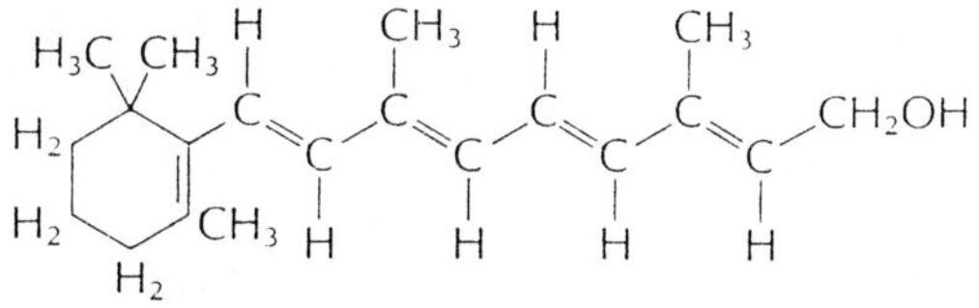

FIGURE 36
Structure of all trans-retinol (vitamin A).

Background/History/Function

The early history of vitamin A has been considered by Rodriquez and Irwin in their "Conspectus of Research on Vitamin A Requirements of Man."[101] Details on the discovery of vitamin A and carotene are interestingly provided in the book entitled *The Newer Knowledge of Nutrition* co-authored by McCollum, Orent-Keiles, and Day.[102] Additional information on the earlier history of vitamin A may be obtained from the book entitled *The Fat-Soluble Vitamins*, edited by H. F. DeLuca and J. W. Suttie.[112] Only a few comments will be provided here. Night blindness, an early symptom of vitamin A deficiency, has been recognized for several thousands of year. The Egyptian Eber's Papyrus circa. 1500 B.C. recommended the use of liver as a treatment.[113]

Prior to 1913, it was believed that all fats were useful in nutrition only as fuel foods. In 1913, McCollum and Davis of Wisconsin observed that rats fed diets containing either butter fat or the ether extractable matter from egg yolk grew rather well.[101-104] In the laboratory of Osborne and Mendel of Yale, similar findings were reported.[105,106]

Osborne, Mendel[107] and McCollum et al.[108] found that green vegetables also had fat-soluble vitamin A activity. Thereabouts, Steenbock of Wisconsin[109] found that certain carotenoids, including carotene, promoted growth in the rat. Subsequently, in 1929, Moore

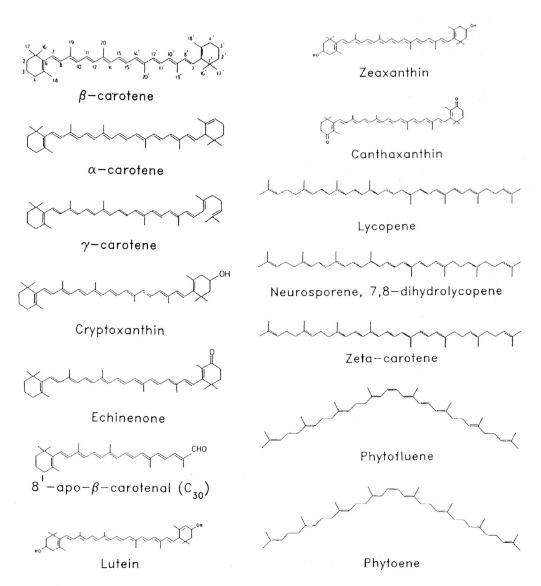

FIGURE 37
Structure of common carotinoids.

demonstrated in the rat the conversion of carotene to vitamin A.[110] In 1931, Karrer and associates[111] determined the structure of vitamin A.

Vitamin A in the form of retinol is essential for vision, growth, and differentiation of epithelial tissue, and is required for bone growth, immunity, reproduction, and embryonic development.[33,179182,202,206] Diseases that cause fat malabsorption such as celiac disease may reduce the absorption of retinol and carotinoids. Liver disease may impair the transport and storage of vitamin A.

Vitamin A Sources

Vitamin A is provided in the diet in two major forms. Pre-formed vitamin A as retinol is obtained from animal sources such as liver, butter, cheese, margarine, dried milk, cream, fortified milk, kidney, and some seafoods. Provitamin A is provided as β-carotene, α-carotene, and other provitamin A carotenoids.[333] Important sources of provitamins A carotenoids are sweet potatoes, pumpkin, squash, carrots, tomatoes, peaches, nectarines, apricots, mangos, lettuce and most greens, broccoli, Brussels sprouts, and asparagus.[25-27,36,37]

Of the approximately 600 identified naturally occurring carotenoids, about 60 have provitamin A activity. Of these, β-catotene is the most important as a provitamin A carotenoid.[28] In the United States, information from the second National Health and Nutrition Examination Survey (NHANES-II), indicated that approximately 25% of the vitamin A (retinol equivalents) was provided by carotenoids and 75% by preformed vitamin A (retinol).[29]

Carotenoids, Nutrition and Measurement

Recent investigation have indicated that the dietary intake of selected carotenoids may help delay or prevent the onset of cataracts, atherosclerosis, certain cancers, macular degeneration and other diseases.[61,66-72,92-94,155-157,198,203-205,325,326] These effects have been suggested to be mediated through the antioxidant properties of certain carotinoids.[91] The antioxidant functions appear to be completely independent of any provitamin A activity. Individual carotinoids may have specific protective effects. Consequently, interest has developed as to the concentrations of the individual carotenoids in the diet and in the plasma. The accompanying table lists the caroteniod concentrations in some selected fruits and vegetables (Table 48).[36,37]

With the development of high performance chromatography methods, the individual carotenoids can be readily quantitated in plasma. Numerous methods have been described for the measurement of only the major carotenoids[39] or complex systems that may measure over 50 different carotenoids in plasma.[38,42,45-47,82,84-90,100] Total plasma carotenoids may be measured by extracting the carotenoids from the plasma samples with petroleum ether. The carotene concentration is determined by measuring the absorption of the extract at 450 nm.[45,79-82]

Carotene levels in plasma are highly variable due to the influences of the foods consumed, age, sex, dietary fat, bioavailability, smoking, drug intake, and other factors.[39-44,52,82] Table 49 provides examples of the concentrations of individual carotenoids found in serum.[38,39]

Prolonged consumption of high amounts of carotenoids may produce carotenemia and carotenodermia in the human.[82,83] Bronzing was observed in adult subjects after 90 days on a daily intake of approximately 30 mg of β-carotene and 12 mg of α-carotene.[38] The carotenemia and carotenodermia disappeared quickly with the discontinuance of the elevated intakes of the carotenoids.

Apgar et al.[48] studied the serum carotenoid concentrations in 493 children (65 to 89 months of age) in Belize. The carotenoids measured were lycopene, α-carotene, β-carotene, β-cryptoxanthin, and lutein/zeaxanthin (Table 49). The measurements were performed by

TABLE 48
Sources of Selected Carotenoids in Some Fruits and Vegetables

Food Item	β-Carotene	α-Carotene	Lycopene	Cryptoxanthin	Leutein and Zeaxanthin
Apricot, canned	1500	0	65	0	2
Avocado, raw	34	0	0	0	320
Broccoli, cooked	1300	1	0	0	1800
Brussels sprouts	480	6	0	0	1300
Cabbage, raw red	15	1	0	0	26
Carrot, cooked	9800	3700	0	0	260
Celery, raw	710	0	0	0	3600
Corn, yellow	51	50	0	0	780
Grapefruit, pink	1310	0	3362	0	0
Green beans	630	44	0	0	740
Greens, collard	5400	0	0	0	16300
Lettuce, iceberg	480	4	0	0	1400
Mango	1300	0	0	54	0
Nectarine	103	0	0	43	15
Orange, canned	100	0	0	149	14
Pears, green	350	16	0	0	1700
Pepper, green	230	11	0	0	700
Pumpkin	3100	3800	0	0	1500
Squash, summer	420	12	0	0	1200
Swiss chard, raw	3647	45	0	0	12000
Tangerine	38	20	0	106	20
Tomato juice	900	0	8580	0	330
Tomato, raw	520	0	3100	0	100
Watermelon, raw	230	1	0	4100	14

From Mangles et al.[36,37]

HPLC using 200 μL of a fasting serum sample.[49] Quality control was obtained through the use of the retinol and β-carotene Standard Reference Material (SRM 968a) obtained from the National Institute of Standards and Technology, Gaithersburg, MD.[49] Currently, Standard Reference Material 968b for fat-soluble vitamins, carotenoids, and cholesterol is available.

Investigators have summarized in their publications data from other literature reports on the concentrations of carotenoids in plasma or serum of children and adults.[49,335] Additional studies have been summarized by Rojas-Hidalgo and Olmedilla.[82] Plasma carotenoids concentrations may be useful as an indicator of vitamin A status. The serum concentrations of β-carotene usually reflects recent dietary intakes. Hence, low carotenoid levels commonly indicate the consumption of a diet low in green and yellow vegetables and fruits.[48,50] For populations with adequate intakes of preformed retinol, low carotenoid intakes are of less concern with regards to vitamin A status. However, their concentration may be influenced by various factors, including age, smoking, sex, illness, bioavailability, alcohol, physiological state and season.[44,82,96-99]

Vitamin A Deficiency

Extensive literature exists on vitamin A deficiency and metabolism.[1,4,32,61,62,101,112,113,123,124,127,130,155,164,169,170,171,179,180-183,187-195,203-206,334] Only a few areas can be noted here that may provide

TABLE 49
Serum Carotenoid Concentrations in Adults (Mean or Median Values)

Carotenoid	Young Adults[a] (n = 15)		Middle-Age Adults[b] (n = 110)		Belize Children[c] (n = 493)	
	µg/dL	nmol/L	µg/dL	nmol/L	µg/dL	nmol/L
α-Carotene	11.6	216	3.4	63	5.0	93
β-Carotene	24.5	456	20.3	378	11.0	205
χ-Carotene	12.6	—	—	—	—	—
δ-Carotene	13.4	—	—	—	—	—
Lycopene	36.2	674	20.0	373	6.0	112
Lutein/Zeaxanthin	25.5	448	18.4	323	13.0	228
Phytofluene	16.1	—	—	—	—	—
Phytoene	8.2	—	—	—	—	—
β-Cryptoxanthin	9.5	172	9.2	166	8.0	145
α-Cryptoxanthin	4.4	—	—	—	—	—
Anhydrolutein	8.6	—	—	—	—	—
Neuroporene	3.6	—	—	—	—	—

[a] Sauberlich et al.[38]
[b] Stacewicz-Sapuntzakis et al.[39,100]
[c] Apgar et al.[48]

an indication of the prevalence of the deficiency problem and some of the factors that influence the affliction.[169-171,179,332] In general, vitamin A is involved in cellular proliferation, differentiation, reproduction, and vision.[179,210,334]

Vitamin A Status

Preterm Infants

Preterm infants are generally considered to be at risk for vitamin A deficiency because their plasma retinol concentrations are usually lower than those of term infants, children, or adults.[77] Plasma concentrations of preterm infants were observed to be 0.087 to 0.72 µmol/L (2.5 to 20.5 µg/dL).[121] Zachman[180] also reported low plasma levels of retinol for premature infants (< 0.70 µmol/L). Retinol-binding protein levels in the serum were lower in the premature infants.[180]

Infants and Children

Children under 5 years of age living in developing countries often suffer from a deficiency of vitamin A.[114-118,172,196] A serious consequence of a deficiency is the development of xerophthalmia, which includes ocular changes ranging from night blindness, conjunctival xerosis to corneal xerosis and ulceration. This may progress to keratomalacia resulting in partial or total blindness. Less than optimal vitamin A status was observed in some Hispanic groups in the United States.[122,197]

Information from the second National Health and Nutrition Examination Survey (NHANES-II), indicated that younger children, aged 4 to 5 years, had lower mean serum vitamin A concentrations than did the older children (9 to 11 years).[123,331] The possibility

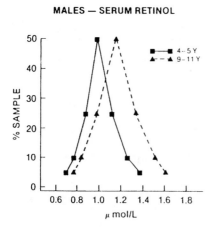
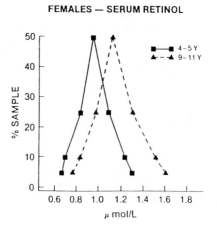

FIGURE 38
Serum retinol distribution curves for males and females aged 4 to 5 and 9 to 11 years in age (NHANES-II, 1976–1980 and HHANES (MA), 1982–1983)[331]

exists that these age differences in vitamin A values are related to physiological changes. Serum vitamin A values for children aged 3 to 11 years of less than < 0.84 μmol/L are considered to indicate less than optimum vitamin A status (Table 50).[123]

TABLE 50
Serum Vitamin A Concentrations of Children
from NHANES-II (1976–1980)

Sex and Age (Years)	No. of Subjects	Serum Vitamin A Concentration 50th percentile (μmol/L)
Males		
4–5	482	1.12
6–8	262	1.16
9–11	333	1.22
Females		
4–5	409	1.09
6–8	279	1.15
9–11	312	1.21

NHANES-II.[123,174,331]

Based on plasma vitamin A levels, little evidence of vitamin A deficiency in the United States was found in the National Health and Nutrition Examination Surveys (NHANES).[62] From the NHANES it was observed that women had plasma vitamin A concentrations 5 to 10% lower than that of men.[163-165]

Adults and Elderly

The Baltimore Longitudinal Study of Aging (Maryland, U.S.A.) studied the effect of vitamin A and E intakes on the plasma concentrations of retinol, β-carotene, and α-tocopherol.[119]

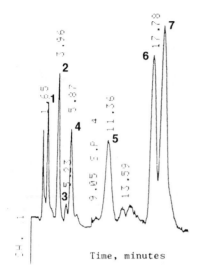

CONSTITUENTS IN HUMAN SERUM

1. RETINOL
2. TOCOL (IS)
3. BETA & GAMMA TOCOPHEROL
4. ALPHA TOCOPHEROL
5. LYCOPENE
6. ALPHA-CAROTENE
7. BETA-CAROTENE

FIGURE 39

HPLC analysis for plasma concentrations of α-carotene, β-carotene, and lycopene. Procedure of Stacewicz-Sapuntzakis et al.[100] was used.

The study involved 200 women and 231 men. Plasma concentrations of retinol were above 0.70 μmol/L, except for two women. Smoking was not significantly related to plasma β-carotene, retinol or α-tocopherol concentrations. Of interest, 8% of the men had an undetectable plasma concentration of β-carotene, but had normal plasma retinol concentrations.

In a study conducted with healthy elderly subjects in Paris, France, concentrations of vitamin A were lower in the elderly men and women than the concentrations found in healthy younger adults.[120] The values observed for vitamin A were 3.06 ± 0.51 μmol/L for the young adult men (n = 40) and 2.79 ± 0.61 μmol/L for the elderly men (n = 40). The young women (n = 40) had plasma vitamin A concentrations of 3.19 ± 0.58 μmol/L compared to concentrations of 2.62 ± 0.68 μmol/L (n = 40) for the elderly women.[120]

A number of other studies have investigated the vitamin A status of institutionalized and non-institutionalized elderly populations.[122,173,174,176] In the study of Lowik et al.,[177] retinol levels of the elderly men and women were lower then the levels of younger adults. Several other studies did not observe any difference in plasma retinol concentration with age.[175,178]

A review of literature reports indicates that plasma retinol concentrations increase from a mean of about 1.22 μmol/L (35 μg/dL) at preschool age to a plateau of about 2.09 μmol/L (60 μg/dL) by age 40 years in men and by age 60 years in women.[162]

Interactions of Vitamin A

General

Vitamin A deficiency has been associated, in addition to visual impairment and blindness, with increased morbidity and mortality.[124,160,226] Thus, vitamin A has been implicated in diarrheal morbidity, respiratory morbidity, immunity, infections, and measles, iron-deficiency anemia,[125] impaired growth, and other conditions.

Serum vitamin A and retinol-binding protein concentrations are lower in patients with diabetes mellitus than those of non-diabetic control subjects.[132] Oral contraceptive agents commonly elevate plasma retinol concentrations. This appears to be associated with an increased concentration of plasma retinol-binding protein.[227] Serum retinol concentrations may decrease in response to trauma or infection.[115,116,336]

Zinc deficiencies can inhibit the synthesis of apo-retinol-binding protein.[127,128,226] In turn, this reduces the amount of the apo-retinol-binding protein available for binding retinol and its secretion into the plasma. Consequently as a result of a zinc deficiency, plasma concentration of retinol and of retinol binding protein can be depressed and could give a false impression of a vitamin A deficiency.[208,209] Similarly, severe protein-energy malnutrition can depress the synthesis of apo-retinol-binding protein resulting in a false low vitamin A status.[128,131,134,135,226]

Vitamin A Status, Immunity, and Infection

In 1923, Daniels et al.[144] observed that rats depleted of vitamin A died of bacterial invasion of the ear and nasal cavities before the appearance of xerophthalmia. During the intervening period, considerable biochemcial and experimental evidence has shown that vitamin A deficiency in the human is associated with decreased resistance to infection. This relationship has been considered in a number of reviews and reports.[145-153,169-171,206] For example, treatment with vitamin A reduces morbidity and mortality in measles.[146,169,171] During marked infections, excretion of retinol in the urine may occur which results in an increased vitamin A requirement.[150,336]

Smoking and Vitamin A Status

A number of factors may affect vitamin A status and plasma concentrations of retinol. Although no significant differences were noted in plasma retinol concentrations of smokers and nonsmokers,[63,64,119] serum concentrations of β-carotene, α-carotene, cryptoxanthin, and lycopene were lower in smokers when compared to nonsmokers.[63-65]

Cancer, Coronary Heart Disease, and Vitamin A Status

Numerous investigations and epidemiologic studies have examined a possible association of carotinoids and vitamin A with the prevention of coronary heart disease and with certain cancers and other diseases.[66-72,76,166] However, β-carotene supplementation was without benefit or harm in altering the incidence of cardiovascular disease or cancer.[67]

Alcohol and Vitamin A Status

Alcohol consumption has little effect on plasma levels of retinol although plasma concentrations of all the carotenoids may be lowered.[20,53] However, chronic alcoholic patients often suffer from night blindness and have lowered plasma retinol levels.[21,22] This may relate to the presence of liver disease and cirrhosis which will impair liver storage of retinol and the production of retinol binding protein.[21,22,30]

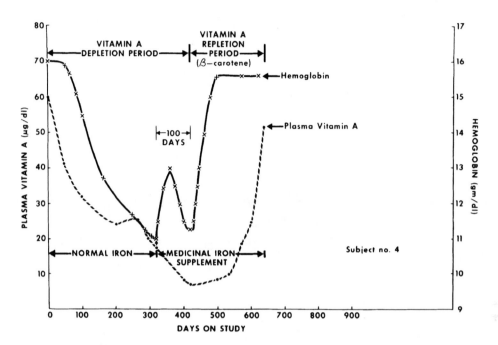

FIGURE 40

Effect of vitamin A and iron supplements on plasma vitamin A and hemoglobin concentrations in a vitamin A-depleted human male volunteer.[136] (With permission.)

Vitamin A and Iron Metabolism

In an experiment with middle-aged men, Hodges et al.[136] induced a vitamin A deficiency by feeding diets deficient or low in vitamin A. During the vitamin A depletion period, the men developed a moderate degree of anemia. The anemia did not respond to medicinal iron but did respond to resupplementation with vitamin A or β-carotene.[136]

This impairment of vitamin A deficiency on iron utilization and the prevalence of anemia has been supported in a number of subsequent studies.[124-126,137,226] In field intervention programs, supplementations of vitamin A have improved hematological indices with decreased anemia in Guatemala,[138,139] Indonesia,[140,141] and Thailand.[142,143] Recently it was reported that vitamin A and β-carotene improved the absorption of nonheme iron from rice, wheat, and corn by the human.[225]

Assessment of Vitamin A Nutritional Status

The following procedures have been used to evaluate vitamin A status:

1. Serum or plasma retinol concentrations
2. Serum retinol-binding protein concentrations
3. Relative-dose-response-measurement
4. Modified relative-dose-response measurement

5. Isotope dilution analysis
6. Clinical assessment: night blindness; dark adaptation; electrorentinograms
7. Histological:
   conjunctival impression cytology
   impression cytology with transfer
8. Liver biopsy

Clinical Assessment

Vitamin A deficiency primarily affects infants and children. In these groups, a severe vitamin A deficiency frequently results in blindness.[160-171,184,185,209] In addition to impaired night blindness and dark adaptation, vitamin A deficiency in the adult may result in anemia, skin lesions (follicular hyperkeratosis) on the arms and thighs as well as in an impaired resistance to infections.[136,186]

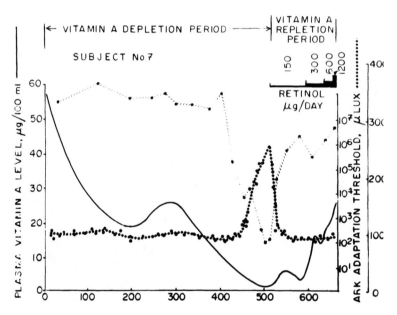

FIGURE 41
The relationship of severity of follicular hyperkeratosis to serum vitamin A concentrations in a vitamin A-depleted human male volunteer.[186] (With permission.)

Although measurement of dark adaptation can serve as a sensitive functional assessment of vitamin A status, the procedure is too involved for routine use. The majority of the vitamin A reserves in the body are present in the liver, but seldom would liver biopsy samples be available for a direct assessment of vitamin A status. Malabsorption conditions, fever, infection, and liver disease may result in low serum levels of retinol. Serum vitamin A concentrations of 1.05 µmol/L (30 µg/dL) or higher are desirable.

Xerophthalmia includes all of the ocular manifestations of vitamin A deficiency. The World Health Organization has classified the eye manifestations of vitamin A deficiency according to their severity as follows.[183]

Classification	Signs
Primary	
X1A	Conjunctival xerosis
X1B	Bitot's spot with conjunctival xerosis
X2	Corneal xerosis
X3A	Corneal ulceration with xerosis
X3B	Keratomalacia

	Signs
Secondary	
XN	Night blindness
XF	Xerophthalmia fundus
XS	Corneal scars

Night blindness (XN) is considered the earliest sign of vitamin A deficiency and is easily corrected with vitamin A supplementations[61,186] Xerosis of the conjunctiva (XIA) is the first visible structural changes in xerophthalmia. Bitot's spots (X1B) usually occur at this stage. This condition may progress to punctuate keratopathy followed by corneal xerosis (X2). Keratomalacia ensues, which represents partial (X3A) or total (X3B) necrosis of the corneal stroma. At this stage the eye may become almost or totally blind. Sommer et al. used the history of blindness as a tool for xerophthalmia (XN) screening of 5925 preschool-age children in Indonesia.[184] A history of nightblindness could be almost as specific and a more sensitive index of vitamin A deficiency then the presence of Bitot's spots (X1B).

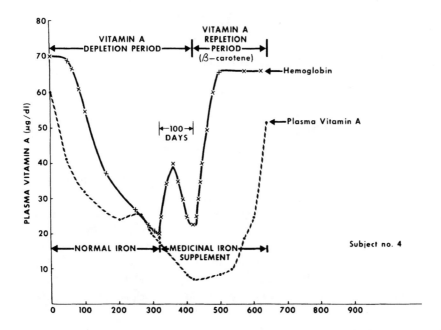

FIGURE 42

The relationship of plasma vitamin A concentrations to the onset of dark adaptation changes and abnormal electroretinograms in a vitamin A-depleted human male volunteer.[186] (With permission.)

The use of rapid dark adaptation time has been summarized by Olson.[274] The test has not been suitable for application with young children, the group most prone to a vitamin A deficiency. In addition, technical problems in administering and evaluation of findings have limited its use. However, several evaluations have been reported.[275-278] Serum vitamin A concentrations > 40 μg/dL predicted normal dark adaptation 95% of the time. A serum concentration of 30 μg/dL predicted normal retinol function 68% of the time, and a level of > 20 mg/dL predicted normal function, 27% of the time.[275,276]

In the Sheffield study on vitamin A requirement,[296] plasma vitamin A did not reach zero levels in the subject, but changes in dark adaptation occurred when plasma vitamin A levels fell below 20 μg/dL.

More recently, pupillary and visual threshold testing has been used as an index of vitamin A status. The tests have been applied to young children in Indonesia[279] and southern India.[280] Pupillary threshold testing was considered to be a noninvasive, valid means of assessing the vitamin A status of a moderately to severely deficient preschool population.[280]

Liver Vitamin A Stores

Inadequate intakes of vitamin A, either as preformed retinol or as active carotenoids, result in a tissue decrease of the vitamin.[186] Since the liver is the major storage organ of vitamin A in the body (90%), the concentration of retinol and its esters in liver tissue is a direct measurement of vitamin A reserves.[186,213-219] This information can be obtained from liver biopsy specimens, but this invasive and complicated procedure is impractical for routine use in population studies; its use can be justified only in special clinical cases. In addition, the uneven distribution of vitamin A in the liver leaves doubt as to the usefulness of this procedure.[224]

Raica et al.,[216] who studied autopsy material obtained mainly from adult subjects, considered a liver vitamin A concentration of less than 40 μg/g to be deficient or low. On this basis 22% of the 369 liver samples studied were low. Similar findings were reported by Hoppner et al.[214,215] and by Underwood et al.,[213] and Olson,[219] who studied infants and children, came to the conclusion that the minimal acceptable vitamin A reserve be considered as 20 μg/g (0.07 μmol/g) of liver.[293] Plasma concentrations of vitamin A decrease markedly when the hepatic reserve have fallen below 0.70 μmol/g liver.[95]

Conjunctival Impression Cytology

Conjunctival impression cytology (CIC) has been used for the assessment of vitamin A status.[257,258,261,273,310] The procedure has been easily performed on children over the age of 3 years, but was more difficult with younger children.[259,260] The CIC technique has been described in detail by Natadisastra et al.[261] and briefly by Kennum.[262] Cellulose acetate filter paper is applied to the inferotemporal bulbar conjunctiva of each eye, removed, and placed in a fixative prior to staining. The preparations are stained for the presence of epithelial cells and goblet cells.

The CIC procedure has been modified and termed "impression cytology with transfer."[273] In the modification, the cells collected on the cellulose acetate filter paper are transferred to a glass slide and then stained directly in one step.[263] The absence of goblet cells and the presence of enlarged, separated epithelial cells in the stained specimen is classified as vitamin A deficient.[262,263] Difficulty may occur in obtaining samples from children under the age of 3 years. Interpretation of borderline specimens and the presence of ocular infections can be difficult. The CIC technique has been utilized in various populations for the detection of subclinical vitamin A deficiency. The populations studied include India,[258] Guatemala,[259,260] Bangladesh,[264] Senegal,[11,265,266] France,[267,268,310] Indonesia,[269,270] South Africa,[271] and Thailand.[272]

When compared to the relative dose response, Rehman et al.[264] felt that the CICy test could not be considered a valid measure of subclinical vitamin A deficiency in the Bangladesh population studied. Gadomski et al.[260] reported that CIC technique failed to detect subclinical vitamin A deficiency that was detected by other biochemical indicators. Interpretation of CICy results have been difficult particularly with borderline cases.

Biochemical Methods for the Assessment of Vitamin A Status

General

Before 1970, the major concern of vitamin A deficiency dwelled on the clinical ocular disease, xerophthalmia. It is now being recognized that a considerably larger population is exposed to the effects of a subclinical vitamin A deficiency.[11] Various reviews have considered procedures for the assessment of vitamin A status.[1,95,179,212,330] The most commonly used biochemical method for evaluating the vitamin A status of individuals and population groups has been the measurement of the concentration of retinol in serum or plasma. Vitamin A and E and carotinoids in plasma samples have been found to be stable for over 2 years when stored at –70°C.[34,35,58,59] All procedures should be performed in very subdued light or with yellow fluorescent lights.

Retinol-Binding Protein and Transthyretin (Prealbumin)

Retinol-binding protein interacts with plasma prealbumin (transthyretin) and normally circulates as a 1:1 molar retinol-binding protein-prealbumin complex.[32,161] The normal concentration of retinol-binding protein in plasma is 40 to 50 µg/mL (1.9 to 2.4 µmol/L) and that of prealbumin of 200 to 300 µg/mL.[129] However, in a study of 144 healthy Swedish children, the median plasma level of prealbumin was 540 µg/L and the median plasma retinol-binding protein level was 30 µg/mL.[133]

After the retinol has been delivered to tissues, the released apo-retinol binding protein is catabolized by the kidney.[130] Both retinol-binding protein and transthyretin (prealbumin) can be measured in serum by radial immunodiffusion assay (commercial assay kits for each are available from The Binding Site, Inc., San Diego, CA). Only 5 µL of sample are required for each analysis. A high correlation exists between plasma retinol concentrations and plasma retinol binding protein concentrations.[154,329]

Retinol-Binding Protein Response Test

Retinol-binding protein is a specific transport protein for vitamin A. When serum vitamin A concentrations are low, retinol-binding concentrations are also low.[247] Retinol-binding protein concentrations, measured by radial immunodiffusion assay, may be used to assess vitamin A status, if protein malnutrition is not present. This simple assay method requires only 20 µL of plasma or serum. Radial immunodiffusion assay kits are available from The Binding Site, San Diego, CA.

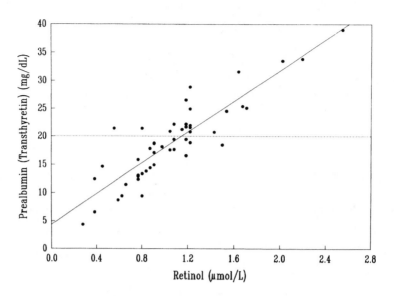

FIGURE 43
Relationship of plasma prealbumin (transthyretin) concentrations and plasma retinol concentrations in men (correlation coefficient = 0.8805).

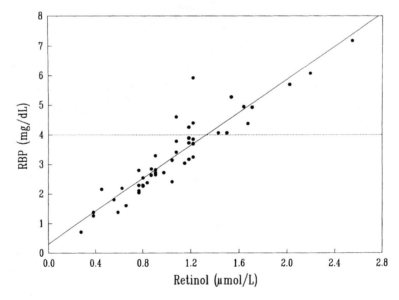

FIGURE 44
Relationship of plasma retinol-binding protein (RBP) concentrations and plasma retinol concentrations in men (correlation coefficient = 0.9264).

Retinol-binding protein assays may serve as the basis for the plasma retinol-binding protein response test.[248,249] The test consists of the measurement of plasma retinol-binding protein concentrations in blood samples obtained just before and approximately 5 hours after an oral dose of 600 to 1000 µg of vitamin A.[248] The percentage increase in plasma retinol-binding protein is calculated. Interpretation of response is somewhat uncertain, but a percentage increase of ≥ 8% along with a low plasma retinol concentration (< 20 µg/dL), was considered compatible with a functional vitamin A deficiency.[248,249] The plasma retinol-binding protein concentration will probably be < 2.0 mg/dL. However, this test requires further evaluation as to applicability, sensitivity, affects of protein and zinc status, and interpretation of results. In addition, the analytical requirements impose demands that may discourage its use.

Relative Dose-Response Assay and the Modified Relative Dose-Response Assay

In recent years, the **relative dose-response assay** and the **modified relative dose-response assay** have been developed and validated as techniques useful in evaluating an individual's vitamin A status.[211,283-285] These two procedures have been briefly summarized by Tanumihardjo.[281,282] The test is based on the observation that during vitamin A deficiency with diminished stores of vitamin A, apo-retinol-binding protein (RBP) accumulates several-fold in the liver.

The principle procedures of the relative dose-response test (RDR) are as follows:[281]

1. A baseline serum vitamin A concentration is obtained on the subject
2. A small oral dose of 450 to 1000 µg (1.57 to 348 µmol) of retinol is given
3. After 5 hours a second blood sample is obtained for serum retinol measurement
4. During this period, some of the administered retinol is taken up by the liver where it combines with some of the excess apo-retinol-binding protein. This is released as holo-retinol-binding protein into the circulation.
5. The amount released into circulation is in proportion to the preexisting deficiency, which results in a rise in the serum retinol concentration.
6. The serum retinol concentrations are determined on the two serum samples obtained.
7. To quantify, the difference between the two serum retinol concentrations is divided by the second retinol concentration and expressed as a percentage. Values above 20% have been considered to indicate low liver stores.[281,293]

The modified relative dose-response assay (MRDR) is similar to the relative dose-response assay,[281] but simpler to perform.[282,289,290] However, the modified procedure requires the availability of 3,4-didehydroretinol, a HPLC system, and at least 200 µl samples of serum or plasma.

The general procedure of the modified relative dose-response assay is as follows:[282]

1. The subject is give a single oral dose of 3,4-didehydroretinol acetate (100 µg/kg bodyweight) dissolved in an oil.
2. A single sample of blood is obtained 4 to 6 hours later. At least 0.5 ml of blood is required to perform the analyses.
3. The retinol and the 3,4-didehydroretinol concentrations in the serum or plasma are measured by HPLC.
4. The 3,4-didehydroretinol/retinol molar ratios can be calculated. It has been suggested for children that 3,4-didehydroretinol/retinol ratios of ≥ 0.06 should be considered to be in a marginal vitamin A status.[282,298,299] However, some investigators have used a cutoff ratio of 0.03.[291]

5. More recently Tanumihardjo et al.[297] have refined the modified relative-dose response test for assessing vitamin A status in a field setting. The main change was in the doses of 3,4-didehydroretinol acetate used.

Several factors can potentially interfere in the relative-dose response test and the modified relative-dose response test that must be considered.[293-295] This includes:

1. Severe protein deficiency could interfere by decreasing liver synthesis of the rapid turnover apo-retinyl-binding protein (12-hr half-life).
2. Effect of infection, inflammation, and trauma may decrease retinol-binding protein levels.[117,150,287,301,307]
3. Liver disease that impairs apo-retinol-binding protein formation.[302]

The relative-dose response assay has been used in various countries in clinical and field vitamin A studies.[285-288,303,309] The modified relative-dose response assay has also received use in a number of studies on the assessment of vitamin A status.[289-292,297,304-306]

Some investigators have reported variable results with the relative dose response test.[180,294,295,298-300,305,306,308] For example, de Pee et al.[299] stated that the modified relative-dose-response test suffered from a relatively large intraindividual variation in the ratio of dehydroretinol to retinol because of vulnerability of the dehydroretinol concentration to laboratory errors and to variations in dosing and absorption. Some of these concerns have been addressed by Olson and Tanumihardjo.[306]

Based upon usage, however, the relative-dose response procedures have been found practical to apply in mildly undernourished children under nonclinical conditions. Serum vitamin A levels of 20 µg/dL or less have invariably been associated with an elevated relative-dose response test.[289] Supplementation with vitamin A reverted the elevated relative-dose response tests to normal. Underwood[211] observed that an abnormal relative-dose response may occur when the plasma vitamin A concentration fell below 30 µg/dL.

Assessment of Vitamin A Status by Isotope Dilution Analysis

The isotope-dilution technique for quantitatively estimating the total body stores of vitamin A was introduced by Furr et al.[223] Deuterated retinol has been used as the stable isotope.[220-223] The procedure is relatively simple.[222] The deuterated-retinol-dilution technique involves the oral administration of a known dose of labeled retinyl acetate. After a period of 18 to 25 days of equilibration, a blood sample is obtained and the plasma retinol extracted and purified by HPLC. The amount of stable isotope in the plasma retinol is measured by mass spectrometry to provide the isotopic ratio.[220-223]

The total body pool of vitamin A can be calculated by the following dilution equation:[222]

$$\text{Total vitamin A} \ = \ \text{dose} \ \times \ \frac{\text{specific activity of dose}}{\text{specific activity of plasma retinol}}$$

The isotope dilution analysis for determining vitamin A status has received only limited use.[220,222] Further refinement in the application of the technique is necessary.[221,337,338] Deterrents to its use have also been commented on by Olson.[220,338] Of concern is the limited availability of the labeled retinyl acetate, the need for high-performance liquid chromatography and mass spectrometry equipment, and the long equilibration time.

Methods for the Measurement of Vitamin A in Plasma or Serum

Colorimetric, Fluorometric, and Spectrophotometric Methods

Retinol can be measured in serum or plasma with the use of microtechniques that employ either fluorometric, spectrophotometric, trifluoracetic acid colorimetric, or high performance liquid chromatographic procedures. Garry[230] and Underwood[234] reviewed many of these procedures as to their accuracy, precision, and difficulties.

The Carr-Price assay, described in 1926, has been the classical method used to determine vitamin A.[231,232] In the Carr-Price reaction, retinol and retinyl esters react with antimony trichloride to give a transient blue color that absorbs at approximately 620 nm.[81] A disadvantage of the method is its sensitivity to moisture which causes turbidity. This problem was overcome by Neeld and Pearson[81,228,229,242] with the use of trifluoroacetic acid in place of antimony trichloride as the chromagen. Trifluoroacetic acid is not sensitive to moisture and the color produced is stable longer. The Neeld-Pearson micro procedure requires only 50 µl of serum. The procedure has proven reliable and has received widespread use.[242] Serum vitamin A concentrations obtained by the colorimetric procedure of Neeld and Pearson[228] correlated closely with the concentrations obtained on the same samples by HPLC (correlation coefficient of 0.997).[242] Serum samples held frozen at –70°C are stable for at least 16 months.[242]

The Bessy-Lowry-Brock-Lopez method[234,235] has been the most widely used spectrophotometric procedure. However, due to technical problems and interference errors, the method has not received wide acceptance. Fluorometric methods for measuring plasma vitamin A are highly sensitive and simple, but require the availability of a quality fluorometer.[230,234,239] Care must be exercised to avoid erroneous results due to interference from fluorescent contaminants, such as phytofluene, that must be removed or avoided.[230,234,236-239] The direct fluorometric method of Futterman et al.[239] is relatively simple, sensitive and useful for application in assessment of vitamin A status in population groups.[240] The direct fluorometric determination is based on the complex of retinol with retinol-binding protein, with the complex having a considerably higher fluorescence than free retinol. Severe hemolysis of samples interfered with the determination of serum retinol by direct fluorometry.[240] This problem can be avoided with the use of HPLC in the analysis for retinol.

High-Performance Liquid Chromatography (HPLC)

HPLC is recommended by the World Health Organization (WHO) for vitamin A assessment in population surveys.[241] The relative dose-response assay and the modified relative dose-response assay are both dependent upon accurate analyses of serum or plasma for retinol and 3,4-didehydroretinol concentrations.

Following the introduction of HPLC for the measurement of vitamin A in serum by De Leenheer et al.[243,244] and Bieri et al.,[245] numerous other HPLC methods for vitamin A assays have been described.[39,49,84-90,154,242,246,311,312,314-323] Most procedures require 100 to 200 µL of serum or plasma.

In our experience, the HPLC method described by Bieri et al.[245,313] has been a reliable, rapid, and easy assay procedure that provides a simultaneous measurement of retinol and α-tocopherol. Depending upon the nature of the sample to be analyzed, retinyl acetate, α-tocopherol acetate, or tocol may be used as internal standards. Echinenone may be used as an internal standard as its presence in sera is unlikely.[45] It is rare in nature where it is found in the sea urchin. We have found tocol to be very satisfactory for this purpose. Standard reference material may be obtained from the National Institute of Standards and Technology, Gaithersburg, MD. Standard reference material (SRM 968b) provides certified values for retinol, retinyl palmitate, α-tocopherol, and trans-β-carotene. Aliquots of plasma pools with established analytical values may be used as quality controls.

Recently, Dreyfuss et al.[324] have provided preliminary information on a procedure to analyze for vitamin A by HPLC in a dried blood spot obtained by finger prick. The retinol values obtained from the blood spots compared quite well with values obtained on plasma samples. The procedure warrants further study. If proven reliable, the procedure would provide for easier collection, transport, and storage of samples and access to younger and more remote populations.

Toxicity of Vitamin A

It is long-recognized that intakes of retinoids in excess of requirements may result in toxic effects termed hypervitaminosis A.[31,55,56,61,73,206,207] Plasma levels retinol above 100 μg/dL (> 3.5 μmol/L) are usually observed.[73] Hypervitaminosis A may occur in both children and adults as a result of overzealous use of retinol, including food fads, and prolonged use of high doses for acne therapy. Intakes more than 7.5 mg of retinol (25,000 IU) is not recommended. Chronic intakes of 15 mg of retinol (50,000 IU) by adults and pregnant women may produce a toxic condition. Studies indicate that excess intakes of preformed vitamin A may be teratogenic and result in birth defects.[23,24,31,73,75] The hypervitaminosis A syndrome appears with headache, vomiting, hair loss, anorexia, desquamation, erythematosis dermatitis, joint pain, chapped lips, and liver damage.[31]

Retinol esters may be found in fasting plasma with an intake of toxic amounts of the vitamin.[56] Total retinyl esters may be measured by HPLC.[56,57] In a study with healthy unsupplemented elderly subjects, their mean plasma concentration of retinol was 2.17 μmol/L and their mean concentration of retinyl esters was 74 nmol/L.[56] Long-term vitamin A supplemental use by elderly has been reported to produce an increase in fasting plasma retinyl esters. These increases have been associated with biochemical evidence of liver damage.[60]

Relationship of Plasma Retinol Levels to Vitamin A Status

Children

Sommer et al.[179,184,185] observed that a significant number of the preschool Indonesian children with mild xerophthalmia had serum vitamin A concentrations above 0.70 μmol/L (20 μg/dL). Lower concentrations of serum retinol were associated with increased severity and prevalence of the deficiency.

National Health and Nutrition Examination Studies (NHANES) indicated that individuals with serum vitamin A concentrations of less than 1.05 μmol/L (30 μg/dL) are suboptimun and are likely to benefit from an increased intake of vitamin A.[174] Similar observations were reported by Flores et al.[250,251] who studied 544 Brazilian children. Their vitamin A status was evaluated by using the relative-dose-response test (RDR).[251,252] The children had serum vitamin A concentrations of 0.80 ± 0.24 µmol/L (23 ± 7 µg/dL).

For the evaluation of serum vitamin A data from the National Health and Nutrition Examination Surveys, Pilch[123,124] used selected low ranges of vitamin A. The ranges were < 0.70 µmol/L (< 20 µg/dL); 0.70 to 0.84 µmol/L (20 to 24 µg/dL); and 0.87 to 1.01 µmol/L (25 to 29 µg/dL). Serum vitamin A levels of < 0.35 µmol/L (< 10 µg/dL) were considered to be likely associated with impairment of functions (e.g., night blindness), while concentrations of 1.05 µmol/L (30 µg/dL) and above would normally represent an adequate vitamin A status. Subsequently, Looker et al.[122] used these guidelines for the interpretation of serum total vitamin A data of the Hispanic Health and Nutrition Examination Survey (Tables 51 to 54).

TABLE 51
Guidelines for the Evaluation of Vitamin A Biochemical Data

| | Less than Acceptable (At Risk) | | | | Acceptable (Low Risk) | |
| | Deficient (High Risk) | | Low (Medium Risk) | | | |
Report	µmol/L	µg/dL	µmol/L	µg/dL	µmol/L	µg/dL
1. ICNND[81,181]						
Plasma retinol:						
All ages	< 0.35	< 10	0.35–0.66	10–19	≥ 0.70	≥ 20
2. Children's Bureau[233]						
Plasma retinol:						
Preschool children	< 0.35	< 10	< 0.70	< 20	≥ 0.70	≥ 20
3. National Nutrition Survey[327]						
Plasma retinol:						
0–5 months	< 0.35	< 10	0.35–0.66	10–19	≥ 0.70	≥ 20
0.5–17 years	< 0.70	< 20	0.70–1.01	20–29	≥ 1.05	≥ 30
Adults	< 0.35	< 10	0.35–0.66	10–19	≥ 0.70	≥ 20
4. NHANES[1,122,123,173-175,252]						
Plasma retinol	< 0.70	< 20	< 1.05	< 30	≥ 1.05	≥ 30
5. Canadian Nutrition Survey[328]						
All Ages: male and female Plasma retinol	< 0.35	< 10	0.35–1.05	10–30	> 1.05	> 30

Additional Special Guidelines:
(a) Modified Relative Dose-Response Assay.[282]
   3,4-didehydroretinol/retinol ratio: ≥ 0.06 indicates marginal or poor vitamin A status.
(b) Relative Dose-Response Assay.[252,281]
   Relative dose-response value ≥ 20% indicates marginal or poor vitamin A status.

Adult Men

In a controlled vitamin A depletion and repletion study with adult men, a daily intake of 1,200 µg of retinol supported a plasma retinol level 1.05 µmol/L (30 µg/dL).[186] A plasma retinol level of 0.70 µmol/L (20 µg/dL) was observed with a daily intake of 600 µg of

TABLE 52

Vitamin A Parameters in Normal Subjects

		Fasting Plasma Concentration			
	Age (Years)	Transthyretin (Prealbumin) (μmol/L)	Retinol (μmol/L)	Retinyl Esters (nmol/L)	Retinol-binding Protein (μmol/L)
Younger Subjects (<50 y)					
Males (*n* = 17)	37 ± 2	5.27 ± 0.16	1.8 ± 0.1	46 ± 11	2.4 ± 0.1
Females (*n* = 11)	33 ± 3	4.77 ± 0.15	1.5 ± 0.1	28 ± 8	2.0 ± 0.1
Older Subjects (≥50 y)					
Males (*n* = 11)	68 ± 2	5.09 ± 0.31	2.0 ± 0.2	57 ± 23	2.8 ± 0.2
Females (*n* = 20)	64 ± 2	4.87 ± 0.20	1.8 ± 0.1	54 ± 11	2.4 ± 0.1

Data from Reference 163.

TABLE 53

Nutritional Status of Institutionalized Elderly

Measurement	Men (*n* = 102)	Women (*n* = 214)
Vitamin A		
μg/dL	61.0 ± 19.8	67.5 ± 21.4
μmol/L	2.13 ± 0.69	2.36 ± 0.75
Transthyretin (Prealbumin)		
mg/L	258 ± 70	265 ± 67
Retinol-binding Protein		
mg/L	50 ± 14	57 ± 24

Data from Reference 173.
Mean ± SD.

TABLE 54

Effect of Vitamin A Supplements on Vitamin A-Related Plasma Biochemical Parameters

	Measurement			
Subjects	Retinol (μmol/L)	Retinol-Binding Protein (μmol/L)	Retinyl Esters (nmol/L)	Carotene (μmol/L)
Young Adults				
Males				
Non-supplement users (*n* = 57)	2.50	2.57	62	2.42
Supplement users (*n* = 39)	2.33	2.63	81	2.99
Females				
Non-supplement users (*n* = 52)	2.08	2.35	57	3.03
Supplement users (*n* = 46)	2.22	2.34	73	3.40
Elderly				
Males				
Non-supplement users (*n* = 116)	2.52	2.92	73	2.60
Supplement users (*n* = 65)	2.56	2.80	108	2.43
Females				
Non-supplement users (*n* = 211)	2.45	2.83	71	2.61
Supplement users (*n* = 170)	2.50	2.77	157	2.68

Adapted from Reference 60.

retinol. This level of intake of retinol was required to normalize the electroretinogram patterns and to cure the observed cutaneous lesions.

From the controlled vitamin A deficiency study of Sauberlich et al.,[136,186] guidelines for evaluating vitamin A data obtained for adults can be derived:

Condition	Plasma Vitamin A Concentration at Time of Occurrence	
	µg/dL	µmol/L
Impaired dark adaptation	3–25	0.10–0.87
Abnormal electroretinograms	4–11	0.14–0.38
Follicular hyperkeratosis	7–37	0.24–1.29
Mild anemia	< 20	< 0.70

Data from 8 volunteer adult male subjects.[136,186]

Summary/Comments

The determination of serum retinol concentrations serves as a practical biochemical test for the assessment of vitamin A nutritional status. Prolonged low dietary intakes of vitamin A correlate with serum retinol levels. Since the vitamin is stored primarily in the liver, low serum concentrations of vitamin A reflect not only a low intake of the nutrient but also depleted liver stores. Serum retinol concentrations above 1.05 µmol/L (30 µg/dL) indicate liver stores of vitamin A. Serum concentrations below this value generally indicate inadequate liver stores of vitamin A, likely to be limited or in the process of being depleted. Serum vitamin A concentrations of 0.35 µmol/L (10 µg/dL) or less are indicative of depleted, or virtually so, liver reserves of the vitamin, with clinical signs or symptoms of a deficiency generally evident.

However, individuals suffering with protein-energy malnutrition with a resulting impairment in the hepatic retinol release and in the serum retinol transport system, low serum vitamin A concentrations may be encountered in the presence of liver stores of vitamin A.[199,200] Similarly, zinc appears to be necessary to maintain normal concentrations of vitamin A in plasma.[201]

Consequently, for some subjects, a zinc deficiency could result in low serum vitamin A concentrations in the presence also of liver stores of the vitamin. Nevertheless, if the functional needs of vitamin A are being impaired by a defective plasma transport system, resulting in a *de facto* deficiency, the condition would still be reflected in low serum vitamin A concentrations. In such instances, serum vitamin A concentrations could be more informative than liver vitamin A concentrations obtained on biopsy material. A vast number of reports exist describing the consequences of vitamin A deficiency. Nevertheless, vitamin A deficiency remains a threat to the vision and health of millions of children worldwide.

References

1. A brief guide to current methods of assessing vitamin A status, A report of the International Vitamin A Consulting Group (IVACG), Underwood, B. A. and Olson, J. A., Eds., The Nutrition Foundation, Inc., Washington D.C., 1994.
2. Nutritional Blindness in Developing Countries, Riboux, C.-A. and Frigg, M., Eds., Swiss Red Cross, Basel, Switzerland, 1997, 105.
3. Global Prevalence of Vitamin A Deficiency, World Health Organization, WHO/NUT/95.3, Geneva, Switzerland, 1995.
4. Underwood, B. A., Blinding malnutrition: a preventable blight on the global society, in *Nutritional Blindness in Developing Countries*, Riboux, C. -A. and Frigg, M., Eds., Swiss Red Cross, Basel, Switzerland, 1997, 13.
5. Frigg, M., Vitamin A – An overview of recent health and survival research, in *Nutritional Blindness in Developing Countries*, Riboux, C. –A. and Frigg, M., Eds., Swiss Red Cross, Basel, Switzerland, 1997, 31.
6. Desai, N. C., Desai, S., and Desai, R., Xerophthalmia clinics in rural eye camps, *Int. Ophthalmology*, 16, 139, 1992.
7. Oomen, H. A. P. C., Vitamin A deficiency, xeraphthalmia and blindness, *Nutr. Rev.*, 32, 161, 1974.
8. Kirkwood, B. R., Ross, D. A., Arthur, P., Morris, S. S., Dollimore, N., Binka, F. N., Shier, R. P., Gyapong, J. O., Addy, H. A., and Smith, P. G., Effect of vitamin A supplementation on the growth of young children in northern Ghana, *Am. J. Clin. Nutr.*, 63, 773, 1996.
9. Katz, J., Khatry, S. K., West, K. P., Humphrey, J. H., Leclerq, S. C., Kimbrough, E., Pradhan, E., Phohkrel, R. P., and Sommer, A., Night blindness is prevalent during pregnancy and lactation in rural Nepal, *J. Nutr.*, 125, 2122, 1995.
10. Fawzi, W. W., Herrera, M. G., Willet, W. C., Nestel, P., El Amin, A., Lipsitz, S., and Mohamed, K. A., Dietary vitamin A intake and the risk of mortality among children, *Am. J. Clin. Nutr.*, 59, 401, 1994.
11. Carlier, C., Etchepare, M., Ceccon, J.–F., and Amedee-Manesme, O., Assessment of the vitamin A status of preschool and school age Senegalese children during a cross-sectional study, *Int. J. Vit. Nutr. Res.*, 62, 209, 1992.
12. Arroyave, G., Mejia, L. A., and Aguilar, J. R., The effect of vitamin A fortification of sugar on the serum vitamin A levels of preschool Guatemalan children: a longitudinal evaluation, *Am. J. Clin. Nutr.*, 34, 41, 1981.
13. Favaro, R. M. D., de Souza, N. V., Batistal, S. M., Ferriani, M. G. C., Desai, I. D., and de Oliveira, J. E. D., Vitamin A status of young children in Southern Brazil, *Am. J. Clin. Nutr.*, 43, 852, 1986.
14. Sivakumar, B., Vitamin A status and requirements in pregnancy, *Nutrition News* (National Institute of Nutrition, Hyderabad, India), 18, 1, 1997.
15. Milton, R. C., Reddy, V., and Naidu, A. N., Mild vitamin A deficiency and childhood morbidity – an Indian experience, *Am. J. Clin. Nutr.*, 46, 827, 1987.
16. Rahmathullah, L., Underwood, B. A., and Thulasiraj, R. D. et al., Reduced mortality among children in southern India receiving a small weekly dose of vitamin A, *N. Engl. J. Med.*, 323, 929, 1990.
17. De Sole, G., Belay, Y., and Zegeye, B., Vitamin A deficiency in southern Ethiopia, *Am. J. Clin. Nutr.*, 45, 780, 1987.
18. Cohen, N., Rahman, H., Mitra, M., Sprague, J., Islam, S., de Regt, E. L., and Jalil, M. A., Impact of massive doses of vitamin A on nutritional blindness in Bangladesh, *Am. J. Clin. Nutr.*, 45, 970, 1987.
19. Northrop-Clewes, C. A., Paracha, P. I., McLoone, U. J., and Thurnham, D. I., Effect of improved vitamin A status on response to iron supplementation in Pakistani infants, *Am. J. Clin. Nutr.*, 64, 694, 1996.
20. Lecomte, E., Grolier, P., Herbeth, B., Pirollet, P., Musse, N., Paille, F., Braesco, V., Siest, G., and Arthur, Y., The relation of alcohol consumption to serum carotenoid and retinol levels: effects of withdrawal, *Int. J. Vit. Nutr. Res.*, 64, 170, 1994.

21. Majumdar, S. K., Shaw, G. K., and Thomson, A. D., Vitamin A utilization status in chronic alcoholic patients, *Int. J. Vit. Nutr. Res.*, 53, 273, 1983.
22. Bvonjour, J. P., Vitamin and alcoholism, IX, Vitamin A, *Int. J. Vit. Nutr. Res.*, 51, 166, 1981.
23. Rothman, K. J., Moore, L. L., and Singer, M. R. et al. Teratogenicity of high vitamin A intake, *N. Eng. J. Med.*, 333, 1369, 1995.
24. Oakeley, G. P. and Erickson, J. D., Vitamin A and birth defects: continuing caution needed, *N. Engl. J. Med.*, 333, 1414, 1995.
25. Paul, A. A. and Southgate, D. A. T., *The Composition of Foods*, McCance and Widdowson's, Elsevier/North Holland, New York, 1978, 418.
26. Handbook No. 8 Series, United States Department of Agriculture, Agricultural Research Service, U.S. Government Printing Office, Washington D.C.
27. Bakemeier, A. H., The potential roles of vitamin A, C, and E and selenium in cancer prevention, *Oncology Nursing Forum*, 15, 785, 1988.
28. Bauernfeind, J. C., Carotenoid vitamin A precursors and analogs in foods and feeds, *J. Agri. Food Chem.*, 20, 456, 1972.
29. Block, G., Dresser, C. M., Hartman, A. M., and Carroll, D. M., Nutrient sources in the American diet: quantitative data from the NHANES II Survey. I. Vitamins and minerals, *Am. J. Epidemiol.*, 122, 13, 1985.
30. Leo, M. A. and Lieber, C. S., Hepatic fibrosis after long-term administration of ethanol and moderate vitamin A supplementation in the rat, *Hepatology*, 3, 1, 1983.
31. Hathcock, J. N., Hattan, D. G., Jenkins, M. Y., McDonald, J. T., Sundaresan, P. R., and Wilkening, V. L., Evaluation of vitamin A toxicity, *Am. J. Clin. Nutr.*, 52, 183, 1990.
32. Goodman, D. S., Plasma retinol-binding protein, in *The Retinoids*, Volumes 1 and 2, Sporn, M. B., Roberts, A. B., and Goodman, D. S., Eds., Academic Press, New York, 1984.
33. Sporn, M. B. and Roberts, A. B., Role of retinoids in differentiation and carcinogenesis, *Cancer Res.*, 43, 3034, 1983.
34. Ahola, I. and Gref, C.–G., Stability of the fatty acid composition and vitamin concentrations in serum samples thawed twice from –70°C, *Clin. Chem.*, 34, 1923, 1988.
35. Craft, N. E., Brown, E. D., and Smith, J. C., Effects of storage and handling conditions on concentration of individual carotenoids, retinol, and tocopherol in plasma, *Clin. Chem.*, 34, 44, 1988.
36. Mangles, A. R., Holden, J. M., Beecher, G. R., Forman, M. R., and Lanza, E., Carotenoid content of fruits and vegetables: An evaluation of analytical data, *J. Am. Diet. Assoc.*, 93, 284, 1993.
37. VERIS, Carotenoids: Fact book, Research Information Service, LaGrange, IL, 1996.
38. Sauberlich, H. E., Weinberg, D. S., Freeberg, L. E., Juan, W.–V., Sullivan, T. R., Tamura, T., and Craig, C. B., Effects of consumption of an umbelliferous vegetable beverage on constituents in human sera, in *Food Phytochemicals for Cancer Prevention: Fruits and Vegetables*, Huang, M.–T., Osawa, T., Ho, C.–T., and Rosen, R. T., Eds., ACS Symposium Series 546, American Chemical Society, Washington D.C., 1994, 258.
39. Stacewicz-Sapuntzakis, M., Bowen, P. E., Kikendall, J. W., and Burgess, M., Simultaneous determination of serum retinol and various carotenoids: their distribution in middle-aged men and women, *J. Micronutrient Analysis*, 3, 27, 1987.
40. Haller, J., Lowick, M. R. H., Ferry, M., and Ferro-Suzzi, A., Nutritional status: blood vitamins A, E, B-6, folic acid, and carotene, *Eur. J. Clin. Nutr.*, 45, 63, 1991.
41. Nierenberg, D. W., Stukel, T. A., Baron, J. A., Dain, B. J., and Greenberg, E. R., Determinants of plasma levels of beta-carotene and retinol, *Am. J. Epidemiol.*, 30, 511, 1989.
42. Cantilena, L. R., Stukel, T. A., Greenberg, E. R., Nann, S., and Nierenberg, D. W., Diurnal and seasonal variation of five carotenoids measured in human serum, *Am. J. Clin. Nutr.*, 55, 659, 1992.
43. Micozzi, M. S, Brown, E. D., Taylor, P. R., and Wolfe, E., Carotenodermia in men with elevated carotinoid intake from foods and β-carotene supplements, *Am. J. Clin. Nutr.*, 48, 1061, 1988.
44. Dimitrov, N. V., Meyer, C., Ullrey, D. E., Chenoweth, E., Michelakis, A., Malone, W., Boone, C., and Fink, G., Bioavailability of β-carotene in humans, *Am. J. Clin. Nutr.*, 48, 298, 1988.
45. Bieri, J. G., Brown, E. D., and Smith, J. C., Determination of individual carotenoids in human plasma by high performance liquid chromatography, *J. Liquid Chromatogr.*, 8, 473, 1985.

46. Khachik, F., Beecher, G. R., and Goli, M. B., and Lusby, W. R., Separation, identification, and quantification of carotenoids in fruits, vegetables and human plasma by high-performance liquid-chromatography, *Pure Applied Chem.*, 63, 71, 1991.
47. Khachik, F., Beecher, G. R., Goli, M. B., Lusby, W. R., and Smith, J. C. Jr., Separation and identification of carotenoids and their oxidation products in the extracts of human plasma, *Anal. Chem.*, 64, 2111, 1992.
48. Apgar, J., Makdani, D., Sowell, A. L., Gunter,. E. W., Hegar, A., Potts, W., Rao, D., Wilcox, A., and Smith, J. C., Serum carotenoids concentrations and their reproducibility in children in Belize, *Am. J. Clin. Nutr.*, 64, 726, 1996.
49. Sowell, A. L., Huff, D. L., Yeager, JP. R., Caudill, S. P., and Gunter, E. W., Simultaneous determination of retinol, α-tocopherol, lutein/zeaxanthin, β-cryptoxanthin, lycopene, α-carotene, trans-β-carotene, and four retinyl esters in serum by reversed-phase high-performance liquid chromatography with multi-wavelength detection, *Clin. Chem.*, 40, 411, 1994.
50. Solomons, N. W. and Bulux, J., Plant sources of provitamin A and human nutriture, *Nutr. Revs.*, 51, 199, 1993.
51. Le Francois, P., Chevassus-Agnes, S., and Ndiaye, A. M., Plasma carotinoids as a useful indicator of vitamin A status, *Am. J. Clin. Nutr.*, 34, 434, 1981.
52. Carughi, A. and Hooper, F. G., Plasma carotenoid concentrations before and after supplementation with a carotenoid mixture, *Am. J. Clin. Nutr.*, 59, 896, 1994.
53. Jacques, P. F., Sulsky, S., Hartz, S. C., and Russell, R. M., Moderate alcohol intake and nutritional status in nonalcoholic elderly subjects, *Am. J. Clin. Nutr.*, 50, 875, 1989.
54. Bilimoria, S., Deczkes, K., Williamson, D., and Rowell, N. R., Hypercarotinaemia in weight watchers, *Clin. Exp. Dermatol.*, 4, 331, 1979.
55. Sommer, A., Large dose vitamin A to control vitamin A deficiency, in *Elevated Dosages of Vitamins, Benefits, and Hazards*, Walter, P., Brubacher, G., and, Stahelin, H., Eds., Hans Huber Publication, Lewison, 1989, 37.
56. Stauber, P. M., Sherry, B., VanderJagt, D. J., Bhagavan, H. N., and Garry, P. J., A longitudinal study of the relationship between vitamin A supplementation and plasma retinol, retinyl esters, and liver enzyme activities in a healthy elderly population, *Am. J. Clin. Nutr.*, 54, 878, 1991.
57. Bankson, D. D., Russell, R. M., and Sadowski, J. A., Determination of retinyl esters and retinol in serum or plasma by normal-phase liquid chromatography: method and applications, *Clin. Chem.*, 33, 35, 1986.
58. Hsing, A. W., Comstock, G. W., and Polk, B. F., Effect of repeated freezing and thawing on vitamins and hormones in serum, *Clin. Chem.*, 35, 2145, 1989.
59. Driskell, W. J., Bashor, M. M., and Neese, J. W., Loss of vitamin A in long-term stored, frozen sera, *Clin. Chem.*, 31, 871, 1985.
60. Krasinski, S. D., Russell, R. M., Otradovec, C. L., Sadowski, J. A., Hartz, S. C., Jacob, R. A., and McGandy, R. B., Relationship of vitamin A and vitamin E intake to fasting plasma retinol, retinol-binding protein, retinyl esters, carotene, α-tocopherol, and cholesterol among elderly people and young adults: increased plasma retinyl esters among vitamin A-supplement users, *Am. J. Clin. Nutr.*, 49, 112, 1989.
61. Ganguly, J., *Biochemistry of Vitamin A*, CRC Press, Boca Raton, FL, 1989, 221.
62. Center for Food Safety and Applied Nutrition, Food and Drug Administration, U.S. Department of Health and Human Services, Assessment of the Vitamin A nutritional status of the U.S. population based on the data collected in the Health and Nutrition Examination Surveys, Washington D.C., FDA, 1985 (FDA 223-84-2059).
63. Pamuk, E. R., Byers, T., Coates, R. J., Vann, J. W., Sowell, A. L., Gunter, E. W., and Glass, D., Effect of smoking on serum nutrient concentrations in African-American women, *Am. J. Clin. Nutr.*, 59, 891, 1994.
64. Paiva, S. A. R., Godoy, I., Vannucchi, H., Favaro, R. M. D., Geraldo, R. C., and Campana, A. O., Assessment of vitamin A status in chronic obstructive pulmonary disease patients and healthy smokers, *Am. J. Clin. Nutr.*, 64, 928, 1996.

65. Albanse, D., Virtamo, J., Taylor, P. R., Rautalahti, M., Pietinen, P., Heinonen, O. P., Effects of supplemental β-carotene, cigarette smoking, and alcohol consumption on serum carotenoids in the Alpha-Tocopherol, Beta-Carotene Cancer Prevention Study, *Am. J. Clin. Nutr.*, 66, 366, 1997.
66. Mayne, S. T., Beta-carotene, carotenoids, and disease prevention, *FASEB J.*, 10, 690, 1996.
67. Hennekens, C. H., Buring, J. E., Manson, J. E., Stampfer, M., Rosner, B., Cook, N. R., Belanger, C., LaMotte, F., Gaziano, J. M., Ridher, P. M., Willett, W., and Peto, R., Lack of effect of long-term supplementation with beta-carotene on the incidence of malignant neoplasms and cardiovascular disease, *N. Engl. J. Med.*, 334, 1145, 1996.
68. Olson, J. A., Carotenoids, vitamin A and cancer, *J. Nutr.*, 116, 1127, 1986.
69. Morris, D. L., Kritchevsky, S. B., and Davis, C. E., Serum carotenoids and coronary heart disease, The lipid research clinics coronary primary prevention trial and follow-up study, *JAMA*, 272, 1439, 1994.
70. The alpha-tocopherol, beta-carotene cancer prevention study group, The effect of vitamin E and beta-carotene on the incidence of lung cancer and other cancers in male smokers, *N. Engl. J. Med., 330, 1029, 1994.*
71. Ziegler, R. G., A review of epidemiologic evidence that carotenoids reduce the risk of cancer, *J. Nutr.*, 119, 116, 1989.
72. Wolf, G., Is dietary β-carotene an anti-cancer agent? *Nutr. Rev.*, 40, 257, 1982.
73. Bendich, A. and Langseth, L., Safety of vitamin A, *Am. J. Clin. Nutr.*, 49, 358, 1989.
74. Ellis, J. K., Russell, R. M., Makraver, F. L., and Schaefer, E. J., Increased risk for vitamin A toxicity in severe hypertriglyceridemia, *Ann. Int. Med.*, 105, 877, 1986.
75. Underwood, B. A., Teratogenicity of vitamin A, in *Elevated Dosages of Vitamins: Benefits and Hazards*, Walter, P., Brubacher, G., and Stähelin, H., Eds., Hans Huber Publication, Lewiston, 1989, 42.
76. VERIS, Efficacy of carotenoids, VERIS Research Summary, VERIS Research Information Service, La Grange, 1997, 11.
77. Koo, W. W. K., Krug-Wispe, S., Succop, P., Tsang, R. C., and Neylan, M., Effects of different vitamin A intakes on very-low-birth-weight infants, *Am. J. Clin. Nutr.*, 62, 1216, 1995.
78. Underwood, B. A., Vitamin A prophylaxis programs in developing countries: past experience and future prospects, *Nutr. Rev.*, 48, 265, 1990.
79. Bessey, O. A., Lowry, O. H., Brock, M. J., and Lopez, J. A., The determination of vitamin A and carotene in small quantities of blood serum, *J. Biol. Chem.*, 166, 177, 1946.
80. Utley, M. H., Brodovsky, E. R., and Pearson, W. N., Hemolysis and reagent purity as factors causing erratic results in the estimation of vitamin A and carotene in serum by the Bessey-Lowry method, *J. Nutr.*, 66, 205, 1958.
81. *Manual for Nutrition Surveys*, Second Edition, Interdepartmental Committee on Nutrition for National Defense, National Institutes of Health, Bethesda, MD, 1963.
82. Rojas-Hidalgo, E. and Olmedilla, B., Carotenoids, *Int. J. Vit. Nutr. Revs.*, 63, 265, 1993.
83. Bendich, A., The safety of β-carotene, *Nutr. Cancer*, 11, 207, 1988.
84. Broich, C. R., Gerber, L. E., and Erdman, J. W., Determination of lycopene, α- and β-carotene and retinyl esters in human serum by reversed-phase high performance liquid chromatography, *Lipids*, 18, 253, 1983.
85. Thurnham, D. I., Smith, E., and Flora, P. S., Concurrent liquid-chromatographic assay of retinol, α-tocopherol, β-carotene, α-carotene, lycopene, and β-cryptoxanthin in plasma, with tocopherol acetate as internal standard, *Clin. Chem.*, 34, 377, 1988.
86. Riso, P. and Porrini, M., Determination of carotenoids in vegetable foods and plasma, *Int. J. Vit. Nutr. Res.*, 67, 47, 1996.
87. Epler, K. S., Ziegler, R. G., and Craft, N. E., Liquid chromatographic method for the determination of carotenoids, retinoids and tocopherols in human serum and in food, *J. Chromatogr.*, 619, 37, 1993.
88. Epler, K. S., Sander, L. C., Ziegler, R. G., Wise, S. A., and Craft, N. E., Evaluation of reversed-phase liquid chromatographic columns for recovery and selectivity of selected carotenoids, *J. Chromatogr.*, 595, 89, 1992.

89. Brown, E. D., Micozzi, M. S., Craft, N. E., Bieri, J. G., Beecher, G., Edwards, B. K., Rose, A., Taylor, P. R., and Smith, J. C. Jr., Plasma carotenoids in normal men after a single ingestion of vegetables or purified β-carotene, *Am. J. Clin. Nutr.*, 49, 1258, 1989.

90. Hess, D., Keller, H. E., Oberlin, B., Bonfanti, R., and Schüep, W., Simultaneous determination of retinol, tocopherols, carotenes and lycopene in plasma by means of high-performance liquid chromatography on reversed phase, *Int. J. Vit. Nutr. Res.*, 61, 232, 1991.

91. Liebler, D. C., Antioxidant reactions of carotenoids, *Ann. N.Y. Acad. Sci.*, 691, 20, 1993.

92. Bendich, A., Biological functions of dietary carotenoids, *Ann. N.Y. Acad. Sci.*, 691, 60, 1993.

93. Hankin, J. H., La Marchand, L., Kolonel, L. N., and Wilkens, L. R., Assessment of carotenoid intakes in humans, *Ann. N.Y. Acad. Sci.*, 691, 68, 1993.

94. Solomons, N. W. and Bulux, J., Effect of nutritional status on carotene uptake and bioconversion, *Ann. N.Y. Acad. Sci.*, 691, 96, 1993.

95. Olson, J. A., Serum levels of vitamin A and carotenoids as reflectors of nutritional status, *J. Natl. Cancer Inst.*, 73, 1439, 1984.

96. Brady, W. E., Mares-Perlman, J. A., Bowen, P., and Stacewicz-Sapuntzakis, M., Human serum carotenoid concentrations are related to physiologic and lifestyle factors, *J. Nutr.*, 126, 129, 1996.

97. Forman, M. R., Beecher, G. R., Muesing, R., Lanza, E., Olson, B., Campbell, W. S., McAdam, P., Raymond, E., Schulman, J. D., and Graubard, B. I., The fluctuation of plasma carotenoid concentrations by phase of the menstrual cycle: a controlled diet study, *Am. J. Clin. Nutr.*, 64, 559, 1996.

98. Yon, L.–C., Forman, M. R., Beecher, G. R., Graubard, B. I., Campbell, W. S., Reichman, M. E., Taylor, P. R., Lanza, E., Holden, J. M., and Judd, J. T., Relationship between dietary intake and plasma concentrations of carotenoids in premenopausal women: application of the USDA-NCI carotenoid food-composition data base, *Am. J. Clin. Nutr.*, 60, 223, 1994.

99. Forman, M. R., Lanza, E., Yong, L.–C., Holden, J. M., Graubard, B. I., Beecher, G. R., Melitz, M., Brown, E. D., and Smith, J. C., The correlation between two dietary assessments of carotenoids intake and plasma carotenoid concentrations: application of a carotenoid food-consumption databsase, *Am. J. Clin. Nutr.*, 58, 519, 1993.

100. Stacewicz-Sapuntzakis, M., Bowen, P. E., and Mares-Perlman, J. A., Serum reference values for lutein and zeaxanthin using a rapid separation technique, *Ann. N.Y. Acad. Sci.*, 691, 207, 1993.

101. Rodriguez, M. S. and Irwin, M. I., A conspectus of research on vitamin A requirements of man, *J. Nutr.*, 102, 909, 1972.

102. McCollum, E. V., Orent-Keiles, E., and Day, H. G., *The Newer Knowledge of Nutrition*, 5th Edition, Macmillan Company, New York, 1939.

103. McCollum, E. V. and Davis, M., The nature of the dietary deficiencies of rice, *J. Biol. Chem.*, 23, 181, 1915.

104. McCollum, E. V. and Davis, M., The necessity of certain lipids in the diet during growth, *J. Biol. Chem.*, 15, 167, 1913.

105. Osborne, T. B. and Mendel, L. B., The influence of butter fat on growth, *J. Biol. Chem.*, 16, 423, 1913.

106. Osborne, T. B. and Mendel, L. B., The influence of cod liver oil and some other fats on growth, *J. Biol. Chem.*, 17, 401, 1914.

107. Osborn, T. B. and Mendel, L. B., The vitamins in green foods, *J. Biol. Chem.*, 37, 187, 1919.

108. McCollum, E. V., Simonds, N., and Pitz, W., The supplementary dietary relationship between leaf and seed as contrasted with combination of seed with seed, *J. Biol. Chem.*, 30, 13, 1917.

109. Steenbock, H., White corn vs. yellow corn and a probable relation between the fat-soluble vitamins and yellow plant pigments, *Science*, 50, 352, 1919.

110. Moore, T., The relation of carotin to vitamin A, *Lancet*, 217, 380, 1929.

111. Karrer, P., Morf, R., and Schopp, K., Vitamin A from fish oil. II. *Helv. Chim. Acta*, 14, 1431, 1931.

112. DeLuca, H. F. and Suttie, J. W., Eds., *The Fat-Soluble Vitamins*, University of Wisconsin Press, Madison, 1970.

113. Wolf, G., A history of vitamin A and retinoids, *FASEB J.*, 10, 1102, 1996.

114. Sommer, A., Tarwotjo, I., and Djunaed, E. et al., Impact of vitamin A supplementation on childhood mortality: a randomized controlled community trial, *Lancet*, 1, 1169, 1986.

115. Samba, C., Galan, P., Luzeau, R., and Amedee-Manesme, O., Vitamin A deficiency in pre-school age Congolese children during malaria attacks. I. Utilization of the impression cytology with transfer in an equatorial country, *Int. J. Vit. Nutr. Res.*, 60, 215, 1990.

116. Ramsden, D. B., Prince, H. P., and Burr, W. A. et al., The inter-relationship of thyroid hormones, vitamin A and their binding protein following acute stress, *Clin. Endrocrinol.*, 8, 109, 1978.

117. Filteau, S. M., Morris, S. S., Abbott, R. A., Tomkins, A. M., Kirkwood, B. R., Arthur, P., Ross, D. A., Gyapong, J. O., and Raynes, J. G., Influence of morbidity on serum retinol of children in a community-based study in northern Ghana, *Am. J. Clin. Nutr.*, 58, 192, 1993.

118. Pirie, A., Vitamin A deficiency and child blindness in the developing world, *Proc. Nutr. Soc.*, 42, 53, 1983.

119. Hallfrisch, J., Muller, D. C., and Singh, V. N., Vitamin A and E intakes and plasma concentrations of retinol, β-carotene, and α-tocopherol in men and women of the Baltimore Longitudinal Study of Aging, *Am. J. Clin. Nutr.*, 60, 176, 1994.

120. Succari, M., Garric, B., Ponteziere, C., Miocque, M., and Cals, M. J., Influence of sex and age on vitamin A and E status, *Age and Aging*, 20, 413, 1991.

121. Woodruff, C. W., Latham, C. B., Mactier, H., and Hewett, J. E., Vitamin A status of preterm infants: correlation between plasma retinol concentration and retinol dose response, *Am. J. Clin. Nutr.*, 46, 985, 1987.

122. Looker, A. C., Johnson, C. L., and Underwood, B. A., Serum retinol levels of persons aged 4–74 years from three Hispanic groups, *Am. J. Clin. Nutr.*, 48, 1490, 1988.

123. Pilch, S. M., Ed., Assessment of the vitamin A nutritional status of the U.S. population based on data collected in the Health and Nutrition Examination Surveys, Federation of American Societies for Experimental Biology, Bethesda, MD, 1985.

124. Underwood, B. A. and Arthur, P., The contribution of vitamin A to public health, *FASEB J.*, 10, 1040, 1996.

125. Bloem, M. W., Interdependence of vitamin A and iron: an important association for programmes of anaemia control, *Proc. Nutr. Soc.*, 54, 501, 1995.

126. Suharno, D., West, C. E., Muhila, Logman, M. H. G. M., de Waart, F. C., Karyadi, D., and Hautvast, J. G. A. J., Cross-sectional study on the iron and vitamin A status of pregnant women in West Java, Indonesia, *Am. J. Clin. Nutr.*, 56, 988, 1992.

127. Smith, J. C. Jr., The vitamin A-zinc connection: a review, *Ann. N.Y. Acad. Sci.*, 355, 62, 1980.

128. Solomons, N. W. and Russell, R. M., The interaction of vitamin A and zinc: implications for human nutrition, *Am. J. Clin. Nutr.*, 33, 2031, 1980.

129. Goodman, D. S., Retinoid-binding proteins in plasma and cells, *Ann. N.Y. Acad. Sci.*, 359, 69, 1981.

130. Ong, D. E., Vitamin A-binding proteins, *Nutr. Rev.*, 43, 225, 1985.

131. Large, S., Neal, G., Glover, J., Thanangkul, O., and Olson, R. E., The early changes in retinol-binding protein and prealbumin concentrations in plasma of protein-energy malnourished children after treatment with retinol and an improved diet, *Br. J. Nutr.*, 43, 393, 1980.

132. Baus, T. K., Tze, W. J., and Leichter, J., Serum vitamin A and retinol-binding protein in patients with insulin-dependent diabetes mellitus, *Am. J. Clin. Nutr.*, 50, 329, 1989.

133. Drott, P., Meurling, S., and Gebre-Medhin, M., Interactions of vitamin A and E and retinol-binding protein in healthy Swedish children — evidence of thresholds of essentially and toxicity, *Scand. J. Clin. Invest.*, 53, 275, 1993.

134. Venkataswamy, G., Glover, J., Cobby, M., and Pirie, A., Retinol-binding protein in serum of xerophthalmic, malnourished children before and after treatment at a nutrition center, *Am. J. Clin. Nutr.*, 30, 1968, 1977.

135. Smith, F. R., Suskind, R., Thanangkul, O., Leitzmann, C., Goodman, D. S., and Olson, R. E., Plasma vitamin A, retinol-binding protein and prealbumim concentrations in protein-calorie malnutrition. III. Response to varying dietary treatments, *Am. J. Clin. Nutr.*, 28, 732, 1975.

136. Hodges, R. E., Sauberlich, H. E., Canham, J. E., Wallace, D. L., Rucker, R. B., Mejia, L. A., and Mohanram, M., Hematopoietic studies in vitamin A deficiency, *Am. J. Clin. Nutr.*, 31, 876, 1978.

137. Mejia, L. A., Vitamin A deficiency as a factor in nutritional anemia, *Int. J. Vit. Nutr. Res.*, (Suppl) 27, 75, 1985.

138. Mejia, L. A. and Chew, F., Hematological effect of supplementing anemic children with vitamin A alone and in combination with iron, *Am. J. Clin. Nutr.*, 48, 595, 1988.

139. Mejia, L. A. and Arroyave, G. The effect of vitamin A fortification of sugar on iron metabolism in preschool children in Guatemala, *Am. J. Clin. Nutr.*, 36, 87, 1982.

140. Suharno, D., West, C. E., Muhilal, Karyadi, D., Hautvast, J. G., A. J., Supplementation with vitamin A and iron for nutritional anaemic in pregnant women in West Java, Indonesia, *Lancet*, 342, 1325, 1993.

141. Semba, R. D., Muhilal, West, K. P., Winget, M., Natadisastra, G., Scott, A., and Sommer, A., Impact of vitamin A supplementation on hematological indicators of iron metabolism and protein status in children, *Nutr. Res.*, 12, 469, 1992.

142. Bloem, M. W., Wedel, M., Egger, R. J., Speek, A. J., Schrijver, J., Saowakontha, S., and Schreurs, W. H. P., Iron metabolism and vitamin A deficiency in children in Northeast Thailand, *Am. J. Clin. Nutr.*, 50, 332, 1989.

143. Bloem, M. W., Wedel, M., van Agtmaal, E. J., Speck, A. J., Saowakontha, S., and Schreurs, W. H. P., Vitamin A intervention: short-term effects of single, oral, massive dose on iron metabolism, *Am. J. Clin. Nutr.*, 51, 76, 1990.

144. Daniels, A. L., Armstron, M. E., and Hutton, M. K., Nasal sinusitis produced by diets deficient in fat-soluble A vitamin, *J. Am. Med. Assoc.*, 81, 828, 1923.

145. Ross, A. C., Vitamin A status: relationship to immunity and the antibody response (Mini review), *PSEBM*, 200, 303,1992.

146. Hussey, G. D. and Klein, M., A randomized, controlled trial of vitamin A in children with severe measles, *N. Engl. J. Med.*, 323, 160, 1990.

147. Rahmathullah, L., Underwood, B. A., Thulasierj, R. D., Milton, R. C., Ramaswamy, K., Rahmathillah, R., and Babu, G., Reduced mortality among children of southern India receiving a small weekly dose of vitamin A, *N. Engl. J. Med.*, 323, 929, 1990.

148. Salazar-Lindo, E., Salazar, M., and Alvarez, J. O., Association of diarrhea and low serum retinol in Peruvian children, *Am. J. Clin. Nutr.*, 58, 110, 1993.

149. Mujibur, M., Majhalanabis, D., Alvarez, J. O., Wahed, M. A., Islam, M. A., Habte, D., and Khaled, M. A., Acute respiratory infections prevent improvement of vitamin A status in young infants supplemented with vitamin A, *J. Nutr.*, 126, 628, 1996.

150. Stephensen, C. B., Alvarez, J. O., Kohatsu, J., Hardmeier, R., Kennedy, J. I. Jr., and Gammon, R. B. Jr., Vitamin A is excreted in the urine during acute infection, *Am. J. Clin. Nutr.*, 60, 388, 1994.

151. Semba, R. D., Muhilal, Ward, B. J., Griffin, D. E., Scott, A. L., Natadisastra, G., West, K. P. Jr., and Sommer, A., Abnormal T-cell subset proportions in vitamin A-deficient children, *Lancet*, 341, 5, 1993.

152. Fawzi, W., Herrera, M. G., Willett, W. C., Nestel, P., El Amin, A., Lipsitz, S., and Mohamed, K. A., Dietary vitamin A intake and the risk of mortality among children, *Am. J. Clin. Nutr.*, 59, 401, 1994.

153. Rahman, M. M., Mahalanabis, D., Alvarez, J. O., Wahed, M. A., Islam, M. A., and Habte, D., Effect of early vitamin A supplementation on cell-mediated immunity in infants younger than 6 months, *Am. J. Clin. Nutr.*, 65, 144, 1997.

154. Viulleumier, J.–P., Keller, H. E., Gysel, D., and Hunziker, F., Clinical chemical methods for the routine assessment of the vitamin status in human populations. I: The fat-soluble vitamins A and E, and β-carotene, *Int. J. Vit. Nutr. Res.*, 53, 265, 1983.

155. Goodman, D. S., Overview of current knowledge of metabolism of vitamin A and caroteinoids, *JNCI*, 73, 1375, 1984.

156. Olson, J. A., Molecular actions of carotenoids, *Ann. N.Y. Acad. Sci.*, 691, 156, 1993.

157. Britton, G., Structure and properties of carotenoids in relation to function, *FASEB J.*, 9, 1551, 1995.

158. Cantilena, L. R., Stukel, T. A., Greenberg, E. R., Nann, S., and Nierenberg, D. W., Diurnal and seasonal variation of five carotenoids measured in human serum, *Am. J. Clin. Nutr.*, 55, 659, 1992.

159. Olmedilla, B., Granado, F., Blanco, I., and Rojas-Hidalgo, E., Seasonal and sex-related variations in six serum carotenoids, retinol, and α-tocopherol, *Am. J. Clin. Nutr.*, 60, 106, 1994.

160. Sommer, A., New imperatives for an old vitamin (A), *J. Nutr.*, 119, 96, 1989.
161. Blomhoff, R., Green, M. H., Berg, T., and Norum, K. R., Transport and storage of vitamin A, *Science*, 250, 399, 1990.
162. Garry, P. J., Hunt, W. C., Bandroschak, J., VanderJagt, D., and Goodwin, J. S., Vitamin A intake and plasma retinol levels in healthy elderly men and women, *Am. J. Clin. Nutr.*, 46, 989, 1987.
163. Johnson, E. J., Drasinski, S. D., and Russell, R. M., Sex differences in postabsorptive plasma vitamin A transport, *Am. J. Clin. Nutr.*, 56, 911, 1992.
164. U.S. Department of Health and Human Sciences, Assessment of the vitamin A nutritional status of the U.S. population based on data collected in the Health and Nutrition Examination Surveys, U.S. Government Printing Office, (FDA publications, 223-84-2059), Washington D.C., 1985.
165. Herboth, B., Zittoun, J., Miravet, L., Reference intervals for vitamins B-1, E, D, retinol, beta-carotene, and folate in blood: usefulness of dietary selection criteria, *Clin. Chem.*, 32, 1756, 1986.
166. Ziegler, R. G. and Subar, A. F., Vegetables, fruits, and carotenoids and the risk of cancer, in *Micronutrients in Health and Disease Prevention*, Bendich, A. and Butterworth, C. E. Jr., Eds., Marcel Dekker, Inc., New York, 1991, 97.
167. Ziegler, R. G., Vegetables, fruits, and carotenoids and the risk of cancer, *Am. J. Clin. Nutr.*, 53, 251S, 1991.
168. Garewal, H. S., Potential role of β-carotene in prevention of oral cancer, *Am. J. Clin. Nutr.*, 53, 294S, 1991.
169. Humphrey, J. H. and West, K. P. Jr., Vitamin A deficiency: role in childhood infection and mortality, in *Micronutrients in Health and in Disease Prevention*, Bendich, A. and Butterworth, C. E. Jr., Eds., Marcel Dekker, New York, 1991, 307.
170. Beaton, G. H., Martorell, R., Aronson, K. J., Edmonsov, B., McCabe, G., Rose, A. C., and Harvey, B., *Effectiveness of Vitamin A Supplementation in the Control of Young Child Morbidity and Mortality in Developing Countries*, A project of the International Nutrition Program, Department of Nutritional Sciences, University of Toronto, Canada, 1993.
171. Gillespie, S. and Mason, J., *Controlling Vitamin A Deficiency*, A report based on the ACC/SCN Consultive Group Meeting on Strategies for the Control of Vitamin A Deficiency, Ottawa, 28–30 July, 1993, Copies obtained from World Health Organization, Geneva, Switzerland.
172. Rankin, J., Green, N. R., Tremper, W., Stacewitz-Sapuntzakis, M., Bowen, P., and Ndiaye, M., Undernutrition and vitamin A deficiency in the Department of Linguere, Louga region of Senegal, *Am. J. Clin. Nutr.*, 58, 91, 1993.
173. Sahyoun, N. R., Otradovec, C. L., Hartz, S. C., Jacob, R. A., Peters, H., Russell, R. M., and McGandy, R. B., Dietary intakes and biochemical indicators of nutritional status in an elderly, institutionalized population, *Am. J. Clin. Nutr.*, 47, 524, 1988.
174. Pilch, S. M., Analysis of vitamin A data from the Health and Nutrition Examination Surveys, *J. Nutr.*, 117, 636, 1987.
175. Garry, P. J., Hunt, W. C., Brandrofchak, J. L., VanderJagt, D., and Goodwin, J. S., Vitamin A intake and plasma retinol levels in healthy elderly men and women, *Am. J. Clin. Nutr.*, 46, 989, 1987.
176. Monget, A. L., Galan, P., Preziosi, P., Keller, H., Bourgeois, C., Arnaud, J., Favier, A., and Hercberg, S., Micronutrient status in elderly people, *Int. J. Vit. Nutr. Res.*, 66, 71, 1996.
177. Lowik, M. R. H., Schrijver, J., Odink, J., van den Berg, H., Wedel, M., and Hermus, R. J. J., Nutrition and aging: nutritional status of "apparently healthy" elderly, (Dutch Nutritional Surveillance System), *J. Am. Coll. Nutr.*, 9, 18, 1990.
178. Vogel, S., Contois, J. H., Tucker, K. L., Wilson, P. W. F., Schaefer, E. J., and Lammi-Keef, C. J., Plasma retinol and plasma and lipoprotein tocopherol and carotenoid concentrations in healthy elderly participants of the Framingham Heart Study, *Am. J. Clin. Nutr.*, 66, 950, 1997.
179. Sommer, A., West, K. P., Olson, J. A., and Ross, A. C., *Vitamin A Deficiency: Health, Survival, and Vision*, Oxford University Press, New York, 1996.
180. Zachman, R. D., Retinol (vitamin A) and the neonate: special problems of the human premature infant, *Am. J. Clin. Nutr.*, 50, 413, 1989.
181. Sauberlich, H. E., Skala, J. H., and Dowdy, R. P., *Laboratory Test for the Assessment of Nutritional Status*, CRC Press, Boca Raton, FL, 1974.

182. Olson, J. A., Vitamin A, retinoids, and carotenoids, in *Modern Nutrition in Health and Disease*, 8th edition, Shils, M. E., Olson, J. A., and Shiuke, M., Eds., Lea & Febiger, Philadelphia, 1994, 287.
183. *Vitamin A Deficiency and Xerophthalmia*, Technical Report Series No. 590, World Health Organization, Geneva, Switzerland, 1976.
184. Sommer, A., Hussaini, G., Muhilal, Tarwatjo, I., Susanta, D., and Saroso, J. S., History of nightblindness: a simple tool for xerophthalmia screening, *Am. J. Clin. Nutr.*, 33, 887, 1980.
185. Sommer, A. and Muhilal, Nutritional factors in corneal xerophthalmia and kertomalacia, *Arch. Ophthalmol.*, 100, 399, 1982.
186. Sauberlich, H. E., Hodges, R. E., Wallace, D. L., Kolder, H., Canham, J. E., Hood, J., Raica, N., and Lowry, L. K., Vitamin A metabolism and requirements in the human studied with the use of labeled retinol, *Vit. Horm.*, 32, 251, 1974.
187. *Vitamin A Deficiency and Its Control*, Bauernfeind, J. C., Ed., Academic Press, New York, 1986.
188. Sklan, D., Vitamin A in human nutrition, *Progress in Food and Nutrition Science*, 11, 39, 1987.
189. Blaner, W. S. and Olson J. A., Retinol and retinoic acid metabolism, in *Retinoids*, 2nd edition, Sporn, M. B., Roberts, A. B., and Goodman, D. S., Eds., Raven Press, New York, 1994, 229.
190. Chytil, F. and Ong, D. E., Intracellular vitamin A binding proteins, *Annu. Rev. Nutr.*, 7, 321, 1987.
191. Norum, K. R. and Bloohoff, R., McCallum Award lecture, Vitamin A absorption, transport, cellular uptake, and storage, *Am. J. Clin. Nutr.*, 56, 735, 1992.
192. Ross, A. C., Overview of retinoid metabolism, *J. Nutr.*, 123, 346, 1993.
193. Soprano, D. R. and Blaner, W. S., Plasma retinol binding protein, in *The Retinoids*, 2nd edition, Sporn, M. B., Roberts, A. B. and Goodman, D. S., Eds., Raven Press, New York, 1994, 257.
194. Olson, J. A., Hypovitaminosis A: Contemporary scientific issues, *J. Nutr.*, 124, 1461S, 1994.
195. Bloomhoff, R., Green, M. H., and Norum, K. R., Vitamin A: physiological and biochemical processing, *Annu. Rev. Nutr.*, 12, 37, 1992.
196. Humphrey, J. H., West, K. P., and Sommer, A., Vitamin A deficiency and attributable mortality among under-5-year-olds, *Bulletin World Health Organization*, 70(2), 225, 1992.
197. Looker, A. C., Johnson, C. L., Woteki, C. E., Yetley, E. A., and Underwood, B. A., Ethnic and racial differences in serum vitamin A levels of children aged 4–11 years, *Am. J. Clin. Nutr.*, 47, 247, 1988.
198. Goodwin, T. W., Metabolism, nutrition, and function of carotenoids, *Annu. Rev. Nutr.*, 6, 273, 1986.
199. Smith, F. R., Goodman, D. S., Zaklama, M. S., Gabr, M. K., El Maraghy, S., and Patwardhan, V. N., Serum vitamin A, retinol-binding protein, and prealbumin-calorie malnutrition. I. A functional defect in hepatic retinol release, *Am. J. Clin. Nutr.*, 26, 973, 1973.
200. Smith, F. R., Goodman, D. S., Arroyave, G., and Viteri, F., Serum vitamin A, retinol-binding protein, and prealbumin concentrations in protein-calorie malnutrition. II. Treatment including supplemental vitamin A, *Am. J. Clin. Nutr.*, 26, 982, 1973.
201. Smith, J. C. Jr., Zinc: a trace element essential in vitamin A metbolism, *Science*, 183, 954, 1973.
202. Combs, G. F. Jr., *The Vitamins: Fundamental Aspects in Nutrition and Health*, Academic Press, New York, 1992, 119.
203. Ross, A. C., *Evaluation of Publicly Available Scientific Evidence Regarding Certain Nutrient-Disease Relationships: 8A Vitamin A and Cancer*, Life Science Research Office, Federation of American Societies for Experimental Biology, Bethesda, MD, 1991.
204. Byers, T. and Perry, G., Dietary carotenes, vitamin C, and vitamin E as protective antioxidants in human cancers, *Annu. Rev. Nutr.*, 12, 139, 1992.
205. Gerster, H., Potential role of beta-carotene in the prevention of cardiovascular disease, *Int. J. Vit. Nutr. Res.*, 61, 277, 1991.
206. Gerster, H., Vitamin A — Functions, dietary requirements and safety in humans, Review, *Int. J. Vit. Nutr. Res.*, 67, 71, 1997.
207. Bauernfeind, J. C., *The Safe Use of Vitamin A*, A report of the International Vitamin A Consultative Groups, The Nutrition Foundation, Washington D.C., 1980.
208. Udomkesmalec, E., Dhanamita, S., Rojroongwasinkul, N., and Smith, J. C., Biochemical evidence suggestive of suboptimal zinc and vitamin A status in schoolchildren in Northeast Thailand, *Am. J. Clin. Nutr.*, 52, 564, 1990.
209. McLaren, D. S., Pathogenesis of vitamin A deficiency, in *Vitamin A Deficiency and Its Control*, Bauernfeid, J. G., Ed., Academic Press, Orlando, FL, 1986, 153.

210. Zile, M. H. and Cullum, M. E., The function of vitamin A: current concepts, *Proc. Soc. Expt. Biol. Med.*, 172, 139, 1983.

211. Underwood, B. A., Hypovitaminosis A and its control, *WHO Bull.*, 56, 525, 1978.

212. Pitt, G. A. J., The assessment of vitamin status, *Proc. Nutr. Soc.*, 40, 173, 1981.

213. Underwood, B. A., Siegel, H., Weisell, R. C., and Dolinski, M., Liver stores of vitamin A in a normal population dying suddenly or rapidly form unnatural causes in New York City, *Am. J. Clin. Nutr.*, 23, 1037, 1970.

214. Hoppner, K., Phillips, W. E. J., Murray, T. K., and Campbell, J. S., Survey of liver vitamin A stores of Canadians, *Can. Med. Assoc. J.*, 99, 981, 1968.

215. Hoppner, K. W. E., Phillips, J., Erdsdy, P., Murray, T. K., and Perrin, K. D., Vitamin A reserves of Canadians, *Can. Med. Assoc. J.*, 101, 84, 1969.

216. Raica, N., Scott, J., Lowry, L., and Sauberlich, H. E., Vitamin A concentrations in human tissues collected from 5 areas in the United States, *Am. J. Clin. Nutr.*, 25, 291, 1972.

217. Flores, H. and deAraujo, C. R. C., Liver levels of retinol in unselected necropsy specimens: a prevalence survey of vitamin A deficiency in Recife, Brazil, *Am. J. Clin. Nutr.*, 40, 146, 1984.

218. Olson, J. A., Gunning, D. B., and Tilton, R. A., Liver concentrations of vitamin A and carotenoids, as a function of age and other parameters, of American children who died of various causes, *Am. J. Clin. Nutr.*, 39, 903, 1984.

219. Olson, J. A., New approaches to methods for the assessment of nutritional status of the individual, *Am. J. Clin. Nutr.*, 35, 1166, 1982.

220. Olson, J. A., Isotope-dilution techniques: a wave of the future in human nutrition, *Am. J. Clin. Nutr.*, 66, 186, 1997.

221. Haskell, M. J., Handelman, G. J., Peerson, J. M., Jones, A. D., Rabbi, M. A., Awal, M. A., Wahed, M. A., Mahalanabis, D., and Brown, K. H., Assessment of vitamin A status by the deuterated-retinol-dilution technique and comparison with hepatic vitamin A concentrations in Bangladeshi surgical patients, *Am. J. Clin. Nutr.*, 66, 67, 1997.

222. Furr, H. C., Isotope dilution analysis, in *A Brief Guide to Current Methods of Assessing Vitamin A Status*, A report of the International Vitamin A Consultive Group (IVACG), The Nutrition Foundation, Inc., Washington D.C., 1994, 31.

223. Furr, H. C., Amedee-Manesme, O., Clifford, A. J., Bergen, H. R. III, Jones, A. D., Anderson, D. P., and Olson, J. A., Vitamin A concentrations in liver determined by isotope dilution assay with tetradeuterated vitamin A and by biopsy in generally healthy adult humans, *Am. J. Clin. Nutr.*, 49, 713, 1989.

224. Olson, J. A., Gunning, D., and Tilton, R., The distribution of vitamin A in human liver, *Am. J. Clin. Nutr.*, 32, 2500, 1979.

225. Garcia-Casal, M. N., Layrisse, M., Solano, L., Baron, M. A., Arguello, F., Llovera, D., Ramirez, J., Leets, I., and Tropper, E., Vitamin A and β-carotene can improve nonheme iron absorption from rice, wheat and corn by humans, *J. Nutr.*, 128, 646, 1998.

226. Mejia, L. A., Vitamin A — nutrient interrelationships, in *Vitamin A Deficiency and Its Control*, Bauernfeeind, J. G., Eds., Academic Press, Orlando, FL, 1986, 69.

227. Gal, L., Parkinson, C., and Kraft, I., Effect of oral contraceptives on human plasma vitamin A levels, *Br. Med. J.*, 2, 436, 1971.

228. Neeled, J. B. Jr. and Pearson, W. N., Macro- and micro-methods for the determination of serum vitamin A using tri-fluoroacetic acid, *J. Nutr.*, 79, 454, 1963.

229. Roels, O. A. and Trout, M., Vitamin A and carotene, in *Standard Methods of Clinical Chemistry*, Cooper, G. R., Ed., Academic Press, New York, 7, 215, 1972.

230. Garry, P. J., Vitamin A, in *Symposium on Laboratory Assessment of Nutritional Status*, Labbe, R. F., Ed., *Clinics in Laboratory Medicine*, 1, 699, 1981.

231. Carr, F. H. and Price, E. A., Color reactions attributed to vitamin A, *Biochem. J.*, 20, 498, 1926.

232. Kaser, M. and Stekol, J. A., A critical study of the Carr-Price reaction for the determination of β-carotene and vitamin A in biological materials, *J. Lab. Clin. Med.*, 28, 904, 1943.

233. *Suggested Guidelines for Evaluation of the Nutritional Status of Pre-school Children*, US Department of Health, Education, and Welfare, Social and Rehabilitation Services, Children's Bureau, Washington D.C., (Document No. 1967-0-275-984), 1967.

234. Underwood, B. A., The determination of vitamin A and some aspects of its distribution, mobilization and transport in health and disease, *World Rev. Nutr. Diet.*, 19, 123, 1974.
235. Bessey, O. A., Lowry, O. H., Brock, M. J., and Lopez, J. A., The determination of vitamin A and carotene in small quantities of blood serum, *J. Biol. Chem.*, 166, 177, 1946.
236. Garry, P. J., Pollack, J. D., and Owen, G. M., Plasma vitamin A assay by fluorometry and use of a silicic acid column technique, *Clin. Chem.*, 16, 766, 1970.
237. Thompson, J. N., Erdody, P., Brien, R., and Murray, T. K., Fluorometric determination of vitamin A in human blood and liver, *Biochem. Med.*, 5, 67, 1971.
238. Thompson, J. N., Erdody, P. A., and Maxwell, W. B., Simultaneous fluorometric determination of vitamins A and E in human serum and plasma, *Biochem. Med.*, 8, 403, 1973.
239. Futterman, S., Swanson, D., and Kalina, R. E., A new, rapid fluorometric determination of retinol in serum, *Investigative Ophthamology*, 14, 125, 1975.
240. Marinovic, A. C., May, W. A., Sowell, A. L., Khan, L. K., Huff, D. L., and Bowman, B. A., Effect of hemolysis on serum retinol as assessed by direct fluorometry, *Am. J. Clin. Nutr.*, 66, 1160, 1997.
241. World Health Organization, Indicators for assessing vitamin A deficiency and their application in monitoring and evaluating intervention programmes, Report of a joint WHO/UNICEF consultation, Geneva, Switzerland, WHO, 1994.
242. Driskell, W. J., Neese, J. W., Bryant, C. C., and Bashor, M. M., Measurement of vitamin A and vitamin E in human serum by high-performance liquid chromatography, *J. Chromatogr.*, 231, 439, 1982.
243. DeRuyter, M. G. M. and de Leenheer, A. P., Determination of serum retinol (vitamn A) by high speed liquid chromatography, *Clin. Chem.*, 22, 1593, 1976.
244. De Leenheer, A. P., de Bevre, V., de Ruyter, M. G. M., and Claeys, A. E., Simultaneous determination of retinol and α-tocopherol in human serum by high-performance liquid chromatography, *J. Chromatogr.*, 162, 408, 1979.
245. Buieri, J. G., Tolliver, T. J., and Catignani, G. L., Simultaneous determination of α-tocopherol and retinol in plasma or red cells by high pressure liquid chromatography, *Am. J. Clin. Nutr.*, 32, 2143, 1979.
246. Oliver, R. W. A. and Kafwembe, E. M., A new spectrophotometric assay for the determination of vitamin A and related compounds in serum, *Int. J. Vit. Nutr. Res.*, 62, 221, 1992.
247. Reddy, V., Mohanram, M., and Raghuramulu, N., Serum retinol-binding protein and vitamin A levels in malnourished children, *Acta Paediatr. Scand.*, 68, 65, 1979.
248. Shenai, J. P., Plasma retinol-binding protein response test, in *A Brief Guide to Current Methods of Assessing Vitamin A Status*, A report of the International Vitamin A Consultive Group (IVAG), Underwood, B. A. and Olson, J. A., Eds., the Nutrition Foundation, Washington D.C., 1994, 16.
249. Shenai, J. P., Rush, M. G., Stahlman, M. T. et al., Plasma retinol-binding protein response to vitamin A administration in infants succeptible to bronchopulmonary dysplasia, *J. Pediatr.*, 116, 607, 1990.
250. Flores, H., Azevedo, M. N. A., Campos, F. A. C. S., Barreto-Lins, M. C., Cavalcanti, A. A., Salzano, A. C., Varela, R. M., and Underwood, B. A., Serum vitamin A distribution curve for children aged 2–6 y known to have adequate vitamin A status: a reference population, *Am. J. Clin. Nutr.*, 54, 707, 1991.
251. Flores, H., Camps, F., Aravjo, C. R. C., and Underwood, B. A., Assessment of marginal vitamin A deficiency in Brazilian children using the relative dose response procedure, *Am. J. Clin. Nutr.*, 40, 1281, 1984.
252. Underwood, B., Methods for assessment of vitamin A status, *J. Nutr.*, 120, 1459, 1990.
253. Karr, M., Mira, M., Causer, J., Earl, J., Alperstein, G., Wood, F., Fett, M. J., and Coakley, J., Age-specific reference intervals for plasma vitamins A, E, and β-carotene and for serum zinc, retinol-binding protein and prealbumin for Sydney children aged 9–62 months, *Int. J. Vit. Nutr. Res.*, 67, 432, 1996.
254. Looker, A. C., Johnson, C. L., Woteki, C. E., Yetley, E. A., and Underwood, B. A., Ethnic and racial differences in serum vitamin A levels of children aged 4–11 years, *Am. J. Clin. Nutr.*, 47, 247, 1988.

255. Lockitch, G., Halstead, A. C., Wadsworth, L., Quigley, G., Reston, L., and Jacobson, B., Age- and sex-specific pediatric intervals and correlations for zinc, copper, selenium, iron vitamins A and E, and related proteins, *Clin. Chem.*, 34, 1625, 1988.

256. Malvy, J. M. D., Mourey, M. S., Carlier, C., Caces, P., Dastalova, L, Montagnon, B., and Amedee-Manesme, O., Retinol, β-carotene and α-tocopherol status in a French population of healthy children, *Int. J. Vit. Nutr. Res.*, 59, 29, 1989.

257. Wittpenn, J. R., Tseng, S., and Sommer, A., Detection of early xerophthalmia by impression cytology, *Arch. Opthalmol.*, 104, 237, 1986.

258. Reddy, V., Rao, V., Arunjyothi, and Reddy, M., Conjunctival impression cytology for assessment of vitamin A status, *Am. J. Clin. Nutr.*, 50, 814, 1989.

259. Kjolhede, C. L., Gadomski, A. M., Wittpenn, J., Bulux, J., Rosas, A. R., Solomons, N. W., Brown, K. H., and Forman, M. R., Conjunctival impression cytology: feasibility of a field trial to detect subclinical vitamin A deficiency, *Am. J. Clin. Nutr.*, 49, 490, 1989.

260. Gadomski, A. M., Kjolhede, C. L., Wittpenn, J., Bulux, J., Rosas, A. R., and Forman, M. R., Conjunctival impression cytology (CIC) to detect subclinical vitamin A deficiency: comparison of CIC with biochemical assessments, *Am. J. Clin. Nutr.*, 49, 495, 1989.

261. Natadisastra, G., Wittpenn, J. R., and West, K. P., Impression cytology for detection of vitamin A deficiency, *Arch. Ophthamol.*, 105, 1224, 1987.

262. Keenum, D., Conjunctival impression cytology, in *A Brief Guide to Current Methods of Assessing Vitamin A Status*, A report of the International Vitamin A Consultative Group (IVACG), Underwood, B. A. and Olson, J. A., Eds., Nutrition Foundation, Inc., Washington D.C., 1994, 19.

263. Carlier, C. and Amedee-Manesme, O., Impression cytology with transfer, in A Brief Guide to Current Methods of Assessing Vitamin A Status, A report of the International Vitamin A Consultative Group (IVACG), Underwood, B. A. and Olson, J. A., Eds., Nutrition Foundation, Inc., Washington D.C., 1994, 22.

264. Rahman, M. M., Mahalanabis, D., Wahed, M. A., Islan, M., Habte, D., Khaled, M. A., Alvarez, J. O., Conjunctival impression cytology fails to detect subclinical vitamin A deficiency in young children, *J. Nutr.*, 125, 1869, 1995.

265. Carlier, C., Coste, J., Etchepare, M., and Amedee-Manesme, O., Conjunctival impression cytology with transfer as a field-applicable indicator of vitamin A status for mass screening, *Int. J. Epidemiology*, 21, 373, 1992.

266. Carlier, C., Moulia-Pelat, J.–P., Ceccon, J.–F., Mourey, M.–S., Fall, M., N'Dianye, M., and Amedee-Manesme, O., Prevalence of malnutrition and vitamin A deficiency in the Diourbel, Fatick, and Kaolack regions of Senegal: feasibility of the method of impression cytology with transfer, *Am. J. Clin. Nutr.*, 53, 66, 1991.

267. Amedee-Manesme, O., Luzeau, R., Wittepen, J. R., Hanck, A., and Sommer, A., Impression cytology detects subclinical vitamin A deficiency, *Am. J. Clin. Nutr.*, 47, 875, 1988.

268. Carlier, C., Mourey, M. S., Luzeau, R., Ellrodt, A., Lemmonier, D., and Amedee-Manesme, O., Assessment of vitamin A status in an elderly French population using impression cytology with transfer, *Int. J. Vit. Nutr. Res.*, 59, 3, 1989.

269. Stoltzfus, R., Miller, K. W., Hakimi, M., and Rasmussen, K. M., Conjunctival impression cytology as an indicator of vitamin A status in lactating Indonesian women, *Am. J. Clin. Nutr.*, 58, 167, 1993.

270. Keenum, D. G., Semba, R. D., Wirasamita, S., Natadisastra, G., Muhilal, West, K. P. Jr., and Sommer, A., Assessment of vitamin A status by a disk applicator for conjunctival impression cytology, *Arch. Ophthalmol.*, 108, 1436, 1990.

271. Coutsoudis, A., Mametja, D., Jinabhai, C. C., and Coovadio, H. M., Vitamin A deficiency among children in a periurban South African settlement, *Am. J. Clin. Nutr.*, 57, 904, 1993.

272. Fuchs, G. J., Ausayakhun, S., Ruckphaopunt, S., Tansuhaj, A., and Suskid, R. M., Relation between vitamin A deficiency, malnutrition, and conjunctival impression cytology, *Am. J. Clin. Nutr.*, 60, 293, 1994.

273. Luzeau, R., Carlier, C., Ellrodt, A., and Amedee-Manesme, O., Impression cytology with transfer: an easy method for detection of vitamin A deficiency, *Int. J. Vit. Nutr. Res.*, 58, 166, 1987.

274. Olson, J. A., Rapid dark adaptation time, in *A Brief Guide to Current Methods of Assessing Vitamin A Status*, A report of the International Vitamin A Consultative Group (IVACG), Underwood, B. A. and Olson, J. A., Eds., Nutrition Foundation, Inc., Washington D.C., 1994, 29.

275. Carney, E. A. and Russell, R. M., Correlations of dark adaptation test results with serum vitamin A levels in diseased adults, *J. Nutr.*, 110, 552, 1980.

276. Vinton, N. E. and Russell, R. M., Evaluation of a rapid test of dark adaptation, *Am. J. Clin. Nutr.*, 34, 1961, 1981.

277. Solomons, N. W., Russell, R. M., and Vinton, N. E. et al., Application of a rapid dark-adaptation test in children, *J. Pediatr. Gastroenterol. Nutr.*, 1, 571, 1982.

278. Duarte Favaro, R. M., Vieira de Souza, N., and Vannucchi, H. et al., Evaluation of rose bengal staining test and rapid dark-adaptation test for the field assessment of vitamin A status of preschool children in southern Brazil, *Am. J. Clin. Nutr.*, 43, 940, 1986.

279. Congdon, N., Sommer, A., Severns, M., Humphrey, J., Friedaman, D., Clement, L., Wu, L.–S.–F., and Natadisastra, G., Pupillary and visual thresholds in young children as an index of population vitamin A status, *Am. J. Clin. Nutr.*, 61, 1076, 1995.

280. Sanchez, A. M., Congdon, N. G., Sommer, A., Rahmathullah, L., Venkataswamy, P. G., Chandravathi, P. S., and Clement, L., Pupillary threshold as an index of population vitamin A status among children in India, *Am. J. Clin. Nutr.*, 65, 61, 1997.

281. Tanumihardjo, S. A., The relative dose-response assay, in *A Brief Guide to Current Methods of Assessing Vitamin A Status*, A report of the International Vitamin A Consultative Group (IVACG), Underwood, B. A. and Olson, J. A., Eds., Nutrition Foundation, Inc., Washington D.C., 1994, 12.

282. Tanumihardjo, S. A., The modified relative dose-response assay, in *A Brief Guide to Current Methods of Assessing Vitamin A Status*, A report of the International Vitamin A Consultative Group (IVACG), Underwood, B. A. and Olson, J. A., Eds., Nutrition Foundation, Inc., Washington D.C., 1994, 14.

283. Loerch, J. D., Underwood, B. A., and Lewis, K. C., Response of plasma levels of vitamin A to a dose of vitamin A as an indicator of hepatic vitamin A reserves in rats, *J. Nutr.*, 109, 778, 1979.

284. Amedee-Manesme, O., Anderson, D., and Olson, J. A., Relation of the relative dose-response to liver concentrations of vitamin A in generally well-nourished surgical patients, *Am. J. Clin. Nutr.*, 39, 898, 1984.

285. Amedee-Manesme, O., Mourey, M. S., Hanck, A., and Therasse, J., Vitamin A relative dose response test: validation by intravenous injection in children with liver disease, *Am. J. Clin. Nutr.*, 40, 286, 1987.

286. Flores, H., Campos, F., Ararrjo, C. R. C., and Underwood, B. A., Assessment of marginal vitamin A deficiency in Brazilian children using the relative dose response procedure, *Am. J. Clin. Nutr.*, 40, 1281, 1984.

287. Campos, F. A. C. S., Flores, H., and Underwood, B. A., Effect of an infection on vitamin A status of children as measured by the relative dose response (RDR), *Am. J. Clin. Nutr.*, 46, 91, 1987.

288. Amatayakul, K., Underwood, B. A., Ruckphaopunt, S., Singkamani, R., Linpisarn, S., Leelapat, P., and Thanangkul, O., Oral contraceptives: effect of long-term use on liver vitamin A storage assessed by the relative dose response test, *Am. J. Clin. Nutr.*, 49, 845, 1989.

289. Tanumihardijo, S. A. and Olson, J. A., The reproducibility of the modified relative dose response (MRDR) assay in healthy individuals over time and its comparison with conjunctival impression cytology (CIC), *Eur. J. Clin. Nutr.*, 45, 407, 1991.

290. Tanumihardjo, S. A., Furr, H. C., Erdman, J. W. Jr., and Olson, J. A., Use of the modified relative dose response (MRDR) assay in rats and its application to humans, *Eur. J. Clin. Nutr.*, 44, 219, 1990.

291. Tanumihardjo, S. A., Koellner, P. G., and Olson, J. A., The modified relative dose response (MRDR) assay as an indicator of vitamin A status in a population of well-nourished American children, *Am. J. Clin. Nutr.*, 52, 1064, 1990.

292. Tanumihardjo, S. A., Muhilal, Yuniar, Y., Permaesih, D., Sulaiman, Z., Karyadi, D., and Olson, J. A., Vitamin A status in preschool-age Indonesian children as assessed by the modified relative-dose-response assay, *Am. J. Clin. Nutr.*, 52, 1068, 1990.

293. Olson, J. A., The reproducibility, sensitivity and specificity of the relative dose response (RDR) test for determining vitamin A status, *J. Nutr.*, 121, 917, 1991.

294. Solomons, N. W., Morrow, F. D., Vasquez, A., Bulux, J., Guerreo, A.–M., and Russell, R. M., Test-retest reproducibility of the relative dose response for vitamin A status in Guatemalan adults: issues of diagnostic sensitivity, *J. Nutr.*, 120, 738, 1990.

295. Morrow, F. D., Guerreo, A.–M., Russell, R. M., Dallal, G., and Solomons, N. W., Test-retest reproducibility of the relative dose response for vitamin A status in Guatemalan adults: issues of diagnostic specificity, *J. Nutr.*, 120, 745, 1990.

296. Hume, E. M. and Krebs, H. H., Vitamin A requirement of human adults: An experimental study of vitamin A deprivation in man, *United Kingdom Medical Research Council*, Special Report Series No. 264, London, 1949.

297. Tanumihardjo, S. A., Cheng, J.–C., Permaesih, D., Muherdiyantiningsih, Rustan, E., Muhilal, Karyadi, D., and Olson, J. A., Refinement of the modified-relative-dose-response test as a method for assessing vitamin A status in a field setting: experience with Indonesia children, *Am. J. Clin. Nutr.*, 64, 966, 1996.

298. Kafwembe, E. M., Sukwa, T. Y., Manyando, C., Mwandu, D., Chipipa, J., and Chipaila, P., The vitamin A status of Zambian children attending an under five clinic as evaluated by the modified dose response (MRDR) test, *Int. J. Vit. Nutr. Res.*, 66, 190, 1996.

299. De Pee, S., Yuniar, Y., West, C. E., and Muhilal, Evaluation of biochemical indicators of vitamin A status in breast-feeding and non-breast-feeding Indonesian women, *Am. J. Clin. Nutr.*, 66, 160, 1997.

300. Olson, J. A., The reproducibility, sensitivity and specificity of the relative dose response (RDR) test for determining vitamin A status, *J. Nutr.*, 121, 917, 1991.

301. Tanumihardjo, S. A., Permaesih, D., Muherdiyantiningsih, Rustan, E., Rusmil, K., Fatah, A., C., Wilbur, S., Muhilal, Karyadi, D., and Olson, J. A., Vitamin A status of Indonesian children infected with *Ascasis lumbricoides* after dosing with vitamin A supplements and albendazole, *J. Nutr.*, 126, 451, 1996.

302. Mobarhan, S., Russell, R. M., Underwood, B. A., Wallingford, J., Mathieson, R. D., and Al-Midani, H., Evaluation of the relative dose response test for vitamin A nutriture in cirrhotics, *Am. J. Clin. Nutr.*, 34, 2264, 1981.

303. Bulux, J., Carranza, E., Castaneda, C., Solomons, N. W., Sokoll, L. T., Morrow, F. D., and Russell, R. M., Studies on the application of the relative-dose-response test for assessing vitamin A status in older adults, *Am. J. Clin. Nutr.*, 56, 543, 1992.

304. Tanumihardjo, S. A., Muherdiyantiningsih, Permaesih, D., Dahro, A. M., Muhilal, Karyadi, D., and Olson, J. A., Assessment of the vitamin A status in lactating and nonlactating, nonpregnant Indonesian women by use of the modified-relative-dose-response (MRDR) test, *Am. J. Clin. Nutr.*, 60, 142, 1994.

305. Tanumihardjo, S. A., Permaesih, D., Dahro, A. M., Rustan, E., Mulilal, Karyadi, D., and Olson, J. A., Comparison of vitamin A status assessment techniques in children from two Indonesian villages, *Am. J. Clin. Nutr.*, 60, 136, 1994.

306. Olson, J. A. and Tanumihardjo, S. A., Evaluation of vitamin A status, *Am. J. Clin. Nutr.*, 67, 148, 1998.

307. Ward, B. J., Humphrey, J. H., Clement, L., and Chaisson, R. E., Vitamin A status in HIV infection, *Nutr. Res.*, 13, 157, 1993.

308. Solomons, N. W., Bulux, J., Russell, R. M., Morrow, F. D., and Dallal, G., Reply to the letter of Dr. Olson, *J. Nutr.*, 121, 919, 1991.

309. Woodruff, C. W., Latham, C. B., Mactier, H., and Hewett, J. E., Vitamin A status of preterm infants: correlation between plasma retinol concentration and retinol dose response, *Am. J. Clin. Nutr.*, 46, 985, 1987.

310. Azais-Braesco, V., Moriniere, C., Guesne, B., Partier, A., Bellenand, P., Baguelin, D., Grolier, P., and Alix, E., Vitamin A status in the institutionalized elderly. Critical analysis of four evaluation criteria: dietary vitamin A intake, serum retinol, relative dose-response test (RDR) and impression cytology with transfer (ICT), *Int. J. Vit. Nutr. Res.*, 65, 151, 1995.

311. Milne, D. B. and Botnen, J., Retinol, α-tocopherol, and α- and β-carotene simultaneously determined in plasma by isocratic liquid chromatography, *Clin. Chem.*, 32, 874, 1986.

312. Zaman, Z., Fielden, P., and Frosst, P. G., Simultaneous determination of vitamin A and E and carotenoids in plasma by reversed-phase HPLC in elderly and younger subjects, *Clin. Chem.*, 39, 2229, 1993.
313. Catignani, G. L. and Bieri, J. G., Simultaneous determination of retinol and α-tocopherol in serum or plasma by liquid chromatography, *Clin. Chem.*, 29, 708, 1983.
314. McCormick, A. M., Napoli, J. L, and DeLuca, H. F., High-pressure liquid chromatography of vitamin A metabolites and analogs, *Meth. Enzymol.*, 67, 220, 1980.
315. MacCrehan, W. A. and Schönerger, E., Determination of retinol, α-tocopherol, and β-carotene in serum by liquid chromatography with absorbance and electrochemical detection, *Clin. Chem.*, 33, 1585, 1987.
316. Katrangi, N., Kaplan, L. A., and Stein, E. A., Separation and quantitation of serum β-carotene and other carotinoids by high performance liquid chromatography, *J. Lipid Res.*, 25, 400, 1984.
317. Nierenberg, D. W. and Nann, S. L., A method for determining concentrations of retinol, tocopherol, and five carotenoids in human plasma and tissue samples, *Am. J. Clin. Nutr.*, 56, 417, 1992.
318. Luo, W., Al-Abdulaly, A. B., Yoon, K., and Simpson, K. L., Rapid determination of blood serum retinol by reverse phase open column chromatography, *Int. J. Vit. Nutr. Res.*, 63, 82, 1993.
319. Kaplan, L. A., Miller, J. A., and Stein, E. A., Simultaneously determined in plasma by isocratic liquid chromatography, *Clin. Chem.*, 32, 874, 1986.
320. Cantilena, L. R. and Nierenberg, D. W., Simultaneous analysis of five carotenoids in human plasma by isocratic high performance liquid chromatography, *J. Micronutr. Anal.*, 6, 127, 1989.
321. Nierenberg, D. W., Serum and plasma beta-carotene levels measured with an improved method of high performance liquid chromatography, *J. Chromatogr. Biomed. Appl.*, 339, 273, 1985.
322. Kaplan, L. A., Stein, E. A., Willett, W. C., Stampfer, M. J., and Stryker, W. S., Reference ranges of retinol, tocopherols, lycopene and alpha- and beta-carotene in plasma by simultaneous high-performance liquid chromatographic analysis, *Clin. Physiol. Biochem.*, 5, 297, 1987.
323. Ito, Y., Ochiai, J., and Saski, R. et al., Serum concentrations of carotenoids, retinol, and alpha-tocopherol in healthy persons determined by high performance liquid chromatography, *Clin. Chim. Acta.*, 194, 131, 1990.
324. Dreyfuss, M. C., Craft, N. E., Yamini, S., Humphrey, J. H., and West, K. P. Jr., Vitamin A analysis in dried blood spots by HPLC, *FASEB J.*, 12 A840, (Abstract No. 4868), 1998.
325. Oshima, S., Sakamoto, H., Ishiguro, Y., and Terao, J., Accumulation and clearance of capsanthin in blood plasma after the ingestion of paprika juice in men, *J. Nutr.*, 127, 1475, 1997.
326. Omenn, G. S., Goodman, G. E., Thomquist, M. D., Barnes, J., Allen, M. R., Glass, A., Keogh, J. P., Meyskens, F. L., Valanis, B., Williams, J. H., Barnhart, S., and Hammar, S., Effects of a combine of beta-carotene and vitamin A on lung cancer and cardiovascular disease, *N. Engl. J. Med.*, 334, 1150, 1996.
327. O'Neal, R. M., Johnson, O. C., and Schaefer, A. E., Guidelines for classification and interpretation of group blood and urine data collected as part of the National Nutrition Survey, *Pediatr. Res.*, 4, 103, 1970.
328. *Nutrition Canada: National Survey*, Information Canada, Ottawa, Canada, 1973.
329. Vahlquist, A., Sjahund, K., Norden, A., Peterson, P. A., Stigmar, G., and Johansson, B., Plasma vitamin A transport and visual dark adaptation in diseases of the intestine and liver, *Scand. J. Clin. Lab. Invest.*, 38, 301, 1978.
330. Maiani, G., Raguzzini, A., Mobarhan, S., and Ferro-Luzzi, A., Vitamin A, *Int. J. Vit. Nutr. Res.*, 63, 252, 1993.
331. Lewis, C. J., McDowell, M. A., Sempos, C. T., Lewis, K. C., and Yetley, E. A., Relationship between age and serum vitamin A in children aged 4–11 yr, *Am. J. Clin. Nutr.*, 52, 353, 1990.
332. Third Report on the World Nutrition Situaton, Chapter 2, ACC/SCN Secretariat, c/o World Health Organization, Geneva, Switzerland, December, 1997, 19.
333. Castenmiller, J. J. M. and West, C. E., Bioavailability and bioconversion of carotenoids, *Annu. Rev. Nutr.*, 18, 19, 1998.
334. Blaner, W. S., Recent advances in understanding the molecular basis of vitamin A action, *Sight and Life Newsletter*, 2, 3, 1998.

335. Winklhoffer-Roob, B. M., van't Hof, M. A., and Shmerling, D. H., Reference values for plasma concentrations of vitamin E and A and carotenoids in a Swiss population from infancy to adulthood, adjusted for seasonal influences, *Clin. Chem.*, 43, 146, 1997.

336. Mitra, A. K., Alvarez, J. O., Guay-Woodford, L., Fuchs, G. J., Wahed, M. A., and Stephensen, C. B., Urinary retinol excretion and kidney function in children with shigellosis, *Am. J. Clin. Nutr.*, 68, 1095,1998.

337. Ribaya-Mercado, J. D., Mazariegos, M., Tang, G., Romero-Abad, M. E., Mena, I., Solomons, N. W., and Russell, R. M., Assessment of total body stores of vitamin A in Guatamalan elderly by the deuterated-retinol-dilation method, *Am. J. Clin. Nutr.*, 69, 278, 1999.

338. Olson, J. A., Vitamin A assessment by the isotope-dilution technique: good news from Guatemala, *Am. J. Clin. Nutr.*, 69, 117, 1999.

Vitamin D

Vitamin D Terminology

Vitamin D: general term used for vitamin D

Ergocalciferol: vitamin D_2

Cholecalciferol: vitamin D_3

Vitamin D: represents vitamin D_2

Vitamin D_2: ergocalciferol molecular weight: 396.63

Vitamin D_3: cholecalciferol molecular weight: 384.62

1,25-dihydroxyvitamin D_3 (calcitriol) represents: 1,25-dihydroxycholecalciferol; 1,25-dihydroxyvitamin D; 1α,25-dihydroxyvitamin D_3; 1α,25-dihydroxycholecalciferol

25-hydroxycholecalciferol represents: 25-hydroxyvitamin D_3 (calcidiol)

Calcitriol: 1,25-dihydroxyvitamin D_3: molecular weight: 416.65

Calcidiol: 25-hydroxyvitamin D_3: molecular weight: 400.65

Converting metric units to International System (SI) units:

Serum 25-hydroxyvitamin D_3: nmol/L × 0.4006 = ng/mL

Serum 1,25-dihydroxyvitamin D_3: pmol/L × 0.4167 = pg/mL

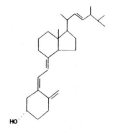

VITAMIN D_2
(ERGOCALCIFEROL)

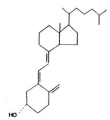

VITAMIN D_3
(CHOLECALCIFEROL)

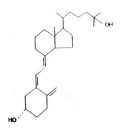

25-HYDROXYVITAMIN D_3
(CALCIDIOL)

1,25-DIHYDROXYVITAMIN D_3
(CALCITRIOL)

FIGURE 45
Structures of several vitamin D active compounds.

Introduction

Vitamin D is required by humans of all ages for maintenance of skeletal integrity and proper utilization of calcium. Since the requirement can be met by the ingestion of vitamin D_2 or vitamin D_3 or in part or entirely by skin exposure to sunlight, biochemical procedures used to evaluate vitamin D status cannot be correlated with dietary intake of the nutrient. As a result of fortification of milk with vitamin D, vitamin D deficiency rickets in children is now rare in the United States, but has been reported in some isolated areas.[98] However, vitamin D deficiency or insufficiency is a problem in the elderly with the occurrence of osteomalacia and osteoporosis.[26,42,43,45-48,69,110,130] The problem is exacerbated in the elderly by their often low consumption of milk and/or by inadequate exposure to sunlight.[130,131] However, the role of vitamin D in the treatment of osteoporosis has been controversial.[26,43,45,67,73,83,110,125,135]

The essentiality of vitamin D throughout life and not just during the growth phase of children is being appreciated. Moreover, in addition to the role of vitamin D in calcium absorption and bone metabolism, other roles for the vitamin appear to be evolving, such as in regulating cell proliferation and differentiation, immune system, and in the treatment of psoriasis.[12,22,27,28,30,39,52,108]

Early studies demonstrated that the consumption of 400 IU (10 µg) of vitamin D daily would prevent rickets and osteomalacia.[113] This level of intake was established as safe. As a result, fortification of foods with vitamin D was adopted and the use of cod-liver oil disappeared. Approximately 14,000 pounds of synthetic vitamin D_2 and vitamin D_3 are produced annually in the United States.[112]

Vitamin D Metabolism

Without vitamin D fortification of foods, such as milk, the dietary intake of vitamin D is small.[38] But even fortified foods may not be a dependable source of vitamin D.[22] The primary source of vitamin D is from the photochemical action of ultraviolet sunlight on the 7-dehydrocholesterol produced in the skin.[12,13,22,23,28,44,108] The vitamin D formed is circulated to the liver where it is converted to 25-hydroxyvitamin D. This metabolite of vitamin D is then converted by the kidney to 1,25-dihydroxyvitamin D, the metabolic active form of vitmain D.[12,22,133] Intestinal absorption of calcium is regulated by the direct action of 1,25-dihydroxyvitamin D on the intestinal mucosal cells.[8,11,12,70] Production of 1,25-dihydroxyvitamin D is increased when the dietary intake of calcium is low or when an increased requirement for calcium exists, such as during lactation or periods of rapid growth. The parathyroid hormone mediates the increased production of 1,25-dihydroxyvitamin D by stimulating the activity of 25-hydroxyvitamin D-1-hydroxylase in the kidney. The serum 1,25-dihydroxyvitamin D level is closely controlled by the serum concentration of calcium and phosphorus. A rise in serum calcium results in a shut down of the parathyroid hormone which in turn shuts down the synthesis of 1,25-dihydroxyvitamin D.[12,70]

Extensive reviews are available that provide details concerning the interactions of calcium, phosphorus, parathyroid hormone and vitamin D and its metabolites.[12,22,26,28,39,45,46,49,52,70,75,93,106,108,109,134]

Vitamin D Deficiency

The kidney produces 1,25-dihydroxyvitamin D_3 (calcitriol). This vitamin D metabolite is associated with the intestinal absorption of calcium.[127] A deficiency of 1,25-dihydroxyvitamin D impairs the absorption of calcium.[3,50] Reduced calcium absorption occurs in the elderly.[14] Hypovitaminosis D as reflected in low serum 25-(OH)-vitamin D levels (<25 nmol/L) occurs frequently in the elderly particularly during the winter period.[6,7,17,28,61,62,63,65,79,126,135]

For example, a sudy was conducted on 3,276 adult Swiss men and women.[65] The study found 6% of the subjects were considered vitamin D deficient with a serum concentration of 25-hydroxyvitamin D of 20 nmol/L or lower. Relatively low concentrations of 25-hydroxyvitamin D (<38 nmol/L) were found in 34% of the population. In a large study conducted among elderly people of Europe (n = 824), 36% of the men and 47% of the women had serum 25-hydroxyvitamin D concentrations below 30 nmol/L.[72]

To prevent vitamin D deficiency and rickets during infancy, daily vitamin D supplementation is commonly used.[59,128] Early studies reported a lack of adequate exposure to sunshine as an important cause of rickets.[10,22] In vitamin D deficiency rickets, elevated levels of 1,25-dihydroxyvitamin D may be observed.[33,34,52]

Vitamin D deficiency in infants should not occur in the United States where dairy products are routinely fortified with vitamin D, and prenatal supplements are prescribed that generally contain vitamin D. However, when milk is not consumed and supplements are not used, cases of vitamin D deficiency may be observed. Vegetarian mothers often have lower concentrations of serum 25-hydroxyvitamin D than nonvegetarian mothers.[35] Breast-fed Black infants are at an increased risk of vitamin D deficiency rickets.[36,37]

Serum concentrations of 25-hydroxyvitamin D (25-hydroxycholecalciferol) remain relatively constant during pregnancy. Infants born of mothers with low serum concentrations of 25-hydroxyvitamin D are likely to have low serum concentrations of this vitamin D metabolite.[14] Infants with iron deficiency anemia have been reported to have low serum 25-hydroxyvitamin D concentrations, although adequate vitamin D was provided. Iron supplementation corrected the condition.[64]

The activity of serum alkaline phosphatase is increased in vitamin D deficiency.[14,63,96] The enzyme also increases during pregnancy, particularly during the third trimester. For example, serum alkaline phosphate activity increased from a level of 3.71 ± 0.58 King-Armstrong units to 8.18 ± 3.25 units during the third trimester.[14]

Blacks living in northern latitudes often have lower serum concentrations of 25-hydroxyvitamin D and thus may be more prone to vitamin D deficiency.[23,24,77,131,132] In another study, no differences were noted between healthy young black and white women with respect to their serum levels of 25-hydroxyvitamin D, 1,25-dihydroxyvitamin D, and parathyroid hormone. However, the black women had a higher bone density than whites.[76]

Pregnancy and lactation may impose an increased requirement for vitamin D, particularly in women with low intakes of milk and live in northern latitudes. Lactating women with a poor vitamin D status have breast milk with low vitamin D levels.[31] Maternal vitamin D deficiency may have adverse effects on the fetus resulting in possible delayed growth and delayed bone ossification.[31,32]

Asian immigrants to Europe have been at risk of developing a vitamin D deficiency, particularly the children and women. An annual oral dosing of these immigrants with 2.5 mg of vitamin D_2 has been effective in maintaining a satisfactory serum concentration of 25-hydroxyvitamin D.[56,57]

The current Recommended Dietary Allowance (RDA) for vitamin D for children and adults is 10 μg per day (400 IU).[58] Excessive intakes of vitamin D may result in hypercalcemia and hypercalciuria that may lead to calcium deposition in soft tissues and to renal and cardiovascular damage. For young children daily intakes as low as 45 μg of vitamin D_3 (cholecalciferol) have resulted in signs of hypervitaminosis D.[59]

Vitamin D and the Elderly

The elderly are often at an increased risk of vitamin D deficiency because of several reasons:[15,22,44,45,47,63,66,74,116,121,130,131,135] (1) elderly absorb vitamin D less efficiently then younger people, (2) elderly produce less vitamin D in the skin because of an age-related decline the contents of the vitamin D procursor, 7-dehydrocholesterol, (3) older people often have less exposure to sunlight and, (4) drug interference in vitamin D utilization. Studies have shown that vitamin D synthesis in the skin is absent or markedly reduced during the winter months in people living above latitude 42°N. This was demonstrated with the marked lowering of 25-hydroxyvitamin D levels in the plasma during the wintertime compared to the summer months (60.6 nmol/L vs. 81.3 nmol/L).[22,25,31,44,130-132] Dietary intakes of vitamin D prevented the fall in plasma 25-hydroxyvitamin D levels. Levels of 25-hydroxyvitamin D serve as an indicator of overall vitamin D status.[17]

McKenna reviewed reports during the period of 1971 on the vitamin D status of 27 regions in the world.[96] Vitamin D status in young adults and the elderly varied widely with the country of residence. Nevertheless, hypovitaminosis D and related abnormalities in bone chemistry were most common in the elderly residents in Europe.[96,116] The vitamin D status of the populations was assessed on the basis of serum 25-hydroxyvitamin D concentrations. A vitamin D deficiency was defined as a serum 25-hydroxyvitamin D level below 25 nmol/L.[97]

Plasma levels of 25 (OH) vitamin D have been reported to fall in elderly males, while 1,25(OH)$_2$ vitamin D levels remained the same when compared with younger subjects.[46] Similar observations have been reported in studies with rats fed low vitamin D diets where their 25 (OH)$_3$ vitamin D levels decreased more rapidly than the 1,25-(OH)$_2$ vitamin D_3 levels.[49] This indicates that low levels of 1,25(OH)$_2$ vitamin D_3 may not alone provide an adequate assessment of a functional vitamin D deficiency.[49]

Assessment of Vitamin D Status

The assessment of vitamin D status may include the following:

1. Serum total calcium and ionized calcium
2. Serum inorganic phosphate
3. Serum alkaline phosphatase[18,29]
4. Serum 25-(OH)-vitamin D[19]
5. Serum 1,25-(OH)$_2$-vitamin D[20,21]
6. Serum parathyroid hormone[52]

Subjects with a vitamin D deficiency commonly have low serum levels of phosphate, 25-hydroxyvitamin D, and 1,25-dihydroxyvitamin D, while serum levels of alkaline phosphatase and parathyroid hormone are elevated. Serum calcium levels may be low to normal.[52]

However, vitamin D status is most commonly assessed by measuring serum concentrations of 25-hydroxyvitamin D, which represents the major circulating vitamin D metabolite.[11-13,72,130-132] Levels of 1,25-dihydroxyvitamin D can be determined but the analysis is somewhat more tedious and expensive to perform.[117] The concentrations of 1,25-dihydroxyvitamin D are considerably lower than those of 25-hydroxyvitamin D (e.g., 69 pmol/L vs. 43 nmol/L),[17] but since it is the biologically active form of vitamin D, its measurement can be informative about vitamin D nutritional status.[117]

Physiological levels of 1,25-dihydroxyvitamin D can exist in the presence of extremely low serum levels of vitamin D or 25-hydroxyvitamin D. The production of 1,25-dihydroxyvitamin D is closely regulated by the serum levels of parathyroid hormone and serum levels of calcium and phosphate.[106] Commonly, vitamin D deficiency has been reflected in rickets and/or substantial reductions in serum 25-hydroxyvitamin D or calcium levels. Hypovitaminosis D has been defined by some investigators as a serum 25-hydroxyvitamin D level below 25 nmol/L (Table 55).[96,97]

Measurement of 25-Hydroxyvitamin D and 1,25-Dihydroxyvitamin D

During the past years numerous procedures have been developed for the measurement of 25-hydroxyvitamin D and for 1,25-dehydroxyvitamin D.[14,50,70,90,100-102] The methods have been based on direct ultraviolet detection following HPLC treatment,[80-82] competitive protein-binding assay,[83-88,90] and radioimmunoassay requiring either tritium or 125 Iodine labeling.[50,89,123]

The concentration of 1,25-dihydroxyvitamin D in serum is normally very low and hence its measurement requires a very sensitive analytical procedure. Many of the earlier procedures required large sample volumes, were tedious to perform, and were subject to technical difficulties.[91,92] Consequently the methods did not permit their general use for vitamin D status assessments.

High performance liquid chromatography procedures have been developed that may in a single serum sample measure the levels of vitamin D_3, 25-hydroxyvitamin D_2, and 25-hydroxyvitamin D_3.[101] Another HPLC procedure permits the measurement of 25-hydroxyvitamin D_2, 25-hydroxyvitamin D_3, 1,25-dihydroxyvitamin D, and 24,25-dihydroxyvitamin D in a single serum sample.[102]

The subsequent development of radioimmunoassays for 25-hydroxyvitamin D and 1,25-dihydroxyvitamin D has provided sensitive, efficient, and practical means for evaluating vitamin D status.[14,39-41,49,50,51,70,123] This has been furthered by the convenience of commercial assay kits available for measurements of 25-hydroxyvitamin D and 1,25-dihydroxyvitamin D. The kits use either a tritiated or a radioiodine tracer, which requires the need for either a scintillation or gamma counter depending upon the tracer employed. Vitamin D_2 and vitamin D_3 forms of 25-hydroxyvitamin D and 1,25-dihydroxyvitamin D are equally measured in their respective assay.

Assay kits for both 25-hydroxyvitamin D and 1,25-dihydroxyvitamin D are available from DiaSorin, Stillwater, MN. Both tritiated and [125]-I tracers were available. An assay kit for measuring 25-hydroxyvitamin D that used a tritium tracer has been available from

Nichols Institute Diagnostics, San Juan Capistrano, CA. Radioimmunoassays kits for 25-hydroxyvitamin D and 1,25-dihydroxyvitamin D measurements using a tritium tracer are available from Amersham Life Sciences, Inc., Arlington, IL.

Total 25-hydroxyvitamin D may be measured in plasma with an ultraviolet detection procedure.[70] The procedure can measure separately 25-hydroxyvitamin D_2 and 25-hydroxyvitamin D_3. However, the method is less sensitive than the competitive protein-binding assay. 25-Hydroxyvitamin D is transported in the blood as a complex with vitamin D binding protein and thus an extraction is performed prior to assay. Serum or plasma (EDTA, heparin) samples may be used and held frozen. Repeated freezing and thawing should be avoided. Determination of 25-hydroxyvitamin D can be useful in evaluating hypocalcemia, hypophosphatemia, and osteopenia.[93]

Serum assays for vitamin D itself are complex and difficult to perform and are seldom considered. Moreover, the vitamin D levels in serum are considerably lower than those of 25-hydroxyvitamin D.

Alkaline Phosphatase

Measurements of serum alkaline phosphatase (actually a group of alkaline phosphatase isoenzymes) have been useful in the investigation of certain bone diseases and as an indirect measure of vitamin D status. The measurement can confirm a clinical diagnosis or as a screening device but will not detect subclinical cases of vitamin D deficiency. Serum alkaline phosphatase activity in osteomalacia is increased but generally is normal in osteoporosis. In rickets, the activity may be two to four times higher than normal levels of adults but return to normal values with vitamin D treatment. Serum alkaline phosphatase activity may be elevated in elderly and in growing children as well as in pregnancy, particularly during the third trimester.[14,63,96]

Previously, measurements of serum alkaline phosphatase activity have been the most reliable and useful biochemical determination for the confirmation of clinically diagnosed rickets. Alkaline phosphatase activity generally rises early with the onset of rickets, even before clinical manifestations. Serum alkaline phosphatase findings must be interpreted with caution since the enzyme is suceptible to alteration by a variety of other disease processes. Increased alkaline phosphatase activity may occur in Paget's disease, hyperparathyroidism, and osteogenic sarcoma. In kwashiorkor or protein-energy malnutrition, serum alkaline phosphatase activity may be depressed and mask a vitamin D deficiency. Although the measurement of this enzyme should not in itself be a sole index for diagnosing vitamin D deficiency, it may be useful as a screening procedure.

Numerous methods are available for the determination of serum alkaline phosphatase activity.[18,29,68,107,118] The manual or automated procedures can be easily performed and require only a small quantity of serum (e.g., Technion Autoanalyzer, Tarrytown, NY). Plasma from heparinized samples may also be used. Several commercial kits are available that are convenient for serum alkaline phosphatase activity measurements. Reference ranges for serum alkaline phosphatase activity are dependent upon the specific analytical procedure used.[29] In the past, serum alkaline phosphatase activities have been expressed in Bodansky, King-Armstrong units, Kind-King units, or International units.[118] Activities are now expressed as U/L.[29] Reference range of 30 to 90 U/L has been established for adults.[17,29,63]

Osteocalcin and Vitamin D

Serum osteocalcin (bone GLA protein) levels are an indicator of bone formation. In a study with elderly women, serum levels of osteocalcin were higher than controls (6 ng/ml vs. 8 ng/ml serum).[78] Osteocalcin levels correlated with lower serum levels of 25-hydroxyvitamin D and the higher parathyroid homone levels. Osteocalcin may be measured by radioimmunoassay for which convenient commercial assay kits are available.[78]

Because other factors and forms of bone disease may influence serum levels of osteocalcin, the use of osteocalcin measurements as a primary method of assessment of vitamin D status may be limited. More likely, osteocalcin measurements may serve as a parameter for monitoring the effects of vitamin D supplementation in bone metabolism, including osteoporosis in the elderly. Kits for the measurement of bone markers such as osteocalcin and forms of procollogen are available from DiaSorin, Inc., Stillwater, MN.

Vitamin D Absorption Test

An intestinal absorption test has been used to evaluate vitamin D status. Subjects are adminstered a standard dose of 25-hydroxyvitamin D_3 (e.g., 10 µg/kg body weight). Serum levels of 25-hydroxyvitamin D_3 are measured 4 and 6 hours later. Levels were depressed in vitamin D deficient elderly subjects.[71]

Vitamin D in Saliva

Levels of 25-hydroxyvitamin D have been measured in saliva, but the diurnal changes observed would preclude its use to assess vitamin D status.[115] Moreover, saliva concentrations of 25-hydroxyvitamin D had no relationship to serum concentrations of 25-hydroxyvitamin D in paired subjects.

Vitamin D Drug Interaction and Toxicity

Elderly often consume a number of medications, some of which may interfere in the absorption and metabolism of vitamin D.[69,95] Impaired absorption of vitamin D may occur with the use cholestyramine or excessive laxatives. Vitamin D metabolism may be interfered with by a number of anticonvulsive drugs, such as phenobarbital, phenytoin, and carbamazepine.[47,69]

Vitamin D and its metabolites are potentially toxic.[53,59,60] 1,25-Dihydroxyvitamin D is a very potent compound and must be used with extreme caution in the treatment of patients with vitamin D deficiency disorders. The activity of 1,25-dihydroxyvitamin D is approximately twelve times more active than 25-hydroxyvitamin D.[52,53] Patients receiving vitamin D treatment should have regular biochemical monitoring of their treatment.[53-56]

Prolonged exposure to sunlight may increase the serum levels of 25-hydroxyvitamin D to about 200 nmol/L. However, regular daily dosing with 0.25 mg of vitamin D (10,000 IU) may result in serum levels of 25-hydroxyvitamin D in excess of 1,000 nmol/L.[53] Hypercalcemic vitamin D toxicity may result from such levels of intake. Whenever serum levels of 25-hydroxyvitamin D above 200 nmol/L are encountered, excessive usage of vitamin D may be suspected.[95] Drinking excessive quantities of fortified milk has resulted in hypervitaminosis D, with elevated serum concentrations of 25-hydroxyvitamin D (731 nmol/L).[114]

Assay Guidelines

Various cut-off values have been applied for evaluating serum 25-hydroxyvitamin D data.[128,129] In a large study conducted during the period of January to March with 823 elderly Europeans, a serum 25-hydroxyvitamin D concentration below 30 nmol/L was considered vitamin D deficient.[72] Vitamin D deficiency in neonates has been defined by Zeghound et al.[128] as a low serum 25-hydroxyvitamin D (calcidiol) concentration of ≤ 30 nmol/L and a high parathyroid hormone concentration of > 60 ng/L (Table 55).

This level appears to have functional significance for vitamin D. Subjects with serum 25-hydroxyvitamin D concentrations below 30 nmol/L were associated with increased bone turnover, secondary hyperparathyroidism, and decreased bone-mass density.[72,103,104] No such associations were seen when the serum concentrations of 25-hydroxyvitamin D were above 30 nmol/L.[72] Bone density can be measured by dual energy X-ray densitometry with instruments such as the Norland X R20 X-ray bone densitometer available from Norland, Fort Atkinson, WI;[103-105,124] also Lunar bone mineral analyzer, Lunar Corp., Madison, WI.

Summary

Serum levels of calcium, phosphate, and alkaline phosphatase are not reliable indicators of vitamin D deficiency. Useful indicators of vitamin D deficiency are the measurement of serum concentrations of 25-hydroxyvitamin D and 1,25-dihydroxyvitamin D. Hypovitaminosis D has been considered to exist when the serum 25-hydroxyvitamin D concentrations is below 30 nmol/L.[72] Serum 25-hydroxyvitamin D concentrations below 12 nmol/L are associated with decreases in serum calcium and phosphate levels and in the calcium-phosphate product.[96] The normal range may vary considerably with season, race, geographic location, and diet.[93,130-132] Serum concentrations of 1,25-dihydroxyvitamin D of 48–100 pmol/L (20 to 40 pg/mL) have been considered normal.

Vitamin D assays permit the monitoring for vitamin D toxicosis in patients receiving vitamin D treatment.[95] The assays can help determine in a patient with impaired calcium metabolism whether it is due to a vitamin D nutritional deficiency, to malabsorption, or to a defective conversion of 25-hydroxyvitamin D to 1,25-dihydroxyvitamin D, or to parathyroid disfunction.

TABLE 55

Literature Values For Serum Vitamin D Parameters

Subjects	25-hydroxy vitamin D (calcidiol) nmol/L	1,25-dihydroxy vitamin D (calcitriol) pmol/L	Reference (Year)
1. Children and Adolescents			
88 boys/76 girls **(Utah)**			124 (1991)
2–5 yr	82 (55–110)	136 (61–238)	
6–8 yr	65 (40–102)	117 (34–243)	
15–16 yr	72 (35–138)	122 (68–275)	
(No differences between sexes)			
2. Children and Young Adults			
Saudi Arabia			120 (1993)
5–10 yr (n = 29)	44.4 ± 14.5	74.9 ± 14.6	
11–15 yr (n = 34)	45.4 ± 7.0	68.6 ± 16.1	
16–25 yr (n = 41)	47.9 ± 10.9	74.4 ± 20.9	
3. Country Reports			
Australia (Postmenopausal women)			126 (1993)
> 70 yr (n = 68)	56.1 ± 3.2		
< 70 yr (n = 365)	64.8 ± 1.3		
Canada (> 65 yr; winter period)			17 (1988)
Men (n = 24)	36.0 ± 2.4	74.1 ± 6.8	
Women (n = 54)	36.1 ± 2.4	108.8 ± 4.6	
Denmark (Normal men and women)			4 (1993)
35 yr (n = 20)	55.2	113.0	
45 yr (n = 38)	63.2	89.8	
55 yr (n = 31)	66.2	94.6	
65 yr (n = 36)	63.2	94.6	
Europe (winter period)			72 (1995)
Elderly men and women			
Vitamin D supplements (n = 29)	54 (median)		
No vitamin D supplement (n = 731)	31 (median)		
France			
Normal adults (40–60 yr; n = 30)	63.6 ± 32.7	79.2 ± 24.3	3 (1987)
Elderly outpatients (74 ± 5 yr; n = 89)	42.9 ± 18.5	56.9 ± 23.0	
Young adults (n = 20)	41.9 ± 15	87.8 ± 20.9	62 (1989)
Institutionalized elderly (80.5 ± 7.2; n = 40)	10.5 ± 4.4	59.8 ± 21.2	
Hong Kong (all Chinese)			
Females (17–40 yr; n = 296)	58 ± 15.5	109 ± 30.7	106 (1994)
Ireland (Winter period)			63 (1985)
Elderly (*n* = 18)	10.0 (< 5.0–58)		
Young adults (n = 28)	33.5 (11.5–98)		
Israel			29 (1989)
Men and women (21–42 yr; n = 97)	61.7 ± 15.2		
Elderly (78 ± 8 yr; n = 338)	33.7 ± 22.2		
The Netherlands			17 (1988)
Nursing home elderly (n = 51)	28 ± 16		
Free-living elderly (n = 52)	38 ± 15		
Switzerland			
Men and women (n = 3,276)	46 (median)		65 (1992)

(continues)

TABLE 55   **(continued)**

Literature Values For Serum Vitamin D Parameters

Subjects	25-hydroxy vitamin D (calcidiol) nmol/L	1,25-dihydroxy vitamin D (calcitriol) pmol/L	Reference (Year)
United Kingdom			
Women (45–65 yr; *n* = 138)	28.8 ± 11.56		67 (1992)
United States			
Normal adults (*n* = 14)		87.8 ± 25.2	117 (1992)
Men (20–94 yr; *n* = 166)	88.5 ± 2.2	64.6 ± 1.6	74 (1990)
Women (20–94 yr; *n* = 114)	82.1 ± 2.3	64.6 ± 1.6	74 (1990)
Men and women (20–40 yr; *n* = 36)	64.2 (24.7–103.6)		89 (1993)
Women (20–80 yr; *n* = 373)	60.2 ± 21.2		119 (1986)
Adult women (*n* = 11)	82.4 ± 19.9	86.6 ± 16.3	122 (1995)
Adolescent women (*n* = 14)	68.9 ± 2.12	90.0 ± 17.8	122 (1995)
Elderly (> 65 yr; *n* = 22) (sunlight deprived)	40.0 ± 4.2	46 ± 5.0	25 (1991)

Suggested Guidelines for Evaluating Vitamin D Status

1. Serum 25-hydroxyvitamin D concentrations (nmol/L)

   acceptable/desired: ≥ 30

   low: < 25

   deficient: ≤ 12

2. Serum 1,25-dihydroxyvitamin D concentration (pmol/L)

   acceptable/desired: 48 to 100

3. Potential vitamin D toxicity

   Serum concentrations of 25-hydroxyvitamin D above 200 nmol/L

References

1. Bullamore, J. R., Wilkinson, R., Gallagher, J. C., Nordin, B. E. C., and Marshall, D. H., Effects of age on calcium absorption, *Lancet*, 2, 535, 1970.
2. Ireland, P. and Fordtran, I. S., Effects on dietary calcium and age on jejunal calcium absorption in humans studied by intestinal perfusion, *J. Clin. Invest.*, 52, 2672, 1973.
3. Chapuy, M.-C. and Meunier, P. J., Calcium and vitamin D supplements: effects on calcium metabolism in elderly people, *Am. J. Clin. Nutr.*, 46, 324, 1987.
4. Rudnicki, M., Thode, J., Jorgensen, T., Heitmann, B. L., and Sorensen, O. H., Effects of age, sex, season and diet on serum ionized calcium, parathyroid hormone and vitamin D in a random population, *J. Int. Med.*, 234, 195, 1993.
5. Zeghoud, F., Ben-Mekhbi, H., Djeghri, N., and Garabedian, M., Vitamin D prophylaxis during infancy: comparison of the long-term effects of three intermittent doses (15, 5, or 2.5 mg) on 25-hydroxyvitamin D concentrations, *Am. J. Clin. Nutr.*, 60, 393, 1994.

6. Freaney, R., McBrinn, Y., and McKenna, M. J., Secondary hyperparathyroidism in elderly people: combined effect of renal insufficiency and vitamin D deficiency, *Am. J. Clin. Nutr.*, 58, 187, 1993.

7. Dubbelman, R., Jonxis, J. H. P., Muskiet, F. A. J., and Saleh, A. E. C., Age-dependent vitamin D status and vertebral condition of white women living in Curacao (The Netherlands Antilles) as compared with their counterparts in The Netherlands, *Am. J. Clin. Nutr.*, 58, 106, 1993.

8. Fraser, D. R., Effects of calcium deficiency on vitamin D metabolism, in *Nutrient Regulation During Pregnancy, Lactation, and Infant Growth*, Allen, L., King, J., and Lonnerdal, B., Eds., Plenum Press, New York, 1994, 237.

9. Klein, G. L. and Simmons, D. J., Nutritional rickets: Thoughts about pathogenesis, *Annu. Med.*, 25, 379, 1993.

10. World Health Organization, Medical assessment of nutritional status: report of an Expert Committee, *WHO*, Technical Report Series No. 377, Geneva, Switzerland, 1966, 31.

11. DeLuca, H. F., The vitamin D story: a collaborative effort of basic science and clinical medicine, *FASEB J.*, 2, 224, 1988.

12. DeLuca, H. F., New concepts of vitamin D functions, *Ann. NY Acad. Sci.*, 669, 57, 1992.

13. Webb, A. R., Pilbeam, C., Hanafin, N., and Holick, M. F., An evaluation of the relative contributions of exposure to sunlight and of diet to the circulating concentrations of 25-hydroxy-vitamin D in an elderly nursing home in Boston, *Am. J. Clin. Nutr.*, 51, 1075, 1990.

14. Sauberlich, H. E., Vitamin indices, in *Laboratory Indices of Nutritional Statues in Pregnancy*, Food and Nutrition Board, National Research Council, National Academy of Sciences, Washington D.C., 1978, 109.

15. Tanka, Y. and DeLuca, H. F., Rat renal 25-hydroxyvitamin D_3 1- and 24-hydroxylases: their *in vivo* regulation, *Am. J. Physiol.*, 246, E168, 1984.

16. Dawson-Hughes, B., USDA Research Center on Aging, Tufts University, personal communication, 1995.

17. Delvin, E. E., Imbach, A., and Copti, M., Vitamin D nutritional status and related biochemical indices in an autonomous elderly population, *Am. J. Clin. Nutr.*, 48, 373, 1988.

18. Bowers, G. N. Jr. and McComb, R. B., A continuous spectrophotometric method for measuring the activity of serum alkaline phosphatase, *Clin. Chem.*, 12, 70, 1966.

19. Delvin, E. E., Dussault, M., and Glorieux, F. H., A simplified assay for serum 25-hydroxy-calciferol, *Clin. Biochem.*, 13, 106, 1980.

20. Eisman, J. A., Hamstra, A. J., Kream, B. E., and DeLuca, H. F., A sensitive, precise and convenient method of determination of 1,25-dihydroxyvitamin D in human plasma, *Arch. Biochem. Biophys.*, 176, 235, 1976.

21. Delvin, E. E. and Glorieux, F. H., Serum 1,25-dihydroxyvitamin D concentrations in hypo-phosphatemic vitamin D resistant rickets, *Calcif. Tissue Int.*, 33, 173, 1981.

22. Holick, M. F., McCallum Award Lecture, 1994, Vitamins - new horizons for the 21st century, *Am. J. Clin. Nutr.*, 60, 619, 1994.

23. Clemens, T. L., Adams, J. S., Henderson, S. L., and Holick, M. F., Increased skin pigment reduces the capacity of the skin to synthesize vitamin D, *Lancet*, 1, 74, 1982.

24. Bell, N. H., Greene, A., Epstein, S., Oexmann, M. J., Shaw, W., and Shary, J., Evidence for alteration of the vitamin D endocrine system in Blacks, *J. Ped.*, 76, 470, 1985.

25. Gloth, F. M. III, Tobin, J. D., Sherman, S. S., and Hollis, B. W., Is the recommended daily allowance for vitamin D too low for the homebound elderly? *J. Am. Geriatr. Soc.*, 39, 137, 1991.

26. Fujita, T., Vitamin D in the treatment of osteoporosis, *Proc. Soc. Expt. Biol. Med.*, 199, 394, 1992.

27. Studzinski, G. P., and Moore, D. C., Sunlight: can it prevent as well as cause cancer? *Cancer Res.*, 55, 4014, 1995.

28. Webb, A. R., and Holick, M. F., The role of sunlight in cutaneous production of vitamin D_3, *Annu. Rev. Nutr.*, 8, 375, 1988.

29. Moss, D. W., Henderson, A. R., and Kachmar, J. F., Enzymes, in *Textbook of Clinical Chemistry*, Teitz, N. W., Ed., W. B. Saunders Company, Philadelphia, 1986, 619, Chapter 5.

30. Baran, D. T., and Sorensen, A. M., Rapid actions of 1α-25-dihydroxyvitamin D_3 physiologic role, *Proc. Soc. Expt. Biol. Med.*, 207, 175, 1994.

31. Specker, B. B., Do North American women need supplemental vitamin D during pregnancy or lactation, *Am. J. Clin. Nutr.*, 59, 484S, 1994.
32. Cockburn, F., Belton, N. R., Purvis, R. J., Gilles, M. M., Brown, J. K., Turner, T. L., Wilkinson, E. M., Forfar, J. O., Barrie, W. J., McKay, G. S., and Pocock, S. J., Maternal vitamin D intake and mineral metabolism in mothers and their newborn infants, *Br. Med. J.*, 231, 1, 1980.
33. Steichen, J. J., Tsang, R. C., Greer, F. R., Ho, M., and Hug, G., Elevated serum 1,25-dihydroxy-vitamin D concentrations in rickets of very low-birth weight infants, *J. Pediatr.*, 99, 293, 1981.
34. Venkataraman, P. S., Tsang, R. J., Buckley, D. D., Ho., M., and Steichen, J. J., Elevation of serum 1,25-dihydroxyvitamin D in response to physiologic doses of vitamin D in vitamin D-deficient infants, *J. Pediatr.*, 103, 416, 1983.
35. Specker, B. L., Tsang, R. C., Ho, M. L., and Miller, D., Effect of vegetarian diet on serum 1,25-dihydroxyvitamin D concentrations during lactation, *Obstet. Gynecol.*, 70, 870, 1987.
36. Bachrach, S., Fisher, J., and Parks, J. S., An outbreak of vitamin D deficiency rickets in a susceptible population, *Pediatrics*, 64, 871, 1979.
37. Edidin, D. V., Levistsky, L. L., Schey, W., Dumbovic, N., and Campos, A., Resurgence of nutritional rickets associated with breast-feeding and special dietary practices, *Pediatrics*, 65, 232, 1980.
38. Provisional table on the vitamin D content of foods, United States Department of Agriculture, Human Nutrition Information Service, HNIS/PT-108, Washington D.C., 1991.
39. Hausaler, M. R., Vitamin D receptors: nature and function, *Annu. Rev. Nutr.*, 6, 527, 1986.
40. Brumbaugh, P. F., Haussler, D. H., Bursac, K. M., and Hausaler, M. R., Filter assay for 1α, 25-dihydroxyvitamin D_3, Utilization of the hormone's target tissue chromatin receptor, *Biochemistry*, 13, 4091, 1973.
41. Reinhardt, T. A., Horst, R. L., Orf, J. W., and Hollis, B. W., A microassay for 1,25-dihydroxyvitamin D not requiring high performance liquid chromatography: application to clinical studies, *Clin. Endocrinol. Metab.*, 58, 91, 1984.
42. Dawson-Hughes, B., Calcium and vitamin D nutritional needs of elderly women, *J. Nutr.*, 126, 1165S, 1996.
43. Holick, M. F., Vitamin D and bone health, *J. Nutr.*, 126, 1159S, 1996.
44. Salamone, L. M., Dallal, G. E., Zantos, D., Makrauer, F., and Dawson-Hughes, B., Contributions of vitamin D intake and seasonal sunlight exposure to plasma 25-hydroxyvitamin D concentration in elderly women, *Am. J. Clin. Nutr.*, 58, 80, 1993.
45. Bikle, D., Role of vitamin D, its metabolites and analogs in the management of osteoporosis, *Clin. of North Am.*, 20, 759, 1996.
46. Orwoll, E. S. and Meier, D. E., Alterations in calcium, vitamin D, and parathyroid hormone physiology in normal men with aging: Relationship to the development of senile osteopenia, *J. Clin. Endocrinol. Metab.*, 63, 1262, 1986.
47. Ryan, C., Eleazer, P., and Egbut, J., Vitamin D in the elderly, *Nutrition Today*, 30, 228, 1995.
48. Thomson, S. P., Wilton, T. J., Hoskinf, D. J., White, D. A., and Pawley, E., Is vitamin D necessary for skeletal integrity in the elderly? *J. Bone Joint Surg.*, 72B, 1053, 1990.
49. Walters, M. R., Kollenkirchen, U., and Fox, J., What is vitamin D deficiency? *Proc. Soc. Expt. Biol. Med.*, 199, 385, 1992.
50. Hollis, B. W. and Pittard, W. B., Improved radioimmunoassay for vitamin D and its use in assessing vitamin D status, *Clin. Chem.*, 31, 1815, 1985.
51. Fraker, L. J., Adami, S., Clemens, T. L., Jones, G., and O'Riordan, J. L. H., Radioimmunoassay of 1,25-dihydroxyvitamin D_3: studies on the metabolism of vitamin D_2 in man, *Clin. Endocrimol.*, 19, 151, 1983.
52. Mankin, H. J., Rickets, osteomalacia, and renal osteodystrophy, an update, *Orthopedic Clin. of North Am.*, 21, 81, 1990.
53. Davies, M., High-dose vitamin D therapy: indications, benefits and hazards in *Elevated Dosages of Vitamins: Benefits and Hazards*, Walter, P., Brubacher, G., and Stahelin, H., Eds., Hans Huber Publication, Toronto, Canada, 1989, 81.
54. Davies, M. and Adams, P. H., The continuing risk of vitamin D intoxication, *Lancet*, ii, 621, 1978.
55. Paterson, C. R., Vitamin D poisoning! Survey of causes in 21 patients with hypercalcaemia, *Lancet*, ii, 1164, 1980.

56. Stephens, W. P., Klimiuk, P. S., Berry J. L., and Mawer, E. B., Annual high dose vitamin D prophylaxis in Asian immigrants, *Lancet*, ii, 1199, 1981.

57. Davies, M., Mawer, E. B., Hann, J. T., Stephens, W. P., and Taylor, J. L., Vitamin D prophylaxis in the elderly: a simple effective method suitable for large populations, *Age and Aging*, 14, 349, 1985.

58. Food and Nutrition Board, National Research Council, *Recommended Dietary Allowances*, 10th edition, National Academy Press, Washington D.C., 1989.

59. American Academy of Pediatrics, The prophylactic requirement and the toxicity of vitamin D, *Pediatrics*, 31, 512, 1963.

60. Mehls, O., Wolf, H., and Wille, L., Vitamin D requirements and vitamin D intoxication in infancy, in *Elevated Dosages of Vitamins: Benefits and Hazards*, Walter, P., Brubacker, G., and Stahelin, H., Eds., Hans Huber Publication, Toronto, Canada, 1989, 87.

61. Lamberg-Allardt, C., Karkkainen, M., Seppanen, R., and Bistrom, H., Low serum 25-hydroxy-vitamin D concentrations and secondary hyperparathyroidism in middle-age white strict vegetarians, *Am. J. Clin. Nutr.*, 58, 684, 1993.

62. Guillemant, S., Guillemant, J., Feteanu, D., and Sebag-Lanoe, R., Effect of vitamin D_3 admin-istration on serum 25-hydroxyvitamin D_3, 1,25-dihydroxyvitamin D_3 and osteocalcin in vitamin D-deficient elderly people, *J. Steroid Biochem.*, 33, 1155, 1989.

63. McKenna, M. J., Freaney, R., Meade, A., and Muldowney, F. P., Hypovitaminosis D and elevated serum alkaline phosphatase in elderly Irish people, *Am. J. Clin. Nutr.*, 41, 101, 1985.

64. Heldenberg, D., Tenenbaum, G., and Weisman, Y., Effect of iron on serum 25-hydroxyvitamin D and 24,25-dihydroxyvitamin D concentrations, *Am. J. Clin. Nutr.*, 56, 533, 1992.

65. Burnand, B., Sloutskis, D., Gianoli, F., Cornuz, J., Rickenbach, M., Paccaud, F., and Burckhardt, P., Serum 25-hydroxyvitamin D: distribution and determinants in the Swiss population, *Am. J. Clin. Nutr.*, 56, 537, 1992.

66. McLaughlin, J. and Holick, M. F., Aging decreases the capacity of human skin to produce vitamin D_3, *J. Clin. Invest.*, 76, 1536, 1985.

67. Khaw, K.-T., Sneyd, M.-J., and Compston, J., Bone density, parathyroid hormone and 25-hydroxyvitamin D concentrations in middle aged women, *BMJ*, 305, 273, 1992.

68. Bowers, G. N. Jr. and McComb, R. B., Measurement of total alkaline phosphatase activity in human serum, *Clin. Chem.*, 21, 1988, 1975.

69. Kumar, R., Osteomalacia, in *Medicine for the Practicing Physician*, 4th edition, Hurst, J. W., Ed., Appleton & Lange, Stamford, 1996, 670.

70. Fraser, D., Jones, G., Kooh, S. W., and Radde, I. C., Calcium and phosphate metabolism, in *Textbook of Clinical Chemistry*, Tietz, N. W., Ed., W. B. Saunders Company, Philadelphia, 1986, chap. 12.

71. Weisman, Y., Schen, R. J., Eisenberg, Z., Edelstein, S., and Harell, A., Inadequate status and impaired metabolism of vitamin D in the elderly, *Isr. J. Med. Sci.*, 17, 19, 1981.

72. vander Wielen, R. P. J., Lowik, M. R. H., van den Berg, H., de Groot, L., CPGM, Holler, J., and Moreiras, O., Serum vitamin D concentrations among people in Europe, *Lancet*, 346, 207, 1995.

73. Dawson-Hughes, B., Harris, S. S., Krall, E. A., Dallal, G. E., and Falconer, G., Rates of bone loss in postmenopausal women randomly assigned to one of two dosages of vitamin D, *Am. J. Clin. Nutr.*, 61, 1140, 1995.

74. Sherman, S. S., Hollis, B. W., and Tobin, J. D., Vitamin D status and related parameters in a healthy population: the effect of age, sex, and season, *J. Clin. Endocrinol. Metab.*, 71, 405, 1990.

75. Manolagas, S. C. and Jilka, R. L., Bone marrow, cytokines, and bone remodeling, Energy insights into the pathophysiology of osteoporosis, *N. Engl. J. Med.*, 332, 305, 1995.

76. Meier, D. E., Luckey, M. M., Wallenstein, S., Clemens, T. L., Orwoll, E. S., and Waslien, C. I., Calcium, vitamin D, and parathyroid hormone status in young white and black women: association with racial diffferences in bone mass, *J. Clin. Endrinol. Metab.*, 72, 703, 1991.

77. Matsuoka, L. Y., Wortsman, J., Haddad, J. G., Kolm, P., and Hollis, B. W., Racial pigmentation and the cutaneous synthesis of vitamin D, *Arch. Dermatol.*, 127, 536, 1991.

78. Pietschmann, P., Woloszczuk, W., and Pietschmann, H., Increased serum osteocalcin levels in elderly females with vitamin D deficiency, *Exp. Clin. Endocrinol.*, 95, 275, 1990.

79. Goldray, D., Mizrahi-Sasson, E., Merdler, C., Edelstein-Singer, M., Algoetti, A., Eisenberg, Z., Jaccard, N., and Weisman, Y., Vitamin D deficiency in elderly patients in a general hospital, *J. Am. Geratr. Soc.*, 37, 589, 1989.

80. Eisman, J. A., Shepard, R. M., and Deluca, H. F., Determination of 25-hydroxyvitamin D_2 and 25-hydroxyvitamin D_3 in human plasma using high-pressure liquid chromatography, *Anal. Biochem.*, 80, 298, 1977.

81. Horst, R. L., Littledike, E. T., Riley, J. L., and Napoli, J. L., Quantitation of vitamin D and its metabolites and their plasma concentrations in five species of animals, *Anal. Biochem.*, 116, 189, 1981.

82. Hollis, B. W. and Frank, N. E., Solid phase extraction system for vitamin D and its major metabolites in human serum, *J. Chromatogr.*, 343, 43, 1985.

83. Haddad, J. G. and Chyu, K. J., Competitive protein-binding radioassay for 25-hydroxy-cholcalciferol, *J. Clin. Endocrinol. Metab.*, 33, 992, 1971.

84. Belsey, R., Deluca, H. F., and Potts, J. T., A rapid assay for 25-OH-vitamin D_3 without preparative chromatography, *J. Clin. Endocrinol. Metab.*, 38, 1046, 1974.

85. Hollis, B. W., Burton, J. H., and Draper, H. H., A binding assay for 25-hydroxycalciferols and 24R,25-dihydroxycalciferols using bovine plasma globulin, *Steriods*, 30, 285, 1977.

86. Offerman, G. and Dittmar, F., A direct protein-binding assay for 25-hydroxycalciferol, *Horm. Metab. Res.*, 6, 534, 1974.

87. Skinner, R. K. and Wills, M. R., Serum 25-hydroxyvitamin D assay, Evaluation of chromatographic and non-chromatographic procedures, *Clin. Chim. Acta*, 80, 543, 1977.

88. Bouillon, R., Van Herch, E., Jans, I., Tan, B. K., Van Baelen, H., and Demoor, P., Two direct (nonchromatographic) assays for 25-hydroxyvitamin D, *Clin. Chem.*, 30, 1731, 1984.

89. Hollis, B. W., Kamerud, J. Q., Selvaag, S. R., Lorenz, J. D., and Napoli, J. L., Determination of vitamin D status by radioimmunoassay with an ^{125}I-labeled tracer, *Clin. Chem.*, 39, 529, 1993.

90. Weisman, Y., Reiter, E., and Root, A., Measurement of 24,25-dihydroxyvitamin D in sera of neonates and children, *J. Pediatr.*, 91, 904, 1977.

91. Oftebro, H., Falch, J. A., Holmberg, I., and Haug, E., Validation of a radioreceptor assay for 1,25-dihydroxyvitamin D using selected ion monitoring GC-MS, *Clin. Chim. Acta*, 176, 157, 1988.

92. Poon, P. M., Mak, Y. T., and Pang, C. P., Gas Chromatographic-mass fragmetographic determination of serum 1-alpha, 25-dihydroxyvitamin D_3, *Clin. Biochem.*, 26, 461, 1993.

93. Mawer, B. E., Clinical implication of measurements of circulating vitamin D metabolites, *Clin. Endocrinol. Metab.*, 9, 63, 1980.

94. Hollis, B. W., Comparison of equilibrium and disequilibrium assay conditions for ergocalciferol, cholecalciferol and their major metabolites, *J. Steroid Biochem.*, 21, 81, 1984.

95. Schwartzman, M. S., and Franck, W. A., Vitamin D toxicity complicating the treatment of senile, postmenopausal, and glucocorticoid-induced osteoporosis, *Am. J. Med.*, 82, 224, 1987.

96. McKenna, M. J., Differences in vitamin D status between countries in young adults and elderly, *Am. J. Med.*, 93, 69, 1992.

97. Parfitt, A. M., Gallagher, J. C., Heaney, R. P., Johnston, C. C., Neer, R., and Whedon, G., Vitamin D and bone health in the elderly, *Am. J. Clin. Nutr.*, 36, 1014, 1982.

98. Lebrun, J. B., Moffatt, M. E. K., Mundy, R. J. T., Sangster, R. K., Postl, B. D., Dooley, J. P., Dilling, L. A., Godel, J. C., and Haworth, J. C., Vitamin D deficiency in a Manitoba community, *Canadian J. Public Health*, 84, 394, 1993.

99. Porteous, C. E., Coldwell, R. D., Trafford, D. J. H., and Makin, H. L. J., Recent developments in the measurement of vitamin D and its metabolites in human body fluids, *J. Steroid Biochem.*, 28, 785, 1987.

100. McGraw, C. A. and Hug, G., Simultaneous measurement of 25-hydroxy, 24,25-dihydroxy-, and 1,25-dihydroxyvitamin D without use of HPLC, *Med. Lab. Sci.*, 47, 17, 1990.

101. Aksnes, L., A simplified high-performance liquid chromatographic method for determination of vitamin D_3, 25-hydroxyvitamin D_2 and 25-hydroxyvitamin D_3 in human serum, *Scand. J. Clin. Lab. Invest.*, 52, 177, 1992.

102. Hummer, L., Rus, B. J., Christiansen, C., and Rickers, H., Determination of mono- and dihydroxyvitamin D metabolites in normal subjects and patients with different calcium metabolic diseases, *Scand. J. Clin. Lab. Invest.*, 45, 611, 1985.

103. Chan, E. L. P., Lau, E., Shek, C. C., MacDonald, D., Woo, J., Leung, P. C., and Swaminathan, R., Age-related changes in bone density, serum parathyroid hormone, calcium absorption and other indices of bone metabolism in Chinese women, *Clin. Endocrinology*, 36, 375, 1992.

104. Nieves, J., Cosman, F., Herbut, J., Shen, V., and Lindsay, R., High prevalence of vitamin D deficiency and reduced bone mass in multiple sclerosis, *Neurology*, 44, 1687, 1994.

105. Sowers, M. D., Wallace, R. B., and Hollis, B. W., The relationship of 1,25-dihydroxyvitamin D and radial bone mass, *Bone & Mineral*, 10, 139, 1990.

106. Ho, S. C., MacDonald, D., Chan, C., Fan, Y. K., Chan, S. S. G., and Swaminathan, R., Determinants of serum 1,25-dihydroxyvitamin D concentration in healthy premenopausal subjects, *Clin. Chemica Acta*, 230, 21, 1994.

107. Wilkinson, J. H., Boutwell, J. H., and Winsten, S., Evaluation of a new system for the kinetic measurement of serum alkaline phosphatase, *Clin. Chem.*, 15, 487, 1969.

108. Reichel, H., Koeffler, H. P., and Norman, A. W., The role of the vitamin D endocrine system in health and disease, *N. Engl. J. Med.*, 320, 980, 1989.

109. Henry, H. L. and Norman, A. W., Vitamin D: metabolism and biological actions, *Annu. Rev. Nutr.*, 4, 493, 1984.

110. Nordin, B. E. C., Baker, M. R., Horsman, A., and Peacock, M., A prospective trial of the effect of vitamin D supplementation on metacarpal bone loss in elderly women, *Am. J. Clin. Nutr.*, 42, 470, 1985.

111. Smith, R., Rickets and osteomalacia, *Human Nutrition: Clinical Nutrition*, 36C, 115, 1982.

112. Holmes, R. P. and Kummerow, F. A., The relationship of adequate and excessive intakes of vitamin D to health and disease, *J. Am. Coll. Nutr.*, 2, 173, 1983.

113. Haddad, J. G., Vitamin D — solar rays, the milky way or both, *N. Engl. J. Med.*, 326, 1213, 1992.

114. Jacobus, C. H., Holick, M. F., Shao, Q., Chen, T. C., Holm, I. A., Kolondney, J. M., Fuleihan, G. E.-H., and Seely, E. W., Hypervitaminosis D associated with drinking milk, *N. Engl. J. Med.*, 326, 1173, 1992.

115. Fairney, A. and Saphier, P. W., Studies on the measurement of 25-hydroxyvitamin D in human salvia, *Br. J. Nutr.*, 57, 13, 1987.

116. Lore, F., Di Cairano, G., and Di Perri, G., Vitamin D status in the extreme age of life, *Annu. Med. Interne.*, 137, 209, 1986.

117. Koyama, H., Prahl, J. M., Uhland, A., Nanjo, M., Inaba, M., Nishizawa, Y., Morii, H., Nishii, Y., and DeLuca, H. F., A new, highly sensitive assay for 1,25-dihydroxyvitamin D not requiring high-performance liquid chromatography: application of monoclonal antibody against vitamin D receptor to radioreceptor assay, *Anal. Biochem.*, 205, 213, 1992.

118. McComb, R. B., Bowers, G. N. Jr., and Posen, S., *Alkaline Phosphatase*, Plenum Press, New York, 1979.

119. Sowers, M. R., Wallace, R. B., Hollis, B. W., and Lemke, J. H., Parameters related to 25-OH-D levels in a population-based study of women, *Am. J. Clin. Nutr.*, 43, 621, 1986.

120. Mohammed, S., Addae, S., Suleiman, S., Adzaku, F., Annobil, S., Kaddoremi, O., and Richards, J., Serum calcium, parathyroid hormone, and vitamin D status in children and young adults with sickle cell disease, *Annu. Clin. Biochem.*, 30, 45, 1993.

121. Lowik, M. R. H., van den Berg, H., Schrijver, J., Odink, J., Wedel, M., and van Houten, P., Marginal nutritional status among institutionalized elderly women as compared to those living more independently (Dutch Nutrition Survelliance System), *J. Am. Coll. Nutr.*, 11, 673, 1992.

122. Weaver, C. M., Martin, B. R., Plawecki, K. L., Peacock, M., Wood, O. B., Smith, D. L., and Wastney, M. E., Differences in calcium metabolism between adolescent and adult females, *Am. J. Clin. Nutr.*, 61, 577, 1995.

123. Hollis, B. W., Kamerud, J. Q., Kurkowski, A., Beaulieu, J., and Napoli, J. L., Quantification of circulating 1,25-dihydroxyvitamin D by radioimmunoassay with ^{125}I-labeled tracer, *Clin. Chem.*, 42, 586, 1996.

124. Chan, G. M., Dietary calcium and bone mineral status of children and adolescents, *AJDC*, 145, 631, 1991.

125. Prince, R., Dick, I., Boyd, F., Kent, N., and Garcia-Webb, P., The effects of dietary calcium deprivation on serum calcitriol levels in premenopausal and postmenopausal women, *Metabolism*, 37, 727, 1988.

126. Need, A. G., Morris, H. A., Horowitz, M., and Nordin, B. E. G., Effects of skin thickness, age, body fat, and sunlight on serum 25-hydroxyvitamin D, *Am. J. Clin. Nutr.*, 58, 882, 1993.

127. Wilz, D. R., Gray, R. W., Dominguez, J. H., and Leman, J. Jr., Plasma 1,25-$(OH)_2$-vitamin D concentrations and net intestinal calcium, phosphate, and magnesium absorption in humans, *Am. J. Clin. Nutr.*, 32, 2052, 1979.

128. Zeghound, F., Vervel, C., Guillozo, H., Walrant-Debray, O., Boutignon, H., and Garabedian, M., Subclinical vitamin D deficiency in neonates: definition and response to vitamin D supplements, *Am. J. Clin. Nutr.*, 65, 771, 1997.

129. Kinyamu, H. K., Gallagher, J. C., Balhorn, K. E., Petranick, K. M., and Rafferty, K. A., Serum vitamin D metabolites and calcium absorption in normal young and elderly free-living women and in women living in nursing homes, *Am. J. Clin. Nutr.*, 65, 790, 1997.

130. Dawson-Hughes, B., Harris, S. S., and Dallal, G. E., Plasma calcidiol, season, and serum parathyroid hormone concentrations in healthy elderly men and women, *Am. J. Clin. Nutr.*, 65, 67, 1997.

131. Norman, A. W., Sunlight, season, skin pigmentation, vitamin D, and 25-hydroxyvitamin D: integral components of the vitamin D endocrine system, *Am. J. Clin. Nutr.*, 67, 1108, 1998.

132. Harris, S. S. and Dawson-Hughes, B., Seasonal changes in plasma 25-hydroxyvitamin D concentrations of young American black and white women, *Am. J. Clin. Nutr.*, 67, 1232, 1998.

133. Norman, A. W., Pleiotropic actions of 1α,25-dihydroxyvitamin D_3: an overview, *J. Nutr.*, 125, 1687S, 1995.

134. Hayes, C. E., Cantorna, M. T., and DeLuca, H. F., Vitamin D and multiple sclerosis, *Soc. Exptl. Biol. Med.*, 216, 21, 1997.

135. Jacques, P. F., Felson, D. T., Tucker, K. L., Mahnken, B., Wilson, P. W. F., Rosenberg, I. H., and Rush, D., Plasma 25-hydroxyvitamin D and its determinants in an elderly population, *Am. J. Clin. Nutr.*, 66, 929, 1997.

Vitamin E (Tocopherols)

α- Tocopherol
molecular weight: 430.7

β- Tocopherol
molecular weight: 416.7

γ- Tocopherol
molecular weight: 416.7

δ- Tocopherol
molecular weight: 402.6

Converting metric units to International System (SI) units:

α-Tocopherol:
$\mu g/mL \times 2.32 = \mu mol/L$

$\mu mol/L \times 0.4307 = \mu g/mL$

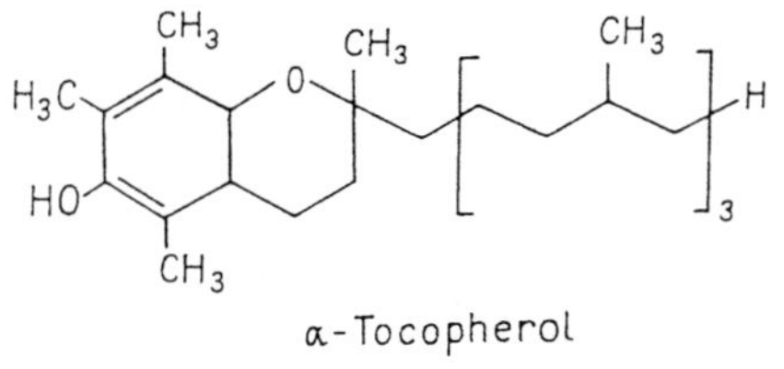

FIGURE 46
Structure of α-tocopherol.

Introduction

The early history of vitamin E has been summarized by H. M. Evans,[68] who with K. S. Bishops, discovered vitamin E in 1922 while at the University of California at Berkeley.[177,178] Evans et al. were the first to isolate α-tocopherol using wheat germ oil as a source of the vitamin.[180]

α-Tocopherol is the major component of the vitamin commonly referred to as vitamin E.[29] Vitamin E is transported in plasma only in the lipoproteins; consequently, plasma vitamin E concentrations are related to the concentrations of plasma lipids.[14,17,52] Vitamin E is the most important lipid-soluble antioxidant and free radical scavenger in the body.[21] In this capacity, vitamin E protects lipids against oxidative damage.[14,20,50,52,58] The mechanism by which vitamin E prevents various metabolic and pathological lesions, such as neurological abnormalities, has not been fully elucidated.

Interest in vitamin E has increased because of its potential health benefit roles such as preventing cancer and atherosclerotic lesions.[36,50,61] In these roles, vitamin E serves as a free radical scavenger.[7,8,62] Evidence from epidemiological studies and biochemical investigations indicate that antioxidants in the diet, particularly vitamin E, may reduce the risk of cardiovascular disease and cancer.[1-7,10,11,45,53-55,57,58,63,176] A number of reviews have evaluated these effects of vitamin E.[1-16,50,59,60,62]

The associations of vitamin E with clinical conditions are numerous. This document permits only a brief mention of these conditions. More information may be obtained from the literature citations noted. The clinical conditions with evidence of a vitamin E association include Alzheimer's disease,[65] Parkinsons's disease,[40] cataracts,[41,88] liver disease,[42] β-thalassemia,[43,46] neuropathies and malabsorption,[47,84-86,139] and genetic disorders.[47]

Sources of Vitamin E

The tocopherol content of foods was summarized in the extensive document of Bauernfeind.[65] Vegetable oils, nuts, seeds, and most grains are good sources of vitamin E. Information on the vitamin E values from the U.S. Department of Agriculture (USDA) handbooks No. 8–1 through 8–12, are available from the U.S. Government Printing Office, Washington D.C. Data from the second Health and Nutrition Examination Survey (NHANES-II) indicate that the mean intake of vitamin E was 9.6 mg/day for men and 5.4 mg/day for women.[69]

Vitamin E serves as a term that includes all tocol and tocotrienol derivatives that qualitatively exhibit the biological activity of α-tocopherol.[19,29,52] α-Tocopherol has the highest biopotency of the tocopherols and the tocotrienols.[29] Tocoherol includes α-, β-, γ-, and δ-tocopherols. Aside from α-tocopherol, only β-tocopherol has significant vitamin E biological activity. α-Tocopherol is properly designated RRR-α-tocopherol. Only plants synthesize vitamin E with vegetable oils serving as a rich dietary source of the vitamin.[19] Safflower oil, sunflower oil, and wheat germ oil are high in α-tocopherol while corn oil and soybean oil contain predominantly γ-tocopherol. Palm oil and cottonseed oil are high in both α-tocopherol and γ-tocopherol. Palm oil is also high in both α-tocotrienol and γ-tocotrienol.[19,126]

Depending upon the source and level of fat in the diet, plasma levels of tocopherols may vary.[159] In general, however, α-tocopherol represent over 90% of the total tocopherols present in the plasma.[25,126,127,160] Even the consumption of oils rich in γ-tocopherol, α-tocotrienol, or γ-tocotrienol had little effect on their level in plasma.[126]

Vitamin E Deficiency

It was not until the 1960s that vitamin E was considered essential for the human.[33] Studies on premature infants with hemolytic anemia demonstrated an association with vitamin E deficiency.[33] Although it is difficult to produce an experimental vitamin E deficiency in the adult human, as demonstrated by the classic studies of Horwitt,[17,19] vitamin E deficiency is now recognized to occur in several clinical conditions.[6,34,35,52,74,83,86]

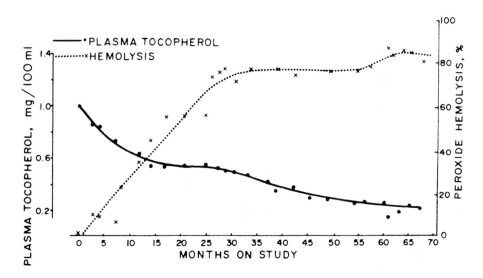

FIGURE 47

Relationship of average plasma tocopherol concentrations to average hydrogen peroxide hemolysis of red blood cells from experimental human subjects on vitamin E-deficient diets (From Horwitt.[66] With permission.)

Vitamin E status has been studied in various groups and populations, that included the elderly,[140] total parenteral nutrition,[141] sickle cell anemia,[142] Italian children,[143] Swedish men and women,[144] smokers,[146] Europe,[147] Japan,[148-150] Australia,[151] Indonesia,[158] and Hispanics.[159] In the European SENECA study,[147] a vitamin E biochemical deficiency was found in seven populations that varied from 0.5 to 24% of the population.

The use of vitamin E supplements has been extensively investigated with regards to the treatment of various chronic diseases.[4,14,52] The diseases studied include Alzheimer's disease,[64] Parkinson's disease, atherosclerosis,[54,57,58,61] ischemic heart disease,[31,87] cataracts,[88] diabetes, total parenteral nutrition, impaired immune function,[14,51,85,88] cancer,[1,5,6] and cholestatic liver disease.[74] A vitamin E deficiency is commonly the result of fat malabsorption or to genetic abnormalities in lipoprotein metabolism.[14,32,49] One genetic abnormality results in a defective hepatic α-tocopherol transfer protein. This abnormality results in impaired transfer of vitamin E to the tissues. This results in a vitamin E deficiency syndrome, which may be characterized ataxia and peripheral neuropathy.[32,74]

Subjects with the genetic disorder abetalipoproteinemia have permitted a clinical description of a vitamin E deficiency.[47,49] These subjects have an inability to transport vitamin E resulting in a vitamin E deficiency. Plasma level of vitamin E are exceedingly low. Autohemolysis occurs as the vitamin E levels in the red cells also become very low. In severe vitamin E conditions, neurological and musculoskeletal abnormalities occur. It has been suggested that plasma vitamin E concentrations should be measured in subjects with peripheral neuropathies or spinocerebellar ataxia.[47,74,86]

Infants and Children

Considerable attention has been given to the vitamin E status of infants and preterm infants.[155,156] The life of the red blood cells of infants and preterm infants is considerably shorter than the red blood cells of normal adults.[153] The infant is born with low levels of vitamin E in the body.[155] Thus, many studies have been directed to the vitamin E needs of the newborn and children.[48,75-77,80-83,88,89,92,135,150,155,158,161-166]

Children who develop vitamin E deficiency commonly exhibit neurological disorders. This may include balance and gait disorders and they may lose the ability to walk.[34,35]

Children with cystic fibrosis are often found to have a vitamin E deficiency.[75,76,79] Vitamin E deficiency may also occur in children with chronic cholestasis.[77,86] Premature infants are recognized as a group with a high risk of vitamin E deficiency.[78,80-82] Plasma vitamin E concentrations of term infants was reported as 1.9 mg/L and for preterm infants only 0.3 mg/L.[80] For comparison, adults had plasma vitamin E concentrations of 9.2 mg/L. Somewhat higher vitamin E concentrations for preterm infants were reported by Gutsher et al.[82] They found that premature infants had total plasma tocopherol concentrations of 2.71 mg/L at the first day of life. Bartolotti et al.[122] found α-tocopherol concentrations in nine newborns to range from 2.0 to 2.8 µg/mL (2.5 ± 0.3 µg/mL). In comparison, adults had α-tocopherol concentrations of that ranged from 7.1 to 12.3 µg/mL (mean: 10.0 ± 2.0 µg/mL). Children in the U.S., aged 1 to 12 years had serum vitamin E concentrations of 5.5 to 6.3 mg/L.[88] Somewhat higher concentrations were reported for children in Japan (6.8 mg/L), Canada (8.2 mg/L), and Austria (8.8 mg/L).[88]

Assessment of Vitamin E Status

General

Several approaches have been used to assess vitamin E status.[185] They include: (1) degree of erythrocyte hemolysis, (2) tocopherol concentrations in serum or plasma, (3) tocopherol concentrations in erythrocytes, lymphocytes, or platelets, and (4) measurement of the production of peroxidation products (e.g., malonaldbyde, TBARS, ethane, and pentane). Measurement of vitamin E stores by liver or adipose tissue biopsies may be informative but are not practical procedures (Tables 56 to 60).[20]

Although measurements of vitamin E concentrations in erythrocytes and platelets can provide a more sensitive indicator of vitamin E status than serum/plasma, or lymphocyte vitamin E measurements, the procedures are more cumbersome and seldom used.[23] Measurement of vitamin E concentrations in plasma and serum are most commonly employed. Methods used are specific, sensitive, and readily performed. Of note, however, platelet vitamin E concentrations are independent of plasma lipid concentrations.[24]

Early Methods

In the past, vitamin E was measured by colorimetric, fluorometric or spectrophotometric methods, and gas-liquid chromatography.[94,95,100,102,103,124,125,128] Many of these methods were based on the Emmerie and Engel oxidative reaction of tocopherols.[101,128,136] For example, in the method of Fabianek et al.,[136] the tocopherol in serum was oxidized by ferric chloride. The pink complex of ferrous ions with 4,7-diphenyl-10,10-phenanthroline (bathophenanthroline) was spectrophotometrically determined.

Thin-layer chromatography was also used prior to the advent of HPLC. With the use of thin-layer chromatography and a spectrophotometric procedure,[1-4] human plasma was reported to have α-tocopherol concentrations of 6.6 to 15.0 (mean 9.6) µg/mL. Human red

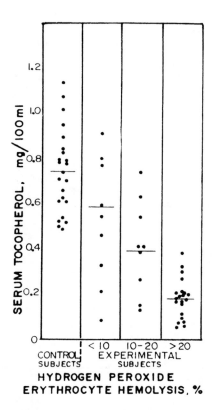

FIGURE 48

Relationship between serum tocopherol concentrations and hydrogen peroxide hemolysis of red blood cells from human subjects. (From Binder and Spiro.[67] With permission.)

TABLE 56
General Guidelines for Interpreting Vitamin E Data[92,128] (For all Age Groups)

	Serum/Plasma α-Tocopherol		Erythrocyte H_2O_2
Classification Category	**μmol/L**	**μg/ml**	**Hemolysis (%)**
Deficient	< 11.6	< 5.0	> 20
Low	11.6–16.2	5.0–7.0	10 to 20
Acceptable	≥ 16.2	≥ 7.0	≤ 10
Normal values (both M and F)			

(a) Plasma α-tocopherol/plasma total lipid ratio (μg/mg)
   Acceptable: $> 0.8 \times 10^{-3}$ [17,150]
(b) Plasma α-tocopherol/plasma cholesterol ratio (μg/mg)
   Acceptable: $> 2.22 \times 10^{-3}$ [56]
(c) Serum/plasma α-tocopherol (μmol/L)
   Acceptable: ≥ 11.6 [181,182]

cells had α-tocopherol concentrations of 0.9 to 1.8 (mean 1.4) μg/mL. Of the total tocopherols, α-tocopherol accounted for approximately 90% in both the red blood cells and in plasma.[104,159]

High Performance Liquid Chromatography (HPLC)

The earlier methods for measuring vitamin E in blood specimens have been replaced by HPLC methods. Various HPLC procedures have been reported; the major difference being

TABLE 57
Some Literature Values for Guidance in Evaluating Vitamin E Status
in Children

Children	Values	References
1. Age 41–54 months ($n = 44$)		
Serum α-tocopherol	6.3 ± 2.6 μmol/L	
	(0.27 ± 0.11 mg/dL)	
Serum α-tocopherol/lipid ratio	1.5 ± 0.72 μmol/g	
2. Age 1–12 years ($n = 39$)		89
Plasma α-tocopherol	13.7 ± 0.69 μmol/L	
	(0.59 ± 0.03 mg/dL)	
α-Tocopherol/cholesterol ratio	3.42 ± 0.20 mg/g	
α-Tocopherol/lipid ratio	1.22 ± 0.06 mg/g	
3. Age 3–11 years ($n = 261$)		150
Plasma α-tocopherol	0.68 ± 12 μg/dL	
Total lipids	513 ± 22 mg/dL	
4. Premature infants ($n = 37$)		150, 162
Postpartum serum α-tocopherol	7.45 ± 3.78 μmol/L	
	(0.321 ± 0.163 mg/dL)	
Plasma α-tocopherol/lipid ratio	1.51 ± 0.02 μg/mg	

TABLE 58
Some Literature Values for Guidance in Interpreting Vitamin E
Data in Adults

Plasma Tocopherol	μmol/L	mg/dL	Reference
1. Men ($n = 30$)			152
α-Tocopherol	27.2 ± 1.0	1.17 ± 0.04	
γ-Tocopherol	3.7 ± 0.3	0.15 ± 0.01	
2. Men ($n = 10$)			154
α-Tocopherol	22.9 ± 1.2	0.99 ± 0.05	
γ-Tocopherol	5.1 ± 0.4	0.21 ± 0.02	
3. Men ($n = 75$)	3.04 ± 7.4	1.31 ± 0.32	111
4. Women ($n = 75$)	29.3 ± 6.7	1.21 ± 0.25	111
5. Adults ($n = 25$)	28.1 ± 5.8	1.21 ± 0.41	112
6. Men			157
Age: 20–40 y ($n = 9$)	19.7 ± 0.7	0.85 ± 0.03	
Age: 60–80 y ($n = 9$)	27.9 ± 1.5	1.20 ± 0.06	
7. Women			157
Age: 20–40 y ($n = 8$)	17.8 ± 0.7	0.77 ± 0.03	
Age: 60–80 y ($n = 8$)	26.3 ± 1.0	1.13 ± 0.04	
8. Young men ($n = 39$)	18.1 ± 3.7	0.78 ± 0.16	149
9. Young women ($n = 17$)	19.0 ± 3.8	0.82 ± 0.16	
10. Elderly men ($n = 26$)	15.1 ± 3.9	0.65 ± 0.17	
11. Elderly women ($n = 43$)	17.6 ± 7.7	0.76 ± 0.33	

the detector used. This includes fluorescence detection,[105,110,111] electrochemical detection,[112-117,183] and UV detection.[106,108,109,118-123] Most of the procedures require only 100 to 200 μg of plasma sample. The procedure of Nierenberg and Lester[38] requires 0.50 mL of plasma, however, the method describes a convenient procedure for the extraction of the vitamin E from plasma.[38,39] HPLC methods are capable of separating and measuring α-, β-, γ-, δ-tocopherols. Vitamin E status is usually related to the α-tocopherol concentrations. HPLC methods are available that permit the quantitation of α-tocopherol in plasma in

TABLE 59
Some Literature Values for Guidance in Interpreting Tocopherol/Lipid Ratios

Tocopherol Ratios	Values	Reference
1. Men (*n* = 113)		151
Plasma α-tocopherol	21.9 μmol/L	
α-Tocopherol/cholesterol ratio	4.51 ± 0.13 mg/g	
2. Women (*n* = 150)		151
Plasma α-tocopherol	23.2 μmol/L	
α-Tocopherol/cholesterol ratio	4.55 ± 0.11 mg/g	
3. Young men (*n* = 39)		149
α-Tocopherol/total lipids ratio	1.85 ± 0.30 μg/mg	
4. Young women (*n* = 17)		149
α-Tocopherol/total lipids ratio	1.90 ± 0.34 μg/mg	
5. Elderly men (*n* = 26)		149
α-Tocopherol/total lipids ratio	1.68 ± 0.40 μg/mg	
6. Elderly women (*n* = 43)		149
α-Tocopherol/total lipids ratio	1.80 ± 0.42 μg/mg	

Erythrocyte Tocopherol	Tocopherol Level	Reference
1. Adults (*n* = 26)	170–180 μg/100 ml of packed cells (mean = 176 ± 9)	148, 150
2. Children (*n* = 261)	179 ± 3 μg/100 ml of packed cells	150

TABLE 60
Vitamin E Findings from the Hispanic Health and Nutrition Examination Survey (HHANES 1982–84)[159]

	Mexican American Survey	
Age (years)	1. Serum α-Tocopherol (μmol/L)	2. Serum α-Tocopherol: Serum Cholesterol ratio (μmol/g × 10^{-3})
4–5 (*n* = 233)	18.0 ± 0.52	—
6–11 (*n* = 1029)	17.1 ± 0.14	—
12–19 (*n* = 1228)	16.0 ± 0.20	—
20–44 (*n* = 1912)	22.4 ± 0.42	4.43
45–74 (*n* = 1202)	29.2 ± 0.59	5.06

Data from the Hispanic Health and Nutrition Examination Survey.[159]

[1] Acceptable > 11.6 μmol/L.

[2] Acceptable > 2.22 × 10^{-3} serum α-tocopherol: serum cholesterol (both male and female) ratio (μmol/g)

approximately 5 minutes. Various internal standards are used including tocol, retinyl acetate, and tocopherol acetate. Vitamin E in plasma or serum is quite stable.[120] Vitamin E remained stable in serum samples stored for at least 16 months at –70°C.[120] In the author's experience, the HPLC procedure of Bieri et al.[91,108] and Driskell et al.[120] have proven to be simple, fast, reliable and suitable for automation.

With the procedure of Bieri et al.,[91,108] if tocol is used instead of α-tocopherol acetate as an internal standard, the assay time can be reduced by several minutes. The procedure of Bieri et al.,[91] has proven to be a reliable HPLC procedure that has received frequent use.[80] The method is sensitive, rapid, and permits the use of several internal standards. Various procedures have been used to extract the tocopherols from plasma prior to injection. As an example,[80] 100 μL of plasma was mixed with 100 μL of anhydrous ethanol containing 5 μg

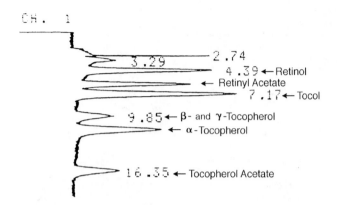

FIGURE 49
HPLC analysis for plasma concentrations of tocopherols and retinol. (Procedure of Beri et al. used).[91,108]

α-tocopherol acetate as an internal standard before extracting with 500 μL of hexane. After vigorous mixing and centrifugation, the hexane layer containing the vitamin E was removed and evaporated under nitrogen. The extract was reconstituted in 400 μL methanol. Similar extraction procedures are used for the measurement of vitamin E concentrations in red blood cells.[80]

Certified reference standards for α-tocopherol have been available from the National Institute of Standards and Technology, Gaithersburg, MD (Standard Reference Material (SRM) 968a).

Plasma Vitamin E Concentrations

Vitamin E circulates in the blood mainly with the low density lipoproteins.[1,17,56,70-72] With normolipemic plasma, a tocopherol concentration of 5 μg/mL (11.6 μmol/L) and above has been considered an acceptable vitamin E status.[17,19,22] To overcome the effects of abnormal plasma lipid concentrations, plasma α-tocopherol levels have been related to several lipid fractions.[19,54] Of the α-tocopherol: individual lipid ratios, the α-tocopherol: cholesterol ratio was the most useful and convenient to perform.[56] A plasma α-tocopherol/cholesterol ratio (μmol/mmol) below 2.2 was associated with clinical signs of a vitamin E deficiency (e.g., neuromuscular disorders and fragility of membranes).[55,56] This is equivalent to 1.11 μmol α-tocopherol/mmol total lipids or to 0.8 mg of α-tocopherol/g total plasma lipids.[42,55,56]

Sokol et al.[42] found in vitamin E-deficient subjects, a ratio of only 0.28 ± 0.08 mg cholesterol/gm total lipids, with a low serum vitamin E level of only 3.2 ± 0.9 μg/mL. Vitamin E–sufficient subjects had a ratio of 1.80 ± 0.13 mg cholesterol/gm total lipids and a serum vitamin E level of 13.5 ± 0.9 μg/mL.

Dimitrov et al.[39] reported in a study with 64 adults, a mean plasma α-tocopherol concentration of 17.2 μmol/L (7.4 μg/mL). In an average adult population, the serum/plasma concentration of vitamin E is reported as approximately 9.5 μg/mL.[22] Helzlsouer et al.[27] reported an average of 11.1 μg/mL of vitamin E in plasma in a group of 70 adults and Knekt et al.[28] in a study of 301 Finnish subjects found plasma vitamin E concentrations of 8.6 μg/mL among men and 10.5 μg/mL among women. Young adults were reported to have plasma levels of α-tocopherol of 17.6 ± 3.11 μmol/L.[126] Plasma levels of γ-tocopherol were 0.65 ± 0.21 μmol/L and δ-tocopherol were 0.24 ± 0.31 μmol/L. There is a tendency for the plasma α-tocopherol concentrations to rise and fall in proportion to the cholesterol, phospholipid, and triglyceride levels in the plasma.[17] From the results of vitamin E deficiency studies, Horwitt[17] considered a ratio of serum tocopherol to total lipids (mg/g) of less than 0.8 to be indicative of a vitamin E deficiency.

The following guidance may be considered regarding the interpretation of plasma α-tocopherol concentrations. A vitamin E deficiency probably exists if (a) the plasma vitamin E concentrations is low and the plasma lipid level is normal or (b) the vitamin E concentration is normal and the plasma lipid level is elevated resulting in a low vitamin E/lipid ratio.

Vitamin E Status: Functional Procedures

Various functional procedures have been used to assess vitamin E status. This includes erythrocyte hemolysis tests, breath pentane production, and malondialdehyde formation.[93,129]

Erythrocyte Hemolysis Test

Depressed plasma α-tocopherol concentrations are associated with an increased susceptibility of the erythrocytes to hemolysis when exposed *in vitro* to dilute solutions of hydrogen peroxide or dialuric acid.[49,73,84,90,128,137-139] This relationship serves as the basis for the erythrocyte hemolysis test. Various modifications of the test have been utilized.[92,138] Basically the test utilizes washed erythrocytes that are incubated with hydrogen peroxide under specified conditions. The hemolysis produced during the incubation is measured. The test is easy to perform and requires only a small amount of blood. The level of hemolysis correlates with the plasma concentration of α-tocopherol.[73]

Malondialdehyde Test

In the malondialdehyde functional test, erythrocytes are incubated *in vitro* with hydrogen peroxide and the malondialdehyde produced and released into the supernatant is measured.[129,131,133] In a controlled study with children, malondialdehyde formation was less than 6% in control children compared to a mean malondialdehyde formation of 41% in vitamin E-deficient children.[129] The control subjects had a mean plasma concentration of vitamin E of 9.8 ± 2.9 µg/mL while the vitamin E-deficient children ($n = 30$) had a mean plasma concentration of vitamin E of only 1.3 ± 1.5 µg/mL.[129] The specificity of the test could be improved by the use of HPLC to quantitate the malondialdehyde.[130]

Breath Ethane and Pentane Test

Lipid peroxidation results in the production of a number of products including ethane and pentane. These gases pass through the lungs into the expired air and can be quantitated. Methods have been described for measuring breath pentane.[132,133] Pentane excretion was significantly higher in vitamin E deficient subjects when compared to the excretion of normal adults. The investigators concluded that the procedure provides for a simple, reproducible, noninvasive method of assessing the role of vitamin E status in reducing or altering lipid peroxidation.[132,134]

In a subsequent study, breath ethane was measured in normal children and in vitamin E deficient children.[135] The breath ethane measurement correlated with other measures of vitamin E status, including serum vitamin E concentrations and erythrocyte peroxide hemolysis tests. The investigators concluded also that the breath ethane test could be useful to screen children for vitamin E deficiency.[135]

Handling of Blood Specimens

Vitamin E is subject to oxidation which can be enhanced by exposure to light, heat, and alkali. To minimize these losses, samples should be handled under amber light and stored at –70°C. Repetitive freezing and thawing of samples should be held to a minimum. Fasting blood samples are preferred in order to reduce the effect of dietary lipids on plasma vitamin E levels. To further minimize this effect, the ratio of plasma tocopherol to total plasma lipid is often employed instead of plasma tocopherol alone.[9,17,19,22,23] To simplify the procedure, the ratio of plasma tocopherol levels to plasma cholesterol levels (or to the sum of cholesterol and triglycerides) has been used.[26] This index allows for a lipid-independent assessment of vitamin E status. For an individual with an average lipid profile, a poor vitamin E status can usually be discerned alone from the plasma α-tocopherol concentrations.

Vitamin E Toxicity

For the normal adult, the toxicity of vitamin E is considered very low.[171,173-175,179,184] Thus, daily dosages of 100 to 300 mg of vitamin E can be considered safe. Oral supplements of 800 mg of α-tocopherol per day for 8 weeks did not produce any adverse side effects.[58] Studies have demonstrated that even higher doses were without adverse effects.[171,172,179] Plasma concentrations of vitamin E are increased considerably with these high supplements of the vitamin.[175]

Children with malabsorption syndromes have been treated with high levels of vitamin E intake with no adverse effects.[14,35,75,77,155] Some toxic effects have been associated with parenterally administered α-tocopherol to infants.[155,165,166] Vitamin E supplements may interfere with the anticlotting effects of vitamin K antagonists (e.g., coumadian, warfarin).[167-169,172]

Summary

Although vitamin E is an essential nutrient for the human, deficiencies of the vitamin are relatively rare. Low plasma vitamin E concentrations have been observed in newborn infants, particularly premature infants, certain malabsorption syndromes, cystic fibrosis patients, with high intakes of polyunsaturated fat,[73] genetic abnormalities, and some diseases. Vitamin E status is commonly evaluated by measurement of plasma or serum concentrations of α-tocopherol with the use of high performance liquid chromatography procedures. Concentrations of less than 11.6 µmol/L (5 µg/mL) indicate a poor vitamin E nutritional status. The plasma α-tocopherol (µmol/L) to plasma cholesterol (mmol/L) ratio is also useful for identifying a vitamin E deficiency. A ratio below 2.2 indicates a risk of vitamin E deficiency. The erythrocyte hemolysis test can be informative and can be easily performed without the need for expensive equipment. Hemolysis occurs when the plasma vitamin E concentration falls below 11.6 µmol/L (5 µg/mL). However, fresh blood cells are required that can limit the use of the test.

References

1. Chow, C. K., Evaluation of publicly available scientific evidence regarding certain nutrient-disease relationships: 8C. Vitamin E and cancer, Report of the Life Sciences Research Office, FASEB, Bethesda, MD, 1991, 46.
2. Reavin, P. D. and Witztum, J. L., Oxidized low density lipoproteins in atherogenesis: role of dietary modification, *Annu. Rev. Nutr.*, 16, 51, 1996.
3. Kushi, L. H., Folsom, A. R., Prineas, R. J., Mink, P. J., Wu, Y., and Bostick, R. M., Dietary antioxidant vitamins and death from coronary heart disease in postmenopausal women, *N. Engl. J. Med.*, 334, 1156, 1996.
4. Gaby, S. K. and Machlin, L. J., *Vitamin Intake and Health*, A scientific review: vitamin E, Marcel Dekker, Inc., New York, 1991, 71.
5. Chen, L. H., Boissouneault, G. A., and Glauert, H. P., Vitamin C, vitamin E and cancer (Review), *Anticancer Res.*, 8, 739, 1988.
6. Chow, C. K., Vitamin E and Cancer, in *Nutrition and Disease Update: Cancer*, Carroll, K. K., and Kritchevsky, D., Eds., AOCS Press, Champaign, IL, 1994, chap. 4.
7. Jialal, I., and Grundy, S. M., Influence of antioxidant vitamins on LDL oxidation, *Ann. N.Y. Acad. Sci.*, 669, 237, 1992.
8. Halliwell, B., Antioxidants in human health and disease, *Annu. Rev. Nutr.*, 16, 33, 1996.
9. Burton, G. W. and Trabu, M. G., Vitamin E: antioxidant activity, biokinetics, and bioavailability, *Annu. Rev. Nutr.*, 10, 357, 1990.
10. Rimm, E. B., Stampfer, M. J., Ascherio, A., Giovannucci, E., Colditz, G. A., and Willett, W. C., Vitamin E Consumption and the risk of coronary heart disease in men, *N. Engl. J. Med.*, 328, 1450, 1993.
11. Stampfer, M. J., Hennekens, C. H., Manson, J. E., Colditz, G. A., Rosner, B., and Willett, W. C., Vitamin E consumption and the risk of coronary disease in women, *N. Engl. J. Med.*, 328, 1444, 1993.
12. Kritchevsky, D., Antioxidant vitamins in the prevention of cardiovascular disease, *Nutrition Today*, 27, 30, 1992.
13. Gaziano, J. M., Manson, J. E., Buring, J. E., and Hennekens, C. H., Dietary antioxidants and cardiovascular disease, *Ann. N.Y. Acad. Sci.*, 669, 249, 1992.
14. Traber, M. G. and Sies, H., Vitamin E in humans: demand and delivery, *Annu. Rev. Nutr.*, 16, 321, 1996.
15. Olson, J. A. and Kabayashi, S., Antioxidants in health and disease: overview, *Proc. Soc. Expt. Biol. Med.*, 200, 245, 1992.
16. Krinsky, N. I., Mechanism of action of biological antioxidants, *Proc. Soc. Expt. Biol. Med.*, 200, 248, 1992.
17. Horwitt, M. K., Harvey, C. C., Dahm, C. H., and Searcy, M. T., Relationship between tocopherol and serum lipid levels for determination of nutritional adequacy, *Ann. N.Y. Acad. Sci.*, 203, 223, 1972.
18. Sheppard, A. J., Pennington, J. A. T., and Weihrauch, J. L., Analysis and distribution of vitamin E in vegetable oils and foods, in *Vitamin E in Health and Disease*, Packer, L. and Fuchs, J., Eds., Marcel Dekker, New York, 1993, 9.

19. Horwitt, M. K., Interrelationship between vitamin E and polyunsaturated fatty acids in adult men, *Vit. Horm.*, 20, 541, 1962.
20. Rautalahti, M., Albanes, D., Hyvonen, L., and Piironen, V., Effect of sample site on retinol, carotenoid, tocopherol, and tocotrienol concentrations of adipose tissue of human breast with cancer, *Annu. Nutr. Metab.*, 34, 37, 1990.
21. Tappel, A. L., Vitamin E and free radical peroxidation of lipids, *Ann. N.Y. Acad. Sci.*, 203, 12, 1972.
22. Machlin, L. J., Vitamin E, in *Handbook of Vitamins*, Machlin, L. J., Ed., 2nd edition, Marcel Dekker, New York, 1991, 99.
23. Lehman, J., Comparative sensitivities of tocopherol levels of platelets, red blood cells, and plasma for estimating vitamin E nutritional status in the rat, *Am. J. Clin. Nutr.*, 34, 2104, 1981.
24. Vatassery, G. T., Krezowski, A. M., and Eckfeldt, J. H., Vitamin E concentrations in human blood plasma and platelets, *Am. J. Clin. Nutr.*, 37, 1020, 1983.
25. Chow, C. K., Vitamin E and blood, *World Rev. Nutr. Diet.*, 45, 133, 1985.
26. Stahelin, H. B., Gey, K. F., Eickholzer, M., Ludin, E., and Brubacher, G., Cancer mortality and vitamin E status, *Ann. N.Y. Acad. Sci.*, 507, 391, 1989.
27. Helzlsouer, K. J., Comstock, G. W., and Morris, J. S., Selenium, lycopene, α-tocopherol, β-carotene, retinol, and subsequent bladder cancer, *Cancer Res.*, 49, 6144, 1989.
28. Knekt, P., Seppanen, R., and Aaran, R. –K., Determinants of serum α-tocopherol in Finnish adults, *Prev. Med.*, 17, 725, 1988.
29. Combs, G. F. Jr., *The Vitamins*, Academic Press, New York, 1992, chapter 7.
30. Burton, G. W., Joyce, A., and Ingold, K. U., Is vitamin E the only lipid-soluble, chain-breaking antioxidant in human blood plasma and erythrocyte membranes, *Arch. Biochem. Biophys.*, 221, 281, 1983.
31. Gey, K. F., Puska, P., Jordan, P., and Moser, U. K., Inverse correlation between plasma vitamin E and mortality from ischemic heart disease in cross-cultural epidemiology, *Am. J. Clin. Nutr.*, 53, 326S, 1991.
32. Sokol, R. J., Vitamin E deficiency and neurological disorders, in *Vitamin E in Health and Disease*, Pacher, L., and Fuchs, J., Eds., Marcel Dekker, New York, 1993, 815.
33. Bieri, J. G., and Farrell, P. M., *Vitamin E. Vit. Horm.*, 34, 31, 1976.
34. Sokol, R. J., Vitamin E deficiency and neurologic disease, *Annu. Rev. Nutr.*, 8, 351, 1988.
35. Sokol, R. J., Vitamin E and neurological function in man, *Free Rad. Biol. Med.*, 6, 189, 1989.
36. Packer, L. and Landrick, S., Introduction to biochemistry and health benefits, *Ann. N.Y. Acad. Sci.*, 570, 1, 1989.
37. Burton, G. W. and Ingold, K. U., Vitamin E as an *in vitro* and *in vivo* antioxidant, *Ann. N.Y. Acad. Sci.*, 570, 7, 1989.
38. Nierenberg, D. W. and Lester, D. C., Determination of vitamins A and E in serum and plasma using a simplified clarification method and high performance liquid chromatography, *J. Chromatogr. Biomed. Appl.*, 375, 275, 1985.
39. Dimitrov, N. V., Meyer, C., Gilliland, D., Ruppenthal, M., Chenoweth, W., and Malone, W., Plasma Tocoperol concentrations in response to supplemental vitamin E, *Am. J. Clin. Nutr.*, 53, 723, 1991.
40. Fahn, S., A pilot trial of high-dose alpha-tocoperol and ascorbate in early Parkinson's disease, *Ann. Neurol.*, 32, S128, 1992.
41. Knekt, P., Heliovaar, M., Rissanen, A., Aroma, A., and Aaran, R.–K., Serum antioxidant vitamins and risk of cataracts, *BMJ*, 305, 1392, 1992.
42. Sokol, R. J., Balistreri, W. F., Hoofnagle, J. H., and Jones, E. A., Vitamin E deficiency in adults with chronic liver disease, *Am. J. Clin. Nutr.*, 41, 66, 1985.
43. Zannos-Mariolea, L., Papagregorius-Theodoridou, M., Costantzas, N., and Matsaniotis, N., Relationship between tocopherols and serum lipid levels in children with β-thalassemia major, *Am. J. Clin. Nutr.*, 31, 259, 1978.
44. Horwitt, M. K., Therapeutic use of vitamin E in medicine, *Nutr. Revs.*, 38, 105, 1980.
45. Losvnczy, K. G., Harris, T. B., and Hanlik, R. J., Vitamin E and vitamin C supplement use and risk of all-cause and coronary heart disease mortality in older persons: the established populations for epidemiology studies of the elderly, *Am. J. Clin. Nutr.*, 64, 190, 1996.

46. Jain, S. K., Vitamin E and membrane abnormalities in red cells of sickle cell disease patients and newborn infants, *Ann. N.Y. Acad. Sci.*, 570, 461, 1989.

47. Kayden, H. J. and Traber, M. G., Neuropathies in adults with or without fat malabsorption, *Ann. N.Y. Acad. Sci.*, 570, 170, 1989.

48. Pereira, C. R., Controversies in neonatal nutrition, *Pediatr. Clinics of North America*, 33, 65, 1986.

49. Muller, D. P. R. and Lloyd, J. K., Effect of large doses of vitamin E on the neurological sequelae of patients with abetalycoproteinemia, *Ann. N.Y. Acad. Sci.*, 393, 133, 1982.

50. Halvoet, P. and Collen, D., Oxidized lipoproteins in atherosclerosis and thrombosis, Review, *FASEB J.*, 8, 1279, 1994.

51. Bendich, A., Vitamin E and immune functions, Review, *Basic Life Sci.*, 49, 615, 1988.

52. Farrel, P. M. and Roberts, R. J., Vitamin E, in *Modern Nutrition in Health and Disease*, Shils, M. E., Olson, J. A., and Shike, M., Eds., Lea & Febiger, Philadelphia, 1994, 326.

53. Stephens, N. G., Parsons, A., Schofield, P. M., Kelly, F., Cheeseman, K., Mitchinson, M. J., and Brown, M. J., Randomised-controlled trial of vitamin E in patients with coronary disease: Cambridge Heart Antioxidant Study (CHAOS), *Lancet*, 347, 781, 1996.

54. Jial, I. and Grundy, S. M., Effect of combined supplementation with α-tocopherol, ascorbate, and Beta-carotene on low-density lipoprotein oxidation, *Circulation*, 88, 2780, 1993.

55. Gey, K. F., Inverse correlation of vitamin E and ischemic heart disease, in *Elevated Dosages of Vitamins: Benefits and Hazards*, Walter, P., Brubacher, G., and Stahelin, H., Eds., Hans Huber Publishers, Lewiston, 1989, 224.

56. Thurnham, D. I., Davies, J. A., Crump, B. J., Situnayake, R. D., and Davis, M., The use of different lipids to express serum tocopherol: lipid ratios for the measurement of vitamin E status, *Annu. Clin. Biochem.*, 23, 514, 1986.

57. Jialal, I. and Grundy, S. M., Effect of dietary supplementation with alpha-tocopherol on the oxidative modification of low density lipoproteins, *J. Lipid Res.*, 33, 899, 1992.

58. Jialal, I., Fuller, C. J., and Huet, B. A., The effect of α-tocopherol supplementation on LDL oxidation, A dose-response study, *Arterioscler. Thomb. Vasc. Biol.*, 15, 190, 1995.

59. Witzum, H. and Steinberg, D., Role of oxidized low density lipoprotein in atherogenesis, *J. Clin. Invest.*, 88, 1785, 1991.

60. Jiirgens, G., Hoff, H. F., Chisolm, G. M. III, and Esterbauer, H., Modification of human serum low density lipoprotein by oxidation: characterization and pathophysiological implications, *Chem. Phys. Lipids*, 45, 315, 1987.

61. Steinberg, D., Antioxidant vitamins and coronary heart disease, *N. Engl. J. Med.*, 323, 1487, 1993.

62. Sies, H., Relationship between free radicals and vitamins: an overview, in *Elevated Dosages of Vitamins: Benefits and Hazards*, Walter, P., Brubacher, G. B., and Stahelin, H. B., Eds., Hans Huber Publishers, Lewiston, 1989, 215.

63. Hodis, H. N., Mack, W. J., LaBree, L., Cashin-Hemphill, L., Sevanian, A., Johnson, R., and Azen, S. P., Serial coronary angiographic evidence that antioxidant vitamin intake reduces progression of coronary artery atherosclerosis, *JAMA*, 273, 1849, 1995.

64. Sano, M., Ernesto, C., Thomas, R. G., Klauber, M. R., Schafer, K. et al., A controlled trial of selegiline, alpha-tocopherol, or both as treatment for Alzheimer's disease, *N. Engl. J. Med.*, 336, 1216, 1997.

65. Bauernfeind, J. C., The tocopherol content of food and influencing factors, *Critical Rev. Food Science and Nutr.*, 8, 337, 1977.

66. Horwitt, M. K., Vitamin E and lipid metabolism in man, *Am. J. Clin. Nutr.*, 8, 451, 1960.

67. Binder, H. J. and Spiro, H. M., Tocopherol deficiency in man, *Am. J. Clin. Nutr.*, 20, 594, 1967.

68. Evans, H. M., The pioneer history of vitamin E, *Vitamins and Hormones*, 20, 379, 1962.

69. Murphy, S. P., Subar, A. F., and Block, G., Vitamin E intake and sources in the United States, *Am. J. Clin. Nutr.*, 52, 361, 1990.

70. Davies, T., Kelleher, J., and Losowsky, M. S., Interrelation of serum lipoprotein and tocopherol levels, *Clin. Chim. Acta*, 24, 431, 1969.

71. Rubenstein, H. M., Dietz, A. A., and Srinavasan, R., Relation of vitamin E and serum lipids, *Clin. Chim. Acta*, 23, 1, 1969.

72. Traber, M. G. and Kayden, H. J., Vitamin E is delivered to cells by the high affinity receptor for low-density lipoprotein, *Am. J. Clin. Nutr.* 40, 747, 1984.

73. Horwitt, M. K., Status of human requirements for vitamin E, *Am. J. Clin. Nutr.*, 27, 1182, 1974.
74. Kayden, H. J., The neurologic syndrome of vitamin E deficiency: a significant cause of ataxia, *Neurology*, 43, 2167, 1993.
75. Sokol, R. J., Butler-Simon, N., Heubi, J. E. et al., Vitamin E deficiency neuropathy in children with fat malabsorption: studies in cystic fibrosis and chronic cholestasis, *Ann. N.Y. Acad. Sci.*, 570, 156, 1989.
76. Wilfond, B. S., Farrell, P. M., Laxova, A., and Mischler, E., Severe hemolytic anemia associated with vitamin E deficiency in infants with cystic fibrosis, *Clinical Pediatrics*, January, 1994.
77. Sokol, R. J., Butler-Simon, N., Conner, C., Heubi, J. E. et al. Multi-center trial of *d*-α-tocopherol polyethylene glycol 1000 succinate for treatment of vitamin E deficiency in children with chronic cholestasis, *Gastroenterology*, 104, 1727, 1993.
78. Oski, F. A., Metabolism and physiologic roles of vitamin E, *Hospital Practice*, 12 (10), 79, 1977.
79. Cynamon, H. A. and Isenberg, J. N., Application of a new test for vitamin E deficiency to cystic fibrosis, *Eur. J. Pediatr.*, 146, 512, 1987.
80. Kelly, F. J., Rodgers, W., Handel, J., Smith, S., and Hall, M. A., Time course of vitamin E repletion in the premature infant, *Br. J. Nutr.*, 69, 631, 1990.
81. Ferlin, M. L. S., Martinez, F. E., Jorge, S. M., Goncalves, A. L., and Desai, I. D., Vitamin E in preterm infants during the first year of life, *Ann. N.Y. Acad. Sci.*, 570, 443, 1989.
82. Gutcher, G. R., Raynor, W. J., and Farrell, P. M., An evaluation of vitamin E status in premature infants, *Am. J. Clin. Nutr.*, 40, 1078, 1984.
83. Mino, M., Clinical uses and abuses of vitamin E in children, *PSEBM*, 200, 266, 1992.
84. Traber, M. G., Schiano, T. D., Steephen, A. C., Kayden, H. J., and Shike, M., Efficacy of water-soluble vitamin E in the treatment of vitamin E malabsorption in short-bowel syndrome, *Am. J. Clin. Nutr.*, 59, 1270, 1994.
85. Kowdley, K. V., Mason, J. B., Meydani, S. N., Cornwall, S., and Grand, R. J., Vitamin E deficiency and impaired cellular immunity related to intestinal fat malabsorption, *Gastroenterology*, 102, 2139, 1992.
86. Sokol, R. J., Kim, Y. S., Hoofnagle, J. H., Heubi, J. E., Jones, E. A., and Balistreri, W. F., Intestinal malabsorption of vitamin E in primary biliary cirrhosis, *Gastroenterology*, 96, 479, 1989.
87. Stephens, N., Anti-oxidant therapy for ischaemic heart disease: where do we stand, *Lancet*, 349, 1710, 1997.
88. Bendich, A., Vitamin E status of U.S. children, *J. Am. Coll. Nutr.*, 11, 441, 1992.
89. Farrell, P. M., Levine, S. L., Murphy, M. D., and Adams, A. J., Plasma tocopherol levels and tocopherol-lipid relationships in a normal population of children as compared to healthy adults, *Am. J. Clin. Nutr.*, 31, 1720, 1978.
90. Horwitt, M. K., Harvey, C. C., Duncan, G. D., and Wilson, W. C., Effects of limited tocopherol intake in man with relationships to erythrocyte hemolysis and lipid oxidations, *Am. J. Clin. Nutr.*, 4, 408, 1956.
91. Bieri, J. G., Tolliver, R. L., and Catignani, G. L., Simultaneous determination of α-tocopherol and retinol in plasma or red cells by high pressure liquid chromatography, *Am. J. Clin. Nutr.*, 32, 2143, 1979.
92. Gordon, H. H., Nitowsky, H. M., and Cornblath, M., Studies of tocopherol deficiency in infants and children, I., Hemolysis of erythrocytes in hydrogen peroxide, *Am. J. Dis. Child*, 90, 669, 1955.
93. Cynamon, H. A., Isenberg, J. N., and Nguyen, C. H., Erythrocyte malondialdehyde release *in vitro:* a functional measure of vitamin E status, *Clin. Chim. Acta*, 151, 169, 1985.
94. Hansen, L. G. and Warwick, W. J., A fluorometric micromethod for serum vitamin A and E, *Am. J. Clin. Pathol.*, 51, 538, 1969.
95. Bieri, J. G., Poulka, R. K. H., and Prival, E. L., Determination of α-tocopherol in erythrocytes by gas-liquid chromatography, *J. Lipid Res.*, 11, 118, 1970.
96. Bunnell, R. H., Vitamin E assay by chemical methods, in *The Vitamins*, Volume VI, 2nd edition, Gyorgy, P. and Pearson, W. N., Eds., Academic Press, New York, 1967, 261.
97. Herting, D. C. and Drury, E. J. E., Plasma tocopherol levels in man, *Am. J. Clin. Nutr.*, 17, 351, 1965.

98. Hashim, S. A. and Schuttringer, G. R., Rapid determination of tocopherol in macro- and microquantities of plasma, Results obtained in various nutrition and metabolic studies, *Am. J. Clin. Nutr.*, 19, 137, 1966.
99. Bieri, J. G. and Privel, E. L., Serum vitamin E determined by thin-layer chromatography, *Proc. Soc. Extl. Biol. Med.*, 120, 554, 1965.
100. Duggan, D. E., Spectrofluorometric determination of tocopherols, *Arch. Biochem. Biophys.*, 84, 116, 1959.
101. Kayden, H. J., Chow, C. K., and Bjornson, L. K., Spectrophotometric method for determination of tocopherol in red blood cells, *J. Lipid Res.*, 14, 533, 1973.
102. Lehman, J. and Slover, H. T., Determination of plasma tocopherols by gas-liquid chromatography, *Lipids*, 6, 35, 1971.
103. Lovelady, H. G., Separation of individual tocopherols from human plasma and red blood cells by thin-layer and gas-liquid chromatography, *J. Chromatogr.*, 85, 81, 1973.
104. Chow, C. K., Distribution of tocopherols in human plasma and red blood cells, *Am. J. Clin. Nutr.*, 28, 756, 1975.
105. Lehmann, J. and Martin, H. L., Improved direct determination of alpha- and gamma-tocopherols in plasma and platelets by liquid chromatography, with fluorescence detection, *Clin. Chem.*, 28, 1784, 1982.
106. Henton, D. H., Merritt, R. J., and Hack, S., Vitamin E measurements in patients receiving intravenous lipid emulsions, *J. Parenterol. Enteral. Nutr.*, 16, 133, 1992.
107. Osterlof, G. and Nyheim, A., The estimation of α-tocopherol in biological material by gas chromatography, *J. Chromatogr.*, 183, 487, 1980.
108. Catignani, G. L. and Bieri, J. G., Simultaneous determination of retinol and α-tocopherol in serum or plasma by liquid chromatography, *Clin. Chem.*, 29, 708, 1983.
109. Milne, D. B. and Botnen, J., Retinol, alpha-tocopherol, lycopene, and alpha- and beta-carotene simultaneously determined in plasma by isocratic liquid chromatography, *Clin. Chem.*, 32, 874, 1986.
110. Epler, K. S., Ziegler, R. G., and Craft, N. E., Liquid chromatographic method for the determination of carotinoids, retinoids and tocopherols in human serum and food, *J. Chromatogr. Biomed. Appl.*, 619, 37, 1993.
111. Vuilleumier, J.-P., Keller, H. E., Gysel, D., and Hunziker, F., Clinical chemical methods for the routine assessment of the vitamin status in human populations. I: The fat-soluble vitamins A and E, and β-carotene, *Int. J. Vit. Nutr. Res.*, 53, 265, 1983.
112. Vandewoude, M., Claeys, M., and Leeuw, I., Determination of α-tocopherol in human plasma by high-performance liquid chromatography with electrochemical detection, *J. Chromatogr. Biomed. Appli.*, 311, 176, 1984.
113. Castle, M. C. and Cooke, W. J., Measurement of vitamin E in serum and plasma by high performance liquid chromatography with electrochemical detection, *Therapeutic Drug Monitoring*, 7, 364, 1985.
114. Chou, P. P., Jaynes, P. K., and Bailey, J. L., Determination of vitamin E in microsamples of serum by liquid chromatography with electrochemical detection, *Clin. Chem.*, 31, 880, 1985.
115. Lang, J. K., Gohil, K., and Packer, L., Simultaneous determination of tocopherols, ubiquinols, and ubiquinones in blood, plasma, tissue homogenates, and subcellular fractions, *Anal. Biochem.*, 157, 106, 1986.
116. Huang, M. L., Burckart, G. J., and Venkateramann, R., Sensitive high-performance liquid chromatographic analyses of plasma vitamin E and vitamin A using amperometric and ultraviolet detection, *J. Chromatogr. Biomed. Appl.*, 380, 331, 1986.
117. Kaempf, D. E., Miki, M., Ogihara, T., Okamoto, R., Konishi, K., and Mino, M., Assessment of vitamin E nutritional status in neonates, infants and children on the basis of α-tocopherol levels in blood components and buccal mucosal cells, *Int. J. Vit. Nutr. Res.*, 64, 185, 1994.
118. Miller, K. W. and Yang, C. S., An isocratic high-performance liquid chromatography method for simultaneous analysis of plasma retinol, α-tocopherol, and various carotenoids, *Anal. Biochem.*, 145, 21, 1985.

119. Stacewicz-Sapuntzakis, M., Bowen, P. E., Kikendall, J. W., and Burgess, M., Simultaneous determination of serum retinol, and various carotenoids: their distribution in middle-aged men and women, *J. Micronutr. Anal.*, 3, 27, 1989.

120. Driskell, W. J., Neese, J. W., Bryant, C. C., and Bashor, M. M., Measurement of vitamin A and vitamin E in human serum by high-performance liquid chromatography, *J. Chromatogr. Biomed. Appl.*, 231, 439, 1982.

121. Chow, F. I. and Omaye, S. T., Use of antioxidants in the analysis of vitamin A and E in mammalian plasma by HPLC, *Lipids*, 18, 837, 1983.

122. Bortolotti, A., Lucchini, G., Barzago, M. M., Stellari, F., and Bonati, M., Simultaneous determination of retinol, α-tocopherol and retinyl palmitate in plasma of premature newborns by reversed-phase high-performance liquid chromatography, *J. Chromatogr. Biomed. Appl.*, 617, 313, 1993.

123. De Leenheer, A. P., De Bevere, V., De Ruyter, M. G. M., and Claeys, A. E., Simultaneous determination of retinol and α-tocopherol in human serum by high-performance liquid chromatography, *J. Chromatogr.*, 162, 408, 1979.

124. Hansen, L. G. and Warwick, W. J., A fluorometric micromethod for serum tocopherol, *Am. J. Clin. Pathol.*, 50, 525, 1968.

125. Thompson, J. N., Erdody, P., and Maxwell, W. B., Simultaneous fluorometric determination of vitamins A and E in human serum and plasma, *Biochem. Med.* 8, 403, 1972.

126. Choudhury, N., Tan, L., and Truswell, A. S., Comparison of palmalein and olive oil: effects on plasma lipids and vitamin E in young adults, *Am. J. Clin. Nutr.*, 61, 1043, 1995.

127. Hayes, K. C., Pronczuk, A., and Liang, J. S., Differences in the plasma transport and tissue concentrations of tocopherols and tocotrienols: observations in humans and hamsters, *Proc. Soc. Exp. Biol. Med.*, 202, 353, 1993.

128. Sauberlich, H. E., Dowdy, R. P., and Skala, J. H., *Laboratory Tests for the Assessment of Nutritional Status*, CRC Press, Boca Raton, FL, 1974.

129. Cynamon, H. A. and Isenberg, J. N., Characterization of vitamin E status in cholestatic children by conventional laboratory standards and a new functional assay, *J. Pediatr. Gastroenterology and Nutr.*, 6, 46, 1987.

130. Esterbauer, H., Lang, J., Zddravec, S., and Slater, T. F., Detection of malondialdehyde by high performance liquid chromatography, in *Methods in Enzymology*, Packer, L., Ed., Academic Press, New York, 1984.

131. Cynamon, H. A., Isenberg, J. N., and Nguyen, C. H., Erythrocyte malondialdehyde release *in vitro*: a functional measure of vitamin E status, *Clinica. Chimaca. Acta*, 151, 169, 1985.

132. Lemoyne, M., Van Gosssum, A., Kurian, R., Ostro, M., Axler, J., and Jeejeebhoy, K. N., Breath pentane analysis as an index of lipid peroxidation: a functional test of vitamin E status, *Am. J. Clin. Nutr.*, 46, 267, 1987.

133. New functional test of vitamin E status in humans, *Nutr. Reviews*, 46, 182, 1988.

134. Shariff, R., Hoshino, E., Allard, J., Prichard, C., Kurian, R., and Jeejeebhoy, K. N., Vitamin E supplementation in smokers, *Am. J. Clin. Nutr.*, 47, 758, 1988 (Abstract).

135. Refat, M., Moore, T. J., Kazui, M., Risby, T. H., Perman, J. A., and Schwarz, K. B., Utility of breath ethane as a noninvasive biomarker of vitamin E status in children, *Pediatr. Res.*, 30, 396, 1991.

136. Fabianek, J., DeFilippi, J., Rickards, J., and Herp, A., Micromethod for tocopherol determination in blood serum, *Clin. Chem.*, 14, 456, 1968.

137. Rose, C. S. and Gyorgy, P., Specificity of hemolytic reaction in vitamin E deficient erythrocytes, *Am. J. Physiol.*, 168, 414, 1952.

138. Stormont, J. M., Hirshberg, E. A., and Davidson, C. S., The peroxide-erythrocyte hemolysis test, Experiences in patients with cirrhosis, jaundice, and polyneuritis, *Am. J. Clin. Nutr.*, 7, 206, 1959.

139. Binder, H. J., Herting, D. C., Hurst, V., Finch, S. C., and Spiro, H. M., Tocopherol deficiency in man, *N. Engl. J. Med.*, 273, 1289, 1965.

140. Panemangalore, M. and Lee, C. J., Evaluation of the indices of retinol and α-tocopherol status in free-living elderly, *J. Gerontology: Biomed. Sci.*, 47, B98, 1992.

141. Thurlow, P. M. and Grant, J. P., Vitamin E and total parenteral nutrition, *Ann. N.Y. Acad. Sci.*, 393, 121, 1982.

142. Broxson, E. Jr., Sokol, R. J., and Githerns, J. H., Normal vitamin E status in sickle hemo-globinopathies in Colorado, *Am. J. Clin. Nutr.*, 50, 497, 1989.

143. Ferro-Luzzi, A., Mobarhan, S., Maiani, G., Scaccini, C., Virgili, F., and Knurman, J. T., Vitamin E status in Italian children subsisting on a Mediterranean diet, *Human Nutr.: Clin. Nutr.*, 38C, 1995, 1984.

144. Ohrvall, M., Tengblad, S., and Vessby, B., Tocopherol concentrations in adipose tissue, Relationship of tocopherol concentrations and fatty acid composition in serum in a reference population of Swedish men and women, *Eur. J. Clin. Nutr.*, 48, 212, 1994.

145. Wei Wo, C. K. and Draper, H. H., Vitamin E status of Alaskan Eskimos, *Am. J. Clin. Nutr.*, 28, 808, 1975.

146. Brown, K. M., Morrice, P. C., Duthie, G. G., Erythrocyte vitamin E and plasma ascorbate concentrations in relation to erythrocyte peroxidation in smokers and nonsmokers: dose response to vitamin E supplementation, *Am. J. Clin. Nutr.*, 65, 496, 1997.

147. Euronut SENECA study, Nutritional status: blood vitamins A, E, B_6, B_{12}, folic acid and carotene, *Eur. J. Clin. Nutr.*, 45, 63, 1991.

148. Mino, M. and Nagamatu, M., An evaluation of nutritional status of vitamin E in pregnant women with respect to red blood cell tocopherol level, *Int. J. Vit. Nutr. Res.*, 56, 149, 1986.

149. Morino, T., Tamai, H., Tanabe, T., Murata, T., Manago, M., Mino, M., and Hirahara, F., Plasma α-tocopherol, β-carotene, and retinol levels in the institutionalized elderly individuals and in young adults, *Int. J. Vit. Nutr. Res.*, 64, 104, 1994.

150. Mino, M., Kitagawa, M., and Nakagawa, S., Red blood cell tocopherol concentrations in a normal population of Japanese children and premature infants in relation to the assessment of vitamin E status, *Am. J. Clin. Nutr.*, 41, 631, 1985.

151. Fenech, M. and Rinaldi, J., The relationship between micronuclei in human lymphocytes and plasma levels of vitamin C, vitamin E, vitamin B_{12}, and folic acid, *Carcinogenesis*, 15, 1405, 1994.

152. Fotouhi, N., Meydani, M., Santor, S., Meydani, S. N., Hennekens, C. H., and Gaziano, J. M., Carotenoid and tocopherol concentrations in plasma, peripheral blood mononuclear cells, and red blood cells after long-term β-carotene supplementation in men, *Am. J. Clin. Nutr.*, 63, 553, 1996.

153. Gross, S. J. and Landaw, S. A., The effect of vitamin E on red cell hemolysis and bilirubinemia, *Ann. N.Y. Acad. Sci.*, 393, 315, 1982.

154. Vatassery, G. T., Kezowski, A. M., and Eckfeldt, J. H., Vitamin E concentrations in human blood plasma and platelets, *Am. J. Clin. Nutr.*, 37, 1020, 1983.

155. Phelps, D. L., Current perspectives on vitamin E in infant nutrition, *Am. J. Clin. Nutr.*, 46, 187, 1987.

156. Bell, E. F., History of vitamin E in infant nutrition, *Am. J. Clin. Nutr.*, 46, 183, 1987.

157. Booth, S. L., Tucker, K. L., McKeown, N. M., Davidson, K. W., Dalla, G. E., and Sadowski, J. A., Relationships between dietary intakes and fasting plasma concentrations of fat-soluble vitamins in humans, *J. Nutr.*, 127, 587, 1997.

158. Bergen, H. R., Natadiastra, G., Muhilal, H., Dedi, A., Karyadi, D., and Olson, J. A., Vitamin A and vitamin E status of rural preschool children of West Java, Indonesia, and their response to oral doses of vitamin A and of vitamin E, *Am. J. Clin. Nutr.*, 48, 279, 1988.

159. Looker, A. C., Underwood, B. A., Wiley, J., Fulwood, R., and Sempos, C. T., Serum α-tocopherol levels of Mexican Americans, Cubans, and Puerto Ricans aged 4–74 years, *Am. J. Clin. Nutr.*, 50, 491, 1989.

160. Behrens, W. A. and Madere, R., Alpha- and gamma-tocopherol concentrations in human serum, *J. Am. Coll. Nutr.*, 5, 91, 1986.

161. Godel, J. C., Vitamin E status of northern Canadian newborns: relation of vitamin E to blood lipids, *Am. J. Clin. Nutr.*, 50, 375, 1989.

162. Schwalbe, P., Büttner, P., and Elmades, I., Development of vitamin E status premature infants after intravenous applications of all-rac-α-tocopherol acetate, *Int. J. Vit. Nutr. Res.*, 62, 9, 1992.

163. Von Mandach, U., Huch, R., and Huch, A., Maternal and cord serum vitamin E levels in normal and abnormal pregnancy, *Int. J. Vit. Nutr. Res.*, 63, 26, 1993.

164. Ronnholm, K. A. R., Dostalova, L., and Siimes, M. A., Vitamin supplementation in very-low-birth-weight infants: long-term follow-up at two different levels of vitamin E supplementation, *Am. J. Clin. Nutr.*, 49, 121, 1989.

165. Bell, E. F. and Filer L. J. Jr., The role of vitamin E in the nutrition of premature infants, *Am. J. Clin. Nutr.*, 34, 414, 1981.

166. Phelps, D. L., The role of vitamin E therapy in high-risk neonates, *Clinics in Perinatology*, 15, 955, 1988.

167. Corrigan, J. J., The effect of vitamin E on warfarin-induced vitamin K deficiency, *Ann. N.Y. Acad. Sci.*, 393, 361, 1982.

168. Bieri, J. G., Effects of excessive vitamin C and E on vitamin A status, *Am. J. Clin. Nutr.*, 26, 382, 1973.

169. Machlin, L. J. and Bendich, A., The use and safety of elevated dosages of vitamin E in adults, in *Elevated Dosages of Vitamins: Benefits and Hazards*, Walter, P., Brubacher, G., Stahelin, H., Eds., Han Huber Publishers, Lewiston, 1989, 56.

170. Mino, M., Use and safety of elevated dosages of vitamin E in infants and children, in *Elevated Dosages of Vitamins: Benefits and Hazards*, Walter, P., Brubacher, G., and Stahelin, H., Eds., Han Huber Publishers, Lewiston, 1989, 69.

171. Kappus, H. and Diplock, A. T., Tolerance and safety of vitamin E: a toxicological position report (Review), *Free Radical Biol. Med.*, 13, 55, 1992.

172. Bendich, A. and Machlin, L. J., Safety of oral intakes of vitamin E, *Am. J. Clin. Nutr.*, 48, 612, 1988.

173. Garewal, H. S. and Diplock, A. T., How 'safe' are antioxidant vitamins, *Drug Safety*, 13, 8, 1995.

174. Hathcock, J. N., *Vitamin and Mineral Safety*, Council for Responsible Nutrition, Washington D.C., 1996.

175. Meydani, S. N., Meydani, M., Rall, L. C., Morrow, F., and Blumberg, J. B., Assessment of the safety of high-dose, short-term supplementation with vitamin E in healthy older adults, *Am. J. Clin. Nutr.*, 60, 704, 1994.

176. Stampfer, M. J. and Rimm, E. B., Epidemiologic evidence for vitamin E in prevention of cardiovascular disease, *Am. J. Clin. Nutr.*, 62, 1365S, 1995.

177. Evans, H. M. and Bishop, K. S., On the existence of a hitherto unrecognized dietary factor essential for reproduction, *Science*, 56, 650, 1922.

178. Mason, K. E., The first two decades of vitamin E, *Fed. Proc.*, 36, 1906, 1977.

179. Salkeld, R. M., Safety and tolerance of high-dose vitamin E administration in man: a review of the literature, F. Hoffman-LaRoche & Co., Basle, Switzerland, unpublished report, January 10, 1975.

180. Evans, H. M., Emerson, O. M., and Emerson, G. A., The isolation from wheat germ oil of an alcohol, α-tocopherol, having the properties of vitamin E, *J. Biol. Chem.*, 113, 319, 1936.

181. Bieri, J. G., Teets, L., Belavady, B., and Andrews, E. L., Serum vitamin E levels in a normal adult population in the Washington D.C. area, *Proc. Soc. Exp. Biol. Med.*, 117, 131, 1964.

182. Harris, P. L., Hardenbrook, E. G., Dean, F. P., Cusack, E. R., and Jensen, J. L., Blood tocopherol values in normal human adults and incidence of vitamin E deficiency, *Proc. Soc. Exp. Biol. Med.*, 107, 381, 1961.

183. MacCrehan, W. A. and Schonberger, E., Determination of retinol, α-tocopherol, and β-carotene in serum by liquid chromatography with absorbance and electrochemical detection, *Clin. Chem.*, 33, 1585, 1987.

184. Diplock, A. T., Safety of antioxidant vitamins and β-carotene, *Am. J. Clin. Nutr.*, 62, 1510S, 1995.

185. Morrissey, P. A., Sheehy, P. J. A., and Gaynor, P., Vitamin E, *Int. J. Vit. Nutr. Res.*, 63, 260, 1993.

Vitamin K

Vitamin K_1 (phylloquinone): present in green plants
molecular weight: 450.68

Vitamin K_2 (menaquinone): produced by bacteria

Converting metric units to International System units (SI):
ng/mL phylloquinone × 2.219 = nmol/L phylloquinone
nmol/L phylloquinone × 0.4507 = ng/mL phylloquinone

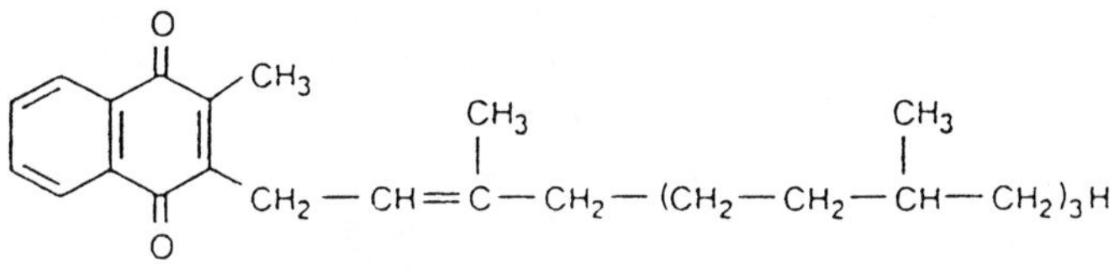

FIGURE 50
Structure of phylloquinone
(vitamin K).

Phylloquinone (Vitamin K_1)

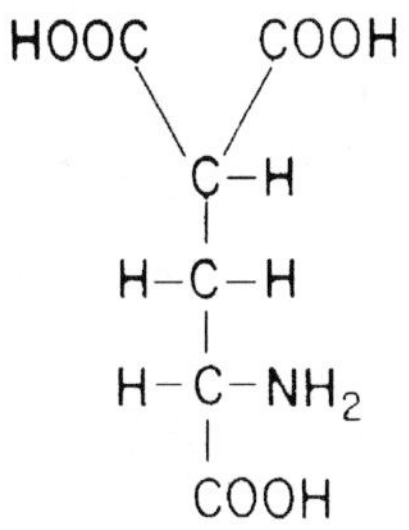

FIGURE 51
Structure of γ-carboxyglutamic
acid (Gla).

Introduction

Vitamin K is one of the fat-soluble vitamins. The history of the discovery of vitamin K and its functions and metabolism have been summarized in various reviews.[5-10,15-18,124,125] In 1929, Henrik Dam of Denmark discovered vitamin K.[17,20-22] Subsequently, vitamin K_1 was isolated from alfalfa by Dam and associates[20-22] and by Doisy and associates in St. Louis, MO.[18-19] The structure was determined to be 2-methyl-3-phytyl-1,4-naphthoquinone (vitamin K_1).[23,24]

All compounds with vitamin K activity contain the 2-methyl-1,4-napthoquinone nucleus. Because vitamin K is light sensitive, precautions need to be taken to protect the vitamin during analysis. In the human, the turnover of vitamin K is rapid with a relatively small total body pool.[12,15,16]

Sources of Vitamin K

Vitamin K_1 (phylloquinone) is synthesized by green plants which can serve as a major source of vitamin K for the human.[11,65] Vitamin K is also present in significant amounts in animal products and most oils.

Vitamin K contents of most food items are listed:[11,65,86,125]

	Vitamin K (μg/100 g)
Vegetables	
Broccoli (raw)	154
Cabbage (raw)	149
Carrots (raw)	13
Cauliflower (raw)	191
Kale (raw)	275
Lettuce (raw)	113
Spinach (raw)	266
Tomatoes (ripe)	23
Fruits	
Oranges (raw)	1
Strawberries (raw)	14
Oils	
Canola oil	830
Soybean oil	200
Cottonseed oil	60
Corn oil	5
Olive Oil	55
Miscellaneous	
Whole wheat flour	1
Lentils (dry)	22
Eggs (whole)	50
Beef liver (raw)	104
Bacon	46
Milk, cow, whole	4
Cheese	35

In general, animal products, including milk, are relatively poor sources of vitamin K. However, another source of vitamin K for the human is the production of vitamin K_2 (menaquinones) by the intestinal flora.[8,9,12,66,85,86] Results of human studies indicate that the menaquinones may account for 75 to 95% of the total hepatic stores of vitamin K on a molar basis.[8,12] However, the usefulness of these stores to the maintenance of vitamin K sufficiency is uncertain.[8]

Vitamin K Deficiency

Vitamin K is essential for the post-translational carboxylation of certain glutamate residues to γ-carboxyglutamate residues in a number of proteins.[5,9,15,124,125] Bacterial flora in the jijunum and ileum may also provide vitamin K. Thus approximately one-half of the vitamin K intake may be provided by bacterial synthesis.[2,3,85,125] Consequently, vitamin K deficiency may occur in adult subjects treated with antibiotics for an extended period.

Other causes of impaired vitamin K function include the use of coumarin anticoagulants (warfarin, coumadin), total parenteral nutrition, liver disease, dietary inadequacies, and megadoses of vitamin E.[36,87,116] The vitamin K-dependent coagulation factors are synthesized in the liver. Hence, liver disease can result in lowered plasma levels of these factors and in reduced response to vitamin K therapy. Younger subjects have been reported to be more sensitive to dietary vitamin K depletion than older subjects.[53] Lower serum levels of vitamin K have been reported to occur in elderly persons.[120] Based on the current U.S. Recommended Dietary Allowance[68] for vitamin K (80 μg/day for adult males and 65 μg/day for adult women), a number of adults in the United States, particularly the younger adults, are not obtaining these allowances.[125]

Clinical Patient

A vitamin K deficiency is associated with a prolonged prothrombin time and ecchymoses (small hemorrhagic spots). When a vitamin K deficiency is suspected, a plasma prothrombin time should be obtained. The normal prothrombin time is two seconds or less beyond the control time. When available, measurement of plasma vitamin K concentrations or of specific clotting factors should be considered. Normally, a prolonged prothrombin time can be corrected in 12 to 24 hours with intravenous vitamin K, administration. Subjects with chronic fat malabsorption are at an increased risk of a vitamin K deficiency, such as with jaundice.

Newborn and Infants

Breast-fed infants commonly have a very poor vitamin K status with low plasma prothrombin concentrations.[3,5,6,15,88,96,97,99] Human milk is a poor source of vitamin K (2 μg/L). Moreover, infants have not established in their intestine an effective flora of vitamin K-synthesizing bacteria. In addition, the neonatal liver is immature with regards to its ability to synthesize prothrombin. Therefore, newborn infants are given vitamin K_1 immediately after birth to prevent hemorragic disease. Hemorragic disease is of significant concern throughout most of the world.[99]

Miscellaneous Conditions

A vitamin K deficiency may be associated with a number of disorders. Subjects with certain chronic forms of gastrointestinal disorders are commonly deficient in vitamin K.[76] Other conditions that pose a risk of a vitamin K deficiency include patients with primary biliary cirrhosis,[77] antibiotic therapy,[3,78] cancer,[79] and long-term hyperalimentation,[3] surgery,[80] and chronic alcoholism.[83] In these disorders, vitamin K deficiency was assessed largely by the presence of abnormal prothrombin (PIVKA-II) in the plasma as measured by a radioimmunoassay.[81,82] Levels of abnormal prothrombin greater than 20 ng per mL of plasma were considered to indicate vitamin K deficiency.[76] The abnormal prothrombin immunoassay (PIVKA-II) was considered approximately 1000-fold more sensitive than the prothrombin time test for the diagnosis of vitamin K deficiency.[76]

Blood Clotting Process

The blood clotting process involves the participation of a number of vitamin K dependent plasma proteins. They include factors II (prothrombin), XII (proconvertin), IX (Christmas factor), and X (Stewart factor), and proteins C, S, Z, and M.[1,5,6,9,36,41,89,111-113]

For these proteins, vitamin K functions in the post-translational carboxylation of certain glutamate residues to γ-carboxyglutamate (Gla) residues.[5,9] All Gla-containing proteins are characterized by a high affinity for calcium. Thus, the γ-carboxyglutamate residues of prothrombin bind calcium to form thrombin. With inadequate vitamin K_1 present, the γ-carboxyglutamate residues do not form and calcium is not bound to the prothrombin and thus blood clotting does not occur. Plasma levels of undercarboxylated prothrombin (PIVKA-II) have been used as a marker of vitamin K deficiency.[118]

Vitamin K and Anticoagulants

In the human, vitamin K deficiency is often associated with the use of anti-coagulants (e.g., warfarin, coumadin) which inhibit vitamin K epoxide reductase.[46-49,87] Subjects receiving anti-coagulant therapy require careful monitoring of their vitamin K status by regular prothrombin (PT) tests.[49,50] The prothrombin time test is responsive to depressions of the vitamin K-dependent clotting factors II, VII, and X. Some of the procedures used to measure prothrombin times have been described by Hirsh et al.[49] and by Dzung et al.[50] Of note, prothrombin times may be influenced by levels of intake of dietary vitamin K, such as of green leafy vegetables. Moreover, prothrombin time tests are a rather insensitive measure of vitamin K status.[51,125]

In a controlled study, a mild vitamin K deficiency was induced in adult subjects by administrating daily 1 mg of warfarin.[51] From the standpoint of assessment of vitamin K status, the most consistent finding with the administration of warfarin was an increase in the concentration of serum under-γ-carboxylated osteocalcin. This was followed by an increased immunochemical detection of plasma under-γ-carboxylated prothrombin (PIVKA-II) (a protein induced by vitamin K absence; des-γ-carboxyglutamic acid prothrombin), and by a decreased urinary excretion of γ-carboxyglutamic acid.[51,122] Patients receiving an anticoagulant (e.g., warfarin, coumadin) for the prophylaxis and treatment of thromboembolic disease commonly have increased plasma levels of PIVKA-II (>1.0 µg/mL).[100]

Other studies have also investigated the effect of dietary restriction of vitamin K on various measures for assessing vitamin K status.[14,52-56,74,125] These studies have indicated that a vitamin K deficiency may result in (a) under-γ-carboxylated prothrombin (PIVKA-II),[54] (b) under-γ-carboxylated osteocalcin,[55] (c) changes in urinary excretion of γ-carboxyglutamic acid,[51,114] or (d) changes in prothrombin activation products.[56] These procedures are more sensitive to vitamin K inadequacies then the measurement of plasma vitamin K-dependent clotting factors.

Vitamin K-Dependent Carboxylase

This specific microsomal carboxylase catalyze the γ-carboxylation of protein-bound glutamate residues.[10,42] This carboxylase is found primarily in the liver, although it has also been shown to be present in kidney, bone, lung, and other tissues. The carboxylation results in a parallel formation of vitamin K-2,3-epoxide.[5] The vitamin K epoxide formed can be recycled back to its biologically active hydroquinone form by the action of specific reductases.[5,10,42-45]

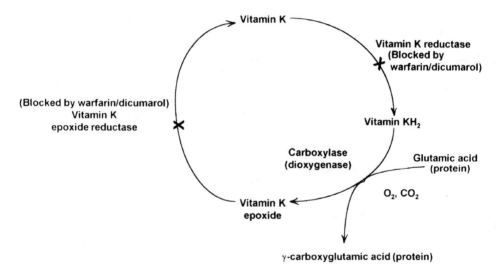

FIGURE 52
Vitamin K metabolic cycle.

Vitamin K and Bone Formation

Vitamin K has a crucial role in normal bone formation.[10,31,32,37,38,92-94,124] Osteocalcin (bone Gla protein) serves as the protein matrix for new bone formations.[39,40] The γ-carboxyglutamic acid in osteocalcin binds calcium ions to provide for normal bone calcification.[38] With inadequate vitamin K_1, γ-carboxylation does not proceed and bone calcification is impaired. The concentrations of vitamin K_1 in serum is related to the serum triglyceride concentrations.[69,93] Plasma vitamin K/plasma triglyceride ratio may be a better index of vitamin K status than plasma vitamin K levels alone. Osteocalcin (bone Gla protein), measured by a radioimmunoassay, can serve as a marker of bone metabolism.[39,40] The upper limit of normal serum total osteocalcin for adult women ($n = 21$; age 21 to 44 y) was 13.9 ng/mL. Normal plasma undercarboxylated osteocalcin was ≤ 1.65 ng/mL.[94] The undercarboxylated osteocalciin was reported to be elevated in elderly women.[94,95] Another vitamin K-dependent bone protein is found in bone, dentin, and cartilage.[7,10,28-31,37] This protein is referred to as the matrix Gla protein.

It has been suggested that the function of osteocalcin in human bone can be compromised by nutritional levels of vitamin K that are still able to support a normal coagulation time.[37] Serum vitamin K testing has been suggested for individuals with osteoporosis, or in women who have relatives with osteoporosis. Subjects with low vitamin K status may following dietary change or vitamin K supplementation be given a repeat testing to evaluate improvement in status. Of interest, patients receiving long-term maintenance therapy with a vitamin K antagonist (warfarin) had normal bone densities.[92] However, it has been reported that low intakes of vitamin K may increase the risk of hip fractures in women.[126] Vitamin K may participate in renal stone and arteriosclerotic plaque formation and in the onset of osteoporosis.[7,10,25-27,90,124]

Methods for the Assessment of Vitamin K Status

Traditional methods for assessing vitamin K status, such as prothrombin tests, and activated partial thromboplastin time, are relatively insensitive for detecting a subclincial vitamin K deficiency.[59,84,100,110,125] Nevertheless, the prothrombin time test is the most common laboratory procedure used to detect potential bleeding problems and to monitor oral anticoagulant therapy.

The newer knowledge as to the functions of vitamin K has permitted the development of sensitive functional procedures to assess vitamin status.[60] With the discovery of γ-carboxyglutamic acid, vitamin K received new nutritional importance. This was enhanced by presence of the vitamin K-dependent carboxylase in diverse tissues.

Previously, based on studies of blood clotting function, vitamin K deficiency was assumed to be uncommon. With the development of analytical procedures capable of direct measurement of vitamin K in blood, the importance of vitamin K status has required reassessment.[117,125] For example, subjects with osteoporosis resulting in femoral or vertebral neck fractures had serum vitamin K_1 levels of only one-third those of age-matched controls.[33,34,120,124] In another report, vitamin K supplementation of osteoporotic subjects reduced calcium loss by 18 to 50%.[35,90] Plasma phylloquinone concentrations appear to reflect dietary intakes of vitamin K (Table 61).[53,62]

TABLE 61
Effect of Phylloquinone Intake on Fasting Plasma Concentrations of Phylloquinone in Humans

Subjects	Phylloquinone Intake (μg/day)	Phylloquinone Concentrations nmol/L Plasma (ng/mL)
Younger (31 years)		
Men ($n = 9$)	119 ± 15	1.06 ± 0.14 (0.48 ± 0.06)
Women ($n = 8$)	103 ± 1.6	1.02 ± 0.11 (0.46 ± 0.05)
Older (70 years)		
Men ($n = 9$)	150 ± 20	1.43 ± 0.23 (0.64 ± 0.10)
Women ($n = 8$)	136 ± 21	1.47 ± 0.20 (0.66 ± 0.09)

Adapted from Reference 75.

Other procedures used to evaluate vitamin K status include the quantitation of serum osteocalcin and undercarboxylated osteocalcin by radioimmunoassay[58,63,119] and measurement of urinary γ-carboxyglutamate (Gla) by derivatization followed by HPLC separation and fluorometric detection.[64] Serum undercarboxylated osteocalcin appears to be a sensitive and functional indicator of vitamin K nutritional status.[51,59,62] In a controlled vitamin K intake study, it was found that the measurement of undercarboxylated osteocalcin, plasma phylloquinone, and urinary γ-carboxyglutamic acid excretion were sensitive markers of vitamin K nutritional status and each responded to changes in the dietary intake of vitamin K. In contrast, prothrombin and blood clotting measures were insensitive to small changes in vitamin K status.[53,62] Undercarboxylated prothrombin (PIVKA-II) measurements appeared to be less sensitive than under-γ-carboxylated osteocalcin as an indicator of vitamin K status.[51,59] Undercarboxylated prothrombin (PIVKA-II) may be measured in citrated plasma with an enzyme-linked immunosorbent assay (American Bioproducts Company, Parsippany, NJ).[67,118]

Determination of Vitamin K

The older methods for the determination of vitamin K in plasma and tissues lacked sensitivity and specificity. Hence, older reported concentrations are often considered unreliable. Currently, HPLC methods are routinely employed with detection of the vitamin K forms by electrochemical techniques,[12,33,70] ultraviolet absorption procedures,[12,13] fluorescence of hydroquinone derivatives,[58] or combined gas chromatography (GC)-mass spectrometry.[71]

For vitamin K analyses, blood samples collected with the use of EDTA are commonly used. Since vitamin K is rapidly destroyed by light, sample handling and analyses must be conducted in a subdued light. It is also very sensitive to alkali. Vitamin K_1, which circulates in the plasma bound to lipoproteins, can be readily extracted. Flocculation of the plasma proteins with ethanol followed by extraction with hexane provides a simple extraction procedure. The use of high-performance liquid chromatography (HPLC) in the measurement of vitamin K forms has been extensively reviewed by Shearer.[13] Information on plasma levels of vitamin K has been dependent upon the results from HPLC procedures. When facilities are available, direct measurements of plasma phylloquinone and phylloquinone-2,3-epoxide may be considered. Both are measured by HPLC with flurometric detection after postcolumn zinc reduction.[57,58] Similar HPLC methods for measuring phylloquinone have been described from other laboratories.[61,101,121] The procedures usually require only 0.5 to 1.0 ml of plasma. The ratio of serum phylloquinone epoxide to phylloquinone has been used as an indicator of vitamin K status.

In general, the various methods provide comparable analytical results when applied to the measurement of phylloquinone in plasma.[2,114,115] Some of these values have been summarized by Shearer et al.[12] With the use of electrochemical detection, plasma concentrations of phylloquinone in normal adults ranged from 0.17 to 0.68 ng/mL (0.38 to 1.51 nmol/L), with a mean of 0.37 ng/mL (0.82 nmol/L).[12] Somewhat higher values were reported with the use of fluormetric detection (e.g., 0.2 to 2.7 ng/mL ; 0.44 to 5.0 nmol/L) (mean 1.3 ng/mL; 2.9 nmol/L).[58,72,73]

Sadowski et al.[114] reported a mean plasma vitamin K concentration for 133 young men and women of 0.98 ± 0.66 nmol/L (0.44 ± 0.30 ng/mL). A group of 199 elderly men and women had a mean plasma vitamin K concentration of 1.13 ± 0.92 nmol/L (0.51 ± 0.37 ng/mL).[114]

Although age, sex, and severe hyperlipidemia may have a variable effect on plasma phylloquinone concentrations, dietary intakes of vitamin K appear to be the strongest determinant of plasma phylloquinone values.[12,73,74] Fasting plasma phylloquinone concentrations have been reported to correlate significantly with dietary intakes of phylloquinone ($r = 0.51$, P = 0.004).[75]

Studies on the Assessment of Vitamin K Status

Sokoll and Sadowski[59] made a detailed comparison of various biochemical indexes used to assess vitamin K nutritional status. For this study, 263 healthy adult subjects (136 females; 127 males) aged 18 to 85 years were used. The measurements performed included plasma phylloquinone and undercarboxylated prothrombin (PIVKA-II) concentrations, urinary γ-carboxylutamic (Gla)-creatinine excretion ratios, and undercarboxylated osteocalcin concentrations. Phylloquinone was determined in EDTA treated plasma by reversed-phase HPLC using postcolumn solid-phase chemical reduction of the phylloquinone to its hydroquinone form, followed by fluorometric detection.[58] Undercarboxylated plasma prothrombin (PIVKA-II) was measured in citrated plasma with an enzyme-linked immunosorbent assay (American Bioproducts Company, Parsippany, NJ). Urinary levels of γ-carboxylglutamic acid (Gla) were determined with an HPLC-fluorometric procedure.[64] Serum osteocalcin and undercarboxylated osteocalcin were quantitated with the use of radioimmunoassay.[63]

The study indicated that undercarboxylated osteocalcin concentrations may serve as a useful marker of vitamin K nutritional status.[90] The measure correlated with both plasma phylloquinone and plasma PIVKA-II concentrations. Aging, sex, and menopause had some influence on plasma phylloquinone concentrations, urinary Gla to creatinine ratio, serum osteocalcin and undercarboxylated osteocalcin concentrations, and plasma PIVKA-II concentrations.[59] Guidelines used for evaluating vitamin K status need to consider these influences.

The Following Values May be Used For Initial Guidance[59]	
Plasma PIVKA-II (undercarboxylated prothrombin):	1.58 μg/L
Plasma Undercarboxylated Osteocalcin:	
women (30 y):	3.3 ± 0.4 μg/L
women (50 y):	1.6 ± 0.2 μg/L
women (70 y):	2.8 ± 0.2 μg/L
men (70 y):	2.0 ± 0.1 μg/L
Plasma Carboxylated Osteocalcin	
women (30)	8.4 ± 0.3 μg/L
women (50)	6.8 ± 0.5 μg/L
men (30)	9.9 ± 0.5 μg/L
men (70)	7.0 ± 0.5 μg/L
Urine Gla-creatinine ratio:	
adult women:	3.83 ± 0.08 μmol/mmol
adult men:	3.16 ± 0.06 μmol/mmol

Guidelines for assessing vitamin K nutritional status can vary considerably between reports. Further studies are necessary to establish reliable criteria for evaluating vitamin K status.

Vitamin K Toxicity

Vitamin K_1 is normally well tolerated.[4-6] However, oral or intramuscular administrations are preferred over intravenous injections. There are no reports of toxic effects from vitamin K_1, the phylloquinone form, when 500 times the RDA have been used. The use of the synthetic menadione (vitamin K_3) may be associated with adverse effects and should be avoided for human use.[4] The upper limit of phylloquinone used in infant formulas has been suggested not to exceed 20 µg/100 kcal.[4]

Of note, high intakes of vitamin E can result in a vitamin K-responsive hemorragic condition.[116,123] Hydantoin anticonvulsants are antagonist of vitamin K and subjects on such medication should have their vitamin K status monitored.[98]

Summary

The most common causes of vitamin K deficiency are malnutrition, antibiotic therapy, oral anticoagulants, and infant hemorrhagic disease.[36,87,96,99] The routinely used coagulation tests are not adequate to detect a biochemcial vitamin K deficiency. A number of sensitive markers of vitamin K deficiency have been investigated. Quantitative measurements of phylloquinone (vitamin K_1) have been extensively used. The methods appears reliable with comparable values observed between laboratories.[114,115]

With further investigations, measurements of plasma PIVKA-II (des-γ-carboxyglutamic acid prothrombin) may prove a sensitive indicator of vitamin K status. However, more readily available means for its measurement are needed.[99] Currently, levels are measured with a specific antibody method.[82] Similarly, urinary excretion of γ-carboxyglutamic acid has promise as an indicator of vitamin K nutritional status. Undercarboxylated osteocalcin measurements also appear useful for vitamin K evaluation. However, for this measurement and for the others noted, further studies are required to establish reliable procedures and suitable guidelines for evaluating vitamin K nutritional status.[51,53,59]

References

1. Harlos, K., Holland, S. K., Boys, C. W. G., Burgess, A. I., Esnouf, M. P., and Blake, C. C. F., Vitamin K-dependent blood coagulation proteins form hetero-dimers, *Nature*, 330, 82, 1987.
2. Rietz, P., Gloor, U., and Wiss, O., Menachinone aus menschlicher Leber und Faulschlamm, *Int. J. Vit. Nutr. Res.*, 40, 351, 1970.
3. Olson, J. A., Recommended dietary intakes (RDI) of vitamin K in humans, *Am. J. Clin. Nutr.*, 45, 687, 1987.
4. Olson, J. A., Upper limits of vitamin A in infant formulas, with some comments on vitamin K, *J. Nutr.*, 119, 1820, 1989.
5. Olson, R. E., Vitamin K, in *Modern Nutrition in Health and Disease*, Shils, M. E., Olson, J. A., and Shike, M., Eds., 8th edition, Lea & Febiger, Philadelphia, 1994, 342.
6. Suttie, J. W., Vitamin K, in *Present Knowledge of Nutrition*, Ziegler, E. E., and Filer, L. J., Eds., 7th edition, ILSI Press, Washington D.C., 1996, 137.

7. Vermeer, C., Jie, K.–S. G., and Knapen, M. H. J., Role of vitamin K in bone metabolism, *Annu. Rev. Nutr.*, 15, 1, 1995.

8. Suttie, J. W., The importance of menaquinones in human nutrition, *Annu. Rev. Nutr.*, 15, 399, 1995.

9. Combs, G. F. Jr., *The Vitamins*, Academic Press, New York, 1992, 419.

10. Dowd, P., Ham, S.–W., Naganathan, S., and Hershline, R., The mechanism of action of vitamin K, *Annu. Rev. Nutr.*, 15, 419, 1995.

11. Weihrauch, J. L. and Bowman, S. A., *Provisional Table on the Vitamin K Content of Foods*, United States Department of Agriculture, Human Nutrition Information Service, Washington D.C., Item No. HNIS/PT-104, June, 1990.

12. Shearer, M. J., McCarthy, P. T., Cramptons, O. E., and Matlock, M. B., The assessment of human vitamin K status from tissue measurements, in *Current Advances in Vitamin K Research*, Suttie, J. W., Ed., Elsevier Science Publishers, New York, 1988, 437.

13. Shearer, M. J., High-performance liquid chromatography of K vitamins and their antagonists, *Adv. Chromatogr.*, 21, 243, 1983.

14. Suttie, J. W., Mummah-Schendel, L. L., Shah, D. V., Lyle, B. J., and Greger, J. L., Vitamin K deficiency from dietary vitamin K restriction in humans, *Am. J. Clin. Nutr.*, 47, 475, 1988.

15. Olson, R. E., The function and metabolism of vitamin K, *Annu. Rev. Nutr.*, 4, 281, 1984.

16. Bjornsson, T. D., Meffin, P. J., Smezey, S. F., and Blaschke, T. F., Disposition and turnover of vitamin K_1 in man, in *Vitamin K Metabolism and Vitamin K-dependent Proteins*, Suttie, J. W., Ed., University Park Press, Baltimore, MD, 1980, 328.

17. Dam, H., Vitamin K, its chemistry and physiology, *Adv. Enzymol*, 2, 285, 1942.

18. Doisy, E. A., Binkley, S. B., and Thayer, S. A., Vitamin K, *Chem. Rev.*, 28, 477, 1941.

19. Binkley, S. B., MacCorquodale, D. W., Thayer, S. A., and Doisy, E. A., The isolation of vitamin K, *J. Biol. Chem.*, 130, 219, 1939.

20. Dam, H., Hemorrhages in chicks reared on artificial diets, A new deficiency disease, *Nature*, 133, 909, 1934.

21. Dam, H., Antihaemorrhagic vitamin of the chick, *Biochem. J.*, 29, 1273, 1935.

22. Dam, H., Antihaemorrhagic vitamin of the chick: occurrence and chemical nature, *Nature*, 135, 652, 1935.

23. Karrer, P., Geiger, A., Ruegger, A., and Saloman, H., Uber nor-α-phyllochinon (nor vitamin K) und ahnlich Verbendungen, *Helv. Chim. Acta*, 22, 1513, 1939.

24. MacCorquodale, D. W., Cheney, L. C., Binkley, S. B., Holcomb, W. F., and McKee, R. W. et al., The constitution and synthesis of vitamin K, *J. Biol. Chem.*, 131, 357, 1939.

25. Gijsbers, B. L., van Haarlem, L. J., Soute, B. A., Ebbeink, R. H., and Vermeer, C., Characterization of Gla-containing protein from calcified human atherosclerotic plaques, *Arteriosclerosis*, 10, 991, 1990.

26. Lian, J. B. and Friedman, P. A., The vitamin K-dependent synthesis of –carboxyglutamic acid by bone microsomes, *J. Biol. Chem.*, 253, 6623, 1978.

27. Knapen, M. H., Hamulyak, K., and Vermeer, C., The effect of vitamin K supplementation on circulating osteocalcin (bone Gla protein) and urinary calcium excretion, *Annu. Int. Med.*, 111, 1001, 1989.

28. Hauschka, P. V., Lian, J. B., and Gallop, P. M., Direct identification of the calcium-binding amino acid, γ-carboxyglutamate, in mineralized tissue, *Proc. Natl. Acad. Sci. USA*, 72, 3925, 1975.

29. Hauschka, P. V., Lian, J. B., and Gallop, P. M., Vitamin K and mineralization, *Trends Biochem. Sci.*, 5, 75, 1978.

30. Price, P. A., Otsuka, A. S., Poser, J. W., Kirstaponis, J., and Raman, N., Characterization of a γ-carboxyglutamic acid-containing protein from bone, *Proc. Natl. Acad. Sci. USA*, 73, 1447, 1975.

31. Gallop, P. M., Lian, J. B., and Heuschka, P. V., Carboxylated calcium-binding proteins and vitamin K, *N. Engl. J. Med.*, 302, 1460, 1980.

32. Osteocalcin: a vitamin K-dependent calcium-binding protein in bone, *Nutr. Rev.*, 37, 54, 1979.

33. Hart, J. P., Shearer, M. J., Klenerman, L., Catterall, A., Reeve, J., Sambrook, P. M., Dodds, R. A., Bitensky, L., and Chayen, J., Electrochemical detection of depressed circulating levels of vitamin K_1 levels in osteoporosis, *J. Clin. Endo. Metab.*, 60, 1268, 1985.

34. Hart, J. P., Catterall, A., Dodds, R. A., Klenerman, L., Chayen, J., Shearer, M. J., and Bitensky, L., Circulating vitamin K_1 levels in fractured neck of femur, *Lancet*, 2, 283, 1984.

35. Tomita, A., Postmenopausal osteoporosis Ca-47 study with vitamin K_2, *Clin. Endocrinol. (Japan)*, 19, 731, 1971.

36. Duncan, A., Coagulation defects, in *Medicine for the Practicing Physician*, 3rd edition, Hurst, J. W., Ed., Butterworth-Heinemann, Boston, 1992, 786.

37. Price, P. A., Role of vitamin K-dependent proteins in bone metabolism, *Annu. Rev. Nutr.*, 8, 565, 1988.

38. Price, P. A., Vitamin K-dependent formation of bone Gla protein (osteocalcin) and its function, *Vit. Horm.*, 42, 65, 1985.

39. Price, P. A. and Nishimoto, S. K., Radioimmunoassay for the vitamin K-dependent protein of bone and its discovery in plasma, *Proc. Natl. Acad. Sci. USA*, 77, 2234, 1980.

40. Price, P. A., Parthemore, J. G., and Deftos, L. J., A new biochemical marker for bone metabolism, *J. Clin. Invest.*, 66, 878, 1980.

41. Stern, D. M., Naworth, P. P., Harris, K., and Esmon, C. T., Culture bovine aortic endothelial cells promote activated protein C-protein S-mediated inactivation of factor Va, *J. Biol. Chem.*, 261, 713, 1986.

42. Suttie, J. W., Vitamin K-dependent carboxylase, *Annu. Rev. Biochem.*, 54, 459, 1985.

43. Friedman, P. A., Shia, M. A., Gallop, P. M., and Griep, A. E., Vitamin K-dependent gamma-carbon-hydrogen bond cleavage and non-mandatory concurrent carboxylation of peptide-bound glutamic acid residues, *Proc. Natl. Acad. Sci. USA*, 76, 3126, 1979.

44. Larson, A. E., Friedman, P. A., and Suttie, J. W., Vitamin K-dependent carboxylase: stoichiometry of carboxylation and vitamin K 2,2-epoxide formation, *J. Biol. Chem.*, 256, 11032, 1981.

45. Hall, A. L., Kloepper, R., Zee-Cheng, R. K.–Y., Chiu, Y. J. D., Lee, F. C., and Olson, R. E., Mechanisms of action of tert-butyl hydroperoxide in the inhibition of vitamin K-dependent carboxylation, *Arch. Biochem. Biophys.*, 214, 45, 1982.

46. Whitlon, D. S., Sadowski, J. A., and Suttie, J. W., Mechanism of coumarin action: significance of vitamin K epoxide reductase inhibition, *Biochemistry*, 17, 1371, 1978.

47. Fasco, M. J., Hildebrandt, E. F., and Suttie, J. W., Evidence that warfarin anticoagulant action involves two distinct reductase activities, *J. Biol. Chem.*, 257, 11210, 1982.

48. Choonara, I. A., Malia, R. G., Haynes, B. P., Hay, C. R., Cholerton, S., Breckenridge, A. M., Preston, F. E., and Park, B. K., The relationship between inhibition of vitamin K 1, 2, 3,-epoxide reductase and reduction of clotting factor activity with warfarin, *Br. J. Clin. Pharmacol.*, 25, 1, 1988.

49. Hirsh, J., Dalen, J. E., Deykin, D., and Poller, L., Oral anticoagulants: mechanism of action, clinical effectiveness, and optimal therapeutic range, *Chest*, 102, 312S, 1992.

50. Dzung, T. L., Weibert, R. T., Sevilla, B. K., Donnelly, K. J., and Rapaport, S. I., The international normalized ratio (INR) for monitoring warfarin therapy: reliability and relation to other monitoring methods, *Annu. Int. Med.*, 120, 552, 1994.

51. Bach, A. U., Anderson, S. A., Foley, A. L., Williams, E. C., and Suttie, J. W., Assessment of vitamin K status of human subjects administered "minidose" warfarin, *Am. J. Clin. Nutr.*, 64, 894, 1996.

52. Allison, P. M., Mummah-Schendel, L. L., Kindberg, C. G., Harms, C. S., Bang, N. U., and Suttie, J. W., Effects of a vitamin K-deficient diet and antibiotics in normal human volunteers, *J. Lab. Clin. Med.*, 110, 180, 1987.

53. Ferland, G., Sadowski, J. A., and O'Brien, M. E., Dietary induced subclinical vitamin K deficiency in normal human subjects, *J. Clin. Invest.*, 91, 1761, 1993.

54. Blanchard, R. A., Furie, B. C., Jorgensen, M., Druger, S. F., and Furie, B., Acquired vitamin K-dependent carboxylation deficiency in liver disease, *N. Engl. J. Med.*, 305, 242, 1981.

55. Price, P. A., Williamson, M. K., and Lothringer, J. W., Origin of the vitamin K-dependent bone protein found in plasma and its clearance by kidney and bone, *J. Biol. Chem.*, 256, 12760, 1981.

56. Bauer, K. A. and Rosenberg, R. D., The pathophysiology of the prethrombotic state in humans: insights gained from studies using markers of hemostatic system activation, *Blood*, 70, 343, 1987.

57. Hirauchi, K., Sakano, T., and Morimoto, A., Measurement of K vitamins in human and animal plasma by high-performance liquid chromatography with fluorometric detection, *Chem. Pharm. Bull.*, 34, 845, 1986.

58. Haroon, Y., Bacon, D. S., and Sadowski, J. A., Liquid-chromatographic determination of vitamin K_1 in plasma with fluorometric detection, *Clin. Chem.*, 32, 1925, 1986.

59. Sokoll, L. J. and Sadowski, J. A., Comparison of biochemical indexes for assessing vitamin K nutritional status in a healthy adult population, *Am. J. Clin. Nutr.*, 63, 566, 1996.

60. Rucker, R. B., Improved functional endpoints for use in vitamin K assessment: important implications for bone disease, *Am. J. Clin. Nutr.*, 65, 883, 1997.

61. Jakob, E. and Elmadfa, I., Rapid HPLC assay for the assessment of vitamins K_1, A, E, and beta-carotene status in children (7–19 years), *Int. J. Vit. Nutr. Res.*, 65, 31, 1995.

62. Sokoll, L. J., Booth, S. L., O'Brien, M. E., Davidson, K. W., Tsaioun, K. I., and Sadowski, J. A., Changes in serum osteocalcin, plasma phylloquinone, and urinary γ-carboxyglutamic acid in response to altered intakes of dietary phylloquinone in human subjects, *Am. J. Clin. Nutr.*, 65, 779, 1997.

63. Sokoll, L. J., O'Brien, M. E., Camilo, M., Sadowski, J. A., Undercarboxylated osteocalcin: development of a method to determine vitamin K status, *Clin. Chem.*, 41, 1121, 1995.

64. Haroon, Y., Rapid assay for gamma-carboxylutamic acid in urine and bone by precolumn derivatization and reverse-phase liquid chromatography, *Anal. Biochem.*, 140, 343, 1984.

65. Booth, S. L., Gennington, J. A., and Sadowski, J. A., Food sources and dietary intakes of vitamin K-1 (phylloquinone) in the American diet: data from the FDA Total Diet Study, *J. Am. Diet. Assoc.*, 96, 149, 1996.

66. Conly, J. M., Stein, K., Worobetz, L., and Rutledge-Harding, S., The contribution of vitamin K2 (menaquinones produced by the intestinal microflora) to human nutritional requirements for vitamin K, *Am. J. Gastroenterol.*, 89, 915, 1994.

67. Francis, J. L., A rapid and simple micromethod for the specific determination of descarboxylated prothrombin (PIVKA-II), *Med. Lab. Sci.*, 45, 69, 1988.

68. *Recommended Dietary Allowances*, 10th Edition, Food and Nutrition Board, National Research Council, National Academy Press, Washington D.C., 1989, 112.

69. Sadowski, J. A., Hood, S. J., Dallal, G. E., and Garry, P. J., Phylloquinone in plasma from elderly and young adults: factors influencing its concentration, *Am. J. Clin. Nutr.*, 50, 100, 1989.

70. Ueno, T. and Suttie, J. W., High-pressure liquid chromatographic-reductive electrochemical detection analysis of serum trans-phylloquinone, *Anal. Biochem.*, 133, 62, 1983.

71. DiMari, S. J., Supple, J. H., and Rapoport, H., Mass spectra of naphthoquinones: vitamin $K_1(20)$, *Am. Chem. Soc.*, 88, 1226, 1966.

72. Mummah-Schendel, L. L. and Suttie, J. W., Serum phylloquinone concentrations in a normal adult population, *Am. J. Clin. Nutr.*, 44, 686, 1986.

73. Lambert, W. E., DeLeenheer, A. P., and Baert, E. J., Wet-chemical post-column reaction and fluorescence detection analysis of the reference interval of endogenous serum vitamin $K_1(20)$, *Ann. Biochem.*, 158, 257, 1986.

74. Suttie, J. W., Kindberg, C. G., Greger, J. L., and Bang, N. U., Effects of vitamin K (phylloquinone) restriction in the human, in *Current Advances in Vitamin K Research*, Suttie, J. W., Ed., Elsevier Science Publishers, New York, 1988, 465.

75. Booth, S. L., Tucker, K. L., McKeown, N. M., Davidson, K. W., Dallal, G. E., and Sadowski, J. A., Relationship between dietary intakes and fasting plasma concentrations of fat-soluble vitamins in humans, *J. Nutr.*, 127, 587, 1997.

76. Krasinski, S. D., Russell, R. M., Furie, B. C., Kruger, S. F., Jacques, P. F., and Furie, B., The prevalence of vitamin K deficiency in chronic gastrointestinal disorders, *Am. J. Clin. Nutr.*, 41, 639, 1985.

77. Kaplan, M. M., Elta, G. H., Furie, B., Sadowski, J. A., and Russell, R. M., Fat-soluble vitamin nutriture in primary biliary cirrhosis, *Gastrenterology*, 95, 787, 1988.

78. Cohen, H., Scott, S. D., Mackie, I. J., Shearer, M., Box, R., Karran, S. J., and Machin, S.–J., The development of hypoprothrombinaemia following antibiotic therapy in malnourished patients with low serum vitamin K_1 levels, *Br. J. Haematol.*, 68, 63, 1988.

79. Conly, J., Suttie, J., Reid, E., Loftson, J., Ramstar, K., and Louie, T., Dietary deficiency of phylloquinone and reduced serum levels in febrile neutropenic cancer patients, *Am. J. Clin. Nutr.*, 50, 109, 1989.

80. Usui, Y., Tanimura, H., Nishimura, N., Kobayasi, N., Okanoue, T., and Ozawa, K., Vitamin K concentrations in the plasma and liver of surgical patients, *Am. J. Clin. Nutr.*, 51, 846, 1990.

81. Blanchard, R. A., Furie, B. C., and Furie, B., Antibodies specific for bound abnormal (des-γ-carboxy) prothrombin, *J. Biol. Chem.*, 254, 12513, 1979.

82. Blanchard, R. A., Furie, B. C., Druger, S. F., Waneck, G., Jorgansen, M. J., and Furie, B., Immunoassay of human prothrombin species which correlate with functional coagulant activities, *J. Lab. Clin. Med.*, 101, 242, 1983.

83. Iber, F. L., Shamszad, M., Miller, P. A., and Jacob, R., Vitamin K deficiency in chronic alcoholic males, *Alcoholism: Clin. Expt. Res.*, 10, 679, 1986.

84. Suttie, J. W., Vitamin K and human nutrition, *J. Am. Diet. Assoc.*, 92, 585, 1992.

85. Lipsky, J. J., Nutritional sources of vitamin K, *Mayo Clin. Proc.*, 69, 462, 1994.

86. Shearer, M. J., Bach, A., and Kohlmeier, M., Chemistry, nutritional sources, tissue distribution and metabolism of vitamin K with special reference to bone health, *J. Nutr.*, 126, 1181S, 1996.

87. Griminger, P., Vitamin K antagonists: the first 50 years, *J. Nutr.*, 117, 1325, 1987.

88. *Vitamin K and Vitamin K-dependent Proteins*, Shearer, M. J., and Seghatchian, M. J., Eds., CRC Press, Boca Raton, FL, 1993, 336.

89. D'Angelo, A., Vigano-D'Angelo, S., Esmon, C. T., and Comp, P. C., Acquired deficiencies of protein S: protein S activity during oral anticoagulation, in liver disease, and in disseminated intravascular coagulation, *J. Clin. Invest.*, 81, 1445, 1988.

90. Binkley, N. C., and Suttie, J. W., Vitamin K nutrition and osteoporosis, *J. Nutr.*, 125, 1812, 1995.

91. Rosen, H. N., Maitland, L. A., Suttie, J. W., Manning, W. J., Glynn, R. J., and Greenspan, S. L., Vitamin K and maintenance of skeletal integrity in adults, *Am. J. Med.*, 94, 62, 1993.

92. Vermeer, C., Gijsbers, B. L. M. G., Cracium, A. M., Groenen-Van Dooren, M. M. C. L., and Knapen, M. H. J., Effects of vitamin K on bone mass and bone metabolism, *J. Nutr.*, 126, 1187S, 1996.

93. Kohlmeier, M., Salomon, A., Saupe, J., and Shearer, M. J., Transport of vitamin K to bone in humans, *J. Nutr.*, 126, 1192S, 1996.

94. Szulc, P., Chaupuy, M.–C., Meunier, P. J., and Delmas, P. D., Serum undercarboxylated osteocalcin is a marker of the risk of hip fracture in elderly women, *J. Clin. Invest.*, 91, 1769, 1993.

95. Plantalech, L., Guillaumont, M., Leclercq, M., and Delmas, P. D., Impaired carboxylation of serum osteocalcin in elderly women, *J. Bone Miner. Res.*, 6, 1211, 1991.

96. Lane, P. A. and Hathaway, W. E., Medical progress: vitamin K in infancy, *J. Pediatr.*, 106, 351, 1985.

97. Bleyer, W. A., Hakami, N., and Shepard, T. H., The development of homeostasis in the human fetus and newborn infant, *J. Pediatr.*, 79, 838, 1971.

98. Evans, A. R., Forrester, R. M., and Discombe, C., Neonatal haemorrhage following maternal anticonvulsant therapy, *Lancet*, 1, 517, 1970.

99. von Kries, R., Grur, F. R., and Suttie, J. W., Assessment of vitamin K status of the newborn infant, Review, *J. Pediatr. Gastroenterol. Nutr.*, 16, 231, 1993.

100. Umeki, S. and Umeki, Y., Levels of a carboxy prothrombin (PIVKA-II) and coagulation factors in warfarin-treated patients, *Med. Lab. Sci.*, 47, 103, 1990,

101. Cham, B. E., Roeser, H. P., and Kamst, T. W., Simultaneous liquid-chromatographic determination of vitamin K_1 and vitamin E in serum, *Clin. Chem.*, 35, 2285, 1989.

102. von Kries, R., Shearer, M. J., and Gobel, U., Vitamin K in infancy, *Eur. J. Pediatr.*, 147, 106, 1988.

103. Geer, F. R., Marshall, S., Cherry, J., and Suttie, J. W., Vitamin K status of lactating mothers, human milk, and breast-feeding infants, *Pediatrics*, 88, 751, 1991.

104. Greer, F. R., Mummah-Schendel, L. L., Marshall, S., and Suttie, J. W., Vitamin K_1 (phylloquinone) and vitamin K_2 (menaquinone) status in newborns during the first week of life, *Pediatrics*, 81, 137, 1988.

105. Motohara, K., Matsukane, I., Endo, F., Kiyota, Y., and Matsuda, I., Relationship of milk intake and vitamin K supplementation to vitamin K status in newborns, *Pediatrics*, 84, 90, 1989.

106. Widdershoven, J., Kollee, L., van Munster, P., Bosman, A.–M., and Monnens, L., Biochemical vitamin K deficiency in early infancy: diagnostic limitation of conventional coagulation tests, *Helv. Paediat. Acta*, 41, 195, 1986.

107. Lambert, W., DeLeenheer, A., Tassaneeyakul, W., and Widdershoven, J., Study of vitamin $K_{1(20)}$ in the newborn by HPLC with wet-chemical post-column reduction and fluorescence detection, in *Current Advances in Vitamin K Research*, Suttie, J. W., Ed., Elsevier Science Publishers, New York, 1988, 509.

108. von Kries, R., Shearer, M. J., Haug, M., Harzer, G., and Gobel, U., Vitamin K deficiency and vitamin K intake in infants, in *Current Advances in Vitamin K Research*, Suttie, J. W., Ed., Elsevier Science Publishers, New York, 1988, 515.

109. Brown, S. G., McHugh, G., Shapleski, J., Wotherspoon, P. A., Taylor, B. J., and Gillett, W. R., Should intramuscular vitamin K prophylaxis for haemorrhagic disease of the newborn be continued? A decision analysis, *NZ. Med. J.*, 102, 2, 1989.

110. Paul, B., Oxley, A., Brigham, K., Cox, T., and Hamilton, P. J., Factor II, VII, IX and X concentrations in patients receiving long term warfarin, *J. Clin. Pathol.*, 40, 94, 1987.

111. Thiel, W., Preissner, K. T., Delvos, U., and Muller-Bergheus, G., A simplified functional assay for protein C in plasma samples, *Blut*, 52, 169, 1986.

112. D'Angelo, S. V., Comp, P. C., Esmon, C. T., and D'Angelo, A., Relationship between protein C antigen and anticoagulant activity during oral anticoagulation and in selected disease status, *J. Clin. Invest.*, 77, 416, 1986.

113. Howard, P. R., Bovill, E. G., Mann, K. G., and Tracy, R. P., A monoclonal-antibody-based radioimmunoassay for measurement of protein C in plasma, *Clin. Chem.*, 34, 324, 1988.

114. Sadowski, J. A., Bacon, D. S., Hood, S., Davidson, K. W., Ganter, C. M., Haroon, Y., and Shepard, D. C., The application of methods used for the evaluation of vitamin K nutritional status in human and animal studies, in *Current Advances in Vitamin K Research*, Suttie, J. W., Ed., Elsevier Science Publishers, New York, 1988, 453.

115. Haroon, Y., Bacon, D. S., and Sadowski, J. A., Chemical reduction system for the detection of phylloquinone (vitamin K_1) and memaquinones (vitamin K_2), *J. Chromatogr.*, 384, 383, 1987.

116. Corrigan, J. J., and Marcus, F. I., Coagulapathy associated with vitamin E ingestion, *JAMA*, 230, 1300, 1974.

117. Price, P. A., Vitamin K nutrition and postmenopausal osteoporosis (editoral), *J. Clin. Invest.*, 91, 1268, 1993.

118. Widdershoven, J., van Munster, P., DeAbreu, R., Bosman, H., van Lith, Th., van der Putten-van Meyel, M., Motohara, K., and Matsuda, I., Four methods compared for measuring des-carboxyprothrombin (PIVKA-II), *Clin. Chem.*, 33, 2074, 1987.

119. Knapen, M. H. J., Hamulysk, K., and Vermeer, C., The effect of vitamin K supplementation on circulating osteocalcin (bone Gla-protein) and urinary calcium excretion, *Annu. Int. Med.*, 111, 1001, 1989.

120. Hodges, S. J., Akesson, K., Vergnaud, P., Obrant, K., and Delmas, P. D., Circulating levels of vitamins K_1 and K_2 decreased in elderly women with hip fracture, *J. Bone Miner. Res.*, 8, 1241, 1993.

121. MacCrehan, W., and Schonberger, E., Determination of vitamin K_1 in serum, in *Methods for Analysis of Cancer Chemopreventive Agents in Human Serum*, Thomas, J. B., and Sharpless, K., Eds., NIST Special Publication 874, National Institute of Standards and Technology, Gaithersburg, MD, 1995, 5-1.

122. Levy, R. J., and Lian, J. B., γ-Carboxyglutamate excretion and warfarin therapy, *Clin. Pharm. Ther.*, 25, 562, 1979.

123. Kappus, H., and Diplock, A. T., Tolerance and safety of vitamin E: a toxicological position report, *Free Radical Biology & Medicine*, 13, 55, 1992.

124. Weber, P., Management of osteoporosis: is there a role for vitamin K, *Int. J. Vit. Nutr. Res.*, 67, 350, 1997.

125. Booth, S. L. and Suttie, J. W., Dietary intake and adequacy of vitamin K, *J. Nutr.*, 128, 785, 1998.

126. Feskanich, D., Weber, D., Willett, W. C., Rockett, H., Booth, S. L., and Colditz, G. A., Vitamin K intake and hip fractures in women: a prospective study, *Am. J. Clin. Nutr.*, 69, 74, 1999.

Carnitine

$$(CH_3)_3\ ^+NCH_2\ CH(OH)\ CH_2COO^-$$
molecular weight: 161.2

Animal products, including dairy products, are usually rich in carnitine (β-hydroxy-γ-N-trimethylaminobutyric acid), while plant materials are generally low.[27,55] Milk contains an appreciable amount of carnitine, with human milk containing 28 to 95 mmoles/L. The intake of carnitine by the average nonvegetarin has been estimated to be 100 to 300 mg/day.[1,27]

Carnitine plays important roles in lipid metabolism, where it participates in trans-esterification reactions.[1,2,57,62,63] Thus, carnitine has an essential role in the transport of long-chain fatty acids from the cytosol into the mitochondria.[1,7] This transport system requires the participation of the mitochondrial enzymes carnitine translocase, carnitine acyl-transferases I and II.[1,4,23,24,34] Carnitine participates also in the metabolism of short-chain and medium-chain organic acids.[1,7,28] Various aspects of carnitine metabolism and requirements have been summarized in a number of reviews.[1,2,5-7,13,22,23,26-28,30,34,55,57,61,63]

Although carnitine was isolated from muscle tissue in 1905[56] and was recognized as a growth factor for the common meal worm, *Tennebrio molitor* (vitamin B_T),[29] a deficiency of carnitine in the human was not considered. The carnitine needs of the human were considered to be provided by its endogenous biosynthesis from methionine and lysine along with dietary sources.[1,11-13,24] This appears to be true for the healthy, well-nourished American adult population.

In 1973, however, a syndrome was described in a human patient that was associated with a carnitine deficiency.[2,3] Subsequent studies have now established numerous other instances of impaired carnitine status.[2,4,5,30,31,33,55,57] Thus, carnitine has been considered a conditionally essential nutrient. A deficiency may result from inherited metabolic disorders and secondary to various clinical situations. This may include premature neonates, inborn errors of carnitine biosynthesis, burn patients, genetic disorders of vitamin B-12 metabolism, and extended vitamin B-12 deficiency.[2,4,8-10,31,33,57]

Hence, a conditional carnitine requirement may result from a number of conditions such as (1) high carnitine requirements of neonates and premature infants,[17-20,23,30,34] (2) excess loss of carnitine as with hemodialysis,[14,34] (3) ability to biosynthesize carnitine reduced,[24,34] and (4) genetic and congenital disorders.[8,9,23,33,34,58]

Low tissue carnitine concentrations may lead to intramuscular lipid accumulation and muscular weakness.[2,30] Dietary carnitine supplements can correct these symptoms.[2,30,58]

Neonates and Infants

Preterm infants have tissue carnitine concentrations lower than normal and may be at risk of developing a carnitine deficiency.[2,5,17,18,23,25] After birth carnitine levels gradually increase in plasma and urine with breast feeding.[19] Carnitine-containing formulas given to infants also increase the carnitine levels in plasma and urine,[19] when compared to the use of carnitine-free formulas. Other studies on the effect of carnitine supplementation in parenterally fed newborn infants have been summarized by Schmidt-Sommerfield and Penn.[20]

In a study with 9 children given low-fat, carnitine-free total parenteral nutrition for up to 10 years, low plasma carnitine concentrations were observed, however, no clinical consequences appeared.[21] The low fat diet may have reduced the carnitine requirement.[25]

Children treated with valproic acid to control seizures or recurrent febrile convulsions have been reported to develop a carnitine deficiency status.[59,60] Plasma carnitine concentrations were depressed and some of the children complained of fatigue.[59] Carnitine supplements corrected the condition.

Vegetarian children, 1 to 17 years of age, were reported to have plasma concentrations of carnitine significantly lower than that of omnivorous children. Plasma carnitine concentrations of omnivorous children were in the same range as that of adults.[13,30,32]

Carnitine Assays

A number of spectrophotometric enzymatic methods that employ carnitine acetyltransferase have been utilized for the measurement of serum carnitine.[35-39,45-47] Sensitive radioisotopic assays have also been used.[18,41-44,54] Modifications of the method of Cederblad and Lindstedt[41] have been frequently used for carnitine measurements. L-carnitine enzymatic assay kits are available for measuring carnitine in urine and plasma or serum. Such convenient kits have been available from Boehringer Mannheim, Indianapolis, IN.

Mitchell[61,64] has reviewed extensively the reports on carnitine concentrations in biological fluids and influencing factors. A number of more recent reports provide additional information on the carnitine concentrations in serum, plasma, and erythrocytes.[64] Some of these reports are summarized in the accompanying tables (Tables 62 to 64).

Toxicity

The toxicity of carnitine appears to be quire low. Chronic hemodialysis patients have significant losses of carnitine from plasma and muscle.[14] Treatment of such patients with intravenous administration of 2 g of carnitine 3 times weekly for 6 months produced no adverse effects.[14] Subsequently, patients received 1g per day of carnitine for 10 months. No adverse effects were observed, but muscle strength improved in 9 of 14 patients.[14] In another study, cardiopathic patients were treated with 2 g daily of L-carnitine for a year.[16] Other pharmacokinetic studies support the safety of carnitine.[15,57]

Summary

Carnitine is biosynthesized from methionine and lysine. Healthy adults can normally synthesize adequate amounts of carnitine to meet their metabolic needs. However, the newborn infant has reduced stores of carnitine and apparently a low capacity for synthesizing

TABLE 62
Some Literature Citations on Carnitine Concentrations in Plasma
of Infants and Children

| Infants and Children | Carnitine | | References |
	Free (μmol/L)	Total (μmol/L)	
1. Plasma			
Neonates			
Preterm (*n* = 53)		2.90 ± 1.8	18
Term (*n* = 72)		22.4 ± 0.8	18
2. Plasma			
(a) Children			
0–2 yr (*n* =20)	33.3 ± 2.0	41.0 ± 2.0	43
2–5 yr (*n* = 20)	29.7 ± 1.0	34.8 ± 0.9	43
2–2 yr (*n* = 20)	33.7 ± 1.7	41.1 ± 2.2	43
(b) Children			
1–6 yr (*n* = 72)	41.7 ± 0.9	54.4 ± 1.2	20, 50
6–10 yr (*n* = 85)	41.4 ± 1.1	56.2 ± 1.2	20, 50
10–17 yr (*n* = 97)	39.4 ± 0.9	53 ± 1.0	20, 50
(c) Children (1-17 yr)			
Males (*n* = 15)	38.7 ± 7.5	46.8 ± 9.1	30, 32
Females (*n* = 14)	34.4 ± 6.3	45.9 ± 5.3	30, 32
3. Plasma			
Male and Females (*n* = 54)			
Age 17–20 yrs		41.6 ± 2.3	48
Age 10–18 yrs	45.3 ± 8.8	43.2 ± 55.9	52

TABLE 63
Some Literature Citations on Carnitine Concentrations in
Plasma of Adults

| Adults | Carnitine | | References |
	Free (μmol/L)	Total (μmol/L)	
1. Serum			
Men (*n* = 23)	34.8–69.5	44.2–79.3	36
Women (*n* = 28)	9.3–53.9	28.1–66.4	36
2. Plasma			
Adults (*n* = 17)	50.6 ± 9.7	62.6 ± 11.7	46
3. Plasma			
Adults			
Males (*n* = 15)	39.9 ± 4.9	49.4 ± 7.3	30, 32
Women (*n* = 15)	32.5 ± 5.3	43.3 ± 5.5	30, 32
Strict Vegetarians			
Males (*n* = 9)	35.8 ± 4.5	46.7 ± 8.1	30, 32
Women (*n* = 9)	27.7 ± 6.6	36.6 ± 83	30, 32
4. Plasma			
Adults			
Males (*n* = 14)	35.4 ± 8.8	43.0 ± 12.3	49
Women (*n* = 14)	31.3 ± 6.1	39.9 ± 12.0	49

carnitine. In addition, a number of patients have a carnitine deficiency as a result of genetic defects that respond to carnitine supplementation. Carnitine deficiency may be identified by the determination of the carnitine levels in blood and urine.

A reference interval used for serum carnitine has been 28 to 70 μmol/L.[35] Plasma total carnitine concentrations of less than 30 μmol/L probably indicate low carnitine status.

TABLE 64

Carnitine Concentrations in Red Blood Cells

1. Red Blood Cells	Carnitine Concentrations (nmol/g Hgb)	References
Preterm ($n = 53$)	240 ± 20	18
Term ($n = 72$)	140 ± 10	18
Adults (348)	160 ± 60	53

2. RBC and Plasma	Plasma Carnitine (μmol/L)	RBC Carnitine (μmol/L)	
Control	47.9 ± 11.7 ($n = 888$)	0.16 ± 0.06 ($n = 346$)	51
65–74 yrs	59.4 ± 15.9 ($n = 18$)	0.23 ± 0.10 ($n = 18$)	51
>75 yrs	61.1 ± 12.1 ($n = 32$)	0.21 ± 0.06 ($n = 38$)	51

References

1. Broquist, H. P., Carnitine, in *Newer Knowledge of Human Nutrition*, Chapter 29, 1994, 459.
2. Kendler, B. S., Carnitine: an overview of its role in preventive medicine, *Preventive Medicine*, 15, 373, 1986.
3. Engel, A. G. and Angelini, C., Carnitine deficiency of human skeletal muscle with associated lipid storage myopathy: a new syndrome, *Science*, 179, 899, 1973.
4. Anonymous, Carnitine metabolism in B-12 deficiency, *Nutr. Rev.*, 47, 89, 1989.
5. Borum, P. R. and Bennett, S. G., Carnitine as an essential nutrient, *J. Am. Coll. Nutr.*, 5, 177, 1986.
6. Rebouche, C. J., Is carnitine an essential nutrient for humans, *J. Nutr.*, 116, 704, 1986.
7. Bremer, J., Carnitine – metabolism and functions, *Physiol. Rev.*, 63, 1420, 1983.
8. Chalmers, R. A., Roe, C. R., Tracey, B. M., Stacey, T. E., Hoppel, C. L., and Millington, D. C., Secondary carnitine insufficiency in disorders of organic acid metabolism: Modulation of Acy-CoA/CoA ratios by L-carnitine *in vivo*, *Biochem. Soc. Trans.*, 11, 724-725, 1983.
9. Roe, C. R., Hoppel, C. L., Stacey, T. E., Chalmers, R. A., Tracey, B. M., and Millington, D. S., Metabolic response to carnitine in methylmalonic aciduria, *Arch. Dis. Child.*, 58, 916, 1983.
10. Frenkel, E. P., Kitchens, R. L., Hersh, L. B., and Frenkel, R., Effect of vitamin B-12 deprivation on the *in vivo* levels of Coenzyme A intermediates associated with propionate metabolism, *J. Biol. Chem.*, 249, 6984, 1974.
11. Cox, R. A. and Hoppel, C. L., Biosynthesis of carnitine and 4-N-trimethylaminobutyrate from 6-N-trimethyllysine, *Biochem. J.*, 136, 1083, 1973.
12. Horne, D. W. and Broquist, H. P., Role of lysine and ε-N-trimethyllysine in carnitine biosynthesis, *J. Biol. Chem.*, 248, 2170, 1973.
13. Broquist, H. P., Carnitine biosynthesis and function, Introductory remarks, *Fed. Proc.*, 41, 2840, 1982.
14. Siami, G., Clinton, M. E., Mrak, R., Griffis, J., and Stone, W., Evaluation of the effect of intravenous L-carnitine therapy on function, structure and fatty acid metabolism of skeletal muscle in patients receiving chronic hemodialysis, *Nephron*, 57, 306, 1991.
15. Uematsu, T., Itaya, T., Nishimoto, M., Takiguchi, Y., Mizuno, A., Nakashima, M., Yoshinobu, K., and Hasebe, T., Phamacokinetics and safety of l-carnitine infused I.V. in healthy subjects, *Eur. J. Clin. Pharmacol.*, 34, 213, 1988.
16. Fernandez, C. and Proto, C., L-carnitine in the treatment of chronic myocardial ischemia, An analysis of three multicenter studies and a bibliographic review (In Italian), *Clinica Terapeutica*, 140, 353, 1996.
17. Shenai, J. P. and Borum, P. R., Tissue carnitine reserves of newborn infants, *Pediatr. Res.*, 18, 679, 1984.

18. Shenai, J. P., Borum, P. R., Mohan, P., and Donlevy, S. C., Carnitine status at birth of newborn infants of varying gestation, *Pediatr. Res.*, 17, 579, 1983.
19. Novak, M., Carnitine supplementation in soy-based formula-fed infants, *Biol. Neonate*, 58, 89, 1990.
20. Schmidt-Sommerfeld, E., and Penn, D., Carnitine and total parenteral nutrition of the neonate, *Biol. Neonate*, 58, 81, 1990.
21. Moukarzel, A. A., Dahlstrom, K. A., Buchman, A. L., and Ament, M. E., Carnitine status of children receiving long-term total parenteral nutrition: A longitudinal prospective study, *J. Pediatr.*, 120, 759, 1992.
22. Borum, P. R., Carnitine, *Annu. Rev. Nutr.*, 3, 233, 1983.
23. Borum, P. R., Possible carnitine requirement of the newborn and the effect of genetic disease on the carnitine requirement, *Nutr. Rev.*, 39, 385, 1981.
24. Broquist, H. P. and Borum, P. R., Carnitine biosynthesis: Nutritional implications, in *Advances in Nutritional Research*, Draper, H. H., Ed., Plenum Press, New York, 1982, 181.
25. Olson, A. L., Nelson, S. E., and Rebouche, C. J., Low carnitine intake and altered lipid metabolism in infants, *Am. J. Clin. Nutr.*, 49, 624, 1989.
26. Giovannini, M., Agostoni, C., and Salari, P. C., Is carnitine essential in children, *J. Int. Med. Res.*, 19, 88, 1991.
27. Combs, G. F. Jr., *The Vitamins*, Academic Press, Inc., New York, 1992, 403.
28. Rebouche C. J. and Paulson, D. J., Carnitine metabolism and function in humans, *Annu. Rev. Nutr.*, 6, 41, 1986.
29. Carter, H. E., Bhattashargya, P. K., Weidman, K. R., and Fraenkel, G., Chemical studies on vitamin B_T, isolation and characterization as carotine *Arch. Biochem. Biophys.*, 38, 405, 1952.
30. Rebouche, C. J., Carnitine function and requirements during the life cycle, *FASEB J.*, 6, 3379, 1992.
31. Engel, A. G., Rebouche, C. J., Wilson, D. M., Glasgow, A. M., Ronche, C. A., and Cruse, R. P., Primary systemic carnitine deficiency. II. Renal handling of carnitine, *Neurology*, 31, 819, 1981.
32. Lombard, K. A., Olson, A. L., Nelson, S. E., and Rebouche, C. J., Carnitine status of lactoovo-vegetarians and strict vegetarian adults and children, *Am. J. Clin. Nutr.*, 50, 301, 1989.
33. An unusual presentation of human carnitine deficiency, *Nutr. Rev.*, 43, 23, 1985.
34. Feller, A. G. and Rudman, D., Role of carnitine in human nutrition, *J. Nutr.*, 118, 541, 1988.
35. Shihabi, Z. K., Oles, K. S., McCormick, C. P., and Penry, J. K., Serum and tissue carnitine assay based on dialysis, *Clin. Chem.*, 38, 1414, 1992.
36. Deufel, T., Determination of L-carnitine in biological fluids and tissue, *J. Clin. Chem. Biochem.*, 28, 307, 1990.
37. Tegelaers, F. P. W., Pickkus, M. G., and Seelen, P. J., Effect of deproteinization and reagent buffer on the enzymatic assay of L-carnitine in serum, *J. Clin. Chem. Biochem.*, 27, 967, 1990.
38. Cederblad, G., Harper, P., and Lindgren, K., Spectrophotometry of carnitine in biological fluids and tissues with a Cobas Bio centrifugal analyzer, *Clin. Chem.*, 32, 342, 1986.
39. Bohmer, T., Rydning, A., and Solberg, H., E., Carnitine levels in human serum in health and disease, *Clin. Chim. Acta*, 57, 55, 1974.
40. Rodriguez-Segade, S., Pena, C. A., Paz, J. M., and Rio, R. O., Determination of L-carnitine in serum and implementation on the ABA-100 and CentrifiChem 600, *Clin. Chem.*, 31, 754, 1985.
41. Cederblad, G. and Lindstedt, S., A method for the determination of carnitine in the picomole range, *Clin. Chim. Acta*, 37, 235, 1972.
42. McGarry, J. D. and Foster, D. W., An improved and simplified radioisotopic assay for the determination of free and esterified carnitine, *J. Lipid Res.*, 17, 277, 1976.
43. De Sousa, C., English, N. R., Stacey, T. E., and Chalmers, R. A., Measurement of L-carnitine and acylcarnitines in body fluids and tissues in children and in adults, *Clin. Chim. Acta*, 187, 317, 1990.
44. Bhuiyan, A. K. M. J., Jackson, S., Turnbull, D. M., Ayseley-Green A., Leonard, T. V., and Bartlett, K., The measurement of carnitine and acyl-carnitines: application to the investigation of patients with suspected inherited disorders of mitochondial fatty acid oxidation, *Clin. Chim. Acta*, 207, 185, 1992.

45. Roe, D. S., Terada, N., and Willington, D. S., Automated analysis for free and short-chain acylcarnitine in plasma with a centrifugal analyzer, *Clin. Chem.*, 38, 2215, 1992.
46. Xia, L.-J. and Folkers, K., Improved methodology to assay carnitine and levels of free and total carnitine in human plasma, *Biochem. Biophys. Res. Comm.*, 176, 1617, 1991.
47. Montgomery, J. A. and Mamer, O. A., Measurement of urinary free and acylcarnitines: quantitative acylcarnitine profiling in normal humans and in several patients with metabolic errors, *Anal. Biochem.*, 176, 85, 1989.
48. Warady, B. A., Borum, P., Stall, C., Millspraugh, J., Taggart, E., and Lum, G., Carnitine status of pediatric patients on continuous ambulatory peritoneal dialysis, *Am. J. Nephrol.*, 10, 109, 1990.
49. Lennon, D. L. F., Shrago, E. R., Madden, M., Nagle, F. J., and Hanson, P., Dietary carnitine intake related to skeletal muscle and plasma carnitine concentrations in adult men and women, *Am. J. Clin. Nutr.*, 43, 234, 1986.
50. Schmidt-Sommerfeld, E., Werner, D., and Penn, D., Carnitine plasma concentrations in 353 metabolically healthy children, *Br. J. Pediatr.*, 147, 356, 1988.
51. Powers, J. S., Folk, M. C., Burger, C., Wilson, P., Stocking, B. J., and Collins, J., Assessment of nutritional status in non-institutionalized elderly, *Southern Med. J.*, 82, 990, 1989.
52. Buchta, R., Nykan, W. L., Broock, R., and Schragg, P., Carnitine in adolescents, *J. Adolescent Health*, 14, 440, 1993.
53. Borum, P. R., Plasma carnitine compartment and red blood cell carnitine compartment of healthy adults, *Am. J. Clin. Nutr.*, 46, 437, 1987.
54. Reichmann, H. and Lindeneirer, N. V., Carnitine analysis in normal human red blood cells, plasma, and muscle tissue, *Eur. Neurol.*, 34, 40, 1994.
55. Mitchell, M. E., Carnitine metabolism in human subjects. I. Normal metabolism, *Am. J. Clin. Nutr.*, 31, 293, 1978.
56. Fraenkel G. and Friedman, S., Carnitine, *Vit. Horm.*, 15, 73, 1957.
57. Mitchell, M. E., Carnitine metabolism in human subjects. III. Metabolism in disease, *Am. J. Clin. Nutr.*, 31, 645, 1978.
58. Mandel, H., Africh, D., Blitzer, M., and Shapira, E., The importance of recognizing secondary carnitine deficiency in organic acidaemias: case report in glutaric acidameia type II, *J. Inherit. Metab. Dis.*, 11, 397, 1988.
59. Van Wouwe, J. P., Carnitine deficiency during valproic acid treatment, *Int. J. Vit. Nutr. Res.*, 65, 211, 1995.
60. Laub, M. C., Paetzke-Brunner, I., and Jaeger, J., Serum carnitine during valproic acid therapy, *Epilepsia*, 27, 559, 1986.
61. Mitchell, M. E., Carnitine metabolism in human subjects II. Values of carnitine in biological fluids and tissues of "normal" subjects, *Am. J. Clin. Nutr.*, 31, 481, 1978.
62. Rebouche, C. J. and Seim, H., Carnitine metabolism and its regulation in microorganisms and mammals, *Annu. Rev. Nutr.*, 18, 39, 1998.
63. Kerner, J. and Hoppel, C., Genetic disorders of carnitine metabolism and their nutritional management, *Annu. Rev. Nutr.*, 18, 179, 1998.
64. Chen, W., Huang, Y.–C., Shultz, T. D., and Mitchell, M. E., Urinary, plasma, and erythrocyte carnitine concentrations during transition to a lactovegetarian diet with vitamin B-6 depletion and repletion in young and adult women, *Am. J. Clin. Nutr.*, 67, 221, 1998.

Choline

Choline (β-hydroxyethyl): trimethyl ammonium hydroxide
   molecular weight: 121.18

Choline chloride
   molecular weight: 139.63

Choline was isolated and identified by Strecker in 1868.[25,26] It has been long recognized as a lipotropic factor. Most species can synthesize their needs for choline. An exception is the need for choline for growth and in prevention of the leg disorder, perosis, in poultry and turkeys.[29] A low-choline diet fed to rats results in fatty infiltration of the liver. Prolonged feeding of a choline deficient diet may result in the development of hepatocarcinomas.[38-41,44]

Under normal conditions, the human has been considered not to require a dietary source of choline.[29,36-38,49] Choline is found widespread in foods, primarily in the form of phosphatidyl choline.[29] An average adult diet provides daily about 800 to 900 mg of choline.[27] Good sources of choline in the diet are beef liver and kidney, ham, most cereals, egg yolk, peanuts, soybean, asparagus, cauliflower, wheat germ, iceberg lettuce, and fish.[29,47]

Choline serves as a precursor for the biological synthesis of lecithin (phosphatidyl-choline), sphingomyelin, and choline plasmalogens. These compounds are essential components of membranes.[28-30] Choline is also the precursor of the neurotransmitter acetylcholine and a methyl donor for betaine formation.[30] Choline metabolism, function, and requirements have been the topics of several extensive reviews.[29,36-38,49]

Determination of Choline

Sensitive and specific methods to measure choline and acetylcholine are available. In 1971, Reid et al.[1] described an enzymatic radioassay for the determination of acetylcholine and choline. The assay had high specificity and sensitivity. Goldberg, McCaman, and Zeisel modified this procedure into a microassay with increased sensitivity to measure choline and acetylcholine in biological specimens.[2,3,8-11] Using a radioenzymatic technique,[2] plasma choline concentrations in normal subjects ranged from 10 to 20 μmol/L.[7] A diet high in choline doubled the plasma choline concentration.[7]

Eckernas and Aquilonius[4] described a simple and rapid method to measure free choline in plasma. Plasma was subjected to ultrafiltration and the choline concentration measured in the filtrate by a radio-enzymatic procedure.[5,6]

High-performance liquid chromatography (HPLC) may be used to isolate choline and related metabolites from blood, plasma and other biological specimens.[12,13,16,18] The separated choline and choline metabolites may be quantitated by colorimetric,[14] radioenzymatic,[2,11,15,19,20] electrochemical detection,[21-24] or mass spectrometric[15-17] techniques. Choline may be determined also with the use of gas chromatography/mass spectrometry.[12,13] The expensive equipment required will exclude many laboratories from using this procedure.

Choline Requirements and Assessment

Adults

In a controlled study, Zeisel et al. [29,30,36,38] fed 16 healthy male volunteers a semi-synthetic diet devoid of choline (Figure 53). Two groups were used: one group was supplemented with choline and the other group remained on the choline deficient diet for three weeks. In the choline-deficient group, plasma choline concentrations decreased an average of 30% during the 21 days of choline deficiency. During this deficiency period, plasma and erythrocyte phosphatidylcholine concentrations decreased 15%. The choline deficient subjects developed incipient liver dysfunction as reflected in the steadily increasing serum alanine aminotransferase activity. The initial plasma choline concentration was 10.5 µmol/L and fell to 7.5 µmol/L at the end of the three week choline depletion period. The investigators concluded that choline was an essential nutrient for the human.[30]

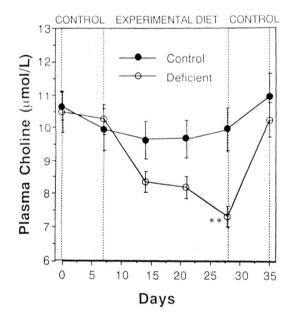

FIGURE 53
The effects of feeding a choline-deficient diet or a choline-supplemented diet on the plasma choline concentrations in healthy male subjects.[30,36] (With permission.)

Malnourished patients ($n = 25$) receiving total parenteral nutrition (TPN) without choline supplementation were observed to have decreasing plasma choline concentrations (from 7.3 ± 1.0 to 4.7 ± 0.5 µmol/L).[45] Plasma choline concentrations increased when the patients received lipid emulsions. Controlled hospitalized patients ($n = 23$) had plasma choline concentrations of 9.7 ± 0.7 µmol/L.[45]

Buchman et al.[46] also observed that most patients who require long-term TPN had plasma free choline concentrations that were below normal. Hepatic aminotransferase abnormalities also occurred in the patients. The hepatic dysfunction was corrected when choline was made available through lecithin supplementation.

These above studies indicate that the adult human has a requirement for a dietary source of choline.[29,30] The essentiality of choline is supported also by the benefits of choline supplements in the treatment of some adults and children with neuropsychiatric and medical problems.[28-35] The Food and Nutrition Board Recommended Dietary Allowance Committee suggests a choline intake of 550 mg/day for adult men and 425 mg/day for adult women.

Infants

Evidence suggests that prematurely born infants or infants of low birth weight may have reduced abilities to synthesize choline. Accordingly, the Committee on Nutrition of the American Academy of Pediatrics, has recommended the addition of choline in special formula diets, such as in infant formulas based on milk substitutes, to a level of at least 7 mg per 100 kcal.[42]

Plasma Choline Concentrations

The free choline concentrations in plasma from healthy fasted adult subjects ($n = 23$) was 10.6 ± 0.4 µmol/L.[4] The free choline concentration in plasma from the umbilical vein at post partum was 24.5 ± 1.9 µmol/L.[4] Children age 4 to 11 years ($n = 8$) had a free choline concentration of 9.7 ± 0.6 µmol/L.[4]

Choline Toxicity

Although the toxicity of choline has not been evaluated in the healthy adult, oral pharmacological doses of up to 20 g per day have been used for periods of several weeks to treat patients with Huntington's disease or tardive dyskinesia.[28] Occasionally patients reported dizziness, nausea, and diarrhea.

Summary

The occurrence of a choline deficiency in the healthy human must be rare, since most ordinary foods contain significant amounts of choline. In addition, the normal person has an endogenous pathway for the *de novo* biosynthesis of the choline moiety that involves an interrelationship between choline, methionine, folate, and vitamin B-12.[43] Kang[43] has noted that supplementation of choline, pyridoxine, folic acid, and vitamin B-12 to maintain serum concentrations above the low normal range may help prevent the development of hyperhomocyst(e)inemia and associated vascular diseases. For adults, the maintenance of a plasma choline concentration of about 10 µmol/L would be desired.[4,45]

References

1. Reid, W. R., Haubrich, O. R., and Krishna, G., Enzymic rdioassay for acetylcholine and choline in brain, *Analyt. Biochem.*, 42, 390, 1971.
2. Goldberg, A. M. and McCaman, R. E., The determination of picomole amounts of acetylcholine in mammalian brain, *J. Neurochem.*, 20, 1, 1973.
3. Goldberg, A. and McCaman, R., in *Choline and Acetylcholine: Handbook of Chemical Assay Methods*, Hanin, I., Ed., Raven Press, New York, 1974.
4. Eckernas, S.–A. and Aquilonius, S.–M., Free choline in human plasma analyzed by a simple radio-enzymatic procedure: age distribution and effect of a meal, *Scand. J. Clin. Invest.*, 37, 183, 1977.
5. Shea, P. A. and Aprison, M. H., An enzymatic method for measuring picomole quantities of acetylcholine and choline in CNS tissue, *Analyt. Biochem.*, 56, 165, 1973.
6. Smith, J. C. and Saelens, J. K., Determination of tissue choline with choline acetyltransferase, *Fed. Proc.*, 26, 296, 1967.
7. Zeisel, S. H., Growdon, J. H., Wurtman, R. J., Magil, S. G., and Logue, M., Normal plasma choline responses to ingested lecithin, *Neurology*, 30, 1226, 1980.
8. Zeissel, S. H., Char, D., and Sheard, N. F., Choline, phosphatidylcholine and sphingomyelin in human and bovine milk and infant formulas, *J. Nutr.*, 116, k 50, 1986.
9. Zeisel, S. H., Formation of unesterified choline by rat brain, *Biochem. Biophys. Acta*, 835, 331, 1985.
10. McCaman, R. E. and Stetzler, J., Radiochemical assay for acetylcholine modification for sub-picomole measurements, *J. Neurochem.*, 28, 669, 1977.
11. Zeisel, S. H. and Wurtman, R. J., Developmental changes in rat blood choline concentration, *Biochem. J.*, 198, 565, 1981.
12. Zeisel, S. H. and da Costa, K. A., Choline: determination using gas chromatography/mass spectrometry, *J. Nutr. Biochem.*, 1, 55, 1990.
13. Pomfret, E. A., daCosta, K. A., Schurman, L. L., and Zeisel, S. H., Measurement of choline and choline metabolite concentrations using high-pressure liquid chromatography and gas chromatography-mass spectrometry, *Annu. Biochem.*, 180, 85, 1989.
14. Barak, A. J. and Tuma, D. J., Determination of free choline and phosphorylcholine in rat liver, *Lipids*, 14, 304, 1979.
15. Sheard, N. F. and Zeisel, S. H., An *in vitro* study of choline uptake by intestine from neonatal and adult rats, *Pediatr. Res.*, 20, 768, 1986.
16. Jope, R. S. and Jenden, D. J., Choline and phospholipid metabolism in the synthesis of acetylcholine in rat brain, *J. Neurosci. Res.*, 4, 69, 1979.
17. Liberato, D. J., Yergey, A. L., and Weintraub, S. T., Separation and quantification of choline and acetylcholine by thermospray liquid chromatography/mass spectrometry, *Biomed. Environ. Mass Spectrom.*, 13, 171, 1986.
18. Liscovitch, M., Freese, A., Blusztajn, J. K., and Wurtman, R. J., High-performance liquid chromatography of water-soluble choline metabolites, *Anal. Biochem.*, 151, 182, 1985.
19. Gilberstadt, M. L. and Russell, J. A., Determination of picomole quantities of acetylcholine and choline in physiologic salt solutions, *Analyt. Biochem.*, 138, 78, 1984.
20. Muma, N. A. and Rowell, P. P., A sensitive and specific radioenzymatic assay for the simultaneous determination of choline and phosphatidylcholine, *J. Neurosci. Meth.*, 12, 249, 1985.
21. Potter, P. E., Meek, J. L., and Neff, N. H., Acetylcholine and choline in neuronal tissue measured by HPLC with electrochemical detection, *J. Neurochem.*, 41, 188, 1983.
22. Barnes, N. M., Costall, B., Fell, A. J., and Naylor, R. J., An HPLC assay procedure of sensitivity and stability for measurement of acetylcholine and choline in neuronal tissue, *J. Pharm. Pharmacol.*, 39, 727, 1987.
23. Damsma, G. and Flentge, F., Liquid chromatography with electrochemical detection for the determination of choline and acetylcholine in plasma and red blood cells: failure to detect acetylcholine in blood of humans and mice, *J. Chromatogr.*, 428, 1, 1988.

24. Kaneda, N., Asamo, M., and Nagatsu, T., Simple method for the simultaneous determination of acetylcholine, choline, noradrenaline, dopamine and serotonin in brain tissue by high-performance liquid chromatography with electrochemical detection, *J. Chromatogr.*, 360, 211, 1986.

25. Strecker, A., *Annu. de Chem. u. Pharm.*, 148, 77, 1868.

26. Strecker, A., Uber einige neue Bestandtheile der Schwengalle, *Annu. de Chem. u. Pharm.*, 123, 353, 1862.

27. Ziesel, S. H., Choline an important nutrient in brain development, liver function and carcino-gensis, *J. Am. Coll. Nutr.*, 11, 473, 1992.

28. Woodbury, M. M. and Woodbury, M. A., Neuropsychiatric development: two case reports about the use of dietary fish oils and/or choline supplementation in children, *J. Am. Coll. Nutr.*, 12, 239, 1993.

29. Ziesel, S. H., Choline deficiency, *J. Nutr. Biochem.*, 1, 332, 1990.

30. Ziesel, S. H., da Costa, K. A., Franklin, P. D., Alexander, E. A., Lamont, J. T., Sheard, N. F., and Beiser, A., Choline, an essential nutrient for humans, *FASEB J.*, 5, 2093, 1991.

31. Wood, J. L. and Allison, R. G., Effects of consumption of choline and lecithin on neurological cardiovascular systems, *Fed. Proc.*, 41, 3015, 1982.

32. Rosenberg, G. S. and Davis, K. L., The use of cholinergic precursors in neuropsychiatric disease, *Am. J. Clin. Nutr.*, 36, 709, 1982.

33. Davis, K. L. and Berger, P., Pharmacological investigations of cholinergic imbalance hypothesis of movement disorders and psychosis, *Biol. Psychiatr.*, 13, 23, 1978.

34. Barbeau, A., Cholinergic treatment in Tourette's syndrome, *N. Engl. J. Med.*, 302, 1310, 1980.

35. Tozaki, Y., Sakai, F., Otomo, E., Kutsazawa, T., Kameyama, M., Omae, T., Fujishima, M., and Sakuma, A., Treatment of acute cerbral infarction with a choline precursor in a multicenter double-blind placebo-controlled study, *Stroke*, 19, 211, 1988.

36. Zeisel, S. H. and Blusztajn, J. K., Choline and human nutrition, *Annu. Rev. Nutr.*, 14, 269, 1994.

37. Zeisel, S. H., Dietary choline: biochemistry, physiology, and pharmacology, *Annu. Rev. Nutr.*, 1, 95, 1981.

38. Zeisel, S. H., Choline, in *Modern Nutrition in Health and Disease*, 8th edition, Shils, M. E., Olsen, J. A. and Shike, M., Eds., Lea & Febiger, Philadelphia, 1994, 449.

39. Copeland, D. H. and Salmon, W. D., The occurrence of neoplasmas in the liver, lungs, and other tissues of rats as a result of prolonged choline deficiency, *Am. J. Pathol.*, 22, 1059, 1946.

40. Salmon, W. D., Copeland, D. H., and Burns, M. J., Hepatomas in choline deficiency, *J. Natl. Cancer Inst.*, 15, 1549, 1955.

41. Newberne, P. M. and Rogers, A. E., Labile methyl groups and the promotion of cancer, *Annu. Rev. Nutr.*, 6, 407, 1986.

42. Committee on Nutrition: Commentary on breast-feeding and infant formulas including proposed standards for formulas, *Pediatrics*, 57, 278, 1976.

43. Kang, S.–S., Treatment of hyperhomocyst(e)inemia: physiological basis, *J. Nutr.*, 126, 1273S, 1996.

44. Salmon, W. D. and Copeland, D. H., Liver carcinoma and related lesions in chronic choline deficiency, *Ann. N.Y. Acad. Sci.*, 57, 664, 1954.

45. Sheard, N. F., Tayek, J. A., Bistrian, B. R., Blackburn, G. L., and Zeisel, S. H., Plasma choline concentrations in humans fed parenterally, *Am. J. Clin. Nutr.*, 43, 219, 1986.

46. Buchman, A. L., Moukarzel, A., Jenden, D. J. et al., Low plasma free choline is prevalent in patients receiving long-term parenteral nutrition and is associated with hepatic amino-transferase abnormalities, *Clin. Nutr.*, 12, 33, 1993.

47. Engel, R. W., The choline content of animal and plant products, *J. Nutr.*, 25, 441, 1943.

48. Life Sciences Research Office, Evaluation of the health aspects of choline chloride and choline bitartrate as food ingredients, Life Sciences Research Office, FASEB, Bethesda, MD, SCOGS-42, 1975.

Inositol (Myo-Inositol)

Inositol (myo-inositol)

molecular weight: 180.16

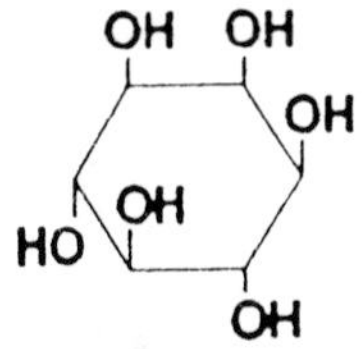

FIGURE 54
Structure of inositol.

The typical U.S. diet provides approximately 1 gram of inositol per day. Most of the inositol is present in plant foodstuffs in the form of phytate. A major source of information on the myo-inositol contents of foods was the report of Clements and Darnell.[18] They analyzed 487 common foods for myo-inositol content by gas chromatography. Although inositol is essential for the mouse, gerbil, and a few other rodents and some fish, its essentiality in the human has been less established.[1-9] Consequently, a Recommended Dietary Allowance for myo-inositol has not been established.[10] Nevertheless, important metabolic roles have been reported for myo-inositol.[1-3] Of particular interest has been the metabolic association of myo-inositol in several clinical conditions such as renal disease, diabetes, and respiratory distress syndrome.[1-4] Pre-term infants with respiratory distress syndrome have been reported to benefit from inositol supplements.[11] The level of myo-inositol in human milk is quite high (1840 ± 451 µmol/L).[4] Although breast-fed infants have a two-fold higher serum concentration of myo-inositol than infants receiving parenteral nutrition or formula, the nutritional significance of these differences require further studies. Infant formulas frequently contain added inositol.[12] Plasma levels of inositol are high in neonates (108 ± 10 µmol/L)[4,13] and continue high through the early months of life.[5] Adult human plasma contains considerable less inositol (52 ± 6 µmol/L).[4] Inositol appears to be relatively nontoxic and is considered by the Food and Drug Administration as a GRAS item.

Myo-inositol can be measured in serum and other samples by a specific enzymatic fluorimetic assay.[6] Analyses have been performed also by gas chromatography and other methods.[14,15] Also available for the measurement of inositol are microbiological assays.[16,17] *Saccharomyces uvarum* (ATCC 9080, formerly *Saccharomyces carlsbergensis* ATCC 9080), has been the most employed assay organism. A standard curve of 0 to 1.0 µg/mL is used that provides adequate sensitivity to measure inositol concentrations in plasma. The assay may be performed also with the use of *Kloeckerra brevis* ATCC 9774 as the test organism.[16]

References

1. Holub, B. J., Metabolism and function of myo-inositol and inositol phospholipids, *Annu. Rev. Nutr.*, 6, 563, 1986.
2. Holub, B. J., The nutritional significance, metabolism, and function of myo-inositol and phosphatidylinositol in health and disease, *Adv. Nutr. Res.*, 4, 107, 1982.
3. Aukema, H. M. and Holub, B. J., Inositol and pyroloquinoline quinone, A. Inositol, in *Modern Nutrition in Health and Disease*, 8th edition, Shils, M. E., Olson, J. A., and Shike, M., Eds., Lea & Febiger, Philadelphia, 1994, 466.
4. Pereira, G. R., Baker, L., Egler, J., Corcoran, L., and Chiavacci, R., Serum myo-inositol concentrations in premature infants fed human milk, formula for infants, and parenteral nutrition, *Am. J. Clin. Nutri.*, 51, 589, 1990.
5. Pereira, G. R., Baker, L., and Egler, J. et al., The effect of gestational age and types of feeding on serum levels of myo-inositol in neonates, *Pediatr. Res.*, 21, 435A, 1987.
6. McGregor, L. C. and Matschinsky, F. M, An enzymatic fluorimetric assay for myo-inositol, *Annu. Biochem.*, 141, 382, 1984.
7. Berridge, M. J., Inositol triphosphate and diacylglycerol: two interacting second messengers, *Annu. Rev. Biochem.*, 56, 159, 1987.
8. Downes, C. P. and Macphee, C. H., Myo-inositol metabolites as cellular signals, *Eur. J. Biochem*, 193, 1, 1990.
9. Ranna, R. S. and Hodin, L. E., Role of phosphinositides in transmembrane signaling, *Physiol. Rev.*, 70, 115, 1990.
10. Institute of Medicine/National Research Council, Recommended Dietary Allowances. 10th edition, National Academy Press, Washington D.C., 1989.
11. Hallman, M., Arjomaa, P., and Hoppu, K., Inositol supplementation in respiratory distress syndrome: relationship between serum concentration, renal excretion, and lung effluent phospholipids, *J. Pediatr.*, 110, 604, 1987.
12. Composition of medical foods for infants, children and adults with metabolic disorders, Ross Products Division, Abbott Laboratories, Columbus, OH 43215, February, 1994.
13. Bromberger, P. and Hallman, M., Myo-inositol in pre-term infants: relationship between intake and serum concentrations, *J. Pediatr. Gastroenterol. Nutr.*, 5, 455, 1986.
14. Eades, D. M., Williamson, J. R., and Sherman, W. R., Rapid analysis of sorbitol, galactitol, mannitol, and myo-inositol mixtures from biological sources, *J. Chromatogr.*, 490, 1, 1989.
15. Palmer, S. and Wakelam, M. J., Mass measurement of inositol phosphates, *Biochim. Biophys. Acta*, 1041, 239, 1989.
16. Difco Supplementary Literature, Difco Laboratories, Detroit, MI, 1972, 445.
17. Atkin, L., Schultz, A. S., Williams, W. L., and Frey, C. N., Yeast microbiological methods for the determination of vitamins, Pyridoxine, *Ind. Eng Chem., Anal. Ed.*, 15, 141, 1943.
18. Clements, R. S. Jr. and Darnell, B., Myo-inositol content of common foods: development of a high-myo-inositol diet, *Am. J. Clin. Nutr.*, 33, 1954, 1980.

Taurine

Taurine (2-aminoethanesulfonic acid)

$H_2N\text{-}CH_2\text{-}CH_2\text{-}SO_3H$

molecular weight: 125.14

Taurine has been recognized since 1827 when it was isolated from ox bile,[35] however, its nutritional importance for the human has remained unclear. Cats and kittens are susceptible to taurine deficiency.[3,4,6-8] The deficiency is associated with retinol degeneration, cardiomyopathy, growth and reproductive failure, fetal malformations, and neutrophil dysfunction.[1-6] The condition may reflect an inadequate synthesis of taurine.[8] An impairment of the transsulfuration pathway may result in an inadequate synethesis of taurine from methionine.[8-10]

In the human, the primary pathway for taurine biosynthesis involves the conversion of methionine to cysteine to cysteine sulfinic acid.[1-3] Cysteine sulfinic acid may then be converted to hypotaurine, which is oxidized to taurine. Cysteine sulfinic acid may also be oxidized to cysteic acid which is then decarboxylated to form taurine. Normally the taurine needs of the human are provided by this biosynthetic system. Several reviews have considered the biochemistry and physiology of taurine.[1-6,9,10]

Although it has been long recognized that taurine participates in the cojugation of bile acids, evidence now exist that taurine participates in other biological roles, including development of the nervous system, neuromodulation, cell membrane stabilization, detoxifications, and osmoregulation.[1,2,8,9,28,34] Other evidence suggests a possible role for taurine use in congestive heart disease, acute hepatitis, cystic fibrosis, and myotonia.[1]

In the human, bile acids are conjugated with either taurine or glycine.[32] Taurocholic acid is superior to glycocholic acid as a detergent. Infants given taurine-free total parenteral nutrition become hypotaurinemic and hypocystinemic. Such infants were observed to have abnormal electroretinograms.[27,28,31,38] Taurine supplements corrected the condition. Fasting plasma taurine concentrations of patient children receiving total parenteral nutrition were only $26 \pm 13\ \mu mol/L$ compared to concentrations of $57 \pm 16\ \mu mol/L$ for the control children. The investigators concluded that children (and possible adults) receiving long-term parenteral nutrition have a nutritional requirement for taurine.[29,30,37-39]

With long-term parenteral nutrition, taurine concentrations of plasma, platelets, lymphocytes, and erythrocytes were reduced by 35 to 49%.[28,29] Thus plasma taurine was reduced from $74 \pm 27\ \mu mol/L$ in the adult controls ($n = 15$) to $34 \pm 16\ \mu mol/L$ ($n = 40$) in the adult patients.

Taurine deficiency is commonly observed in children with cystic fibrosis[22,23] and with cholestasis.[39] Taurine supplements (30 mg/kg/day) increased the urinary excretion of taurine, but did not significantly increase the plasma taurine concentrations. Plasma and platelet taurine concentrations have been reported to be lower in insulin-dependent diabetes.[24] Thus, the plasma taurine concentrations in the controls ($n = 34$) was $93.3 \pm 6.3\ \mu mol/L$ versus $65.6 \pm 31\ \mu mol/L$ in the diabetic patients ($n = 39$). Supplements of 500 mg of taurine three times a day raised the plasma taurine concentrations to 126.8 ± 12 μmol/L. Plasma taurine concentrations have been observed to be uniformly low in patients after intensive chemotherapy and/or radiation.[25] The clinical significance of this effect is not clear.

Strict vegetarians (vegans) have low plasma taurine concentrations compared to the levels of nonvegetarian controls subjects (e.g., 45 ± 7 versus 58 ± 16 μmol/L, respectively).[26] Urinary excretion of taurine was lower for the vegetarians when compared to that of the nonvegetarian controls (e.g., 266 ± 279 versus 903 ± 580 μmol/day, respectively).[26] The vegetarian diets provided only negligible amounts of taurine. Generally, taurine is found only in foods of animal origin.[1] Taurine is present in high concentrations in the retina and in human breast milk.

Assessment of Taurine Status

Satisfactory methods to assess the status of taurine in the body are not available. At present, the most reliable accurate evaluation of status is the use of plasma and whole blood taurine concentrations. Whole-blood taurine values would appear to be the best single measure.[16]

For normal human subjects, whole blood taurine may range from 164 to 318 μmol/L with a mean concentration of 225 ± 38 μmol/L.[16] The normal range of taurine in plasma is considered to range form 35 to 60 μmol/L (mean: 44 ± 9 μmol/L; $n = 70$).[16] Hence, plasma taurine concentrations below 30 μmol/L may suggest the onset of taurine depletion.[2,16] What plasma concentration of taurine corresponds to a taurine deficiency in the human is uncertain.[2] Nevertheless, plasma taurine concentrations in low-birth-weight infants are low. Plasma taurine concentrations were found to range from 16 to 34 μmol/L between the third and seventh postnatal week.[17]

Measurement of Taurine

A comparison was made of high-performance capillary electrophoresis (HPCE), high performance liquid chromatography (HPLC), and automated amino acid analyzer for the measurement of taurine and related sulfur compounds in blood and urine.[18] Comparable results were obtained with the three methods. HPCE provides a quick, simple, and sensitive alternative to the use of an automated amino acid analyzer.

Automatic amino acid analyzers have been commonly used to quantitate taurine levels in plasma. Using this method, normal adults were found to have plasma taurine concentrations of 45 ± 4 nmol/L.[19] Certain precautions must be applied in the preparation of the plasma samples to avoid overestimation of the taurine concentrations.[20]

Hayes et al.[11] studied the effect of taurine supplements on the plasma and platelet taurine concentrations and platelet aggregation in the human. Taurine was measured by the HPLC method of Stables and Siegal[12] using fluorescence detection. Several other sensitive HPLC methods for measuring taurine in biological fluids are available.[13-15] Collecting blood samples with EDTA as the anticoagulant is recommended.[16]

Effect of Taurine Supplementation on Plasma and Platelet Taurine Concentration ($n = 5$)

Diet	Plasma Taurine (μmol/L)	Platelet Taurine (μmol/10^{10} platelets)
Basal diet	50 ± 2	1.31 ± 0.06
Basal + 400 mg taurine	71 ± 3	2.10 ± 0.08
Basal + 1600 mg taurine	74 ± 4	2.80 ± 0.10

Adapted from Reference 11.

Summary

Although taurine has been considered a conditional essential nutrient,[8] more recent investigations have established its importance in a number of roles, including fetal development, neurologic development, and in the vision process.[2,36,37] Thus pre-term and low-birth-weight infants may benefit from taurine supplementation.[37,38] Plasma concentrations below 30 μmol/L probably indicates an inadequate taurine status. Some of the infant formulas and commercial modified medical food preparations are fortified with taurine. Commonly, 100 g of the dry nutritional preparation is fortified with 60 mg of taurine.[30,33,37,38]

References

1. Kendler, B. S., Taurine: an overview of its role in preventive medicine, *Preventive Med.*, 18, 79, 1989.
2. Hayes, K. C. and Trautwein, E. A., Taurine, in *Moderin Nutrition in Health and Disease*, Shils, M. E., Olson, M. A., and Shike, M., Eds., Lea & Febiger, Philadelphia, 1994, 477.
3. Hayes, K. C. and Sturman, J. A., Taurine in metabolism, *Annu. Rev. Nutr.*, 1, 401, 1981.
4. Hayes, K. C., Taurine requirements in primates, *Nutr. Rev.*, 43, 65, 1985.
5. Sturman, J. A. and Hayes, K. C., The biology of taurine in nutrition and development, *Adv. Nutr. Rev.*, 3, 231, 1980.
6. Hayes, K. C., Taurine nutrition, *Nutr. Res. Rev.*, 1, 99, 1988.
7. Knopf, K., Sturman, J. A., Armstrong, M., and Hayes, K. C., Taurine: an essential nutrient for the cat, *J. Nutr.*, 108, 773, 1978.
8. Gaull, G. E., Taurine as a conditionally essential nutrient in man, *J. Am. Coll. Nutr.*, 5, 121, 1986.
9. Wright, C. E., Tallan, H. H., and Lin, Y. Y., Taurine: biological update, *Annu. Rev. Biochem.*, 55, 427, 1986.
10. Jacobsen, J. G. and Smith, L. H., Biochemistry and physiology of taurine derivatives, *Physiol. Rev.*, 48, 423, 1968.
11. Hayes, K. C., Pronczuk, A., Addesa, A. E., and Stephan, Z. F., Taurine modulates platelet aggregation in cats and humans, *Am. J. Clin. Nutr.*, 49, 1211, 1989.
12. Stabler, T. V. and Siegel, A., Rapid liquid-chromatographical fluorometric method for taurine in biological fluids involving prederivation with fluorescamine, *Clin. Chem.*, 27, 1771, 1981.
13. Trautwein, E. A. and Hayes, K. C., Evaluating taurine status: determination of plasma and whole blood taurine concentration, *J. Nutr. Biochem.*, 2, 571, 1991.
14. Larsen, B. R., Grosso, D. S., and Chang, S. Y., A rapid method for taurine quantitation using high performance liquid chromatography, *J. Chromatogr. Sci.*, 18, 233, 1980.

15. Porter, D. W., Banks, M. A., Castravova, V., and Martin, W. G., Reversed-phase high-performance liquid chromatography technique for taurine quantitation, *J. Chromatogr.*, 454, 311, 1988.
16. Trautwein, E. A. and Hayes, K. C., Taurine concentrations in plasma and whole blood in humans: estimation of error from intra- and interindividual variation and sampling techniques, *Am. J. Clin. Nutr.*, 52, 758, 1990.
17. Zelikovic, I., Chesney, R. W., Friedman, A. L., and Ahlfors, C. E., Taurine depletion in very low birth weight infants receiving prolonged total parenteral nutrition: role of renal immaturity, *J. Pediatr.*, 116, 301, 1990.
18. Jellum, E., Thorsrud, A. K., and Time, E., Capillary electrophoresis for diagnosis and studies of human disease, particularly metabolic disorders, *J. Chromatogr.*, 559, 455, 1991.
19. Tachiki, K. H., Hendrie, H. C., Kellams, J., and Aprison, M. H., A rapid column chromatographic procedure for the routine measurement of taurine in plasma of normal and depressed patients, *Clin. Chim. Acta*, 75, 455, 1977.
20. Connolly, B. M., and Goodman, H. O., Potential sources of errors in caution-exchange chromatographic measurement of plasma taurine, *Clin. Chem.*, 26, 508, 1980.
21. Goodman, H. O. and Shinkabl, Z. K., Automated analysis for taurine in biological fluids and tissues, *Clin. Chem.*, 33, 835, 1987.
22. Thompson, G. N., and Tomas, F. M., Protein metabolism in cystic fibrosis: responses to malnutrition and taurine supplementation, *Am. J. Clin. Nutr.*, 46, 606, 1987.
23. Thompson, G. N., Assessment of taurine deficiency in cystic fibrosis, *Clin. Chim. Acta*, 171, 233, 1988.
24. Franconi, F., Bennardini, F., Mattana, A., Miceli, M., Ciuti, M., Mian, M., Gironi, A., Anichini, R., and Seghieri, G., Plasma and platelet taurine are reduced in subjects with insulin-dependent diabetes mellitus: effects of taurine supplementation, *Am. J. Clin. Nutr.*, 61, 1115, 1995.
25. Desai, T. K., Maliakkal, J., Kinzie, J. L., Ehrinpreis, M. N., Luk, G. D., and Cejka, J., Taurine deficiency after intensive chemotherapy and/or radiation, *Am. J. Clin. Nutr.*, 55, 708, 1992.
26. Laidlaw, S. A., Shultz, T. D., Cesschino, J. T., and Kopple, J. D., Plasma and urine taurine levels in vegans, *Am. J. Clin. Nutr.*, 47, 660, 1988.
27. Rudman, D. and Williams, P. J., Nutrient deficiencies during total parenteral nutrition, *Nutr. Rev.*, 43, 1, 1985.
28. Geggel, H. S., Ament, M. E., Heckenlively, J. R., Martin, D. A., and Kopple, J. D., Nutritional requirements for taurine in patients receiving long-term parenteral nutrition, *N. Engl. J. Med.*, 312, 142, 1985.
29. Vinton, N. E., Laidlow, S. A., Ament, M. E., and Kopple, J. D., Taurine concentrations in plasma, blood cells, and urine of children undergoing long-term total parenteral nutrition, *Pediatr. Res.*, 21, 399, 1987.
30. Vinton, N. E., Laidlaw, S. A., Ament, M. E., and Kopple, J. D., Taurine concentrations in plasma and blood cells of patients undergoing long-term parenteral nutrition, *Am. J. Clin. Nutr.*, 44, 398, 1986.
31. Lombardini, J. B., Taurine: retinol function, *Brain Res. (Brain Res. Rev.)*, 16, 151, 1991.
32. Heird, W. C., Sulfur-containing amino acids in parenteral nutrition, in *Parenteral Nutrition in the Infant Patient*, Filer, L. J., and Leathem, W. D., Eds., Abbott Laboratories, Publishers, North Chicago, IL.
33. Ready reference: *Composition of Medical Foods for Infants, Children and Adults with Metabolic Disorders*, Ross Products Division, Abbott Laboratories, Columbus, OH, 1994.
34. Sturman, J. A., Nutritional taurine and central nervous system development, *Ann. N. Y. Acad. Sci.*, 477, 196, 1986.
35. Tiedemann, F. and Gmelin, L., Einige new Bestandtheile der Galle des Achsen, *Annu. Physik Chem.*, 9, 326, 1827.
36. Sturman, J. A., Taurine in development, *J. Nutr.*, 118, 1169, 1988.
37. Gaull, G. E., Taurine in pediatric nutrition: review and update, *Pediatrics*, 83, 433, 1989.
38. Ament, M. E., Geggel, H. S., Heckenlively, J. R., Martin, D. A., and Kopple, J., Taurine supplementation in infants receiving long-term total parenteral nutrition, *J. Am. Coll. Nutr.*, 5, 127, 1986.
39. Howard, D. and Thompson, D. F., Taurine: an essential amino acid to prevent cholestasis in neonates, *Annu. Pharmacotherapy*, 26, 1390, 1992.

Section III

Minerals

Body Electrolytes

Macrominerals

Trace Elements

Ultratrace Elements

Sodium, Potassium, and Chloride

Sodium
atomic weight: 23.00

Potassium
atomic weight: 39.10

Chloride
atomic weight: 35.45

units: 1 mmol/L = 1 mEq/L

The classical study of McCance first described the effect of a sodium chloride deficiency in the normal human adult.[1] A salt-free diet along with sweating were used to produce the deficiency. The deprivation led to aberrations of flavor, weakness, cramps, lassitude, severe cardiorespiratory distress on exertion, negative nitrogen balance, and weight loss.[1] The signs and symptoms of the deficiency were largely reversed within 24 hours after the consumption of sodium chloride.

A dietary deficiency of sodium normally would not occur;[2,3,4,50,53] however, with heavy and continuous sweating the body may become depleted of sodium.[5,6] Sodium retention may be impaired in certain medical conditions, including chronic diarrhea, use of diuretics, trauma, and renal disease.[7-9,26-28] Hyponatremia (decreased plasma sodium levels) is caused most commonly by either retention of water or a loss of sodium.[8,9,26-28,47,48] Increased plasma sodium concentrations (hypernatremia) may occur in conditions where body water loss is disproportionate to the body sodium loss or with inadequate intake of water.[7,9,27,28,47] Increased urinary excretion of sodium (hypernatriuria) may occur with the development of hyponatremia, adrenal failure, and diuretic usage. Low dietary intakes of sodium may be reflected in hyponatriuria.

Assessment

The main electrolytes in the body are the cations, sodium and potassium, and the anion, chloride. Phosphate is also important because of its buffering capacity. High concentrations of potassium and phosphate are present in the intracellular fluid, while the extracellular fluid contains high levels of sodium and chloride. Cell membranes, along with the kidney, regulate the transfer of electrolytes to and from the plasma. Thus, red blood cells are high in potassium and low in sodium. The presence of some hemolysis in samples has little effect on plasma sodium values, but hemolysis will give rise to falsely high plasma potassium values.

Plasma samples are preferred for potassium analysis. Serum potassium levels may be 0.1 to 0.7 mmol/L higher than that of plasma because of the release of potassium from the platelets during coagulation.

In the United States, as high as 40% of the Black Americans over age 50 years and 20% of the White Americans of the same age may have high blood pressure. It is recognized that the presence of high blood pressure may double the risk of death from heart attack, stroke, kidney disease, and other illnesses.[12] Blood pressure as low as 130/85 mmHg may be desirable.[67,68] Although genetic factors provide an important contribution to the occurrence or lack of occurrence of high blood pressure, sodium chloride (salt) has been implicated as a possible causal factor.[22,23,53] Regardless, a low sodium intake may ameliorate hypertension in many patients. Consequently, considerable attention is now given to the dietary intake of salt and its implications (Tables 65 and 66).[13,25,44,49,53,67,68]

TABLE 65
Reference Values for Sodium Assessment

Sample	Sodium Concentration mmol/L (mEq/L)	References
Plasma/Serum		
Normal	135 (136–146)	8
Abnormal		
Hyponatremia	< 130	8
Hypernatremia	≥ 150	7
Infants	Slightly lower than adults	17
Pregnancy (Plasma/Serum)		
Gestation	mmol/L	45
Week 15–18	135 (132–139)	
Week 27–30	136 (134–138)	
Week 35–38	137 (134–140)	
Urine Excretion (The Netherlands)		69
Men (*n* = 376)	167 ± 66	
Women (*n* = 440)	137 ± 56	
Urine Excretion (Japan)		60
Males	232 ± 6	
Female	186 ± 7	
Urine Excretion (Ireland)		59
Male	168 ± 45	
Female	134 ± 49	
Urine Excretion (U.S.A.)	Sodium level in the diet	57
Adult women	2000 mg/day 3500 mg/day	
Sodium excretion (mg/24 hr)	1945 ± 127 3412 ± 128	
Urine Sodium Excretion (Diet-Dependent)		
Adult males and females	100–150 mmol/g creatinine	58
Adult males	170–255 mmol/L urine	16
Sweat		
Normal	10–40 mmol/L	16
Cystic fibrosis	> 70 mmol/L	16

Potassium

Potassium occurs in a large number of foods. Consequently a dietary deficiency of potassium in the healthy individual is very unlikely. However, populations with a general low intake of potassium appear to have an increased incidence of various cardiovascular problems and an

TABLE 66
Reference Values for Potassium Assessment

Sample	Potassium Concentration mmol/L (mEq/L)	References
Plasma/Serum		17
Normal (plasma)	4.4 ± 0.3	
Non-pregnant women (plasma)	4.26 ± 0.13	
Normal adults (serum)	3.5–5.0	14
Hypokalemia (Serum)		14
Low	< 3.5	
Mild	3.0–3.5	
Severe	< 2.5	
Hyperkalemia (Serum)		15
Abnormal	> 5.0	
Emergency state	> 6.5	
Normal Adults		
Serum	3.5–5.0	
Plasma	3.5–4.5	
Newborn (serum)	3.7–5.9	
Pregnancy (Serum)		
Gestation		45
Week 15–18	3.4 (3.2–3.6)	
Week 27–30	3.5 (3.4–3.7)	
Week 35–38	3.6 (3.4–3.8)	
Urine Potassium Excretion		
Hypokalemia	< 20 mmol/L urine	14
Adults on average diet	25–125 mmol/day (40–60 mmol/g creatinine)	16, 57
Urine Excretion (The Netherlands)		
Men (*n* = 376)	79 ± 24 mmol/24 hrs.	69
Female (*n* = 440)	66 ± 19 mmol/24 hrs.	69
Urine Excretion (Japan)		
Adult males	59 ± 2 mmol/24 hrs.	60
Adult females	53 ± 2 mmol/24 hrs.	60
Urine Excretion (Ireland)		
Males (*n* = 92)	90 ± 26 mmol/24 hrs.	59
Females (*n* = 64)	65 ± 24 mmol/24 hrs.	59
Urine Excretion (U.S.A.)		58
Males	20 ± 11 mmol/g creatinine	
Females	21 ± 11 mmol/g creatinine	
Sweat	5–17 mmol/L	16
(Higher levels with cystic fibrosis)		

TABLE 67
Reference Values for Chloride Assessment

Samples	Chloride Concentration mmol/L (mEq/L)	References
Serum		
Normal	103 ± 3.0 (range 99–110 mmol/L)	11
Serum		
Non-pregnant women	104.7 (range 105–110 mmol/L)	17
Urine		
Chloride levels of < 10 mmol/L are abnormal and require medical attention.		

increased frequency of hypertension.[67] Low serum levels of potassium usually reflect reduced total body potassium. Potassium is located primarily intracellularly, with only 2% found in the intracellular fluid. Plasma levels of potassium are usually maintained quite constant with normal renal function.[47]

Serum potassium concentrations generally parallel body potassium stores. Hypokalemia (low serum potassium) is considered present when the serum potassium level is less than 3.5 mmol/L (3.5 mEq/L).[14] Hypokalemia usually occurs in a clinical setting such as with the use of laxatives or diurectics.[14] It is estimated that hypokalemia and hyperkalemia affects approximately 2% of normal healthy adults and 20 to 80% of subjects who are receiving diurectics.[51,55,56] A decrease in extracellular potassium may result in irritability, muscle weakness, and eventually to paralysis and impaired cardiac performance.[14]

In a study conducted on a population of elderly men and women (*n* = 381), 20% were found to have low concentrations of erythrocyte potassium and 2% had low levels of plasma potassium.[56] Plasma measurements of potassium provide little information as to the potassium nutritional status. Wide variations in dietary intake are generally not reflected in changes in potassium concentrations in the plasma or serum. The potassium homeostasis is closely regulated by potassium excretion by the kidney.

Hyperkalemia (elevated serum potassium; above 5.0 mmol/L) requires clinical attention dictated by the elevated serum levels of potassium and by abnormal electrocardiograms. Nutritional status has limited involvement in the problem, although the consumption of foods high in potassium need to be avoided (e.g., fruits, juice, potatoes, and potato chips.)

Sample Preparation for Sodium and Potassium Determinations

Plasma is preferred (sodium and ammonium heparin) for potassium determination. Separate plasma or serum from cells as soon as possible. Serum potassium levels maybe slightly higher than plasma because of release of potassium in the platelets during coagulation. Avoid hemolysis which will increase the potassium level in serum or plasma.

Because of the low level of sodium present in the red blood cells, some hemolysis can be tolerated without significantly influencing plasma or serum sodium values.

Both sodium and potassium concentrations in plasma or serum may be determined by flame emission spectrophotometry, by ion-selective electrode methods or atomic absorption spectrophotometry: usually flame emission spectrophotometry or ion-selective electrode methods are employed.[35] Both procedures have been incorporated into commerical automated analyzer systems that permit rapid analyses of large numbers of samples.[9] Commercial sodium chloride and potassium chloride standards are available that are based on standard reference materials (SRMs) available from the National Institute of Standards and Technology, Gaithersburg, MD, 20899. More detailed information on the methods for determining potassium and sodium are available eleswhere.[9]

Urine Measurements of Sodium and Potassium

Measurement of the urinary excretion of sodium and potassium have been used as an indirect estimation of sodium and potassium intake.[57,58] Urinary excretions of sodium and potassium represent 85 to 95% of the ingested sodium and potassium. Despite the use of various urine collection methods (e.g., morning urine samples, 24-hr collection, or multiple 24-hr urine collection), urine analyses for sodium and potassium have not been a practical or reliable means of assessing sodium and potassium intakes.[58,59] Difficulties are commonly encountered in collecting 24-hr urine samples. Multiple urine collections are required to characterize an individuals intake of sodium and potassium. For estimating the mean excretion of sodium or potassium of a population group, single 24-hr urine collections have been useful.[59] Correlations between dietary intake information and urinary excretion values for sodium and potassium have been low.[57,58] Relating sodium and potassium excretion to urinary creatinine excretion have also been used for the assessment of sodium and potassium intake.[60-66]

Although urinary creatinine excretion is fairly constant,[62-64] the use of a casual urine collection has not been a satisfactory substitute for a 24-hr urine collection.[61] This relates in part to the observation that urinary excretions of sodium and potassium have a circadian rhythm.[60] Attempts have been made to minimize this effect through the use of the second morning voided urine sample.[60]

Chloride

The occurrence of a chloride deficiency is unlikely in view of its widespread presence in the diet and its ready absorption. However, a diet-related chloride deficiency was observed in healthy infants fed inadvertantly diets containing only 1 to 2 mmol/L (1 to 2 mEq/L) of diet preparation.[18-20,46] In contrast, the American Academy of Pediatrics recommends a minimum of 10.4 mEg/L for infant formulas.[21]

Chloride represents the main inorganic anion in the extracellular fluid compartment. Chloride is an essential component of gastric juices and in the maintenance of fluid and electrolyte balance (Table 67).

On a nutritional basis, chloride should be considered along with sodium and potassium since nearly all dietary chloride occurs as sodium chloride. Additionally, the homeostatic control of chloride is closely related to potassium homeostasis. Thus, conditions that may lead to sodium and/or potassium deficiency would very likely result in a chloride deficiency as well. Chloride is also ubiquitous in nature and not easily considered along conventional nutritional lines.

Literature concerning analytical methodology for chloride is voluminous, perhaps because of the difficulty involved in obtaining accurate and precise measurements. The older gravimetric technique of precipitation as silver chloride had many limitations when considered on biological sample basis, including differences in organic matter content, possible loss of chloride during ashing procedures, and lack of completeness of extraction. Automated analyzers are available that use the spectrophotometric procedure (e.g., Technicon Instrument Corp.) of Zall et al.[10] Chloride is commonly measured in plasma, serum, urine or sweat. Various procedures are currently used, including mercurimetric titration, spectrophotometric methods, coulometric-amperometric titrations, and ion-selective electrode methods. The mercurimetric titration procedure may be applied to measurement of chloride in sweat samples collected on filter paper or gauze. The coulometric-amperometric titration methods and ion-selective methods can be adapted also to measure chloride levels in sweat samples. The technique results in the indirect determination of chloride through a coupled reaction. Mercuric thiocyanate is reacted with chloride to release thiocyanate which is subsequently reacted with ferric iron to form a red complex which is measured photometrically. Despite the indirectness of the assay, it has been used quite successfully. Using this procedure, chloride can be determined in plasma, serum, and urine.

The average serum chloride concentration in a group of "normal" subjects has been reported[11] as 103 ± 3.0 mmol/L (103 ± 3.0 mEq/L). A normal range for serum chloride based on numerous literature reports would appear to be 99 to 110 mmol/L (99 to 110 mEq/L).

A review of the older techniques that have been tried for the determination of chloride is available.[24]

Toxicity

Excessive intakes of sodium chloride may result in edema and hypertension. Normally with an adequate intake of water, the kidney will excrete the excess sodium.[53] For the healthy individual, excess dietary intakes of potassium are stored inside the cells and then eventually removed by urinary excretion.[53]

Sodium, Potassium, and Chloride

Sodium and potassium can be considered together on an analytical basis since the most widely used assay methods for each is flame photometry or use of ion-selective electrodes.[35] These methods can be used to determine sodium and potassium in plasma and urine, usually in a matter of minutes and without the necessity of chemical separations which are required in many of the wet chemical techniques. Additional advantages to the flame photometric method include: (a) the ability to determine both sodium and potassium on a very small sample; (b) the two elements may be determined without the supervision of an experienced chemist; (c) it is highly specific; and (d) accuracy and sensitivity are usually equal, and frequently exceed, those of the chemical techniques.

There are limitations to flame photometry. The equipment is more expensive than the equipment required in the chemical methods. This limitation becomes much less important if the number of samples to be processed is large as would be obtained in a large-scale survey for determining nutritional status. Another limitation of flame photometry is that the method gives an answer which is not absolute, but relative, to a standard solution; and herein lies the limitation. In order to truly compare the sample with the standard, the standard should be in the same matrix (similar in composition) as the sample. This is necessary to compensate for any spectrophotometric interferences or enhancements which might occur.[29-31,37,38,40] The preparation of such standards may be quite time consuming. However, this limitation has largely been overcome with the availability of commercially prepared standards of sodium chloride and potassium chloride and the use of reference methods for the determination of sodium potassium, and chloride.[29-34,38,40] Both flame emission spectrophotometry and ion-selective electrodes permit the simultaneous determination of sodium, potassium, and chloride on the same sample.[36] Clinical automated analyzers are available for both procedures that permit quick analyses of large sample number (e.g.,

Beckman Instruments, Instrumentation Laboratories, NOVA Biomedical, Eastman Kodak, Technicon Instruments).[29,30,36-39]

Potassium and sodium ion-selective field effect transistors have been studied as to their use in the measurement of sodium and potassium ions in whole blood.[41,42] This analytical procedure was found to be highly promising.[41] A portable hand-held analyzer has also been developed for the rapid bedside measurement of sodium, potassium and chloride (i-STAT Portable Clinical Analyzer; i-STAT Corp., Princeton, NJ).[52] An evaluation study indicated that the device was generally suitable for point-of-care testing in a clinical setting.[52]

Patient point-of-care testing for whole blood potassium levels may also employ the STAT K system (PD Technologies Inc., Westlake Village, CA).[51] The instrument uses disposable ion-selective electrodes. An evaluation of this handheld analyzer was found to be accurate, precise, and rapid and compared favorably with analyses obtained in a central clinical laboratory.[51]

Platelet levels of sodium and potassium have been proposed to provide a better index of intracellular cautions or total body ion status than serum/plasma, or erythrocyte concentrations. A relatively simple procedure has been reported for the isolation of platelets and the determination of their sodium and potassium levels by flame photometry.[43] Normal sodium and potassium concentrations were observed to be 1.3 ± 0.6 and 4.5 ± 1.5 µmol 10^8 cells, respectively. The usefulness of the assay in the clinical environment requires further study.

Various procedures have been studied for the assessment of the dietary intake of sodium and potassium.[57,58] Food consumption information has been unreliable because of the widespread and variable levels of sodium in food items, discretionary and non-discretionary intakes of sodium, contributions from drinking water, medications, and other soruces.[53] To overcome some of these influences, individual food consumption data have been collected for 7 to 10 day periods using dietary diary-interview techniques.[53,57,58] Other procedures have also been attempted to assess dietary sodium intakes.[57]

Guidelines for normal plasma levels of electrolytes have been quite variable between laboratories presumably due to methodological differences and the quality of the reference standards used. This has been reduced with the use of commercially prepared standards of KCl and NaCl. Certified reference materials (SRM) for sodium, potassium, and chloride analyses are also available from the National Institute of Standards and Technology, Gaithersburg, MD, 20899.

Serum or plasma concentrations of sodium below 135 mmol/L (135 mEq/L) are classified as hyponatremia.[8] Hypernatremia is defined as an increase in serum or plasma sodium concentrations to above 150 mmol/L (150 mEq/L).[7] Hypernatremia may be caused by an inadequate intake of water and dehydration.

Summary

Attaching nutritional significance to fluctuations in serum sodium and potassium levels is difficult and probably inconclusive due to variations resulting from certain pathological states. However, a deficiency might be anticipated in specific cases in which excessive loss of sodium and potassium have occurred, such as in prolonged use of diuretics, diarrhea, chronic renal failure, vomiting, profuse sweating, etc. The ubiquity of sodium and potassium in nature probably renders meaningless their consideration from a conventional nutritional point of view. Conversely, their nutritional importance is increased under the conditions mentioned above where a deficiency may be induced, or, in cases in which salt tablets have been ingested to maintain osmotic equilibrium.

Nevertheless, information on the intake of sodium may have important implications because of its associations with hypertension. Urinary measurements of sodiums can serve as an indicator of level of salt intake. Hyponatremia may occur with low intakes of sodium. Elderly are frequently found to have low erythrocyte potassium levels. The electrolytes, sodium, potassium, and chloride, are of major consideration in the clinical environment where conditions such as hypokalemia and hyperkalemia are encountered. The availability of ion-selective electrodes, flame emission spectrometry, or coulometric-amperometric procedures permit the simultaneous measurement of the electrolytes. Automated clinical analyzers are available that permit the rapid analyses of sodium, potassium, and chloride on large sample numbers. Portable analyzers are available for bedside measurement of electrolyes.

References

1. McCance, R. A., Experimental sodium chloride deficiency in man, *Proceedings of the Royal Society of London, series B-Biological Sciences*, 119, 245, 1935-1936.
2. *Nutrition Monitoring in the United States*, An update report on nutrition monitoring, Life Sciences Research Office, Federation of American Societies for Experimental Biology, U. S. Department of Health and Human Services, Hyattsville, Publication No. (PHS) 89-1255, 1989.
3. Page, L. B., Epidemiologic evidence on the etiology of human hypertension and its possible prevention, *Am. Heart J.*, 91, 527, 1976.
4. NRC (National Research Council), *Diet and Health: Implications for Reducing Chronic Disease Risk*, Report of the Committee on Diet and Health, Food and Nutrition Board, National Academy Press, Washington D.C., 1989.
5. Conn, J. W., The mechanism of acclimatization to heat, *Adv. Int. Med.*, 3, 373, 1949.
6. Consolazio, C. F., Matoush, L. O., Nelson, R. A., Harding, R. S., and Canham, J. E., Excretion of sodium, potassium, magnesium and iron in human sweat and the relation of each to balance and requirements, *J. Nutr.*, 79, 407, 1963.
7. Oh, M. S. and Carroll, H. J., Hypernatremia, in *Medicine for the Practicing Physician*, 4th ed., Hurst, J. W., Ed., Appleton & Lange, Stamford, 1996, 1411.
8. Carroll, H. J. and Oh, M. S., Hyponatremia, in *Medicine for the Practicing Physician*, 4th ed., Hurst, J. W., Ed., Appleton & Lange, Stamford, 1996, 1404.
9. *Textbook of Clinical Chemistry*, Tietz, N. W., Ed., W. B. Saunders, Philadelphia, 1986, 1172.
10. Zall, D. M., Fisher, D., and Garner, M. Q., Photometric determination of chlorides in water, *Anal. Chem.*, 28, 1665, 1956.
11. Frank, H. A., and Carr, M. H., "Normal" serum electrolytes with a note on seasonal and menstrual variation, *J. Lab. Clin. Med.*, 49, 246, 1957.
12. Abernethy, J. D., Sodium and potassium in high blood pressure, *Food Technology*, 57, 1979.
13. Hall, W. D. Jr., Mild, moderate, severe, and resistant hypertension, in *Medicine for the Practicing Physician*, 4th ed., Hurst, J. W., Ed., Appleton & Lange, Stamford, 1996, 1080.
14. Delaney, V., and Preuss, H. G., Hypokalemia, in *Medicine for the Practicing Physician*, 4th ed., Hurst, J. W., Ed., Appleton & Lange, Stamford, 1996, 1429.
15. Delaney, V., and Preuss, H. G., Hyperkalemia, in *Medicine for the Practicing Physician*, 4th ed., Hurst, J. W., Ed., Appleton & Lange, Stamford, 1996, 1433.
16. *Clinical Guide to Laboratory Test*, Tietz, N. W., Ed., W. B. Saunders, Philadelphia, 1983.
17. *Laboratory Indices of Nutritional Status in Pregnancy*, Food and Nutrition Board, National Research Council, National Academy of Sciences, Washington D.C., 1978.

18. Grossman, H., Duggan, E., McCamman, S., Welchert, E., and Hellerstein, S., The dietary chloride deficiency syndrome, *Pediatrics*, 66, 366, 1980.
19. Rodriquez-Soriano, J., Vallo, A., Castillo, G., Oiveros, R., Cea, J. M., and Balzategui, M. J., Biochemical features of dietary chloride deficiency syndrome: a comparative study of 30 cases, *J. Pediatr.*, 103, 209, 1983.
20. Roy, S. and Arant, B. S., Hypokalemic metabolic alkalosis in normotensive infants with elevated plasma renin activity and hyperaldosteronism: role of dietary chloride deficiency, *Pediatrics*, 67, 423, 1981.
21. American Academy of Pediatrics, *Pediatric Nutrition Handbook*, 2nd edition, American Academy of Pediatrics, Elk Grove Village, 1985.
22. Tobian, L. Jr., The relationship of salt to hypertension, *Am. J. Clin. Nutr.*, 32, 2739, 1979.
23. National Research Council, *Diet and Health: Implications for Reducing Chronic Disease Risk*, Report of the Committee on Diet and Health, Food and Nutrition Board, National Academy Press, Washington D.C., 1989.
24. Armstrong, G. W., Gill, H. H., and Rolf, R. F., The halogens, in *Treatise on Analytical Chemistry, Part II, Analytical Chemistry of the Elements*, Vol. 7, Kolthoff, I. M., and Elving, P. J., Eds., Interscience Publishers, New York, 1961, 335.
25. *Nutrition Monitoring in the United States*, Life Science Research Office, Federation of American Societies for Experimental Biology, U. S. Department of Health and Human Services, Hyattsville, 1989.
26. Subramanian, D. and Ayus, J. C., Case report: severe symptomatic hyponatremia associated with lisinopril therapy, *Am. J. Med. Sci.*, 303, 177, 1992.
27. Oh, M. S. and Carroll, H. J., Disorders of sodium metabolism: hypernatremia and hyponatremia, *Critical Care Med.*, 20, 94, 1992.
28. Votey, S. R., Peters, A. L., and Hoffman, J. R., Disorders of water metabolism: hyponatremia and hypernatremia, *The Emergency Medicine Clinics of North America*, 7, 749, 1989.
29. Kulpmann, W. R., Maibaum, P., and Sonntag, O., Analyses with KODAK-Ektachem, Accuracy control using reference method values and the influence of protein concentration. I. Electrolytes, *J. Clin. Chem. Clin. Biochem.*, 28, 825, 1990.
30. Kulpmann, W. R., Influence of protein on the determination of sodium, potassium and chloride in serum by Extachem DT 60 with DTE module; evaluation with special attention to a possible protein error by flame atomic emission spectrometry and ion-selective electrodes; proposals to their calibration, *J. Clin. Chem. Clin. Biochem.*, 27, 815, 1989.
31. Burnett, D., Ayers, G. J., Rumjen, S. C., and Woods, T. F., Sodium measurements in the presence of paraproteins by four direct ISE methods and flame photometry compared, *Annu. Clin. Biochem.*, 25, 102, 1988.
32. Velapoldi, R. A., Paule, R. C., Schaffer, R., Mandel, J., Murphy, T. J., and Gramlich, J. W., *Standard Reference Materials*: A reference method for the determination of chloride in serum, NBS Special Publication, 1979, 260-67.
33. Velapoldi, R. A., Paule, R. C., Schaffer, R., Mandel, J., Machlan, L. A., and Gramlich, J. W., *Standard Reference Materials*: A reference method for the determination of potassium in serum, NBS Special Publication, 1979, 260-64.
34. Velapoldi, R. A., Paule, R. C., Schaffer, R., Mandel, J., Machlan, L. A., and Gramlich, J. W., *Standard Reference Materials*: A reference method for the determination of sodium in serum, NBS Special Publication, 1978, 260-60.
35. Worth, H. G. J., A comparison of the measurement of sodium and potassium by flame photometry and ion-selective electrode, *Annu. Clin. Biochem.*, 22, 343, 1985.
36. Guagnellini, E., Spagliard, G., Berandi, G., and Stella, P., Reliability of 1L Monarch ion-sensitive electrode module for sodium, potassium, and chloride determinations, *Clin. Chem.*, 34, 746, 1988.
37. Cowell, D. C. and McGrady, P. M., Direct-measurement ion-selective electrodes: analytical error in hyponatremia, *Clin. Chem.*, 31, 2009, 1985.
38. Weisberg, L. S., Pseudohyponatremia: a reappraisal, *Am. J. Med.*, 86, 315, 1989.
39. Baadenhuijsen, H., Bayer, P. M., Keller, H., Knedel, M., Montalbetti, N., Vassault, A., Bablok, W., Poppe, W., and Stoeckmann, W., Multicentre evaluation of the Boehringer Mannheim/Hitachi 717 Analysis System, *J. Clin. Chem. Clin. Biochem.*, 28, 261, 1990.

40. Russell, L. J., Smith, S. C. H., and Buckley, B. M., Plasma sodium and potassium measurement: minimising ISE-flame differences using specimens from patients, *Annu. Clin. Biochem.*, 25, 96, 1988.

41. Thompson, J. M., Smith, S. C. H., Cramb, R., and Hutton, P., Clinical evaluation of sodium ion selective field effect transistors for whole blood assay, *Annu. Clin. Biochem.*, 31, 12, 1994.

42. Thompson, J. M., Emmett, C., Smith, S. C. H., Cramb, R., and Hutton, P., Comparison of potassium ISFETs with the Radiometer KNA1 and the Corning 902 ion-selective electrode analyzers for whole blood potassium ion estimation, *Annu. Clin. Biochem.*, 26, 274, 1989.

43. Touyz, R. M. and Milne, F. J., A method for determining total magnesium, calcium, sodium and potassium contents of human platelets, *Miner. Electrolyte Metab.*, 17, 173, 1991.

44. Weinsier, R. L., Salt and the development of essential hypertension, *Preventive Med.*, 5, 7, 1976.

45. Moniz, C. F., Nicolaides, K. H., Bamforth, F. J., and Rodeck, C. H., Normal reference ranges for biochemical substances relating to renal, hepatic, and bone function in fetal and maternal plasma throughout pregnancy, *J. Clin. Pathol.*, 38, 468, 1985.

46. Schwartz, R. B., The infant formula fiasco: the lack that will lead to a law, *Am. Council on Science and Health (ACSH)*, 1, 1, 1980.

47. Oh, M. S., Water, electrolyte, and acid-base balance, in *Modern Nutrition in Health and Disease*, 8 edition, Vol. 1, Shils, M. E., Olson, J. A., and Shike, M., Eds., Lea & Febiger, Philadelphia, 1994, 112.

48. Natkunam, A., Shek, C. C., and Swaminathan, R., Hyponatremia in a hospital population, *J. Med.*, 22, 83, 1991.

49. Food and Nutrition Board, Sodium-restricted diets and the use of diuretics, National Academy of Sciences, Washington D.C., 1979.

50. Haycock, G. B., The influence of sodium on growth in infancy, *Pediatr. Nephrol.* 7, 871, 1993.

51. Bishop, M. S., Husain, I., Aldred, M., and Kost, G. J., Multisite point-of-care potassium testing for patient-focused care, *Arch. Pathol. Lab. Med.*, 118, 797, 1994.

52. Erickson, K. A. and Wilding, P., Evaluation of a novel point-of-care system, the i-STAT portable clinical analyzer, *Clin. Chem.*, 39, 283, 1993.

53. Fregly, M. J., Sodium and potassium, *Annu. Rev. Nutr.*, 1, 69, 1981.

54. Zull, D. N., Disorders of potassium metabolism, *Emerg. Med. Clin. North Am.*, 7, 771, 1989.

55. Szerlip, H. M., Weiss, J., and Singer, I., Profound hyperkalemia without electrocardiographic manifestations, *Am. J. Kidney Dis.*, 7, 461, 1986.

56. Toultou, Y., Godard, J.-P., Ferment, O., Chastang, C., Proust, J., Bogdan, A., Ouzeby, A., and Toultou, C., Prevalence of magnesium and potassium deficiencies in the elderly, *Clin. Chem.*, 33, 518, 1987.

57. Sowers, M. and Stumbo, P., A method to assess sodium intake in populations, *J. Am. Dietet. Assoc.*, 86, 1196, 1986.

58. Kretsch, M. J., Sauberlich, H. E., and Skala, J. H., Nutritional status assessment of marines before and after the installation of the "multi-restaurant" food service system at the Twenty-nine Palms Marine Corps Base, California, Institute Report No. 192, Letterman Army Institute of Research, Presidio of San Francisco, 1984.

59. Shortt, C., Flynn, A., and Morrissey, P. A., Assessment of sodium and potassium intakes, *Eur. J. Clin. Nutr.*, 42, 605, 1988.

60. Kawasaki, T., Itoh, K., Uezono, K., and Sasaki, H., A simple method for estimating 24 hr. urinary sodium and potassium excretion from second morning voiding urine specimens in adults, *Clin. Exptl. Pharmocol. Physiol.*, 20, 7, 1993.

61. Watson, R. L. and Langford, H. G., Pilot studies of sodium, potassium, and calcium excretion, *Am. J. Clin. Nutr.*, 23, 290, 1970.

62. Arroyave, G. and Wilson, D., Urinary excretion of creatinine of children under different nutritional conditions, *Am. J. Clin. Nutr.*, 9, 170, 1961.

63. Liu, K., Dyer, A. R., Cooper, R. S., Stamler, R., and Stamler, J., Can overnight urine replace 24-hour urine collections to assess salt intake? *Hypertension*, 1, 529, 1979.

64. Pollack, H., Creatinine excretion as index for estimating urinary excretion of micronutrients or their metabolic and products, *Am. J. Clin. Nutr.*, 23, 865, 1970.

65. Pietinen, P. I., Findley, T. W., Causen, J. D., Finnerty, F. A., and Altschul, A. M., Studies in community nutrition: estimation of sodium output, *Preventive Med.*, 5, 400, 1976.

66. Milne, F. J., Gear, J. S. S., Laidley, L., Ritchie, M., and Schulty, E., Spot urinary electrolyte concentrations and 24 hour excretion, *Lancet*, 2, 1135, 1980.

67. Food and Nutrition Board, National Research Council, *Diet and Health*, National Academy Press, Washington D.C., 1989.

68. Public Health Service, U. S. Department of Health and Human Services, *The Surgeon General's Report on Nutrition and Health*, DHHS (PHS) Publication No. 88-50210, U. S. Government Printing Office, Washington D.C., 1988.

69. Brug, J., Lowik, M. R. H., van Binsbergen, J. J., Odink, J., Eggers, R. J., and Wedel, M., Indicators of iodine status among adults: Dutch nutrition surveillance system, *Annu. Nutr. Metab.*, 36, 129, 1992.

Calcium

Calcium
atomic weight: 40.08

$mEq/L \times 0.5 = mmol/L$; $mg/dL \times 0.25 = mmol/L$

$mmol/L \times 2 = mEq/L$; $mmol/L \times 4.0 = mg/dL$

Approximately 1% of the body calcium is present in the intracellular structures, cell membrane, and extracellular fluids. When inadequate calcium is absorbed or present in the diet, the calcium levels of these tissues and fluids are maintained by calcium removed from bone. Blood levels of calcium are maintained within narrow limits.[99] This control is the result of interplays with numerous factors, including 1,25-dihydroxycholecalciferol, parathyroid hormone, calcitonin, phosphorus, protein, estrogen, and other.[10,11,12,60]

In addition to its essential role in bone health,[5,70,73] calcium has a regulatory role in many metabolic processes including blood coagulation, muscle contraction, nerve conduction, heart contraction, and secretion of hormones.[10,52-55,60] As an example, in the case of the blood coagulation cascade, calcium is essential for factors VII, VIII, IX, prothrombin, fibrinogen, and platelet aggregation.

Osteoporosis

Interest in calcium nutritional status has increased as investigations have indicated an association of an adequate intake of calcium with a lowered risk of osteoporosis and of essential hypertension.[27,30,31,32,41,55,59,70,73,78,88,89] Bone disease, especially osteoporosis, is very common in elderly populations particularly in women.[93,99] With more people reaching an advanced age, bone health has become an important concern in the United States.

When the mass of bone mineral per unit volume of bone has significantly decreased beyond what it was at normal maturity, an osteoporotic condition exits.[30,55,70] The National Institute of Arthritis, Diabetes, and Digestive and Kidney Diseases estimates that at least 15 million Americans have some degree of osteoporosis. Adequate intake of calcium throughout life is probably the best way for people to protect themselves from the risk of osteoporosis.[22,58]

Calcium absorption may be decreased with age, in malabsorption syndromes, celiac disease, Crohn's disease, diabetes, chronic renal failure, montropical sprue, hypoparathyroidism, and primary biliary cirrhosis.[2,35] Increased absorption may occur with hyperparathyroidism.[2] Dietary fiber and phytate may decrease calcium absorption.[2] However, vitamin D is the major regulator of calcium absorption from the intestine.[3,4] With a vitamin D deficiency, calcium absorption is decreased.[3,4]

Osteoporosis represents a condition that relates to past long-term calcium losses, where bone resorption exceeds bone formation.[70] Bone loss is an accompaniment of the aging process. Bone remodeling is a constant process involving bone resorption and bone formation.

Biochemical markers have been proposed to study the bone resorptive process.[106-108,110] They include urinary measurements of calcium, 4-hydroxyproline, deoxypridinoline, and pyridinium cross-linking amino acids (pyridinoline).[44,45,50,87]

Elevated urinary levels of pyridinium cross-links are associated with elevated bone loss. Measurement of pyridinium cross-links can be used for the early diagnosis of osteoporosis before the disease has advanced to the stage of bone fractures. Early detection may permit effective treatment of osteoporosis. A commercial immunoassay test (Pyrilinks-D) is available for the measurement of pyridinium cross-links in urine (Metra Biosystems, Inc., Mountain View, CA). Bone formation may be studied with the use of serum biochemical markers such as osteocalcin (bone gla protein), bone-specific alkaline phosphatase, and carboxyterminal telopeptide of type I collagen.[37,40,42-44,46-49,108] High serum alkaline phosphatase reflects increased bone modeling.[24] These biochemical measurements, along with bone density determinations, are valuable in determining the effectiveness of therapy in the treatment of osteoporosis.[110] However, these procedures have had limited practical application in the assessment of calcium nutritional status. Intestinal absorption of calcium declines with age, partly as a result of declining efficiency of vitamin D metabolism.[7,22,76,77,86,94] Thus, men and women of over 50 years have been advised to increase their intake of calcium and of vitamin D.[7,22,74] Post-menopausal women commonly have bone loss which may lead to an osteoporotic condition.[8,38,74,78,93,96]

However, young people have also been advised to increase their intake of calcium.[33,73-75] Thereby, they can maximize the peak bone attained in the second and third decade, and protect against osteoporosis of late years.[7,22,74,75,95] Physical exercise may also increase bone mass.[12,73]

Rickets, osteomalacia, or osteoporosis may occur in infants and elderly subjects as a result of insufficient exposure to sunlight and/or to insufficient intake of vitamin D.[10-12,72] Osteomalacia is often due to a lack of adequate amounts of calcium and phosphorus in extracellular fluids.[85] This is commonly due to a decrease in the efficiency of calcium and mineral absorption from the intestine. A number of causes can be involved in the impaired calcium absorption such as a vitamin D deficiency, impaired conversion of vitamin D to its active metabolite, 1,25-dihydroxyvitamin D, drug interferences, low sunlight exposure, and renal failure.[72] Parathyroid hormone (parathormone) is produced by the parathyroid glands. The hormone increases serum levels of calcium and decreases serum levels of phosphorus. Increased parathyroid hormone levels in serum will cause bone to release stored calcium and phosphorus.

In a deficiency of 1,25-dihyroxycholecalciferol (calcitriol), intestinal absorption of calcium is reduced and serum levels of calcium may decrease. Serum calcium levels can be influenced by serum albumin levels, since a considerable amount of calcium in serum is bound to albumin. Hence, if serum albumin levels are above or below normal, corrections in the serum calcium level are made.[5,6,51] A normal serum albumin level is considered 40 g/L. Thus for a serum albumin level above 40 g/L, 8 mg/L of calcium is subtracted for each 10 g of serum albumin above the normal serum albumin level. If the albumin level is below normal, 8 mg/L of calcium is added for each 10 g/L of serum albumin.

Hypocalcemia

Hypocalcemia as seen in the clinic is rarely caused by a dietary deficiency of calcium, but rather by disorders of calcium metabolism, most commonly with hypoparathyroidism.[60,66,69]

Plasma total calcium concentration below 2.18 mmol/L (87 mg/L) is regarded as hypocalcemia.[66,69] The condition is usually corrected with the administration of calcium and vitamin D.[60,61,66] Hypocalcemia is often associated with hypoalbuminemia.[66] Hypocalcemia may occur also as a result of vitamin D deficiency, particularly in breast-fed infants that are not exposed to sunlight nor receiving vitamin D supplements (infantile rickets or osteomalacia).[60]

In patients with renal failure, where the production of 1,25-dihydroxy vitamin D is decreased, intestinal absorption of calcium is impaired that results in hypocalcemia. Signs and symptoms of hypocalcemia are usually present when the serum levels of ionized calcium fall below 0.63 mmol/L (25 mg/L; 1.25 mEq/L).[60] Patients with hypocalcemia may have weakness and fatigue, associated with neuromuscular symptoms, along with depression, cardiac abnormalities and other signs and symptoms.[60,66,69]

Hypercalcemia

Hyperparathyroidism is the most common cause of hypercalcemia.[71] When hypercalcemia occurs, calcitonin is released by the thyroid gland, which promotes the uptake of calcium by bone and induces blockage of bone resorption or breakdown.[10,60,66,68]

Parathyroid hormone (parathormone) released by the parathyroid glands may increase serum levels of calcium while decreasing serum levels of phosphorus. Increased production of parathyroid hormone will increase the release of calcium from the bone.[10,60] The majority of the cases of hypercalcemia (70 to 80%) are the result of hyperparathyroidism or malignancies.[59,60,66,68] The parathyroid hormone can be measured with the use of immunoradiometric assays.[60,66,68,71] Hypercalcemia is considered to exist when the plasma calcium level is greater than 2.6 mmol/L (105 mg/L).[66,71] Other causes of hypercalcemia include use of thiazide diuretics, vitamin A toxicity, vitamin D toxicity, thyrotoxicosis, and immobilization.[60,66,68,71] The patient with hypercalcemia may manifest neuropychiatric changes (depression) and serious cardiovascular conditions.[66,71]

Calcium Determination

An older method of determining calcium in serum was that of Clark and Collip[62] and of Kramer-Tisdall[63] wherein calcium is precipitated as the oxalate, the precipitate dissolved in acid, and resultant solution titrated with permanganate. The time-consuming titration procedures have been replaced with rapid automated procedures that commonly use the o-cresolphthalein complexone method.[60,66,68] Commercial clinical laboratory instruments are available that permit the completion of a calcium determination within 10 minutes on approximately 20 μL of serum (e.g., Technicon Instruments, Beckmann, Dupont, Abbott, Eastman Kodak, Hycel).[64,66]

Other sensitive and accurate methods are available to measure serum and urine calcium concentrations. Flame photometry and atomic absorption spectroscopy are often used.[65,68,109] Atomic absorption spectrophotometry provides greater precision but because of high sensitivity, sample dilution may be required. Standard reference materials (SRM) for calcium measurements in serum and urine are available from the National Institute of Science and Technology, Gaithersburg, MD.

Normal total serum calcium concentrations fall within a narrow range of about 2.10 to 2.55 mmol/L (85 to 105 mg/L; 4.25 to 5.25 mEq/L).[51,66,69] Values for children are slightly higher (2.20 to 2.70 mmol/L). Serum calcium levels maybe slightly depressed in pregnancy, mainly in the late stages. Nutritional interpretation of sera calcium data is extremely difficult due to the highly developed homeostatic control system. In fact, blood calcium is controlled so closely that, should it vary outside the normal range, one might suspect pathological problems before nutritional aspects.

Serum is the preferred sample for total calcium determination. Many anticoagulates can interfere with calcium determinations such as complexing with or precipitating the calcium in the sample. In addition stored serum samples are more reliable because with plasma samples, calcium may coprecipitate with fibrin. For the determination of ionized calcium, other precautions must be applied in the collection and handling of whole blood or plasma samples.[68,79,80,97,100] A number of clinical instruments are available for the measurement of ionized calcium in whole blood as well in serum or plasma (e.g., Nova Biomedical, Waltham, MA; Radiometer, Copenhagen, Denmark).[59,79-81,90,92-100]

The normal total serum concentration of calcium for the adult is 2.10 to 2.55 mmol/L (84 to 102 mg/L; 4 to 5 mEq/L).[51] For the adult, the normal concentration of ionized calcium as determined by ion selective electrodes is 1.12 to 1.23 mmol/L (44.8 to 49.2 mg/L; 2.24 to 2.46 mEq/L).[57,60,92] No difference in ionized calcium levels were noted between normal men and women.[100,102] Ionized calcium levels are considered to reflect calcium metabolism better than total serum levels.[90,92,97,98] For example, a significant decrease of serum ionized calcium regardless of the total calcium level may result in an increase in neuromuscular irritability which may lead to tetany. Serum ionized calcium levels have been useful in following hypocalcemia in critically ill surgical patients (Tables 68 to 74).[98]

TABLE 68
Reference Serum Calcium Concentrations

Group	Serum Calcium mmol/L (mg/L)	References
Adolescent (n = 21)	2.40 ± 0.2 (96 ± 8)	95, 103
Adults (n = 15)	2.45 ± 0.17 (98 ± 7)	
Elderly (age 75)		
Men and women (n = 89)	2.34 ± 0.08 (94 ± 3)	105
Definition:		
Hypocalcemia	< 2.18 mmol/L serum (< 85 mg/L)	66
Hypercalcemia	> 2.6 mmol/L serum (> 105 mg/L)	

TABLE 69
Serum Calcium Biochemical Parameters in Children

Parameter	Age (years) 2–5	9–11	15–16	References
Total calcium (mmol/L)	2.4 (22–2.7)	2.3 (1.6–2.8)	2.3 (1.6–2.7)	96, 101
Alkaline phosphatase (IU/L)	123 (60–220)	100 (33–222)	63 (21–155)	
25-(OH)-vitamin D (nmol/L)	82 (55–110)	68 (32–112)	72 (35–138)	
1,25-(OH)$_2$-vitmain D (pmol/L)	136 (61–238)	112 (46–294)	122 (68–275)	

n = 164.

TABLE 70

Calcium Biochemical Parameters for Young Girls

		Reference
Ages 8–13 (*n* = 370)		
Serum calcium (mmol/L)	2.40 ± 0.004	24
Urinary calcium (mmol/day)	2.06 ± 0.06	
Urinary calcium: creatinine	0.35 ± 0.01	
Calcium intake (mmol/day)	23.69	

TABLE 71

Calcium Levels in Serum and Urine in Adolescent and Adult Females

Parameters	Adolescent (*n* = 14)	Adults (*n* = 11)	References
Serum calcium (mg/L)	96 ± 4	96 ± 4	1
Urinary calcium (mg/day)	106 ± 44	204 ± 73	
Calcium intake (mg/day)	1332 ± 17	1349 ± 30	
Urinary calcium (mmol/day)			
Women		4.55 (1.25–10)	11
Men		6.22 (1.25–12.5)	11

TABLE 72

Effect of Age on Calcium Biochemical Parameters (Median Values)

	Age (Years)			
	<40	**50–59**	**70–79**	
Parameter	(*n* = 46)	(*n* = 52)	(*n* = 52)	References
Serum calcium (mg/dL)	9.46	9.46	9.46	104
Serum osteocalcium (mg/dL)*	5.45	6.65	7.86	
Serum alkaline phosphatase (IU/L)	20.9	24.7	28.6	
Urinary calcium (mg/24-hrs)	136	157	136	104

* Bone gla protein.

TABLE 73

Calcium Biochemical Parameters During Pregnancy

	Week of Pregnancy (n = 344)			
	15–18	**27–30**	**35–38**	**Reference**
Plasma calcium (mmol/L)	2.42	2.30	2.24	45
	(2.30–2.55)	(2.21–2.40)	(2.19–2.20)	
Plasma alkaline phosphatase (IU/L)	80	120	145	
	(4.3–110)	(90–150)	(80–200)	
Plasma phosphate (mmol/L)	1.05	1.02	1.00	
	(0.91–1.15)	(0.90–1.10)	(0.95–1.10)	

TABLE 74

Total Calcium and Ionized Calcium Levels in Serum From Various Population Groups

| | Serum Calcium | | |
| | Total | Ionized | |
Subject	(mmol/L)	(mmol/L)	References
Male (1–20 yr)	—	1.30	92
Females (1–20 yr)	—	1.30	92
Young women ($n = 66$)	2.40	1.21	99
Young men ($n = 69$)	2.41	1.48	99
Men ($n = 54$)	—	1.26 ± 0.04	102
Women ($n = 73$)	—	1.24 ± 0.05	102
Normal adult ($n = 149$)	2.43 ± 0.02	1.18 ± 0.006	100
Normal adults	2.5 (2.3–2.75)	1.18 (1.1–1.28)	84
Women			
Premenopausal ($n = 66$)	2.40 ± 0.01	1.21 ± 0.005	93
Postmenopausal ($n = 305$)	2.43 ± 0.004	1.20 ± 0.002	93
Elderly (80 ± 8 yr) ($n = 558$)	2.28 ± 0.12	1.24 ± 0.07	90
Geriatric Patients			
Men ($n = 116$)	2.28 (1.94–2.55)	1.23 (1.09–1.43)	81
Women ($n = 442$)	2.28 (1.83–2.84)	1.24 (0.95–1.63)	81

Bone Density Measurements and Calcium Status

The calcium requirement has been difficult to ascertain.[23,78,88,91] Often emphasis has been placed on dietary calcium intake, while the actual need for calcium is dependent on its absorption.[9-11,31] The bioavailability of calcium from various sources can be evaluated with the use of calcium absorption tests. However, calcium balance studies are necessary to arrive at the daily need for the mineral.[1,11,29,78,91] From the standpoint of nutritional assessment, the level of calcium intake that provides a calcium balance may serve as a state of calcium adequacy. Despite the many influencing factors and the difficulties and costs encountered, balance studies have been exceedingly valuable in determining the calcium requirement of the human.[9,10,78,83] Nevertheless, balance studies do not provide information on the extent to which calcium may have been lost in the past. Techniques are available that can provide information on bone mineral loss, such as single-photon absorptiometry[13] and dual-energy, x-ray absorptiometry (DEXA).[14,35,38,40,84]

For routine assessment of calcium status, calcium balance studies and bone density measurements are not practical. Bone mineral density changes have been followed over several years with the use of dual-energy, x-ray absorptiometry (e.g., Lunar DPX-L dual-energy x-ray absorptiometer (DEXA), Lunar Corp, Madison, WI).[14,24,25,35,38,40,84] Bone mass and bone mineral density measurements are useful in determining the effects of dietary calcium intake and of long-term calcium supplementation on bone density, particularly in the prevention and treatment of postmenopausal osteoporosis in women.[14-21,26-28,38] Thus, dual-energy, x-ray absorptiometry can provide information on the long-term calcium status, but the measurement cannot provide the information needed for clinical patient care, when the physiologic roles of calcium come into consideration.[84]

Urinary Excretion of Calcium

With adults, urinary excretion of calcium correlates with calcium intake.[23] In growing individuals, this relationship becomes uncertain because of the variable fraction of absorbed calcium that is retained in the skeletal compartment rather than excreted.[10,24,25] Obligatory urinary losses of calcium occur even under condition of low dietary intake and low calcium status.[35] Calcium excretion in the urine increases in postmenopausal women.[99]

Urinary excretion of calcium ranges from 2.5 to 6.0 mmol/day (100 to 240 mg/day), with considerable variation among normal subjects.[10] Dietary intakes of protein above the RDA[11] may also increase the urinary excretion of calcium.[56] Urinary excretion and absorption of calcium has been reported to increase during pregnancy.[39] Osteomalacia seen in elderly women is mainly the result of low vitamin D intake and an inadequate exposure to sunlight. Such patients commonly have low 24-hr urinary calcium levels (< 50 to 70 mg).

Because of the numerous factors that may influence the absorption and excretion of calcium, measurement of urinary excretion levels have not been a reliable index of dietary calcium deficiency.[9,10] A number of methods have been used to determine urinary calcium levels, including atomic absorption spectrometry and fluorimetric and colorimetric procedures.[82]

Calcium Toxicity

Calcium intakes up to 2500 mg/day have been considered safe for normal people. Only in rare disease conditions may elevated calcium intakes have an adverse effect.[34] High intakes of calcium are occasionally related to an increase in renal stones.[36]

Summary

A calcium deficiency is difficult to assess.[84] It develops slowly and is associated with a number of factors, such as dietary, endocrine, age, genetic, and clinical conditions. Serum calcium levels are closely controlled by the body over a wide range of intakes. Thus, serum or blood calcium concentrations outside of normal would be suspect of a pathological problem before that of a nutrition concern. A simple reliable laboratory technique for monitoring the adequacy of calcium intake does not exist.

However, it is possible to assess long-term calcium nutritional status by periodic measurements of bone density by photon densitometry or by dual-energy, x-ray absorptiometry (DEXA). The measurements can assess the body stores of calcium and the effects of long-term increased intakes of dietary calcium on these stores.

References

1. Weaver, C. M., Martin, B. R., Plawecki, K. L., Peacock, M., Wood, O. B., Smith, D. L., and Wastney, M. E., Differences in calcium metabolism between adolescent and adult females, *Am. J. Clin. Nutr.*, 51, 577, 1995.
2. Allen, L. H., Calcium bioavailability and absorption: a review, *Am. J. Clin. Nutr.*, 35, 783, 1982.
3. DeLuca, H. F., Recent advances in the metabolism of vitamin D, *Annu. Rev. Physiol.*, 43, 199, 1981.
4. Bikle, D. D., Calcium absorption and vitamin D metabolism, Clinics in Gastroenterol., 12, 379, 1983.
5. Chambers, J. K., Metabolic bone disorders: Imbalances of calcium and phosphorus, *Nursing Clinics of North America*, 22, 861, 1987.
6. Iqbal, S. J., Giles, M., Ledger, S., Nanji, N., and Howl, T., Need for albumin adjustments of urgent total serum calcium, *Lancet*, II, 1477, 1988.
7. Rowe, P. M., New U.S. recommendations on calcium intake, *Lancet*, I, 1559, 1994.
8. Prince, R., Dick, I., Boyed, F., Kent, N., and Garcia-Webb, P., The effects of dietary calcium deprivation on serum calcitriol levels in premenopausal and postmenopausal women, *Metabolism*, 37, 727, 1988.
9. Charles, P., Calcium absorption and calcium bioavailability, *J. Int. Med.*, 231, 161, 1992.
10. Allen, L. H., and Wood, R. J., Calcium and phosphorus, in *Modern Nutrition in Health and Disease*, Shils, M. E., Olson, J. A., and Shike, M., Eds., 8th edition, Lea & Febiger, Philadelphia, 1994, 144.
11. *Recommended Dietary Allowances*, 10th edition, Food and Nutrition Board, National Research Council, National Academy Press, Washington D.C., 1989.
12. Toss, G., Effect of calcium intake vs. other life-style factors on bone mass, *J. Internal Med.*, 231, 181, 1992.
13. Abrams, S. A., Schanter, R. J., and Garza, C., Bone mineralization in former very low birth weight infants fed either human milk or commercial formula, *J. Pediatr.*, 112, 956, 1988.
14. Reid, I. R., Ames, R. W., Evan, M. C., Gamble, G. D., and Sharpe, S. J., Long-term effects of calcium supplementation on bone loss and fractures in postmenopausal women: a randomized controlled trial, *Am. J. Med.*, 98, 331, 1995.
15. Welton, D. C., Kemper, H. C. G., Post, G. B., and Van Staveren, W. A., A meta-analysis of the effect of calcium intake on bone mass in young and middle age females and males, *J. Nutr.*, 125, 2802, 1995.
16. Sowers, M. R. and Galuska, D. A., Epidemiology of bone mass in premenopausal women, *Epidemiol. Rev.*, 15, 374, 1993.
17. Arnaud, C. D. and Sanchez, S. D., The role of calcium in osteoporosis, *Annu. Rev. Nutr.*, 10, 397, 1990.
18. Avioli, L. V. and Heaney, R. P., Calcium intake and bone health, *Calcif. Tissue Int.*, 48, 221, 1991.
19. Heaney, R. P., Nutritional factors in osteoporosis, *Annu. Rev. Nutr.*, 13, 287, 1993.
20. Kanis, J. A. and Passmore, R., Calcium supplementation in the diet, II, *Br. Med. J.*, 298, 205, 1989.
21. Kanis, J. A., Calcium requirements for optimal skeletal health in women, *Calcif. Tissue Int.*, 49, 533, 1991.
22. Optimal calcium intake, *NIH Consensus Statement*, Vol. 12, No. 4, June 6–8, 1994.
23. Nordin, B. E. C. and Marshall, D. H., Dietary requirements for calcium, in *Calcium in Human Biology*, Nordin, B. E. C., Ed., ILSI Human Nutrition Reviews, Springer-Verlag, Berlin, 1988, 447.
24. Matkovic, V., Ilich, J. Z., Andon, M. B., Hsieh, L. C., Tzagournis, M. A., Lagger, B. J., and Goel, P. K., Urinary calcium, sodium, and bone mass of young females, *Am. J. Clin. Nutr.*, 62, 417, 1995.
25. Matkovick, V., Fontana, D., Tominac, C., Goel, P., and Chesnut, C. H., Factors which influence peak bone mass formation: a study of calcium balance and the inheritance of bone mass in adolescent females, *Am. J. Clin. Nutr.*, 52, 878, 1990.
26. Sambrook, P. N., The treatment of postmenopausal osteoporosis, *N. Engl. J. Med.*, 333, 1495, 1995.
27. Calcium update: osteoporosis and hypertension, *Dairy Council Digest*, 58, 13, 1987.

28. Horowitz, M., Weshart, J. M., Goh, D., Morris, H. A., Need, A. G., and Nordin, B. E. C., Oral calcium suppresses biochemical markers of bone resorption in normal men, *Am. J. Clin. Nutr.*, 60, 965, 1994.

29. Selby, P. L., Calcium requirements — a reappraisal of the methods used in its determination and their application to patients with osteoporosis, *Am. J. Clin. Nutr.*, 60, 944, 1994.

30. Bronner, F., Calcium and osteoporosis, *Am. J. Clin. Nutr.*, 60, 831, 1994.

31. Weaver, C. M., Calcium bioavailability and its relation to osteoporosis, *Proc. Soc. Exp. Biol. Med.*, 200, 157, 1992.

32. Barger-Lux, M. J. and Heaney, R. P., The role of calcium intake in preventing bone fragility, hypertension, and certain cancers, *J. Nutr.*, 124, 1406S, 1994.

33. Andon, M. B., Lloyd, T., and Matkovick, V., Supplementation trials with calcium citrate malate: evidence in favor of increasing the calcium RDA during childhood and adolescence, *J. Nutr.*, 124, 1412S, 1994.

34. Heaney, R. P., Gallagher, J. C., Parfitt, A. M., and Whedon, G. D., Calcium nutrition and bone health in the elderly, *Am. J. Clin. Nutr.*, 36, 986, 1982.

35. Weaver, C. M., Age related calcium requirements due to changes in absorption and utilization, *J. Nutr.*, 124, 1418S, 1994.

36. Curhan, G. C., Willett, W. C., Rimm, E. B., and Stampfer, M. J., A prospective study of dietary calcium and other nutrients and the risk of symptomatic kidney stones, *N. Engl. J. Med.*, 238, 833, 1993.

37. Deftos, L. J., Bone protein and peptide assays in the diagnosis and management of skeletal disease, *Clin. Chem.*, 37, 1143, 1991.

38. Dawson-Hughes, B., Dallal, G. E., Krall, E. A., Sadowski, L., Sahyoun, N., and Tannenbaum, S., A controlled trial of the effect of calcium supplementation on bone density in postmenopausal women, *N. Engl. J. Med.*, 323, 878, 1990.

39. Cross, N. A., Hillman, L. S., Allen, S. H., Krause, G. F., and Vieira N. E., Calcium homeostasis and bone metabolism during pregnancy, lactation, and postweaning: a longitudinal study, *Am. J. Clin. Nutr.*, 61, 514, 1995.

40. Kleerehoper, M., Bone mass, bone remodeling, and biochemical markers, *Clinical Lab. News*, 5 (Nov.), 1994.

41. Hamet, P., The evaluation of the scientific evidence for a relationship between calcium and hypertension, *J. Nutr.*, 125, 311S, 1995.

42. Delmas, P. D., Christiansen, C., Mann, K. G., and Price, P. A., Bone Gla protein (osteocalcin) assay standardization report, *J. Bone Miner. Res.*, 5, 5, 1990.

43. Gertz, B. J., Shao, P., Hanson, D. A., Quan, H., Harris, S. T., Genant, H. K., Chesnut, C. H., III, and Eyre, D. R., Monitoring bone resorption in early postmenopausal women by an immunoassay for cross-linked collagen peptides in urine, *J. Bone Miner. Res.*, 9, 135, 1994.

44. Hanson, D. A., Weis, M. A., Singer, F. R., Eyre, D. R., Bollen, A. M., and Maslan, S. L., A specific immonoassay for monitoring human bone resorption: quantitation of type I collagen cross-linked N-telopeptides in urine, *J. Bone Miner. Res.*, 7, 1251, 1992.

45. Harvey, R. D., McHardy, K. C., Reid, I. W., Paterson, F., Bewsher, P. D., Duncan, A., and Robin, S. P., Measurement of bone collagen degradation in hyperthyroidism and during thyroxine replacement therapy using pyridinium cross-links as specific urinary markers, *J. Clin. Endocrin. Metab.*, 72, 1189, 1991.

46. Haslin, C., Mosekilde, L., Risteli, J., Eriksen, E. F., Melkko, J., Risteli, L., and Charles, P., Effect of a combined estrogen-gestagen regimen of serum levels of the carboxy-terminal propeptide on human type I procollagen in osteoporosis, *J. Bone Miner. Res.*, 6, 1295, 1991.

47. Kanzaki, S., Hosoda, K., Moriwake, T., Tanaka, H., Kubo, T., Inoue, M., Higuchi, J., Yamaji, T., and Seino, Y., Serum propeptide and intact molecular osteocalcin in normal children and children with growth hormone (GH) deficiency: a potential marker of bone growth and response to GH therapy, *J. Clin. Endocrinol. Metab.*, 75, 1104, 1992.

48. Masters, P. W., Jones, R. G., Purves, D. A., Cooper, E. H., and Cooney, J. M., Commercial assays for serum osteocalcin give clinically discordant results, *Clin. Chem.*, 40, 358, 1994.

49. Orwoll, E. S. and Deftos, L. J., Serum osteocalcin (BEF) levels in normal men: a longitudinal evaluation reveals an age-associated increase, *J. Bone Miner. Res.*, 5, 259, 1990.

50. Sehlemmer, A., Hassager, C., Jensen, S. B., and Christiansen, C., Marked diurnal variation in urinary excretion of pyridinium cross-links in premenopausal women, *J. Clin. Endocrin. Metab.*, 74, 476, 1992.
51. Tietz, N. W., *Clinical Guide to Laboratory Tests*, W. B. Saunders, Ed., Philadelphia, 1983, 92.
52. Klee, C. B. and Vanaman, T. C., Calmodulin, Review, *Adv. Protein Chem.*, 35, 213, 1982.
53. Wasserman, R. H. and Fullmer, C. S., Calcium transport proteins, calcium absorption, and vitamin D, *Annu. Rev. Physiol.*, 45, 375, 1983.
54. Reichardt, L. F. and Kelly, R. B., A molecular description of nerve terminal function, *Annu. Rev. Biochem.*, 52, 871, 1983.
55. Avioli, L. V., Calcium and osteoporosis, *Annu. Rev. Nutr.*, 4, 471, 1984.
56. Kerstetter, J. and Allen, L. H., Dietary protein increases urinary calcium, *J. Nutr.*, 120, 134, 1990.
57. Nielsen, F. H., Studies on the relationship between boron and magnesium which possibly affects the formation and maintenance of bones, *Magnesium Trace Elem.*, 9, 61, 1990.
58. Gaby, A. R. and Wright, J. V., Nutrition and osteoporosis, *J. Nutr. Med.*, 1, 63, 1990.
59. Frasher, D., Jones, G., Kooh, S. W., and Radde, I. C., Calcium and phosphate metabolism, in *Textbook of Clinical Chemistry*, Tietz, N. W., Ed., W. B. Saunders, Philadelphia, 1986, 1317.
60. DeCristofaro, J. B. and Tsang, R. C., Calcium, *Emergency Med. Clinics of North Am.*, 4, 207, 1986.
61. Juan, D., Hypocalcemia differential diagnosis and mechanisms, *Arch. Int. Med.*, 139, 1166, 1979.
62. Clark, E. P. and Collip, J. B., A study of the Tisdall method for the determination of blood serum calcium with a suggested modification, *J. Biol. Chem.*, 63, 461, 1925.
63. Kramer, B. and Tisdall, F. F., A simple technique for the determination of calcium and magnesium in small amounts of serum, *J. Biol. Chem.*, 47, 475, 1921.
64. Gilbert, R. K., Calcium analysis in clinical laboratories; according to the survey program of the College of American Pathologists, *Lab. Med.*, 2, 21, 1977.
65. Zettner, A. and Seligson, D., Application of atomic absorption spectrophotometry in the determination of calcium in serum, *Clin. Chem.*, 10, 869, 1964.
66. Bourke, E. and Delaney, V., Assessment of hypocalcemia and hypercalcemia, *Clinics Lab Med.*, 13, 157, 1993.
67. Endres, D. B., Villanueva, R., Sharp, C. F. Jr., and Singer, F. R., Measurement of parathyroid hormone, *Endocrinol. Metab. Clin. North Am.*, 18, 611, 1989.
68. Fraser, D., Jones, G., Kooh, S. W., and Radde, I. C., Calcium and phosphate metabolism, in *Textbook of Clinical Chemistry*, Tietz, N. W., Ed., Saunders, Philadelphia, 1986, 1317.
69. Umpierrez, G. E., Hypocalcemia and hypoparathyroidism, in *Medicine for the Practicing Physician*, Hurst, J. W., Ed., 4th edition, Appleton & Lange, Stamford, 1996, 662.
70. Heaney, P. R., Osteoporosis, in *Medicine for the Practicing Physician*, Hurst, J. W., Ed., 4th edition, Appleton & Lange, Stamford, 1996, 666.
71. Downs, R. W. Jr., Hypercalcemia and hyperparathyroidism, in *Medicine for the Practicing Physician*, Hurst, J. W., Ed., 4th edition, Appleton & Lange, Stamford, 1996, 655.
72. Kumar, R., Osteomalacia, in *Medicine for the Practicing Physician*, Hurst, J. W., Ed., 4th edition, Appleton & Lange, Stamford, 1996, 670.
73. Ulrich, C. M., Georgiou, C. C., Snow-Harter, C. M., and Gillis, D. E., Bone mineral density in mother-daughter pairs: relations to lifetime excercise, life-time milk consumption, and calcium supplements, *Am. J. Clin. Nutr.*, 63, 72, 1996.
74. Dawson-Hughes, B., Calcium and vitamin D nutritional needs of elderly women, *J. Nutr.*, 126, 1165S, 1996.
75. Anderson, J. J. B., Calcium, phosphorus and human bone development, *J. Nutr.*, 126, 1153S, 1996.
76. Holick, M. F., Vitamin D and bone health, *J. Nutr.*, 126, 1159S, 1996.
77. Calvo, M. S. and Park, Y. K., Changing phosphorus content of the U.S. diet: potential for adverse effects on bone, *J. Nutr.*, 126, 1168S, 1996.
78. Nordin, B. E. C., Horsman, A., Marshall, D. H., Simpson, M., and Waterhous, G. M., Calcium requirement and calcium therapy, *Clinical Orthopaedics and Related Research*, 140, 216, 1979.
79. Uldall, A., Fogh-Anderson, N., Thode, J., Boink, A. B. T. J., Kofstad, J., Larsson, L., Narvanen, S., Pedersen, K. O., and Weber, T., Measurement of ionized calcium with five types of instruments, An external quality assessment, *Scand. J. Clin. Lab. Invest.*, 45, 255, 1985.

80. Wandrup, J., Critical analytical and clinical aspects of ionized calcium in neonates, *Clin. Chem.*, 35, 2027, 1989.
81. Sorva, A., Elfving, S., Pohja, P., and Tilvis, R. S., Assessment of calcaemic status in geriatric hospital patients: serum ionized calcium versus albumin-adjusted total calcium, *Scand. J. Clin. Lab. Invest.*, 48, 489, 1988.
82. Gowans, E. M. S. and Fraser, C. G., Five methods for determining urinary calcium compared, *Clin. Chem.*, 32, 1560, 1986.
83. Spencer, H. and Kramer, L., The calcium requirement and factors causing calcium loss, *Federation Proc.*, 45, 2758, 1986.
84. Weaver, C. M., Assessing calcium status and metabolism, *J. Nutr.*, 120, 1470, 1990.
85. Okonofua, F., Alabi, Z. O., Thomas, M., Bell, J. L., and Dandona, P., Rickets in Nigerian children: a consequence of calcium malnutrition, *Metabolism*, 40, 209, 1991.
86. Fujita, T., Aging and calcium as an environmental factor, *J. Nutr. Sci. Vitaminol.*, 31, S15, 1985.
87. Shapses, S. A., Robins, S. P., Schwartz, E. I., and Chowdhurg, H., Short-term changes in calcium but not protein intake alter the rate of bone resorption in healthy subjects as assessed by urinary pyridinium cross-link excretion, *J. Nutr.*, 125, 2814, 1995.
88. Spencer, H. and Kramer, L., Osteoporosis, calcium requirement, and factors causing calcium loss, *Clinics in Geriatric Med.*, 3, 389, 1987.
89. Young, E. W., Bukoski, R. D., and McCarron, D. A., Calcium metabolism in experimental hypertension, *Proc. Soc. Expt. Biol. Med.*, 187, 123, 1988.
90. Sorva, A., Elfving, S., Sievers, G., and Tilvis, R. S., Calcemic status of geriatric patients: a longitudinal study, *Gerontology*, 38, 87, 1992.
91. Nordin, B. E. C., Polley, K. J., Need, A. G., Morris, H. A., and Marshall, D., The problem of calcium requirements, *Am. J. Clin. Nutr.*, 45, 1295, 1987.
92. Toffaletti, J., Ionized calcium: Part I, *Clin. Chem. News*, July, 10, 1989.
93. Nordin, B. E. C. and Morris, H. A., The calcium deficiency model for osteoporosis, *Nutr. Rev.*, 47, 65, 1989.
94. Ravaglia, G., Forti, P., Pratelli, L., Maioli, F., Scali, C. R., Bonini, A. M., Tedilo, S., Marasti, N., Pizzoferrato, A., and Gasbarrini, G., The association of aging with calcium active hormone status in men, *Age and Aging*, 23, 127, 1994.
95. Chan, G. M., Dietary calcium and bone mineral status of children and adolescents, *AJDC*, 145, 631, 1991.
96. Heaney, R. P., Effect of calcium on skeletal development, bone loss, and risk of fractures, *Am. J. Med.*, 91, 5B-23S, 1991.
97. Vanstapel, F. J. and Lissens, W. D., Free ionized calcium — a critical review, *Annu. Clin. Biochem.*, 21, 339, 1984.
98. Zaloga, G. P., Chernow, B., Cook, D., Snyder, R., Clapper, M., and O'Brian, J. T., Assessment of calcium homeostasis in the critically ill surgical patient, *Annu. Surg.*, 202, 587, 1985.
99. Nordink, B. E. C., Calcium homeostasis, *Clin. Biochem.*, 23, 3, 1990.
100. White, T. F., Farndon, J. R., Conceicao, S. C., Laker, M. F., Ward, M. K., and Kerr, D. N. S., Serum calcium status in health and disease: a comparison of measured and desired parameters, *Clin. Chim. Acta*, 157, 199, 1986.
101. Mohammed, S., Addae, S., Sulerman, S., Adzaku, F., Annobil, S., Kaddoumi, O., and Richards, J., Serum calcium, parathyroid hormone, and vitamin D status in children and young adults with sickle cell disease, *Annu. Clin. Biochem.*, 30, 45, 1993.
102. Rudnicki, M., Thode, J., Jorgensen, T., Heitmann, B. L., and Sorensen, O. H., Effects of age, sex, season and diet on serum ionized calcium, parathyroid hormone and vitamin D in a random population, *J. Internal Med.*, 234, 195, 1993.
103. Chan, G. M., McMurry, M., Westover, K., Englebert-Fenton, K., and Thomas, M. R., Effects of increased dietary calcium intake upon calcium and bone mineral status of lactating adolescent and adult women, *Am. J. Clin. Nutr.*, 46, 319, 1987.
104. Kotowicz, M. A., Melton, L. J. III, Cedel, S. L., O'Fallon, W. M., and Riggs, B. L., Effect on age on variables relating to calcium and phosphorus metabolism in women, *J. Bone Miner. Res.*, 5, 345, 1990.

105. Chapuy, M.-C., Chapuy, P., and Meunier, P. J., Calcium and vitamin D supplements: effects on calcium metabolism in elderly people, *Am. J. Clin. Nutr.*, 46, 324, 1987.
106. Colwell, A., Russell, G. G., and Eastell, R., Factors affecting the assay of urinary 3-hydroxy pridinium crosslinks of collagen as markers of bone resorption, *Eur. J. Clin. Invest.*, 23, 341, 1993.
107. Delmas, P. D., Clinical use of biochemical markers of bone remodeling in osteoporosis, Bone, 13, S17, 1992.
108. Rus, B. J., Biochemical markers of bone turnover in diagnosis and assessment of therapy, *Am. J. Med.*, 91, 5B, 1991.
109. *Analytical Methods for Atomic Absorption Spectrophotometry*, Perkin-Elmer Corporation, Norwalk, CT, 1982.
110. Kleerekoper, M., Evaluating and managing osteoporosis, *Clin. Lab. News*, December, 6, 1997.

Phosphorus

Phosphorus

atomic weight: 30.97 (mmol/L × 30.97 = mg/L)

About 80 to 88% of the body's phosphorus is found in bones and teeth where, mainly as hydroxyapatite, it has a structural role. The remaining phosphorus is located in the soft tissues and extracellular fluids. A major portion of the phosphorus that is located intracellularly is bound to lipids (phospholipids) and protein (phosphoproteins). A small fraction of phosphorus, referred to as inorganic phosphate (Pi), functions in high-energy transfer reactions. Most phosphate in serum or plasma is present as the "inorganic phosphate." Phosphorus absorption is intimately associated with vitamin D and calcium metabolism, calcitonin actions, and indirect influence of parathyroid hormone.[38] Vitamin D enhances phosphorus absorption although not absolutely essential for its absorption. Phosphorus has essential roles in the formation of triose and hexose phosphates in carbohydrate metabolism and in energy storage in the form of adenosine triphosphate (ATP) and creatine phosphate.[6] Phosphorus has many regulatory roles. For example, cyclic adenosine phosphate (CAMP) serves as a secondary messenger in the action of various hormones.

Because of the widespread presence of phosphorus in foods, a dietary deficiency of phosphorus would be very rare. An unusual phosphorus status is generally associated with a clinical or abnormal condition such as metabolic defects, inherited genetic defects, and tumors.[1,7,32,33,40,41] Thus, childhood hypophosphatemic rickets is frequently caused by a genetically related defect in renal tubular resorption of filtered phosphorus.[7] The presence of a tumor may also produce hypophosphatemia in adults.[1] Some early total parenteral nutrition preparations were phosphate-free and their use led to reports of acute, symptomatic hypophosphatemia.[35]

Hypophosphatemia

A serum phosphate level of less than 0.80 mmol (25 mg/L) indicates hypophosphatemia.[14] Normally, because of feedback systems, phosphorus homeostasis as well as calcium homeostasis are regulated within narrow limits.[6] Absorbed phosphate is readily excreted in the urine under the influence of parathyroid hormone. The average serum phosphate level of the normal adult is 1.0 to 1.5 mmol/L (35 mg/L; range 25 to 40 mg/L). Children 1 to 10 years of age have levels of 1.49 mmol/L (46 mg/L). Higher serum phosphate levels occur in premature infants [2.55 mmol/L (79 mg/L)] and full-term infants [1.97mmol/L (61 mg/L)].[3] Elevated serum alkaline phosphatase activity may also occur.[4,24,25,27,28] Premature infants fed exclusively human milk require additional phosphorus to avoid the development of hypophosphatemic rickets.[4,24,25,29-31] Laboratory procedures usually measure only the inorganic phosphate fraction in plasma or serum.[14-17] Thus, phosphorus values and reference ranges are commonly expressed as plasma inorganic phosphate (Pi).[14-17]

Phosphorus Measurements

Measuring phosphorus levels in the serum is essentially the only procedure available to evaluate phosphorus status. However, the interpretation of phosphorus levels is difficult because of the numerous factors that may influence the serum level.[41] Hypophosphatemia may result from chronic use of aluminum-containing antacids.[5,41] Insulin therapy, rickets, hyperparathyroidism, and malabsorption may result in hypophosphatemia. Rapid intravenous infusion of glucose in hospitalized patient may result in lowered serum phosphate levels.[6]

Abnormal plasma phosphate values may not reflect the body phosphate state of depletion. In starvation, the tissue catabolism releases phosphate to maintain an apparent normal plasma phosphate level. Hence, it is essential that adequate phosphate be provided in the nutritional preparations used to treat the starvation patient. Thereby, an acute intracellular phosphate depletion is avoided. Plasma phosphate (Pi) concentrations in infants are higher than that of adults. The values fall until 20 years of age and then remain essentially constant from then on. Levels in adult males tend to be slightly higher than those of adult females.

Chronic primary hypophosphatemia may result in muscle weakness, in skeletal deformities with resulting pain, malaise, and in growth retardation.[6,41] Phosphate depletion may result in an increased rate of red blood cell hemolysis and in lowered tissue levels of organic phosphoric acid esters, such as ATP.[6] Serum phosphate levels lower than < 0.30 mmol/L (9.3 mg/L) are usually associated with the occurrence of red blood cell fragility and hemolysis.[8-10] Hypophosphatemia usually results in an elevated serum alkaline phosphatase activity.

Hyperphosphatemia

Serum phosphate concentrations greater than 1.5 mmol/L (47 mg/L) indicate hyperphosphatemia. For children, hyperphosphatamia is associated with levels above 2.0 mmol/L (62 mg/L).[40] Several disease conditions may result in increased plasma/serum concentrations of phosphate. Such may occur with hypervitamosis D, hypoparathyroid disease, or renal failure.[6,40]

Serum Phosphate Determination

Only serum or heparinized plasma should be used since EDTA and other anticoagulants interfere with the color reaction of the assay.[14-17] Hemolysis must be avoided as erythrocytes contain about seven times more phosphate than plasma.[23] Frozen serum samples may be stored for several months before analyses.

Nearly all methods for the assay of inorganic phosphate utilize the principle introduced by Fiske and Subba Row in 1925.[18-20,26] Manual procedures for measuring phosphate in plasma have been adapted to automated applications (e.g., Technicon Autoanalyzer, SMAC Technicon Instruments and E. I. Du Pont Instrument Products).[19,20]

Serum or heparinized plasma samples may be used. The proteins are precipitated by trichloroacetic acid and the protein-free filtrate is mixed with ammonium phosphomolybdate. This complex is reduced to a blue colored complex with semidine HCl (N-phenyl-p-phenylenediamine HCl)and the color produced measured spectrophotometrically.[17]

The average normal range for serum phosphorus in the adult human appears to be 0.81 to 1.29 mmol/L (25 to 45 mg/L). In infants, serum phosphorus is somewhat higher at 1.60 to 2.10 mmol/L (50 to 65 mg/L). A small downward trend in serum phosphate appears to be associated with pregnancy.[36]

The number of factors that have been reported to alter plasma or serum phosphorus is too great to be within the scope of this review concerning methodology.[41] However, it would be germane to the discussion here to mention a few of the more prominent factors which effect serum or plasma phosphorus since they might be suspect should the assay produce data which are outside the normal range. Some of these factors have been summarized.[19] Blood inorganic phosphorus in rickets of children is markedly reduced. Vitamin D treatment of the disease will normalize the blood phosphorus picture. In persons with healing fractures, plasma phosphorus may be increased. In children, there appears to be a seasonal variation in plasma phosphorus; it rises during the summer and declines during the winter. This phenomenon is perhaps related, through the action of vitamin D, to solar ultraviolet radiation. In hypervitaminosis D, plasma levels of phosphorus as well as those of calcium may be elevated due to their increased intestinal absorption. In the diabetic, plasma phosphate levels may be quite variable since insulin injections tend to decrease the phosphorus in plasma. The information presented here is merely to show that the interpretation of laboratory test data for phosphorus from a nutritional point of view may be extremely difficult (Tables 75 and 76).

TABLE 75
Reference Values for Inorganic Phosphate in Serum Samples

Age	Concentrations of Inorganic Phosphate	
	mmol/L	mg/L
7 Days	2.16 ± 0.06	67 ± 2
14 Days	2.32 ± 0.03	72 ± 1
0–2 years	1.20–2.23	37–69
2–5 years	0.97–2.13	30–66
4–9 years	1.23–1.81	38–56
10–15 years		
Male	1.03–1.74	32– 54
Female	1.07–1.71	33–53
14–20 years		
Male	0.78–1.49	24–46
Female	0.84–1.49	26–46
40 years		
Male	0.78–1.36	24–42
Female	0.84–1.39	26–43
< 60 years		
Male	0.74–1.20	23–36
Female	0.90–1.32	28–41
> 70 years		
Male	0.65–1.26	20–39
Female	0.94–1.55	29– 48

From References 19, 20, and 39.

TABLE 76
Reference Values for Phosphorus Assessment

Sample	Phosphorus Concentration		Reference
	mmol/L	mg/L	
Military personnel			37
Serum			
Male	1.38 ± 0.02	42.7 ± 5.4	
Females	1.31 ± 0.02	40.2 ± 6.1	
Urine	mmol/g creatinine	mg/g creatinine	37
Male	22.6 ± 6.7	700 ± 209	
Female	22.5 ± 7.4	698 ± 229	

Toxicity

Excess intake of phosphate salts may have a cathartic effect. Otherwise phosphates appear safe and are rapidly removed from the body by urinary excretion. However, excessive intakes of phosphorus may block the hydroxylation of 25-hydroxyvitamin D to form 1,25-dihydroxyvitamin D. This may result in hypocalcemia.[34]

Urinary Phosphate

The mean intake of phosphorus is approximately 1,500 mg per day for the adult male and about 1,000 mg per day for the adult female.[2] The healthy kidney can excrete high loads of phosphate and thereby prevent hyperphosphatemia. The average individual in the United States excretes in the urine 600 to 800 mg of phosphate per day.[11] With a phosphate depletion state, the urinary excretion of phosphate approaches zero.[12,13] With renal failure plasma phosphate concentrations may rise. Measurement of urinary phosphate levels is of limited value. Phosphate levels reflect closely the dietary intake of phosphate, hence, day-to-day excretion may vary considerably.[37] However, a generally low intake of phosphate will be reflected in a low excretion level that may be of assessment value. Excessive intake of phosphate will be reflected in hyperphosphaturia.[21,22] Urine phosphate levels over 1,300 mg/24 hours (41.9 mmol) are considered high.

Summary

For the general population a dietary deficiency of phosphorus would be exceedingly rare. A phosphorus deficiency is usually the result of an abnormal metabolic conditions such as inherited genetic defects, hypoparathyroid disease, renal failure, or hypervitaminosis D. A phosphorus deficiency is characterized by hypophosphatemia, hypophosphaturia, hypercalciuria, and an elevated serum alkaline phosphatase activity. To evaluate the phosphorus status of a subject, serum or plasma phosphate concentrations are usually determined. Measurement of serum alkaline phosphatase activity or urinary concentrations of phosphate or of calcium may be useful but are less reliable predictors. Because of various interactions, the data must be evaluated with care.

References

1. Hanukoglu, A., Chalew, S. A., Sun, C. J., Dorfman, H. D., and Bright, R. W., Surgically curable hypophosphatemic rickets, *Clin. Pediatrics*, 28, 321, 1989.
2. *Recommended Dietary Allowances*, 10th edition, Food and Nutrition Board, National Research Council, National Academy Press, Washington D.C., 1989.
3. *Fundamentals of Clinical Nutrition*, Weinsier, R. L. and Morgan, S. L., Eds., Mosby, St. Louis, MO, 1993.
4. Rowe, J. C., Wood, D. H., Rowe, D. W., and Raisz, L. G., Nutritional hypophosphatemic rickets in a premature fed breast milk, *N. Engl. J. Med.*, 299, 293, 1979.
5. Lotz, M., Zisman, E., and Bartter, F. C., Evidence of a phosphorus-depletion syndrome in men, *N. Engl. J. Med.*, 278, 409, 1968.
6. Berner, Y. N. and Shike, M., Consequence of phosphate imbalance, *Annu. Rev. Nutr.*, 8, 121, 1988.
7. Rasmussen, A. and Anast, C., Familial hypophosphatemic rickets and vitamin D dependent rickets, in The Metabolic Basis of Inherited Disease, 5th edition, Stanbury, J. B., Wyngarden, J. B., Fredrickson, D. S., Goldstein, J. L., and Brown, M. S., Eds., McGraw-Hill Book Co., New York, 1983, 1743.
8. Jacob, H. S. and Amsden, T., Acute hemolytic anemia with rigid cells in hypophosphatemia, *N. Engl. J. Med.*, 285, 1446, 1971.
9. Lichtman, M. A., Miller, D. R., and Cohen, J., Reduced red cell glycolysis, 1,2-diphosphoglyc-erate and adenosine triphosphate concentration and increased hemoglobin-oxygen affinity caused by hypophosphatemia, *Annu. Int. Med.*, 74, 562, 1971.
10. Klock, J. C., Williams, H. E., and Metzer, W. C., Hemolytic anemia and somatic cell dysfunction in severe hypophosphatemia, *Arch. Int. Med.*, 134, 360, 1974.
11. Lau, K., Phosphate disorders, in *Fluids and Electrolytes*, Kokko, J. P. and Tanner, R. L., Eds., Saunders, Philadelphia, 1986, 398.
12. Dominguez, J. H., Gray, R. W., and Seean, J. Jr., Dietary phosphate deprivation in women and men: effect on mineral and acid balances, parathyroid hormone, and the metabolism of 25-OH-vitamin D, *J. Clin. Endocrinol. Metab.*, 43, 1056, 1976.
13. Sheldon, G. F. and Grzyb, S., Phosphate depletion and repletion, Relation to parenteral nutrition and oxygen transport, *Annu. Surg.*, 182, 683, 1975.
14. Keating, F. R., Jones, J. D., and Elveback, L. R. et al., The relation of age and sex to distribution of values in healthy adults of serum calcium, inorganic phosphorus, magnesium, alkaline phosphatase, total proteins, albumin, and blood ureas, *J. Lab. Clin. Med.*, 73, 825, 1969.
15. Cheng, M. H., Lipsey, A. I., and Blanco, V. et al., Microchemical analyses for 13 constituents of plasma from healthy children, *Clin. Chem.*, 25, 692, 1976.
16. Cherian, A. G. and Hill, J. G., Percentile estimates of reference values for fourteen chemical constituents in sera of children and adolescents, *Am. J. Clin. Nutr.*, 69, 24, 1978.
17. Garber, C. C. and Miller, R. C., Revisions of the 1963 semidine HCl standard method for inorganic phosphorus, *Clin. Chem.*, 29, 184, 1983.
18. Fiske, C. H. and Subba Row, Y., The colorimetric determination of phosphorus, *J. Biol. Chem.*, 66, 375, 1925.
19. *Textbook of Chimical Chemistry*, Tietz, N. W., Ed., W. B. Sanders Co., Philadelphia, 1986.
20. *Clinical Guide to Laboratory Tests*, Tietz, N. W., Ed., W. B. Sanders Co., Philadelphia, 1983.
21. Nordin, B. E. C. and Frasev, R., Assessment of phosphate excretion, *Lancet*, 1, 947, 1960.
22. Thalassinos, N. C., Leese, B., and Latham, S. C. et al., Urinary excretion of phosphate in normal children, *Arch. Dis. Child.*, 45, 269, 1970.
23. Kay, H. D., The distribution of phosphorus compounds in the blood of certain mammals, *J. Physiol.* (London), 65, 374, 1928.
24. Rowe, J., Rowe, D., and Horak, E. et al., Hypophosphatemia and hypercalciuria in small premature infants fed human milk: evidence for inadequate dietary phosphorus, *J. Pediatr.*, 104, 112, 1984.

25. Carey, D. E., Rowe, J. C., Goetz, C. A., Horak, E., Clark, R. M., and Goldberg, B., Growth and phosphorus metabolism in premature infants fed human milk, fortified human milk, or special premature formula, *AJDC*, 141, 511, 1987.

26. Gomori, G., A modification of the colorimetric phosphorus determination for use with the photoelectric colorimeter, *J. Lab. Clin. Med.*, 27, 955, 1942.

27. Bowers, G. N. and McComb, R. B., Measurement of total alkaline phosphatase activity in human serum, *Clin. Chem.*, 21, 1988, 1975.

28. Kovar, I., Mayne, P., and Barltrop, D., Plasma alkaline phosphatase activity: a screening test for rickets in preterm infants, *Lancet*, 1, 308, 1982.

29. Kovar, I. Z., Mayne, P. D., and Robbe, I., Hypophosphatemic rickets in the preterm infant: hypocalcemia after calcium and phosphorus supplementation, *Arch. Dis. Child.*, 58, 629, 1983.

30. Rowe, J. C. and Carey, D. E., Phosphorus deficiency syndrome in very low birth weight infants, *Pediatr. Clin. North America*, 34, 997, 1987.

31. Atkinson, S. A., Calcium and phosphorus requirements of low birth weight infants: a nutritional and endocrinological perspective, *Nutr. Rev.*, 41, 69, 1983.

32. Fiaccadori, E., Coffrini, E., Fracchia, C., Rampulla, C., Montagna, T., and Borghetti, A., Hypophosphatemia and phosphorus depletion in respiratory and peripheral muscles of patients with respiratory failure due to COPD, *Chest*, 105, 1392, 1994.

33. Knochel, J. P., The clinical status of hypophosphatemia, *N. Engl. J. Med.*, 313, 447, 1985.

34. DeLuca, H., Some new concepts emanating from a study of the metabolism and function of vitamin D, *Nutr. Rev.*, 38, 169, 1980.

35. Rudman, D. and Williams, P. J., Nutrient deficiencies during total parenteral nutrition, *Nutr. Revs.*, 43, 1, 1985.

36. *Laboratory Indices of Nutritional Status in Pregnancy*, Food Nutrition Board, National Research Council, National Academy of Sciences, Washington D.C., 1978.

37. Kretsch, M. J., Sauberlich, H. E., and Skala, J. H., Nutritional status assessment of marines before and after the installation of the "multi-restaurant" food services system at the Twentynine Palms Marine Corps Base, California, Institute Report No. 192, Letterman Army Institute of Research, Presidio of San Francisco, 1984.

38. Allen, L. H. and Wood, R. J., Calcium and phosphorus, in *Modern Nutrition in* Health *and Disease*, Volume 1, 8th edition, Shils, M. E., Olson, J. A., and Shike, M., Eds., Lea & Febiges, Philadelphia, 1994, 144.

39. Greer, F. R., Calcium, phosphorus, and magnesium: how much is too much for infant formulas, *J. Nutr.*, 119, 1846, 1989.

40. Bourke, E., and Berlyne, G. M., Hyperphosphatemia, in *Medicine for the Practicing Physician*, 4th edition, Hurst, J. W., Ed., Appleton & Lange, Stamford, CT, 1996, 1442.

41. Bourke, E., and Berlyne, G. M., Hypophosphatemia, in *Medicine for the Practicing Physician*, 4th edition, Hurst, J. W., Ed., Appleton & Lange, Stamford, CT, 1996, 1445.

Magnesium

Magnesium

atomic weight: 24.32

1 mmol/L = 2mEq/L = 24.3 mg of magnesium

mmol/L × 2.433 = mg of magnesium/dL

The adult body contains 20 to 30 grams of magnesium, with over half of it present in the bones in combination with bicarbonate and phosphate. The remainder is present in the cellular space of the soft tissues, primarily in muscle. Of the total amount of magnesium in the body, only 120 mg is found in the serum. Over 300 enzyme systems are activated by magnesium. Hence, the element has significant roles in all major anabolic and catabolic processes in the body, including protein, lipid, and carbohydrate metabolism.[39]

Metabolism

Magnesium and calcium metabolism are closely related mainly through the action of the parathyroid hormone.[48,111] Magnesium and calcium levels in the blood are increased by parathyroid hormone. The ionized forms of magnesium and calcium exert a negative regulator feedback effect on the parathyroid gland. Since magnesium has a cofactor function for the parathyroid, magnesium deficiency may impair the production of the parathyroid hormone.[1-4] The cardiovascular system is also highly dependent on ionized magnesium (Mg^{2+}). Ionized magnesium passes through the cell membrane rather quickly and thus appears that intracellular and extracellular magnesium reservoirs are in a dynamic state of equilibrium. Thus, the measurement of Mg^{2+} in plasma, serum, or whole blood would reflect the dynamic intracellular-extracellular magnesium homeostasis.

Magnesium Deficiency

The first description of magnesium deficiency as a specific entity in man demonstrated that it was indistinguishable from hypocalcemic tetany except by chemical analysis.[43] In magnesium deficiency, serum magnesium was markedly reduced. A magnesium deficiency has also been induced experimentally in adult human volunteers.[33,64,78] The subjects developed deficiency signs, some as early as 24 to 26 days on the magnesium deficient diet. The signs observed were irritability, muscle weakness, nausea, and mental derangement.[33]

Hypomagnesemia may occur with inadequate dietary intake of magnesium, malabsorption, alcohol addition,[102,104-106] diarrhea, renal loss (e.g., with uses of diuretics), and other conditions.[31,32,61,63,74,76,77,79,80] Hypermagnesemia is considered when the serum magnesium level is greater than 1.25 mmol/L (2.5 mEq/L).[69,71] Hypomagnesemia is frequently accompanied by hypocalcemia and hypokalemia.[76] Hypermagnesemia may occur with renal failure or the use of magnesium-containing medications (e.g., laxatives and antacids)[23,25,39,79,80] Hypomagnesemia is considered a serious risk factor for hypertension, cardiac arrhythmias, stroke, and heart failure.[8,9,23-26,32,34,62,63,72,76,87,105-108] Hypomagensemia has been reported to occur in 25 to 75% of patients with diabetes mellitus.[12,70,107] Abnormal serum magnesium levels were found in 29% of patients entering an intensive care unit.[13] Magnesium supplements have been reported to decrease the severity of leg cramps in pregnant women, elderly, and diabetics.[75]

Clinical studies have reported that abnormal magnesium levels were the most frequently abnormal analyte observed in pediatric patients in an intensive care unit.[6,63] Hypomagnesemia has been defined as a serum concentration of magnesium of < 0.62 mmol/L to <0.75 mmol/L (<1.25 mEg/L to <1.5 mEg/L).[10,11,23] Normal serum magnesium levels range from 0.75 to 1.25 mmol/L (1.5 – 2.5 mEq/L.[23]

National Health and Nutrition Examination Survey

The first National Health and Nutrition Examination Survey (NHANES-I)[53] conducted between 1971 and 1974, obtained serum magnesium information on a U.S. population sample involving 15,820 persons.[42] The data obtained from this large survey can serve as normative serum magnesium values for the U.S. population. Serum magnesium concentrations of the 18 to 74 years group ranged between 0.75 and 0.95 mmol/L (1.50 and 1.91 mEq/L) with a mean of 0.85 mmol/L (1.70 mEq/L).

The mean serum magnesium levels decreased in both sexes from age 1 to ages 12 to 24 years. Both white females and males had higher serum magnesium levels than black females and black males of the same age. For example, for males at age 24 to 34 years, the mean serum magnesium level for blacks was 0.83 mmol/L (1.66 mEq/L) compared to 0.85 mmol/L (1.72 mEq/L) for whites.[42]

Evaluation of Magnesium Status

There are numerous published procedures for the determination of magnesium in serum and plasma.[36,41,52,80,83,88-90,105] Perhaps one of the oldest procedures is the gravimetric technique of McCrudden in which magnesium is precipitated as magnesium ammonium phosphate.[109] This procedure or some modification, is still often used. One of the major modifications measures magnesium indirectly through a colorimetric determination of the precipitated phosphate.

Automated colorimetric or fluorometric methods for magnesium measurements have proven useful in the clinical laboratories, although atomic absorption spectroscopy procedures are probably more reliable.[40,41,66,79,81,89,91,103] Total serum or plasma concentrations of magnesium can be determined rapidly with the use of flame and atomic absorption spectroscopy and by inductively coupled plasma emission spectroscopy.[36,44,45,82,85,86,110] Serum or plasma samples require only a 50-fold dilution with water prior to analysis.[44] Particular attention must be given to the standards employed and the use of quality control serum samples. Magnesium standard reference materials are available from the National Institute

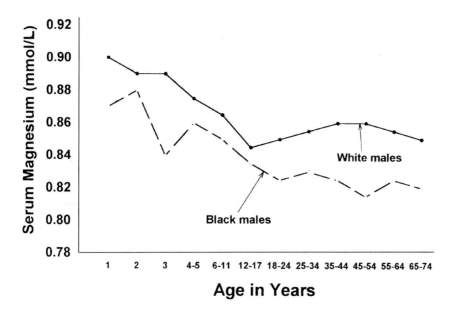

FIGURE 55
Effect of age and race on the serum concentrations of magnesium in males. (Lowenstein and Stanton.[42] With permission.)

for Standards and Technology, Gaithersburg, MD. Hemolysis must be prevented in the blood processing as the erythrocytes contain considerably more magnesium than the serum.

Total and ultra-filterable plasma magnesium measurements have been used in the evaluation of magnesium status.[5,7,37] Extracellular ionized magnesium (Mg^{2+}), the filterable fraction, has been considered the biologically active magnesium fraction.[5] The total serum magnesium levels are not always a reliable reflection of intracellular or total body magnesium stores. Thus, a normal serum magnesium level can occur in the presence of a total body magnesium deficiency.[76,92] The free-ionized magnesium concentrations in serum and plasma have been considered a better indicator of magnesium status.[5] With the availability of magnesium selective electrodes, measurement of the free ionized magnesium levels in serum, plasma, and whole blood can be easily performed.[5,35,37] The electrodes have been incorporated into commercially available instruments such as the NOVA Biomedical Stat Profile 8 Analyzer (NOVA Biomedical, Waltham, MA) and the KONE Microlyte 6 Instrument (KONE Instruments, SF-02320 Espoo, Finland).[5,35,105]

Unfiltered serum ionized magnesium values obtained by the ion-selective magnesium electrode correlated highly with the ultrafiltered serum magnesium values obtained by atomic absorption spectroscopy.[5] In general, 71% of the total magnesium is present in the plasma as ionized magnesium.[5] In healthy subjects, the ionized magnesium levels in plasma or serum fell within the narrow range of 0.53 to 0.67 mmol/L.[5,51] Practical methods are not available to measure intracellular ionized magnesium.[38,80] However, preliminary investigations indicate that the determination of intracellular free magnesium in red blood cells may be feasible with nuclear magnetic resonance techniques.[64,78,80,105] The mean red blood cell ionized magnesium was reported as 178 ± 6.3 μmol/L.[78] The red blood cell ionized magnesium levels correlated with serum magnesium concentrations ($r = 0.54$)

The usefulness of measuring ionized magnesium levels in serum as an indicator of magnesium deficiency status or for diagnostic purposes in medical care settings requires

TABLE 77
Reference Values for Magnesium Assessment

Analysis	Author/Reference

1. Magnesium Values for Children (0.5–16 yrs)

Serum: 0.65–0.99 mmol/L (mean: 0.89) — Geven et al. (1990)/100
Mononuclear cells: 22.1–76.3 μmol/g protein (mean: 37.1)
Erythrocyte magnesium: 5.23–8.08 μmol/g erythrocytes
  (mean: 6.42)

2. Serum Magnesium Levels During Pregnancy

Period	mmol/L	(mEq/L)	Author/Reference
Initial	0.80	1.61	Reynolds (1978)/47
1st trimester	0.75	1.51	
2nd trimester	0.71	1.42	
3rd trimester	0.70	1.39	

3. Magnesium Levels in Blood Mononuclear Cells

Magnesium Level		Author/Reference
μmol/g protein	fmol/cell	
63 ± 10	4.0 ± 0.9	Urdal and Lanmark/94
73 ± 16	5.4 ± 1.9	Sjogren et al./21
59 ± 14	3.3 ± 0.9	Elin and Johnson/112
—	2.9 ± 0.6	Elin and Hosseini/93
—	2.8 ± 0.6	Reinhart et al./95
55	—	Ryzen et al./99

4. Ionized Magnesium by Ion-Selective Magnesium Electrode (n = 23)

Whole Blood	Plasma	Serum	
Mg^{2+} (mmol/L)			Author/Reference
0.60 ± 0.005	0.59 ± 0.008	0.58 ± 0.006	Altura and Altura (1991/92)/5

5. Magnesium Load (Infusion) Test Following Intravenous Load of 30 mmol of $MgCl_2$

Normal	5–6% retention (24-hr)	Rasmussen et al. (1988)/85
Magnesium deficient	31–57% retention (24-hr)	Rasmussen et al. (1988)/85

further study. Preliminary studies indicate that ionized magnesium measurements in serum may have application with renal transplant, cardiac, obstetrical, and asthmatic patients.[5,105] Currently, total serum magnesium analyses appear to be the most accessible, practical, and expeditious method for identifying magnesium abnormalities.[63,79]

Serum magnesium levels decrease from 7 to 12% as pregnancy proceeds. The decline probably reflects uncompensated dilution due to increasing plasma volume.[46,47] Measurements of magnesium levels in red blood cells or in mononuclear blood cells have been used to assess magnesium status.[58] A number of studies have failed to find a correlation between red blood cells and mononuclear blood cells magnesium concentrations or between serum and red blood cell magnesium concentrations in normal individuals.[59] However, in a more recent controlled magnesium deficiency study, with normal subjects, serum hypomagnesemia occurred in all subjects which correlated significantly with a decrease in red blood cell intracellular free (ionized) magnesium levels as determined by nuclear magnetic

TABLE 78
Additional Reference Values for Magnesium Assessment

Study			Reference
Serum Magnesium (adult)			
1. Normal	0.75–1.25 mmol/L	Delaney and Preuss, 1992	23
	(1.5 to 2.5 mEq/L)		
2. Normal	0.8–1.3 mmol/L	Rasmussen et al. 1988	85
	(1.6–2.6 mEq/L)		
3. Normal	0.85 ± 0.004 mmol/L	Singh et al. 1989	68
4. NHANES Survey	0.75–0.96 mmol/L	Lowenstein and Stanton, 1986	42
18–74 years old	(mean: 0.85 mmol/L)		
	(1.50–1.92 mEq/L)		
Hypomagnesemia (serum)			
	< 0.62–0.75 mmol/L	Delaney and Preuss, 1992	23
	(< 1.25–< 1.5 mEq/L)	Whang et al. 1984	10
		Boyd, et al. 1983	11
Hypermagnesemia (serum)			
	> 1.25 mmol/L	Preuss and Delaney, 1992	69
	(> 2.5 mEq/L)	Van Hook, 1991	71
Erythrocyte magnesium (adult)			
	1.88 ± 0.12 mmol/L	Howard, 1990	107

resonance.[54] Similarly, in a study of the prevalence of magnesium deficiency in the elderly, magnesium assays of the red blood cells were a better indicator of magnesium status than that of plasma assays.[67] About 20% of the elderly population studied had low concentrations of red blood cell magnesium, while 10% had low plasma magnesium values.

Tissue Magnesium Levels

Approximately 99% of the magnesium in the body is in the intracellular phase. Hence, the determination of intracellular magnesium has been considered a better indicator of total magnesium status.[16] Normal serum levels of magnesium may exist even when the intracellular pool of magnesium has been significantly depleted.[15] Consequently, serum magnesium levels usually do not correlate with intracellular magnesium status, but only with the interstitial phase.[14] However, practical methods are not available to measure intracellular magnesium concentrations.[38] Some studies indicate that muscle biopsies may provide this information, but such specimens cannot be routinely obtained.[18,21,92,101]

Magnesium status has been evaluated also by measuring magnesium levels in erythrocytes and leucocytes.[14,18,22,64,94,95,97-100] Magnesium levels of leucocytes were proposed as an index of intracellular magnesium status.[96] However, the procedures have not always been satisfactory.[16,18-21,30,92,97]

The magnesium content of mononuclear cells isolated by a Ficoll-Hypaque procedure did not correlate with magnesium concentrations of plasma or red blood cells.[93,95,97] However mononuclear cell concentrations of magnesium correlated significantly with muscle biopsy concentrations of magnesium.[101] Regardless, the usefulness of mononuclear cell magnesium determinations need further evaluation with patient populations, particularly those with specific diseases known to have an association with magnesium aberrations.[18,97]

Compared to other magnesium assessment procedures, the amount of blood volume required and the increased time needed for sample preparation, along with technical difficulties limits the use of magnesium analyses of mononuclear cells.

Magnesium Loading Test

The magnesium loading test has been used by a number of investigators to assess the magnesium status in various patient groups.[16,27-30,65,85] In general, the procedure involves the continuous intravenous infusion of isotonic saline magnesium sulfate (30 mmol) solution over a period of 8 hours.[16] In some reports magnesium chloride (30 mmol) have been infused over a period of 12 hours.[16,30] Urine is collected from the start of the infusion for 24 hours and the magnesium content measured by atomic absorption spectrophotometry. Magnesium status is evaluated on the basis of the 24-hr retention of the magnesium infused. Normal subjects retain about 5 to 6% of the load.[16] Magnesium deficient patients may retain from 31 to 57% of the magnesium load.

The intravenous magnesium loading test can be a useful procedure in the estimation of a magnesium deficiency. To avoid variability, the test must be conducted in a standardized manner.[16] The procedure is time-consuming, invasive, and expensive to perform. Consequently the load test can be useful in a clinical setting, but not practical for general use to evaluate magnesium status.

Urine Magnesium Levels

The kidney serves as the primary excretory pathway for absorbed magnesium. Approximately 2 to 5 mmol of magnesium are excreted daily.[48] However, the kidney can efficiently retain magnesium when dietary intakes of the mineral are suboptimun.[49,84] Although a dietary deficiency of magnesium can occur, it will more likely be observed in association with disease states, such as abnormal cardiovascular conditions, prolonged diarrhea, malabsorption, diuretic therapy, or hypercalcemia.[24,39,48,50,61,63]

If dietary information on magnesium intake is available, urinary levels of magnesium can be useful. Urinary magnesium excretion levels above the dietary intake may suggest renal tubular dysfunction while a low urinary output may indicate a malabsorption problem. In a study with over 4,000 adult men and women, a strong positive association between dietary magnesium intakes and urinary excretion of magnesium was observed.[73] Twenty-four hour urine collections and 24-hr food records were used in the study.

Magnesium Toxicity

Subjects with renal disease should avoid the use of magnesium-containing medications. In these subjects, elevated serum concentrations of magnesium may occur with the prolonged use of magnesium-containing cathartics or antiacids.[25,60]

Summary

The assessment of magnesium status has been difficult and has been dependent largely on total magnesium levels in the serum. Although these determinations can be readily performed, the interpretation of the results have often been uncertain, since serum magnesium levels do not always reflect intracellular or total body magnesium levels.[87] Ionized magnesium levels in serum appear to be a more useful indicator of magnesium deficiency status and for diagnostic purposes in the clinical environment.

With the availability of magnesium selective electrodes, measurements of serum levels of free ionized magnesium can be easily performed. This measurement should receive increased application in patient care for the assessment of magnesium status. A practical approach to evaluating a magnesium status involves the determination of the serum magnesium level and urinary magnesium excretion, which may then be followed by performing a magnesium load test.[87,105] With the increased recognized importance of magnesium in clinical settings, the inclusion of serum magnesium determinations in clinical chemistry profiles would appear to be justified.[1-4,39,63,79,80,87]

References

1. Loughead, J. L., Mimouni, F., Tsang, R. C., and Khoury, J. C., A role for magnesium in neonatal parathyroid gland function, *J. Am. College Nutr.*, 10, 123, 1991.
2. Anast, C. S., Winnacker, J. C., Forte, L. R., and Burns, T. W., Impaired release of parathyroid hormone in magnesium deficiency, *J. Clin. Endocrinol. Metab.*, 42, 707, 1976.
3. Seelig, M., Cardiovascular consequences of magnesium deficiency and loss: pathogenesis, prevalence, and manifestations — magnesium and chloride loss in refractory potassium repletion, *Am. J. Cartel.*, 63, 4G, 1989.
4. Polanic, J. E., Magnesium: metabolism, clinical importance, and analysis, *Clin. Lab. Sci.*, 4, 105, 1991.
5. Altura, B. T. and Altura, B. M., Measurement of ionized magnesium in whole blood, plasma, and serum with a new ion-selective electrode in healthy and diseased human subjects, *Magnesium Trace Elem.*, 10, 90, 1991/92.
6. Broner, C. W., Hypermagnesemia and hypocalcemia as predictors of high mortality in critically ill pediatric patients, *Crit. Case Med.*, 18, 921, 1990.
7. Zaloga, G. P., A simple method for determining physiologically active calcium and magnesium concentrations in critically ill patients, *Crit. Care Med.*, 15, 813, 1987.
8. Altura, B. M., Role of magnesium in the etiology of cardiovascular disease, *Clin. Chem.*, 35, 1054, 1989.
9. Magnesium deficiency and ischemic heart disease, *Nutr. Rev.*, 46, 311, 1988.
10. Whang, R., Oei, T. O., Aikawa, J. K., Watanabe, A., Vannatta, J., Freyer, A., and Markanich, M., Predictors of clinical hypomagnesemia: hypokalemia, hypophosphatemia, hyponatremia, and hypocalcemia, *Arch. Int. Med.*, 144, 1794, 1984.
11. Boyd, J. C., Bruns, D. E., and Wills, M. R., Frequency of hypomagnesemia in hypokalemic states, *Clin. Chem.*, 29, 178, 1983.
12. Durlach, J. and Collery, P., Magnesium and potassium in diabetes and carbohydrate metabolism: review of the present status and recent results, *Magnesium*, 3, 315, 1984.
13. Reinhart, R. A. and Desbiens, N. A., Hypomagnesemia in patients entering ICU, *Crit. Care Med.*, 13, 506, 1985.
14. Elin, R. J., Assessment of magnesium status, *Clin. Chem.*, 33, 1965, 1987.

15. Dyckner, T. and Wester, P. O., The relation between extra- and intracellular electrolytes in patients with hypokalemic and/or diuretic treatment, *Acta Med. Scand.*, 204, 269, 1978.
16. Gullestad, L., Midtvedt, K., Dolva, L. O., Norseth, J., and Kjekshus, J., The magnesium loading test: reference values in healthy subjects, *Scand. J. Clin. Invest.*, 54, 23, 1994.
17. Wallach, S., Cahill, L. N., Roger, F. H., and Jones, H. C., Plasma and erythrocyte magnesium in health and disease, *J. Lab. Clin. Med.*, 59, 195, 1962.
18. Elin, R. J., Status of the mononuclear blood cell magnesium assay, *J. Am. Coll. Nutr.*, 6, 105, 1986.
19. Alfrey, A. C., Miller, N. C., and Butkus, D., Evaluation of body magnesium stores, *J. Lab. Clin. Med.*, 84, 153, 1974.
20. Dyckner, T. and Wester, P. O., Skeletal muscle magnesium and potassium determinations: correlations with lymphocyte contents of magnesium and potassium, *J. Am. Coll. Nutr.*, 4, 619, 1985.
21. Sjogen, A., Floren, C. H., and Nilsson, A., Magnesium and potassium status in healthy subjects as assessed by analysis of magnesium and potassium in skeletal muscle biopsies and magnesium in mononuclear cells, *Magnesium*, 6, 91, 1987.
22. Ryan, M. P., Ryan, M. F., and Counihan, T. B., The effect of diuretics on lymphocyte magnesium and potassium, *Acta Med. Scand.*, 647, 153, 1980.
23. Delaney, V. and Preuss, H. G., Hypomagnesemia, in *Medicine for the Practicing Physician*, 4th edition., Hurst, J. W., Ed., Appleton & Lange, Stamford, 1996, 1439.
24. Shils, M. E., Magnesium in health and disease, *Annu. Rev. Nutr.*, 8, 429, 1988.
25. Rude, R. K. and Singer, F. R., Magnesium deficiency and excess, *Annu. Rev. Med.*, 32, 245, 1981.
26. Whelton, P. G. and Klag, M. J., Magnesium and blood pressure: review of the epidemiology and clinical trial experience, *Am. J. Cardiol.*, 63, 26G, 1989.
27. Bohmer, T. and Mathiesen, B., Magnesium deficiency in chronic alcoholic patients uncovered by an intravenous loading test, *Scand. J. Clin. Lab. Invest.*, 42, 633, 1982.
28. Gullestad, L., Dolva, L. O., Waage, A., Falch, D., Fagerthun, H., and Kjekshus, J., Magnesium deficiency diagnosed by an intravenous loading test, *J. Clin. Lab. Invest.*, 52, 245, 1992.
29. Holm, C. N., Jepsen, J. M., Sjogaard, G., and Hessob, I., A magnesium load test in the diagnosis of magnesium deficiency. *Human Nutrition: Clin. Nutrition*, 41C, 301, 1987.
30. Sjogren, A., Floren, C. H., and Nilsson, A., Evaluation of magnesium status in Crohn's disease as by intracellular analysis and intravenous magnesium infusion, *Scan. J. Gastroenterol*, 23, 555, 1988.
31. Leary, W. P. and Reyes, A. J., Diuretic-induced magnesium losses, *Drugs*, 28 (suppl. 1), 182, 1984.
32. Toffaletti, J., Hypomagnesemia involved in host of disorders, *CCN*, 8, 1987.
33. Shils, M. E., Experimental production of magnesium deficiency in man, *Ann. N. Y. Acad. Sci.*, 162, 847, 1969.
34. Orlov, M. V., Brodsky, M. A., and Douban, S., A review of magnesium, acute myocardial infarction and arrhythmia, *J. Am. College Nutr.*, 13, 127, 1994.
35. Lewenstam, A., Blomqvist, N., and Ost, J., Characterization, standardizing and experiences with KONE ISE for Mg^{2+}, *Scand. J. Clin. Lab. Invest.*, 54 (suppl. 217), 37, 1994.
36. Fernandez, F. J. and Kahn, H. L., Clinical methods for atomic absorption spectroscopy, *Clin. Chem. Newslett.*, 3, 24, 1971.
37. Altura, B. T., Dell'Orfano, K., Barbour, R. L., Yeh, Q., Young, C. C., Hiti, J., Welch, R., Shirey, T., and Altura, B. M., Ionized magnesium (IMg^{2+}): characteristics of a new ion selective electrode (ISE) for Mg whole blood (WB), plasma (PL) and serum (S), *FASEB J.*, 5, A1309, 1991.
38. Murphy, E., Measurement of intracellular ionized magnesium, *Miner. Electrolyte Metab.*, 19, 250, 1993.
39. Shils, M. E., Magnesium, in *Modern Nutrition in Health and Disease*, Volume 1, 8th edition, Shils, M. E., Olson, J. A., and Shike, M., Eds., Lea & Febiger, Philadelphia, 1994, 164.
40. Toffaletti, J., Abrams, B., Bird, C., Schwing, M., Clinical validation of an automated thin-film reflectance method for measurement of magnesium in serum and urine, *Magnesium*, 7, 84, 1988.
41. Alcock, N. W., Development of methods for the determination of magnesium, *Ann. N. Y. Acad. Sci.*, 162, 707, 1969.

42. Lowenstein, F. W. and Stanton, M. F., Serum magnesium levels in the United States, *J. Am. Coll. Nutr.*, 5, 399, 1986.
43. Vallee, B. L., Wacker, W. E. C., and Ulmer, D. D., The magnesium-deficiency tetany syndrome in man, *N. Engl. J. Med.*, 262, 155, 1960.
44. Willis, J. B., The analysis of biological materials by atomic-absorption spectroscopy, *Clin. Chem.*, 11, 251, 1965.
45. Willis, J. B., Determination of calcium and magnesium in urine by atomic absorption spectroscopy, *Anal. Chem.*, 33, 556, 1961.
46. De Jorge, F. B., Delascio, D., de Ulhoa Cintra, A. B., and Antunes, M. L., Magnesium concentration in the blood serum of normal pregnant women, *Obstet. Gynecol.*, 25, 253, 1965.
47. Reynolds, W. A., Electrolytes in pregnancy, in *Laboratory Indices of Nutritional Status in Pregnancy*, National Academy Sciences, Washington D.C., 1978, 8.
48. Wester, P. O., Magnesium, *Am. J. Clin. Nutr.*, 45, 1305, 1987.
49. Shils, M. E., Experimental human depletion, *Medicine*, 48, 61, 1969.
50. Seelig, M. S., Magnesium deficiency in the pathogenesis of disease, Plenum Press, New York, 1980.
51. Altura, B. T. and Altura, B. M., Measurement of ionized magnesium in whole blood plasma and serum with a new novel ion-selective electrode, *Magnesium Trace Elem.*, 9, 311, 1990.
52. Hansen, H. L. and Freier, F. F., The measurement of serum magnesium by atomic absorption spectrophotometry, *Am. J. Med. Tech.*, 33, 158, 1967.
53. National Center for Health Statistics: Plan and Operation of the Health and Nutrition Examination Survey, United States, 1971-1974, by H. W. Miller, Vital and Health Statistics, Series 1 Nos. 10a and 10b, DHEW Pub. No. (HRA) 77-1310, Government Printing Office, Washington D.C., 1973.
54. Toffaletti, J., Mg may play role in CHD, *CCN*, 1990.
55. Iseri, L. T., Allen, B. J., and Brodsky, M. A., Mg therapy of cardiac arrythmias in critical care medicine, *Magnesium*, 8, 299, 1989.
56. Rasmussen, H. S., Clinical intervention studies on magnesium in myocardial infarction, *Magnesium*, 8, 316, 1989.
57. Wallach, S., Availability of body magnesium during magnesium deficiency, *Magnesium*, 7, 262, 1988.
58. Elin, R. J., Laboratory tests for the assessment of magnesium status in humans, *Magnesium Trace Elem.*, 10, 172, 1991.
59. Elin, R. J., Magnesium in health and disease, *Dis. Mon.* 34, 165, 1988.
60. Mordes, J. P. and Wacker, E. E. C., Excess magnesium, *Pharmacol. Rev.*, 29, 273, 1978.
61. Caddell, J. L., Magnesium in prenatal care and infant health, *Magnesium Trace Elem.*, 10, 229, 1991.
62. Weinsier, R. L. and Norris, D., Recent developments in the etiology and treatment of hypertension: dietary calcium, fat, and magnesium, *Am. J. Clin. Nutr.*, 42, 1331, 1985.
63. Whang, R., Hampton, E. M., and Whang, D. D., Magnesium homeostasis and clinical disorders of magnesium deficiency, *Annu. Pharmacotherapy*, 28, 220, 1994.
64. Rude, R. K., Stephen, A., and Nadler, J., Determination of red blood cells intracellular free magnesium by nuclear magnetic resonance as an assessment of magnesium depletion, *Magnesium Trace Elem.*, 10, 117, 1991.
65. Ryzen, E., Elbaum, N., Singer, F. R., and Rude, R. K., Parenteral magnesium tolerance testing in the evaluation of magnesium deficiency, *Magnesium*, 4, 137, 1985.
66. Kulpmann, W. R., Maibaum, P., and Sonntag, O., Analyses with the KODAK-Ektachem. Accuracy control using reference method values and the influence of protein concentration. I. Electrolytes, *J. Clin. Chem. Clin. Biochem.*, 28, 825, 1990.
67. Toultou, Y., Godard, J. -P., Ferment, O., Chastang, C., Proust, J., Bogdan, A., Auzeby, A., and Toultou, C., Prevalence of magnesium and potassium deficiencies in the elderly, *Clin. Chem.*, 33/4, 518, 1987.
68. Singh, A., Day, B. A., De Bolt, J. E., Trostmann, U. H., Bernier, L. L., and Deuster, P. A., Magnesium, zinc, and copper status of U.S. Navy SEAL trainees, *Am. J. Clin. Nutr.*, 49, 695, 1989.

69. Preuss, H. G. and Delaney, V., Hypermagnesemia, in *Medicine for the Practicing Physician*, 4th edition, Hurst, J. W., Ed., Butterworth-Heinemann, Boston, 1996, 1437.

70. Crook, M., Couchman, S., Tutt, P., and Swaminathan, R., Erythrocyte, plasma total, ultrafilterable and platelet magnesium in type 2 (non-insulin dependent) diabetes mellitus, *Diabetes Research*, 27, 73, 1994.

71. Van Hook, J. W., Endocrine crises, Hypermagnesemia, *Critical Care Clinics*, 7, 215, 1991.

72. Altura, I. M. and Altura, B. T., Interactions of Mg and K on blood vessels - aspects in view of hypertension, Review of present status and new findings, *Magnesium*, 3, 175, 1984.

73. Kesteloot, H. and Joossens, J. V., The relationship between dietary intake and urinary excretion of sodium, potassium, calcium, and magnesium: Belgian Interuniversity Research on Nutrition and Health, *J. Human Hypertension*, 4, 527, 1990.

74. Martin, B. J., McAlpine, J. K., and Devine, B. L., Hypomagnesemia in elderly digitalized patients, *Scottish Med. J.*, 33, 273, and 324, 1988.

75. Dahle, L. O., Berg, G., Hammar, H., Hurtig, M., and Larsson, L., The effect of oral magnesium substitution on pregnancy-induced leg cramps, *Am. J. Obstet Gynecol.*, 173, 175, 1995.

76. Berkelhammer, C. and Bear, R. A., A clinical approach to common electrolyte problems, Hypomagnesemia, *Can. Med. Assoc. J.*, 132, 360, 1985.

77. Cunningham, J. J., Anbar, R. D., and Crawford, J. D., Hypomagnesemia: A multifactorial complication of treatment of patients with severe burn trauma, *J. Parenteral Enteral Nutr.*, 11, 364, 1987.

78. Ryzen, E., Servis, K. L., De Russo, P., Kershaw, A., Stephen, T., and Rude, R. K., Determination of intracellular free magnesium by nuclear magnetic resonance in human magnesium deficiency, *J. Am. Coll. Nutr.*, 8, 580, 1989.

79. Whang, R. and Ryder, K. W., Frequency of hypomagnesemia and hypermagnesemia, *JAMA*, 263, 3063, 1990.

80. Quamme, G. A., Laboratory evaluation of magnesium status, Renal function and free intracellular magnesium concentration, *Clin. Lab. Med.*, 13, 209, 1993.

81. Barbour, H. M. and Davidson, W., Studies on measurement of plasma magnesium: Application of the Margon dye method to the "Monarch" centrifugal analyzer, *Clin. Chem.*, 34, 2103, 1988.

82. Nixon, D. E., Moyer, T. P., Johnson, P., McCall, J. T., Ness, A. B., Fjerstad, W. H., and Wehde, M. B., Routine measurement of calcium, magnesium, copper, zinc, and iron in urine and serum by inductively coupled plasma emission spectroscopy, *Clin. Chem.*, 32, 1660, 1986.

83. West, P., Rapid measurement of serum magnesium with a kit, *Clin. Chem.*, 30, 1426, 1984.

84. Quamme, G. A., Magnesium homeostasis and renal magnesium handling, *Miner. Electrolyte Metab.*, 19, 218, 1993.

85. Rasmussen, H. S., McNair, P., Goransson, L., Balslov, S., Larsen, O. G., and Aurup, P., Magnesium deficiency in patients with ischemic heart disease with and without acute myocardial infarction uncovered by an intravenous loading test, *Arch. Int. Med.*, 148, 329, 1988.

86. Roberts, N. B., Furelough, D., McLoughlin, S., and Taylor, W. H., Measurement of copper, zinc, and magnesium in serum and urine by DC plasma emission spectrometry, *Annu. Clin. Biochem.*, 22, 533, 1985.

87. Ryan M. F., The role of magnesium in clinical biochemistry: an overview, *Annu. Clin. Biochem.*, 28, 19, 1991.

88. Tsang, W. M., Howell, M. J., and Miller, A. L., A simple enzymatic method for the measurement of magnesium in serum and urine on a centrifugal analyzer, *Annu. Clin. Biochem.*, 25, 162, 1988.

89. Pesce, M. A., Bodourian, S. H., and Hills, L. P., Fluorometric measurement of serum magnesium with a centrifugal analyzer, *Clin. Chim. Acta*, 136, 137, 1984.

90. Deuster, P. A., Trostmann, U. H., Bernier, L. L., and Dolev, E., Indirect vs direct measurement of magnesium and zinc in erythrocytes, *Clin. Chem.*, 33, 529, 1987.

91. Liedtke, R. J. and Kroon, G., Automated calmagite compleximetric measurement of magnesium in serum, with sequential addition of EDTA to eliminate endogenous interference, *Clin. Chem.*, 30, 1801, 1984.

92. Reinhart, R. A., Magnesium metabolism, A review with special reference to the relationship between intracellular content and serum levels, *Arch. Int. Med.*, 148, 2415, 1988.

93. Elin, R. J. and Hasseini, J. M., Magnesium content of mononuclear blood cells, *Clin. Chem.*, 31, 377, 1985.
94. Urdal, P. and Landmark, K., Measurement of magnesium in mononuclear blood cells, *Clin. Chem.*, 35, 1559, 1989.
95. Reinhart, R. A., Marx, J. J. Jr., Haas, R. G., and Desbiens, N. A., Intracellular magnesium of mononuclear cells from venous blood of clinically healthy subjects, *Clinica. Chimica. Acta*, 167, 187, 1987.
96. Ross, R., Seelig, M., and Berger, A., Isolation of leukocytes for magnesium determination, in *Magnesium in Health and Disease*, Cantin, M., and Seelig, M. S., Eds., Spectrum Publications, New York, 1980, 7.
97. Martin, B. J., Lyon, T. D. B., Walker, W., and Fell, G. S., Mononuclear blood cell magnesium in older subjects: evaluation of its use in clinical practice, *Annu. Clin. Biochem.*, 30, 23, 1993.
98. Girardin, E. and Paunier, L., Relationship between magnesium, potassium and sodium concentrations in lymphocytes and erythrocytes from normal subjects, *Magnesium*, 4, 188, 1985.
99. Ryzen, E., Elkayam, U., and Rude, R. K., Low blood mononuclear cell magnesium in intensive care unit patients, *Am. Heart J.*, 3, 475, 1986.
100. Geven, W. B., Vogels-Mentink, G. M., Willems, J. L., de Boo, T., Lemmens, W., and Monnens, L. A. H., Reference values of magnesium and potassium in mononuclear cells and erythrocytes of children, *Clin. Chem.*, 36, 1323, 1990.
101. Sjogren, A., Floren, C. -H., and Nilsson, A., Measurement of magnesium in mononuclear cells, *Sci. of the Total Environment*, 42, 77, 1985.
102. Shane, S. R. and Flink, E. B., Magnesium deficiency in alcohol addiction and withdrawal, *Magnes. Trace Elem.*, 10, 263, 1991.
103. Ratge, D., Kohse, K. P., and Wisser, H., Measurement of magnesium in serum and urine with a random access analyzer by use of a modified xylidyl blue-1 procedure, *Clin. Chim. Acta*, 159, 197, 1986.
104. Flink, E. B., Magnesium deficiency in alcoholism, *Alcoholism: Clinical and Exptl. Res.*, 10, 590, 1986.
105. Elin, R. J., Magnesium: the fifth but forgotten electrolyte, *Am. J. Clin. Pathol.*, 102, 616, 1994.
106. Reinhart, R. A., Magnesium deficiency: recognition and treatment in the emergency medicine setting, *Am. J. Emerg. Med.*, 10, 78, 1992.
107. Howard, J. M. H., Magnesium deficiency in peripheral vascular disease, *J. Nutritional Med.*, 1, 39, 1990.
108. Fischer, P. W. F., Belonje, B., and Giroux, A., Magnesium status and excretion in age-matched subjects with normal and elevated blood pressures, *Clin. Biochem.*, 26, 207, 1993.
109. McCrudden, F. H., Magnesium ammonium phosphate method for magnesium in food, urine, and feces, *J. Biol. Chem.*, 7, 83, 1909.
110. Wacker, W. E. C. and Vallee, B. L., A study of magnesium metabolism in acute renal failure employing a multichannel flame spectrometer, *N. Engl. J. Med.*, 257, 1254, 1957.
111. Shils, M. E., Magnesium, calcium, and parathyroid hormone interactions, *Ann. N.Y. Acad. Sci.*, 355, 165, 1980.
112. Elin, R. J., and Johnson, E., A method for determination of the magnesium content of blood mononuclear cells, *Magnesium*, 1, 115, 1982.

Iron

Converting metric units to International System (SI) units:

Serum iron as $\mu g/dL \times 0.179 = \mu mol/L$ iron

Serum total iron binding capacity: iron as $\mu g/dL \times 0.179 = \mu mol/L$ iron

Iron as $\mu mol/L \times 5.585 = \mu g/dL$ iron

atomic weight: 55.85

History of Iron Deficiency

The history of iron deficiency and its treatment goes back several thousand years. The therapeutic use of iron by the Egyptians was recorded as early as 1500 B.C. Romans and Greeks used iron in medical concoctions to restore health to the infirm.[8] The disease "chlorosis" or "green sickness" was recognized by 1500 A.D. The disease affected adolescent females in particular and was characterized by a greenish-yellow discoloration of the skin.[9] The therapeutic value of treating the condition with iron was recognized by Syndenham in 1681.[8] By the end of the nineteenth century, chlorosis was described as anemia. But despite the long recognition of the essentiality of iron and the voluminous studies and reports on the subject, nutritional iron deficiency remains a major public health problem in developing countries as well as in the industrialized countries.[184]

Iron deficiency has been the subject of excellent reviews.[10-22,188] Iron deficient erythropoiesis has been defined as a state in which the supply of iron is inadequate to support optimal erythropoiesis in the developing red cell mass.[1] In 1991, the World Health Organization estimated that over 1.3 billion people suffer from anemia, mainly due to an iron deficiency.[23] for example, in the Caribbean area, iron deficiency may be present in up to 76% of the children 0 to 1 year of age.[97] Nutritional anemia in the South Asian countries accounts for nearly one-half of all anemic persons in the world.[185]

Dietary Sources of Iron

Beef, poultry, clams, oysters, fish, lamb, liver, and pork, are good sources of iron. Most of the iron in these items is present as heme iron, which has a high bioavailability. Other reasonable good sources of dietary iron, present as non-heme iron, include eggs, dried legumes, cane molasses, cocoa, green vegetables, and whole-wheat (or enriched) flour and bread. Vegetarians maintained on a planned well-balanced vegetarian diet have an adequate iron status.[162]

Iron Deficiency and Metabolism

A number of abnormalities have been associated with an iron deficiency. Nonspecific symptoms of a deficiency include decreased exercise tolerance, fatigue, and pallor. Subjects may have headaches, weakness, dyspnea, and palpitations.[21,51,99,188]

Iron is a constituent of hemoglobin, myoglobin, cytochromes, and a number of other proteins which function in the utilization, transport, and storage of oxygen. Some of the other iron-containing proteins are peroxidase, ribonucleotide reductase, monoamine oxidase, and alpha-glycerophosphate dehydrogenase.[20,98] When the dietary intake of iron is insufficient, storage iron is depleted before a fall in hemoglobin and other iron dependent compounds occurs.

Iron is a necessary structural and functional component of hemoglobin and myoglobin.[8,15,20] Iron absorption occurs primarily in the duodemum. The amount of iron absorbed is affected by the source of dietary iron, heme iron being better absorbed than non-heme iron. Absorption of non-heme iron is affected by ascorbic acid and valency state.[164-166] Low absorption of iron from the diet can be a contributing cause of iron deficiency in developing countries.[162,167] Parasitic infections may also increase the demand for iron. The infections are often present in the populations of the developing countries and include malaria, hookworms, *Trichuris trichiura,* and *Ascaris lumbricoides.*[163] Iron is stored as ferritin or hemosiderin in the bone marrow, liver, and spleen.[56,98]

The consequences of iron deficiency are well recognized.[14,16-18,24,25,57,94,99,188] For instances, Viteri has detailed the consequences of iron deficiency during pregnancy.[91] Iron deficiency in developing countries contribute to reduced work output and to increased morbidity and mortality.[56,57] Impaired cognitive performance has been frequently reported with iron deficiency. It may occur at any age, but particularly with children.[19,24,99-105,190]

Laboratory measurements are available to evaluate the three phases of iron deficiency.[66,93] In Phase I a decrease in iron stores occurs. This is reflected in a fall in the concentration of serum ferritin and an increase in erythrocyte protoporphyrin levels. Phase 2 is associated with a decrease in serum iron and mean corpuscular volumes and with an elevation in total iron-binding capacity. In Phase 3, the production of hemoglobin and other iron containing proteins decrease gradually resulting in anemia.

Laboratory Procedures for the Assessment of Iron Status

In 1964, Bainton and Finch[1] stated that "in the past, the presence of hypochromia and microcytosis of the circulating red cells has been considered essential for the diagnosis of iron deficiency anemia." However, it was soon apparent that the recognition of an iron deficiency was in need of more specific, sensitive, and immediate measurements. Consequently, over the next several decades a number of useful laboratory procedures has been developed for this purpose.[47,48,81]

General

A number of articles have summarized procedures used to assess iron status.[48,66,92,93,96] It is difficult to judge an iron deficiency condition in a patient on the basis of signs and

TABLE 79
Summary of Guidelines Useful for Assessing Iron
Nutritional Status*

Deficiency Criteria for Parameters of Iron Status	
Measurement/Age (year)	Deficiency State
Hemoglobin	
0.5–10 yr	<110 g/L
11–15 years old	
males	<120 g/L
females	<115 g/L
>15 years old	
males	<130 g/L
females	<120 g/L
Pregnancy	<110 g/L
Hematocrit	
0.5–4 years old	<32%
5–10 years old	<33%
11–15 years old	
males	<35%
females	<34%
>15 years old	
males	<40%
females	<36%
Serum Iron - >15 years old	<60 µg/dL
Total iron binding capacity	>400 µg/dL
Transferrin saturation	
0.5–4 years old	<12%
5–10 years old	<14%
>10 years old	<16%
Erythrocyte protoporphyrin	
0.5–4 years old	>80 µg/dL RBC
>4 years old	>70 µg/dL RBC
Serum ferritin	
0.5–15 years old	<10 µg/L
>15 years old	<12 µg/L
Serum transferrin receptor [76,80,85]	>8.5 mg/L
Iron overload [84,116]	
Plasma ferritin	>400 µg/L
Plasma iron	≥175 µg/dL
Transferrin saturation	>60%

* Adapted from Reference 48.

symptoms presented. Hence, laboratory measurements are essential. Measurements used
to diagnose an iron deficiency anemia include hemoglobin, hematocrit, serum iron, total
iron-binding capacity (TIBC), transferrin saturation, serum ferritin, erythrocyte protoporphyrins, and serum transferrin receptors (Tables 79 to 84).

Transferrin measurements are relatively insensitive and are prone to assay variability.
Plasma iron levels or transferrin saturation levels are useful for screening purposes. However, their usefulness is compromised by the large number of clinical disorders which
induce secondary changes in plasma iron transport.[81] Serum transferrin receptor assays
provide more reliable information on iron status since non-nutritional factors and chronic
diseases have little effect on transferrin receptor status.

Interpretation of the results of analyses for hematocrit, hemoglobin, and other blood iron
parameters of iron deficiency require consideration of several characteristics of the subject,
such as age, sex, physiological state, race, smoking, and altitude. The accompanying tables
have considered some of these parameters.

TABLE 80
Centers for Disease Control and Prevention: Smoking
Adjustments for Hemoglobin (Hb) and Hematocrit (Hct) Values

Characteristic	Hb (g/L)	Hct (%)
Nonsmokers	0.0	0.0
Smokers (all)	+ 3.0	+ 1.0
½–1 pack/day	+ 3.0	+ 1.0
1–2 packs/day	+ 5.0	+ 1.5
>2 packs/day	+ 7.0	+ 2.0

From Reference 174.

TABLE 81
Effect of Inflammation on Iron Status

Diagnosis	Hemoglobin (g/L)	Ferritin (μg/L)	TfR (mg/L)	Transferrin (g/L)
Iron deficiency and anemia (*n* = 13)	91 ± 4	37	5.8 ± 1.0	2.2 ± 0.2
Inflammation anemia (*n* = 10)	101 ± 3	280	2.6 ± 0.2	1.8 ± 0.2
Iron deficiency anemia (*n* = 11)	88 ± 5	15	6.7 ± 1.1	3.2 ± 0.4

Data from Reference 78.

TABLE 82
Literature Values for Transferrin Receptor (TfR) Assays

Subject	TfR Assay Values	Reference
1. Adults		
Plasma transferrin receptor		
Normal (*n* = 19)	1.7 ± 0.5 mg/L	88
With anemia of chronic disease (*n* = 17)	1.6 ± 0.4 mg/L	88
2. Adult Males and Females		
Plasma transferrin receptor (*n* = 608)	3.63 mg/L (mean)	87
Serum transferrin receptor (*n* = 579)	3.87 mg/L (mean)	87
3. Infants (9–15 m)		
Plasma transferrin receptor (*n* = 485)	4.4 ± 1.1 mg/L	90
4. Adults		
Plasma ferritin (*n* = 396)	43.2 μg/L	87
Serum ferritin (*n* = 402)	44.1 μg/L	87

TABLE 83
WHO Criteria for the Diagnosis of Anemia

Determination	Levels considered anemic or iron-deficient
Hemoglobin (g/L venous blood)	
Children aged 6 months–6 years	<110
Children aged 6–14 years	<120
Adult males	<130
Adult females; nonpregnant	<120
Adult females; pregnant	<110
Serum Iron (μg/100 ml)	
Adults	<50
Transferrin Saturation (%)	
Adults	<15%

Adapted from WHO Technical Report.[63,173]

TABLE 84

Pregnancy: Hemoglobin and Hematocrit Cutoff Values

Gestation (weeks)	12	16	20	24	28	32	36	40
Trimester	1	2	2	2	3	3	3	Term
Mean Hg (g/L)	122	118	116	116	118	121	125	129
5th percentile Hb values (g/L)	110	106	105	105	107	110	114	119
Equivalent 5th percentile Hct values (%)	33.0	32.0	32.0	32.0	32.0	33.0	34.0	36.0

Based on pooled data from four European surveys of healthy women taking iron supplements.[174-178]

A manual that provides a detailed description of the laboratory methods that are commonly used for evaluating iron status in epidemiological surveys has been prepared by the Nutrition Foundation, Washington D.C. in December 1985.[48] The majority of the procedures described are applicable to individual patients as well. Each procedure is introduced with a description of the principle involved along with practical notes, precautions, standards, and references.

The procedures presented include (1) hemoglobin determinations, (2) packed cell volume (PCV), (3) serum iron and iron-binding capacity, (4) erythrocyte protoporphyrin, and (5) serum ferritin. Several other reports have reviewed the diagnostic methods available for assessing iron status.[92,157]

Hematocrit

The packed cell volume of whole blood (hematocrit) is often used as a diagnostic for nutritional iron deficiency. The hematocrit is lowered due to insufficient hemoglobin formation resulting in microcytic hypochromic red blood cells. This measurement alone is not entirely conclusive in detection of iron deficiency although useful in the overall diagnosis. The hematocrit represents the percentage of packed red cells in whole blood. This is a standard clinical procedure available in all clinical laboratories.

Hemoglobin

In whole blood, hemoglobin concentration has been determined by a variety of methods including gasometric measurement of oxygen capacity and carbon monoxide capacity and colorimetric determination of chemically induced derivatives of hemoglobin including oxyhemoglobin, carboxyhemoglobin, acid hematin, and cyanmethemoglobin. Automated instruments have been developed by different manufacturers which are based on some of these methods.

Values are expressed as grams of hemoglobin per liter of blood. This simple colorimetric procedure is a standard clinical procedure available in all clinical laboratories. Hemoglobin measurements are easily performed with the time-tested Drabkin spectrophotometric procedure.[140] Feraudi and Mejia[169] have determined hemoglobin and hematocrit values with the use of blood collected on paper discs. The procedure was suitable for use in field studies. Drabkin's reagent was used. Convenient commercial kits are also available.

Hemoglobin, hematocrit, mean cell volume, white blood count may be obtained on 40 μL of whole blood with the use of a Coulter counter (Coulter Corporation, Hialeah, FL). Hemoglobin concentrations and/or hematocrit values are relatively insensitive indices that detect only the more severe states of iron deficiency.

Ferritin

Serum or plasma ferritin values have been a very useful measurement for assessing iron nutritional status.[45,48,49,66-68,81,161] The measurement is simple, inexpensive, requires only a small sample, is highly specific, and frozen stored samples are stable. The ferritin cutoff values for iron deficiency are well established. A value of < 12 μg/L is observed only with depleted iron stores.[45,161] A low ferritin level in association with a reduced hemoglobin or hematocrit value provides unequivocal evidence of iron deficiency anemia.[45,121]

A spot ferritin assay has been reported for use in field studies.[189] A 20 μL sample of serum is dried on filter paper and stored frozen. However, the filter paper serum samples could be stored at room temperature for up to 4 weeks.

Plasma ferritin levels can be obtained with the use of radioimmunoassay, enzymeimmuno-assay, or chemiluminescent assay procedures. Commercial assay kits are available for these determinations (e.g., NEN/Dupont, Boston, MA; Bio-Rad, Hercules, CA; and DiaSorin, Stillwater, MN). Capillary blood samples are suitable for measurements of circulating ferritin.[160] Various conditions can produce an increase in the plasma ferritin concentration, including inflammation, tissue damage, and neoplastic disease.[161,187] A markedly elevated plasma ferritin level may be indicative of iron overload.

Herbert et al.[171] reported that the measurement of serum ferritin iron provides for an accurate assessment of iron status. Moreover, the assay for serum ferritin iron is more sensitive and specific than conventional tests for iron status. Normal ferritin iron levels were reported as 20.4 ± 2.2 ng/mL. Serum ferritin levels of 5.3 ± 0.7 ng/mL were associated with an iron deficiency, while levels of 68.1 ± 12.6 ng/mL were indicative of iron overload.

Erythrocyte Protoporphyrin Measurements

Iron deficiency limits the rate of hemoglobin synthesis, giving rise to elevated protoporphyrin levels in the blood. The rise in free erythrocyte protoporphyrin usually occurs before anemia becomes discernable. Hence, free erythrocyte protoporphyrin measurements provide a sensitive early indication of iron depletion.[48,141,147-150,151a]

Erythrocyte protoporphyrins are commonly measured by an extraction procedure[142,144] or by using a hematofluorometer.[145,146,151-153] The extraction method is somewhat tedious and thus less widely used. However, it should be remembered that the extraction procedure measures total erythrocyte protoporphyrin while the hematofluorometer measures primarily zinc protoporphyrin. Interpretation of the data may require different guidelines for the two methods. Controls for erythrocyte protoporphyrin measurements and for zinc protoporphyrin measurements have been available from Kaulson Laboratories, Inc. (KLI), 687-693 Bloomfield Avenue, West Caldwell, NJ.

Zinc protoporphyrin measurements require the use of a dedicated, but portable, hematofluorometer.[145,146,151,151a] Such an instrument is available from AVIV Biomedical, Lakewood, CO. Another hematofluorometry system is available from Helena Labs, Beaumont, TX (Proto Flor Z System).[153] Only 25 μL of blood is required to perform the measurement. The zinc protoporphyrin values obtained per gram of hemoglobin may be converted to μg erythrocyte protoporphyrin per liter of red blood cells or to erythrocyte protoporphyrin per gram of hemoglobin. Zinc protoporphyrin assays were found to have a greater sensitivity than hematocrit determinations in identifying children with iron deficiency.[153]

The following guides have been suggested for evaluating erythrocyte protoporphyrin values.[48] Values higher than these were considered indicative of iron deficiency.

Age of Subjects	Erythrocyte Protoporphyrin (µg)		
	/g hemoglobin	/L erythrocytes	/L whole blood
0.5–4 yr	2.8	800	280
> 4 yr	2.4	700	280

Lead poisoning may increase erythrocyte protoporphyrin levels.[149,150] Consequently elevated erythrocyte protoporphyrin values may warrant follow-up studies to determine whether the cause is due to iron deficiency or lead poisoning.[48,149] Erythrocyte protoporphyrin levels may increase in infection and in inflammatory diseases.[141,151,152]

Transferrin Receptor (TfR) Measurements

Anemia may be the result of vitamin B-12 or folacin deficiency as well as from non-nutritional causes such as malaria, hookworms, sickle cell anemia, and other genetically inherited disorders and chronic disease.[50-56] Serum transferrin receptor measurements can assist in identifying the role of iron status in these conditions (Table 82).[76,78,83]

Plasma serum TfR analyses can be performed by using an ELISA technique.[75,83] Commercial TfR immunoassay kits are available that require only 100 µL or serum or plasma. (Quantikine™ human TfR ELISA kits; R&D Systems, 614 McKinley Place, NE, Minneapolis, MN 55413). The serum or plasma may be aliquoted and stored at –20°C. Reference TfR values were obtained on serum and plasma samples from 1,000 apparently healthy donors. These analyses resulted in a normal range of TfR concentration of 0.85 to 3.05 mg/L. The mean ± SD was 1.54 ± 0.43 mg/L plasma or serum. Using this kit, Punnonen et al.[88] reported in patients with iron-deficiency anemia a serum TfR concentration of 5.3 ± 1.8 mg/L, while controls had a concentration of 1.7 ± 0.5 mg/L. Patients with anemia due to chronic disease had concentrations of 1.6 ± 0.4 mg/L.

Serum TfR levels are reported to be independent of age and sex.[70] Recently, children were reported to have higher concentrations of serum TfR than adults.[191] Normal TfR of 5.00 ± 1.10 µg/L were reported by Cazzola and Beguin.[82] Ferguson et al.[76] found for normal controls a mean TfR value of 5.36 ± 0.82 mg/L of serum, compared with 13.91 ± 4.63 mg/L in 20 patients with iron deficiency. Subjects with anemia of chronic disease averaged 5.65 ± 1.91 mg/L.[76,85] Serum transferrin receptor levels above 8.5 mg/L have been considered evidence of iron deficiency.[80] Measurement of serum transferrin receptor concentrations can be a sensitive index of iron deficiency in pregnancy.[80] Pregnancy per se did not influence serum TfR concentrations.[80] The serum transferrin receptor (TfR) assay can provide information about the severity of tissue iron deficiency.[21,73-76,87,186] The usefulnesss of the serum TfR assay has been reviewed by Reguin[73] and by Cook et al.[21,74]

Serum TfR concentrations increase progressively with advancing tissue iron deficiency. In contrast, serum ferritin levels fall dramatically with depletion of storage iron. An improtant advantage of serum TfR measurements is its ability to distinguish iron deficiency anemia from anemia of chronic disease, such as infection and inflammation.[78] This ability has been utilized in a number of studies. For example, an investigation of postpartum women in Jamaica, West Indies, revealed that anemia (Hb <120 g/L) was present in 37% of the subjects.[77] However, assessment by serum TfR assay, only 13% were iron deficient. Numerous other investigators have empolyed the serum TfR assay in the assessment of iron nutritional status.[79-81,84,87-90] Pettersson et al.[78] found that serum TfR measurements, though not superior to serum ferritin measurements, can help to distinguish between anemia of inflammation and iron-deficiency anemia and to identify iron-deficiency in patients with chronic inflammation.

Serum Iron and Total Iron-Binding Capacity (TIBC) and Transferrin

Marked biological variations can occur in **serum iron** and total **iron binding** capacity values. Serum iron values are elevated in the morning and decrease in the afternoon and evening. Hence, morning fasting samples are preferred.

Serum iron and TIBC are measured by standard colorimetric methods. The color reagents used include Ferrozine, TPTZ, bathophenanthroline and bathophenanthroline sulfonate. Atomic absorption spectrometry analyses of serum iron are not recommended because any hemoglobin present will erronously increase serum iron values.

Colormetric kits for measuring serum iron and total iron binding capacity (TIBC) have been available from DiaSorin, Stillwater, MN; Sigma Diagnostics, St. Louis, MO; and from Technicon, Tarrytown, NY; Stanbio Laboratory of San Antonio, TX, also has simple manual kits available for serum iron and total iron binding capacity measurements. From this information, transferrin saturation (percent) is calculated by dividing the serum iron value by TIBC value and multiplying the results by 100.[92,157]

A number of commercial instruments are available for serum iron measurements. The reliability of these instruments for this purpose has been evaluated by Tietz et al.[5] The concentrations of serum transferrin can be measured by enzyme immunoassay[168] or with the use of radial immunodiffusion (RID) kits. Such kits have been available from Kamiya Biomedical Company, Seattle, WA. RID kits have also been available from Binding Site, San Diego, CA.

Factors Influencing the Interpretation of Hematological Data

Racial

The prevalence of iron deficiency is dependent upon the values of normalcy applied. This has been of concern in evaluating hematological data for black versus whites. A number of investigators have observed differences in hemoglobin levels between blacks and whites.[30-34] Reports have indicated hemoglobin values for blacks that are 4 or 9 g/L less than whites. The reason for this apparent difference has received considerable study and may relate to a number of factors, including nutritional, iron status, single gene thalassemia, genetic, environmental, and smoking. But if the difference between blacks and whites is inherent, then separate standards would need to be applied to certain hematological values (e.g., hemoglobin, hematocrit, MCV, MCH) for each race and perhaps for other population groups. Boston et al.[32] concluded from an evaluation of their data that whites had an average of 0.5 g/dL hemoglobin higher than age matched blacks.

Reeves et al.[35] studying 1-yr-old black and white infants found that the black infants had a median hemoglobin level that was 3 g/L lower than that of whites. For other age groups, blacks had an average hemoglobin level of 5 g/L lower than age matched whites.[32,35] If this racial characteristic is considered,[40] then by current standards about 10% of normal blacks would be erroneously designated anemic.[33]

Additional reports based on several United States nutrition surveys support the observation that the mean hemoglobin levels of blacks are lower than those of whites.[36,38,39,42] The studies appear to indicate that the differences are not in iron status but may relate to genetic and environmental determinants.[37,38,40] However, in well-fed military personnel, hemoglobin values of the black males were only 2.7 g/L lower than that of whites.[41]

Based on the summary of studies reported on hemoglobin levels for black and white,[38] a hemoglobin level of 5.0 g/L lower for black than that of whites appears reasonable. This appears to be generally applicable to all ages and to both sexes. Based on limited data, hemoglobin levels of Oriental subjects were comparable to those of Caucasians.

Smoking

It is well known that cigarette smoking will cause an increase in hemoglobin concentrations.[43] Nordenberg et al.[43] evaluated data from the second National Health and Nutrition Examination Survey. They found that women smokers had a mean hemoglobin level of 137 ± 0.4 g/L, while the mean hemoglobin level for never-smokers of 133 ± 0.5 g/L. For the men, the mean hemoglobin level for smokers was 156 ± 0.4 g/L, while the mean hemoglobin level of never-smokers in men was 152 ± 0.5 g/L. This would indicate that the minimum hemoglobin cutoff values should be adjusted upward to compensate for the masking effect of smoking.[143] Application of current standards would underestimate the prevalence of anemia among smokers. It has been suggested by Nordenberg et al.[43] that in the clinical sitting a single uniform upward adjustment of 4 g/L of hemoglobin be applied to all smokers.

Altitude

In addition to age, sex, physiological status, and other noted factors, altitude influences hemoglobin and hematocrit values. The increase in hemoglobin and hematocrit levels are well-recognized for people dwelling in Denver (5,280 ft.), Colorado Springs (5,900 ft.), Aspen (7,853 ft.), and Leadville, Colorado (10,152 ft.). Much of Bolivia has an average height of 12,000 feet. LaPaz, the capital, is at an altitude over 3,632 meters (12,000 ft.). Residents of LaPaz had a mean hemoglobin level of 171 ± 12 g/L.[180] The mean hematocrit value was 49.4 ± 3.1%. Consequently, adjustments of the altitude effect on hemoglobin and hematocrit levels have been attempted. The accompanying tables represent some of these attempts (Table 93 to 96).

Comments

Interpretation of the results of analyses for hematocrit, hemoglobin, and serum iron parameters of iron deficiency requires consideration of several characteristics of the subjects, e.g., age, sex, and physiological state. Certain criteria that have been proposed or utilized for the diagnosis of anemia are summarized in the accompanying tables. Difficulties have been encountered in establishing "normal" hemoglobin and hematocrit levels.[59-68]

Iron Deficiency in Population Groups

Infants and Children

Iron deficiency is particularly prevalent among infants and young children because of large iron needs associated with rapid growth.[111,113,114] Iron deficiency compromises physical growth and mental development in children.[17,21,24,25,98,100,106-108] Commonly iron deficiency is established in infants by measuring hemoglobin concentrations, total iron-binding capacity, transferrin saturation, serum iron concentrations, and ferritin concentrations.[48,92,156]

In a study on 62 healthy boys (11.7 ± 0.04 yrs age) the concentration of serum TfR was 3.8 mg/L (2.3 to 6.3 mg/L).[86] No signs of iron deficiency were noted based on other iron-related laboratory measurements. Yeung and Zlotkin[90] obtained plasma TfR data on 485 healthy infants 9 to 15 mo of age that can be useful as a reference standard for healthy infants. The following is a summary of their findings:

Hematologic Measure	Value
Hemoglobin (g/L)	126.8 ± 14.8
Free erythrocyte protoporphyrin (µg/L plasma)	45.8 ± 29.3
Ferritin (µg/L plasma)	12.9 ± 10.5
Transferrin receptor (mg/L plasma)	4.4 ± 1.1 (3–6.55)
n = 485 healthy infants 9–15 mo of age.	

From Reference 90.

Women and Pregnancy

The consequences of iron deficiency in women during pregnancy are numerous.[91,112,115] It has been estimated that 47% of the women of reproductive age in developing countries have poor iron status,[26] which is higher during pregnancy.[27] Poor iron status may be reflected in reduced levels of energy and productivity, reproductive failure, and impaired immune function.[26] Serum ferritin measurements can provide information as to the iron status during pregnancy.[110] In the United States, approximately 25% of pregnant women are iron deficient.[45,109] Of the young women aged 15 to 19 yrs, 14% were estimated as iron deficient. Overall, approximately 6 to 11% of the women of reproductive age were considered iron deficient.

Adolescents

Because of the high growth of the boys and girls and the start of menstruation by the girls, a higher prevalence of iron deficiency is observed in this group in developing countries.[28] The following are examples of the estimated prevalence of anemia among adolescents: Africa, girls 45%, boys 57%; Latin America, girls 12%, boys 22%; India, 55%; Cameroon, 32%; and Nepal, 42%.[27,29]

Iron Deficiency in the Elderly

In general, the iron status of the elderly in the United States is satisfactory.[66,135,136] A low incidence of anemia has been reported for institutionalized elderly.[135] Six percent were anemic and 6% had low transferrin saturation values. Iron deficiency in non-institutionalized American elderly has been estimated to range from 1 to 6%.[66,136] Iron deficiency in the elderly is often difficult to establish because chronic disease often associated with the elderly may mimic or mask a deficiency.[46,158,136,138,139] Connor and Beard[137] have summarized diagnostic criteria for iron deficiency in the elderly. A plasma ferritin level of <12 μg/L in the elderly has been considered indicative of an iron deficiency.[158] However, some elderly subjects with ferritin concentrations of up to 75 μg/L had evidence of iron deficiency.[158]

Iron Status in Volunteer Blood Donors

In the United Kingdom, volunteer blood donors are required to pass a copper sulfate screening test performed on a fingerstick capillary blood specimen.[2] Over a 30-month period, 0.24% of the males and 2.8% of the females failed the copper sulfate screening test. The volunteer was not accepted if a drop of their blood failed to fall to the copper sulfate solution (specific gravity of 1.054 for men and 1.053 for women). On follow-up studies, the majority of the volunteers who failed were iron deficient.[2]

Similar findings were noted in female volunteer blood donors in Connecticut with the use of the copper sulfate screening test.[3] Donation was deferred in 3.1% of the volunteers. The majority of the deferred volunteers were found to be iron deficient. Ferritin and zinc protoporphyrin levels were used to assess the iron stores.[3,4]

Iron Assessment of Populations

Skikne et al.[83] suggested that the iron status of a population can be fully assessed by using serum ferritin as a measure of iron stores, serum TfR as a measure of mild tissue iron deficiency, and hemoglobin concentration as a measure of advance iron deficiency. In a controlled study, Skikne et al.[83] observe the following results:

Laboratory Analyses Conducted on Subjects Before and After Iron Depletion

Measurement	Initial (n = 14)	After Iron Depletion by Phlebotomies (n = 14)
Hemoglobin (g/L)	14.5 ± 2.1	12.0 ± 2.2
Serum iron (μg /dL)	78 ± 54	32 ± 22
TIBC (μg/dL)	347 ± 117	413 ± 139
Saturation (%)	23 ± 18	8 ± 7
Serum ferritin (μg/L)	40 (16–103)	9 (4–18)
TfR (mg/L)	5.34 ± 2.18	8.77 ± 4.54

From: Reference 83.

National Health and Nutrition Examination Surveys

Results of the National Health and Nutrition Examination Surveys (NHANES) provided an extensive assessment of iron nutritional status of the United States (Tables 85 to 92).[44-46,49,93,95]

NHANES-II

For the NHANES–II, conducted during 1976 to 1980, the following reference normal values were used:[44,66]

1. Serum iron/iron-binding capacity: >16%
2. Mean corpuscular volume: >80 fl
3. Erythrocyte protoporphyrin: <75 μg/dL red blood cells

Using these reference values, the prevalence of anemia was: infants, 5.7%; teenage girls, 5.9%; young women, 5.8%; and elderly men, 4.4%.[44,45,65-68,95] Anemia among low income whites and Hispanic women during the third trimester of pregnancy was about 25%. Iron deficiency predominated as the cause of deficiency. The information on the elderly men may be misleading because of the incidence of inflammatory disease which may elevate serum ferritin concentrations and depress total iron binding capacity.[44,45,66] Approximately 6% of the Americans are in state of iron deficiency, while about 1% have an iron overload.[6,7]

NHANES-III

The NHANES-III was conducted during the period of 1988—1994. Although some changes were made in methodology and laboratory cutoff values used, the conduct of survey was similar to NHANES-II.[96] Overall iron deficiency in the United States has declined over the past 20 years. Nevertheless, in the United States, iron deficiency remains a relatively prevalent nutritional condition in toddlers and women of childbearing age.[96] Based on the survey findings, it was estimated that 700,000 toddlers have an iron deficiency. Similarly, 9 to 11% of adolescent and young adult women had an iron deficiency, with 2 to 5% exhibiting iron deficiency anemia.[96]

Iron Overload/Iron Toxicity

Up to 10% of Caucasians may carry homozygous and heterozygous forms of iron load diseases.[120-126,134] Hemochromatosis is a syndrome of iron overload.[56,58,84,98-134,183] The overloading occurs because of an increased absorption of iron. Hemochromatosis results in cirrhosis of the liver, enlargement of the heart, damage to the pancreas, and in skin pigmentation.[62,117,118,134] The reported adverse effects of dietary iron and iron stores in coronary heart disease has not been supported by other investigations.[126-133] With proper therapeutic treatment, the condition can be controlled. Serum iron, transferrin saturation and serum ferritin level measurements are useful as screening tests for hereditary hemochromatosis and for following the effectiveness of therapeutic treatments.[58,116,119,120,125] This is exemplified by the findings of Skikne and Cook.[120]

TABLE 85

Guidelines Used for the Interpretation of Blood Data from the National Nutrition Survey (Ten-State), 1968–70 [65,182]

Age (Years)	Sex	Determination									
		Hemoglobin (g/L)			Hematocrit (%)			Serum Iron (μg/dL)		Transferrin Saturation (%)	
		High Risk	Medium Risk	Low Risk	High Risk	Medium Risk	Low Risk	High Risk	Low Risk	High Risk	Low Risk
<2	M–F	<90	90–99	≥100	<28	28–30	≥31	<30	≥30	<15	≥15
2–5	M–F	<100	100–109	≥110	<30	30–33	≥34	<40	≥40	<20	≥20
6–12	M–F	<100	100–114	≥115	<30	30–35	≥36	<50	≥50	<20	≥20
13–16	M	<120	120–129	≥130	<37	37–39	≥40	<60	≥60	<20	≥20
	F	<100	100–114	≥115	<31	31–35	≥36	<40	≥40	<15	≥15
>16	M	<120	120–139	≥140	<37	37–43	≥44	<60	≥60	<20	≥20
	F	<100	100–119	≥120	<31	31–37	≥38	<40	≥40	<15	≥15

M = males; F = females.

Adapted from the reports of O'Neal et al.[182] and the Ten-State Survey.[65]

TABLE 86

National Health and Nutrition Evaluation Survey-I (1971-74): Percentile Cuts (25th percentile) for Hemoglobin Values by Age, Sex, and Race

	Hemoglobin (g/L)				Hematocrit Values (%)			
	Male		Female		Male		Female	
Age Group (Years)	White	Black	White	Black	White	Black	White	Black
1	115	96	114	111	35	32	35	34
2–3	119	115	118	114	35	35	35	35
4–5	121	115	121	117	36	35	36	35
6–11	127	119	126	120	37	36	37	37
12–14	135	123	129	125	39	37	38	38
15–17	144	138	131	122	43	41	39	38
18–44	151	147	131	123	44	44	39	38
45–54	151	143	133	128	44	43	40	40
55–64	147	140	135	125	43	42	40	39
65–74	146	132	133	123	43	41	40	38

Mean data from NHANES-I

TABLE 87

National Health and Nutrition Evaluation Survey–II: Hemoglobin and Hemotocrit Criteria for Children, Men, and Non-Pregnant Women

Age (Years)/Sex	Hb (g/L)	Hct (%)
Both sexes		
1–1.9	110	33.0
2–4.9	112	34.0
5–7.9	114	34.5
8–11.9	116	35.0
Female		
12–14.9	118	35.5
15–17.9	120	36.0
≥18	120	36.0
Male		
12–14.9	123	37.0
15–17.9	126	38.0
≥18	136	41.0

NHNES-II.[46,49,174]

TABLE 88

Summary of the National Health and Nutrition Evaluation Survey-II Criteria of Iron Deficiency

Measure	Deficient Values
Hemoglobin (g/L)	
Men	<130
Women	<120
Serum iron (μg/dL)	<50
Transferrin Saturation (%)	<16
Erythrocyte protoporphyrin (μg/dL RBC)	>70
Serum ferritin (μg/L)	<12

From NHANES-II.[95]

TABLE 89

National Health and Nutrition Evaluation Survey – II: Cutoffs for Abnormal Values of Iron Status Indicaters used in the Analysis of Data from NHANES-II

Age (Years)	Serum Ferritin (µg /L)	Transferrin Saturation %	Erythrocyte Protoporphyrin (µg/dL RBC)	MCV fl
1–2	—	<12	>80	<73
3–4	<10	<14	>75	<75
5–10	<10	<15	>70	<76
11–14	<10	<16	>70	<78
15–74	<12	<16	>70	<80

From Reference 45.

TABLE 90

Cutoffs for Serum Ferritin Values Indicative of Iron Overload in Adults used in NHANES-II

Age Group	Serum Ferritin Indicative of Iron Overload	
	Males (µg/L)	Females (µg/L)
20–44 years	>200	>150
45–64 years	>300	>200
65–74 years	>400	>300

From Reference 45.

TABLE 91

National Health and Nutrition Evaluation Survey-III: Hemoglobin Cutoff Values Derived from Data of NHANES-III (1988-1994).

Sex and Age (year)	No. of Subjects	Hemoglobin	
		Mean (SD) (g/L)	Cutoff Value (g/L)
Both Sexes			
1–2	876	122.0 (7.34)	<110
3–5	1741	124.4 (7.57)	<112
6–11	2032	130.9 (7.92)	<118
Female			
12–15	516	134.3 (9.27)	<119
16–19	405	133.7 (8.21)	<120
20–49	2799	134.8 (9.12)	<120
50–69	1486	136.5 (9.82)	<120
≥70	1137	135.6 (10.86)	<118
Male			
12–15	545	142.4 (10.0)	<126
16–19	581	152.9 (10.03)	<136
20–49	3651	153.0 (9.68)	<137
50–69	1632	150.1 (10.64)	<133
≥70	1139	145.3 (12.87)	<124

From References 96 and 174.

TABLE 92

Centers for Disease Control and Prevention: National Health and Nutrition
Evaluation Survey-III. Cutoff Values for Laboratory Tests of Iron Status

Age (Years)	Transferrin Saturation (%)	Serum Ferritin (μg/L)	Erythrocyte Protoporphyrin (μmol/L RBCs)
1–2	<10	<10	>1.42 (80 μg/dL RBC)
3–5	<12	<10	>1.24 (70 μg/dL RBC)
6–11	<14	<12	>1.24
12–15	<14	<12	>1.24
≥16	<15	<12	>1.24

From Reference 96 and 174.

TABLE 93

Altitude Effect on Mean Blood Hemoglobin and Hematocrit Values at Various Ages

Subjects		Altitude			
		Sea Level to 200 Meters[a]		1550 Meters (Denver, CO)[b]	
Age	Sex	Hemoglobin (g/L)	Hematocrit (%)	Hemoglobin (g/L)	Hematocrit (%)
2 months	M–F	133	38.9	114	33.4
6 months	M–F	123	36.2	125	36.9
1 year	M–F	116	35.2	126	37.8
2 years	M–F	117	35.5	129	38.2
4 years	M–F	126	37.1	131	39.0
6 years	M–F	127	37.9	133	39.6
8 years	M–F	129	38.9	134	40.3
10 years	M–F	130	39.0	136	40.8
12 years	M–F	134	39.6	139	41.6
20–40 years	M	158	47.9	168	49.4
	F	141	42.9	146	43.2

[a] From Reference 170.
[b] From Reference 171.

TABLE 94

Centers for Disease Control and
Prevention Altitude Adjustments for
Hemoglobin (Hb) and Hematocrit
(Hct) Cutoffs

Altitude (ft)	Hb g/dL	Hb g/L	Hct (%)
<3000	0.0	0.0	0.0
3000–3999*	+0.2	+2.0	+0.5
4000–4999*	+0.3	+3.0	+1.0
5000–5999*	+0.5	+5.0	+1.5
6000–6999*	+0.7	+7.0	+2.0
7000–7999	+1.0	+10.0	+3.0
8000–8999	+1.3	+13.0	+4.0
9000–9999	+1.6	+16.0	+5.0
>10000	+2.0	+20.0	+6.0

* Based on data from CDC Pediatric
Nutrition Surveillance System.[174,179]

TABLE 95

Guide to Interpretation of Hemoglobin (g/L) According to Altitude, Age, Sex, and Term of Pregnancy

Age	Sex	0 to 2499			2500 to 4999			5000 to 7499			7500+		
		High Risk	Medium Risk	Low Risk	High Risk	Medium Risk	Low Risk	High Risk	Medium Risk	Low Risk	High Risk	Medium Risk	Low Risk
3–11 mo	M-F	<90	90–95	≥96	<92	92–97	≥98	<94	94–99	≥100	<95	96–101	≥102
12–35 mo	M-F	<95	95–102	≥103	<97	97–104	≥105	<99	99–106	≥107	<101	101–108	≥109
3–11 yr.	M-F	<101	101–110	≥111	<103	103–112	≥113	<105	105–114	≥115	<107	107–116	≥117
12–17 yr.	M	<119	119–138	≥139	<121	121–140	≥141	<123	123–142	≥143	<125	125–144	≥145
12–17 yr.	F	<108	108–117	≥118	<110	110–119	≥120	<112	112–121	≥122	<114	114–123	≥124
18–44 yr.	M	<121	121–140	≥141	<123	123–142	≥143	<125	125–144	≥145	<127	127–146	≥147
18–44 yr.	F	<101	101–110	≥111	<103	103–112	≥113	<105	105–114	≥115	<107	107–116	≥117
45–64 yr.	M-F	<111	111–125	≥126	<113	113–127	≥128	<115	115–129	≥130	<117	117–131	≥132
> 65+ yr.	M-F	<109	109–123	≥124	<111	111–125	≥126	<113	113–127	≥128	<115	115–129	≥130
Pregnant Women													
1st Trimester		<101	101–110	≥111	<103	103–112	≥113	<105	105–114	≥115	<107	107–116	≥117
2nd Trimester		<96	96–105	≥106	<98	98–107	≥108	<100	100–109	≥110	<102	102–111	≥111
3rd Trimester		<91	91–105	≥106	<93	93–107	≥108	<95	95–109	≥110	<97	97–111	≥111

From Central American and Panama Nutrition Survey.[64,181]

Altitude in feet.

TABLE 96

Guide to Interpretation of Hematocrit (%) According to Altitude, Age, Sex, and Term of Pregnancy[a]

Age	Sex	0 to 2499			2500 to 4000			5000 to 7499			7500+		
		High Risk	Medium Risk	Low Risk	High Risk	Medium Risk	Low Risk	High Risk	Medium Risk	Low Risk	High Risk	Medium Risk	Low Risk
3–11 mo	M–F	<26.5	26.5–27.9	≥28.0	<27.0	27.0–28.5	≥28.6	<27.6	27.6–29.1	≥29.2	<28.2	28.2–29.7	≥29.8
12–35 mo	M–F	<28.8	28.8–30.9	≥31.0	<29.4	29.4–31.5	≥31.6	<30.0	30.0–32.1	≥32.2	<30.6	30.6–32.7	≥32.8
3–11 yr.	M–F	<30.1	30.1–32.8	≥32.9	<30.7	30.7–33.4	≥33.5	<31.3	31.3–34.0	≥34.1	<31.9	31.9–34.6	≥34.7
12–17 yr.	M	<34.9	34.9–40.5	≥40.6	<35.5	35.5–41.0	≥41.1	<36.1	36.1–41.6	≥41.7	<36.6	36.6–42.2	≥42.3
12–17 yr.	F	<31.7	31.7–34.3	≥34.4	<32.2	32.2–34.9	≥35.0	<32.8	32.8–35.5	≥35.6	<33.4	33.4–36.1	≥36.2
18–44 yr.	M	<35.5	35.5–41.0	≥41.1	<36.1	36.1–41.6	≥41.7	<36.6	36.6–42.2	≥42.3	<37.2	37.2–42.8	≥42.9
18–44 yr.	F	<29.6	29.6–32.2	≥32.3	<30.2	30.2–32.8	≥32.9	<30.8	30.8–33.4	≥33.5	<31.4	31.4–34.0	≥34.1
45–64 yr.	M–F	<32.6	32.6–36.6	≥36.7	<33.1	33.1–37.2	≥37.3	<33.7	33.7–37.8	≥37.9	<34.3	34.3–38.4	≥38.5
≥65 yr.	M–F	<32.0	32.0–36.1	≥36.2	<32.6	32.6–36.6	≥36.7	<33.1	33.1–37.2	≥37.3	<33.7	33.7–37.8	≥37.9
Pregnant Women													
1st Trimester		<29.6	29.6–32.2	≥32.3	<30.2	30.2–32.9	≥33.0	<30.9	30.9–33.5	≥33.6	<31.5	31.5–34.1	≥34.2
2nd Trimester		<28.2	28.2–30.9	≥31.0	<28.8	28.8–31.5	≥31.6	<29.4	29.4–32.0	≥32.1	<30.0	30.0–32.6	≥32.7
3rd Trimester		<26.7	26.7–30.8	≥30.9	<27.4	27.4–31.5	≥31.6	<27.9	27.9–32.0	≥32.1	<28.5	28.5–32.6	≥32.7

a From Central America and Panama Nutrition Survey.[64,181]

Altitude in feet.

A serum ferritin level above 200 µg/L in females is suspect of an iron overload.[62,84] Serum ferritin levels above 700 µg/L are usually associated with symptommatic hemochromatosis. The prevalence of iron deficiency is considerably higher than iron overload. Iron deficiency is estimated to be about 1,000 times more frequent than iron overload.[62] Bolan et al.[116] used the following guidelines to screen for hemochromatosis. Patients with values above these guidelines were considered to suffer from hemochromatosis.

Measure	Value
Serum iron concentration	≥ 180 µg/dL
Transferrin saturation	≥ 62%
Serum ferritin	≥ 400 µg/L

Summary

The consequences of an iron deficiency are well known, particularly during pregnancy and early childhood. The impaired cognitive performance and decreased work capacity that may occur with an iron deficiency at any age is particularly disconcerting.

Although a number of laboratory procedures exist for evaluating iron nutritional status, a simple hemoglobin or hematocrit determination performed on a regular basis would identify the more advanced cases of iron deficiency or anemia. Plasma iron levels and transferrin saturation levels are useful for screening purpose but can be misleading because of influences by other clinical disorders. Ferritin assays, which have become more commonly available, will provide information on body iron stores and even distinguish iron deficiency anemia from other causes, such as folacin or vitamin B-12 deficiency.

Serum transferrin receptor assays, although less available, provide information about the severity of tissue iron deficiency. Infection, inflammation, and most other clinical disorders do not influence the serum transferrin receptor assays.

For the anemic patient, the therapeutic response to iron remains the best test for proving the presence of an iron deficiency.

References

1. Bainton, D. F. and Finch, C. A., The diagnosis of iron deficiency, *Am. J. Med.*, 37, 62, 1964.
2. Lloyd, H., Collins, A., Walker, W., Fail, B., and Hamilton, P. J., Volunteer blood donors who fail the copper sulfate screening test, *Transfusion*, 28, 467, 1988.
3. Morse, E. E., Cable, R., Pisciotto, P., Kakaiya, R., and Kiraly, T., Evaluation of iron status in women identified by copper sulfate screening as ineligible to donate blood, *Transfusion*, 27, 238, 1987.
4. Schifman, R. B., Rivers, S L., Finley, P. R., and Thies, C., RBC zinc protoporphyrin to screen blood donors for iron deficiency anemia, *JAMA*, 248, 2012, 1982.
5. Tietz, N. W., Rinker, A. D., and Morrison, S. R., When is a serum iron really a serum iron, The status of serum iron measurements, *Clin. Chem.*, 40, 546, 1994.
6. Herbert, V., Iron disorders can mimic anything, so always test for them, *Blood Rev.*, 3, 125, 1992.
7. Herbert, V., Everyone should be tested for iron disorders, *J. Am. Diet. Assoc.*, 92, 1502, 1992.

8. London, I. M., Iron and heme, crucial carriers and catalysts, in *Blood Pure and Eloquent*, Wintrobe, M. M., Ed., McGraw-Hill, New York, 1980, 171.

9. Osler, W., *The Principles and Practice of Medicine*, Appleton Press, New York, 1892, 686.

10. Finch, C. A. and Cook, J. D., Iron deficiency, *Am. J. Clin. Nutr.*, 39, 471, 1984.

11. Group of European Nutritionists, *Nutritional Status Assessment of Individuals and Population Groups*, Fidana, F., Ed., Perugia, Italy, 1984.

12. Arthur, C. K. and Isbister, J. P., Iron deficiency misunderstood, misdiagnosed and mistreated, *Drugs*, 33, 171, 1987.

13. Charoenlarp, P., Dhanamitta, S., Kaewvichit, R., and Silprasert, A. et al., A WHO collaborative study on iron supplementation in Burma and Thailand, *Am. J. Clin. Nutr.*, 47, 280, 1988.

14. Bailey, L. B. and Cerda, J. J., Iron and folate nutriture during life cycle, *Wld. Rev. Nutr. Diet.*, 56, 56, 1988.

15. Food and Nutrition Board, *Recommended Dietary Allowances*, 10th edition, National Research Council, National Academy Press, Washington D.C., 1989.

16. Brown, E. B., Iron metabolism: A 40-year overview, *Am. J. Med.*, 87, 3–3SN, 1989.

17. Baynes R. D. and Bothwell, T. H., Iron deficiency, *Annu. Rev. Nutr.*, 10, 133, 1990.

18. *Nutritional Anemias*, Fomon, S. J. and Zlotkin, S., Eds., Raven Press, New York, 1992.

19. Yip, R., Iron deficiency: contemporary scientific issues and international programmatic approaches, *J. Nutr.*, 124, 1479S, 1994.

20. Fairbanks, V. F., Iron in medicine and nutrition, in *Modern Nutrition in Health and Disease*, 8th edition, Shils, M. E., Olson, J. A., and Shike, M., Eds., Lea & Febiger, Philadelphia, 1994, 185.

21. Cook, J. D., Skikne, B. S., and Baynes, R. D., Iron deficiency: The global perspective, in *Progress in Iron Research*, Hershko, C. et al., Eds., Prenum Press, New York, 1994, 219.

22. Green, R., Microcytic hypochromic anemias, in *Medicine for the Practicing Physician*, 4th edition, Hurst, J. W., Ed., Appleton & Lange, Stamford, 1996, 814.

23. *National Strategies for Overcoming Micronutrient Malnutrition*, WHO, World Health Organization, Geneva, Switzerland, 1991.

24. Pollitt, E., Effects of iron deficiency on mental development: methodological consideration and substantive findings, in *Nutritional Anthropology*, Johnston, F., Ed., Alan R. Liss, New York, 1987.

25. Latham, M. C., Stephenson, L. S., Kinoti, S. N., Zaman, M. S., and Kurz, K. M., Improvements in growth following iron supplementation in young Kenyan school children, *Nutrition*, 6, 159, 1990.

26. Levin, H., Pollitt, E., Galloway, R., and McGuire, J., Micronutrient deficiency disorders, in *Disease Control Priorities in Developing Countries*, Jamison, D., Mosley, H., Measham, A., and Babadilla, J. L., Eds., Oxford University Press, New York, 1993.

27. DeMaeyer, E. and Adiels-Tegman, M., The prevalence of anemia in the world, *World Health Statistics Quarterly*, 38, 302, 1985.

28. Brabin, L. and Brabin, B. J., The cost of successful adolescent growth and development in girls in relation to iron and vitamin A status, *Am. J. Clin. Nutr.*, 55, 955, 1992.

29. Kurz, K. M. and Johnson-Welch, C., *The Nutrition and Lives of Adolescents in Developing Countries*, International Center for Research on Women, Washington D.C., 1994.

30. Bazzano, G., Chou, A. C., Mohr, D., Boston, E., and Willis, J. R., A biracial study of children's response to oral iron supplements, in *Iron Fortification*, Bazzano, G. S., Ed., Touro Research Institute, New Orleans, 1986, 31.

31. Bazzano, G., Chou, A. C., Mohr, D., Boston, E., and Willis, J. R., A biracial study of children's response to oral iron supplements, in *Iron Fortification*, Bazzano, G. S., Ed., Touro Research Institute, New Orleans, 1986, 47.

32. Boston, E., Willis, J. R., Mohr, D., Bazzano, G., and Chou, A. C., Descriptive indices of a black/white population measured for hematological parameters, in *Iron Fortification*, Bazzano, G. S., Ed., Touro Research Institute, New Orleans, 1986, 59.

33. Dallman, P. R., Barr, G. D., Allen, C. M., and Shinefield, H. R., Hemoglobin concentration in White, Black, and Oriental children: Is there a need for separate criteria in screening for anemia, *Am. J. Clin. Nutr.*, 31, 377, 1978.

34. Frerichs, R. R., Webber, L. S., Shinivasan, S. R. et al., Hemoglobin levels in children from biracial Southern community, *Am. J. Clin. Nutr.*, 67, 841, 1977.

35. Reeves, J. D., Driggers, D. A., Lo, E. Y. T., and Dallman, P. R., Screening for anemia in infants: evidence in favor of using identical hemoglobin criteria for Blacks and Caucasians, *Am. J. Clin. Nutr.*, 34, 2154, 1981.

36. Owen, Y. O., Should there be a different definition of anemia in black and white children, *Am. J. Public Health*, 67, 865, 1977.

37. Jackson, R. T., Separate hemoglobin standards for blacks and whites: a critical review of the case for separate and unequal hemoglobin standards, *Medical Hypotheses*, 32, 181, 1990.

38. Perry, G. S., Byers, T., Yip, R., and Margen, S., Iron nutrition does not account for the hemoglobin differences between blacks and whites, *J. Nutr.*, 122, 1417, 1992.

39. Johnson-Spear, M. A. and Yip, R., Hemoglobin differences between black and white women with comparable iron status: justification for race-specific anemia criteria, *Am. J. Clin. Nutr.*, 60, 117, 1994.

40. Jackson, R. T. and Jackson, F. L. C., Reassessing "hereditary" interethnic differences in anemia status, *Ethnicity & Disease*, 1, 26, 1991.

41. Jackson, R. T., Sauberlich, H. E., Skala, J. H., Kretsch, M. J., and Nelson, R. A., Comparison of hemoglobin values in black and white male U.S. Military personnel, *J. Nutr.*, 113, 165, 1983.

42. Jackson, R. T., Hemoglobin comparisons between African American and European American males with hemoglobin values in the normal range, *J. Human Biol.*, 4, 313, 1992.

43. Nordenberg, D., Yip, R., and Binkin, N. J., The effect of cigarette smoking on hemoglobin levels and anemia screening, *JAMA*, 264, 1556, 1990.

44. Dallman, P. R., Yip, R., and Johnson, C., Prevalence and causes of anemia in the United States, 1976 to 1980, *Am. J. Clin. Nutr.*, 39, 437, 1984.

45. Expert Scientific Working Group, Summary of a report on assessment of the iron nutritional status of the United States population, *Am. J. Clin. Nutr.*, 42, 1318, 1985.

46. Yip, R., Johnson, C., and Dallman, P. R., Age-related changes in laboratory values used in the diagnosis of anemia and iron deficiency, *Am. J. Clin. Nutr.*, 39, 427, 1984.

47. *Guidelines for the Eradication of Iron Deficiency Anemia*, A report of the International Nutritional Anemia Consultative Group (INACG), The Nutrition Foundation, New York, 1977.

48. *Measurement of Iron Status*, A report of the International Nutritional Anemia Consultative Group (INACG), The Nutrition Foundation, Washington D.C., 1985.

49. *Assessment of the Iron Nutritional Status of the U.S. Population Based on Data Collected in the Second National Health and Nutrition Examination Survey*, 1976–80, Life Sciences Research Office, Federation of American Societies for Experimental Biology, Bethesda, MD, 1984.

50. Sears, A., Anemia of chronic disease and anemia of uremia, in *Medicine for the Practicing Physician*, 3rd edition, Hurst, J. W., Ed., Butterworth-Heinemann, Boston, 1992, 842.

51. Eckman, J. R., Iron deficiency anemia, in *Medicine for the Practicing Physician*, 3rd editon, Hurst, J. W., Ed., Butterworth-Heinemann, Boston, 1992, 846.

52. Eckman, J. R., Thalassemias, in *Medicine for the Practicing Physician*, 3rd editon, Hurst, J. W., Ed., Butterworth-Heinemann, Boston, 1992, 848.

53. Herbert, V. and Das, K. C., Anemias due to nuclear maturation defects (megaloblastic anemias), in *Medicine for the Practicing Physician*, 3rd editon, Hurst, J. W., Ed., Butterworth-Heinemann, Boston, 1992, 851.

54. Eckman, J. R., Hemoglobinopathies, in *Medicine for the Practicing Physician*, 3rd edition, Hurst, J. W., Ed., Butterworth-Heinemann, Boston, 1992, 865.

55. Eckman, J. R., Sickle cell anemia, in *Medicine for the Practicing Physician*, 3rd editon, Hurst, J. W., Ed., Butterworth-Heinemann, Boston, 1992, 867.

56. Marx, J. J. M., Iron deficiency in developed countries: prevalence, influence of lifestyle factors and hazards of prevention, *Eur. J. Clin. Nutr.*, 51, 491, 1997.

57. Cook, J. D. and Lynch, S. R., The liabilities of iron deficiency, *Blood*, 68, 803, 1986.

58. Eckman, J. R., Hemochromatosis, in *Medicine for the Practicing Physician*, 3rd editon, Hurst, J. W., Ed., Butterworth-Heinemann, Boston, 1992, 882.

59. Garby, L., Irnell, L., and Werner, I., Iron deficiency in women of fertile age in a Swedish community, III. Estimation of prevalence based on response to iron supplementation, *Acta Med. Scand.*, 185, 113, 1969.
60. Cook, J. D., Finch, C. A., and Smith, N. J., Evaluation of the iron status of a population, *Blood*, 48, 449, 1976.
61. Ballman, P. R., Reeves, J. D., Driggers, D. A., and Lo, E. Y. T., Diagnosis of iron deficiency: The limitations of laboratory tests in predicting response to iron treatment in 1 year old infants, *J. Pediatr.*, 99, 376, 1981.
62. Finch, C. A. and Huebers, H., Perspectives in iron metabolism, *N. Engl. J. Med.*, 306, 1520, 1982.
63. Waters, A. H., Anemia and normality, in *Metabolic Adaptation and Nutrition*, PAHO Scientific Publication No. 222, Pan American Health Organization, Washington D.C., 1971, 105.
64. Viteri, F. E., DeTuna, V., and Guzman, M. A., Normal haematological values in Central American population, *Br. J. Haematol.*, 23, 189, 1972.
65. *Ten-State Nutrition Survey Reports* (1968-70), I-V, Centers for Disease Control and Prevention, Atlanta, GA.
66. Assessment of iron nutrition, in *Nutrition Monitoring in the United States*, Chapter 6, Life Sciences Research Office, Federation of American Societies for Experimental Biology, U.S. Government Printing Office, Washington D.C., (DHHS Publication No. PHS-89-1255).
67. *Assessment of the Iron Nutritional Status of the U.S. Population Based on Data Collected in the Second National Health and Nutrition Examination Survey*, 1976–80, Life Sciences Research Office, Pilch, S. M. and Senti, F. R., Eds., Federation of American Societies for Experimental Biology, Bethesda, MD, 1984.
68. U.S. Department of Health and Human Sciences, 1988, *The Surgeon General's Report on Nutrition and Health*, DHHS Publication No. (PHS)88-50210, Public Health Services, U.S. Government Printing Office, Washington D.C.
69. Kohgo, Y., Structure of transferrin and transferrin receptor, *Acta Haematol. J.*, 49, 1627, 1986.
70. Kohgo, Y., Nishisato, T., Kondo, H., Tsushima, N., Nitsu, Y., and Usushizaki, L., Circulating transferrin receptor in human serum, *Br. J. Haematol.*, 64, 277, 1986.
71. Huebers, H. A. and Finch, C. A., The physiology of transferrin and transferrin receptors, *Physiol. Rev.*, 67, 520, 1987.
72. Ward, J. H., The structure, function, and regulation of transferrin receptors, *Invest. Radiol.*, 22, 74, 1987.
73. Beguin, Y., The soluble transferrin receptor: Biological aspects and clincial usefulness as quantitative measure of erythroporiesis, *Haematologica*, 77, 1, 1992.
74. Cook, J. D., Skikne, B. S., and Baynes, R. D., Serum transferrin receptor, *Annu. Rev. Med.*, 44, 63, 1993.
75. Flowers, C. H., Skikne, B. S., Covell, A. M., and Cook, J. D., The clinical measurement of serum transferrin receptor, *J. Lab. Clin. Med.*, 114, 368, 1989.
76. Ferguson, B. J., Skikne, B. S., Simpson, K. M., Baynes, R. D., and Cook, J. D., Serum transferrin receptor distinguishes the anemia of chronic disease from iron deficiency anemia, *J. Lab. Clin. Med.*, 119, 385, 1992.
77. Jackson, R. T., Dorah, J., Simmons, W., and Thomas, M., A comparison of transferrin receptor with other iron assessment measures in an upper-income post partum Jamaican sample, *Ecology of Food and Nutrition*, 34, 105, 1995.
78. Pettersson, T., Kivivuori, S. M., and Siimes, M. A., Is serum transferrin receptor useful for detecting iron-deficiency in anaemic patients with chronic inflammatory disease, *Br. J. Rheumatology*, 33, 740, 1994.
79. Kuvibidila, S., Yu, L. C., Ode, D. L., Warrier, R. J., and Mbele, V., Assessment of iron status of Zairean women of childbearing age by serum transferrin receptor, *Am. J. Clin. Nutr.*, 60, 603, 1994.
80. Carriago, M. T., Skikne, B. S., Finley, B., Cutler, B., and Cook, J. D., Serum transferrin receptor for the detection of iron deficiency in pregnancy, *Am. J. Clin. Nutr.*, 54, 1077, 1991.
81. Cook, J. D. and Skikne, B. S., Iron deficiency: definition and diagnosis, *J. Int. Med.*, 226, 349, 1989.

82. Cazzola, M. and Beguin, Y., New tools for clinical evaluation of erythron function in man, *Br. J. Haematol.*, 80, 278, 1992.
83. Skikne, B. S., Flowers, C. H., and Cook, J. D., Serum transferrin receptor: a quantitative measure of tissue iron deficiency, *Blood*, 75, 1870, 1990.
84. Bayness, R. D., Cook, J. D., Bothwell, T. H., Friedman, B. M., and Meyer, T. E., Serum transferrin receptor in hereditary hemochromatosis and African siderosis, *Am. J. Hematol.*, 45, 288, 1994.
85. Cook, J. D., Baynes, R. D., and Skikne, B. S., The physiological significance of circulating transferrin receptors, in *Nutrient Regulation During Pregnancy, Lactation, and Infant Growth*, Allen, L., King, J., Lonnerdal, B., Eds., Plenum Press, New York, 1994, 119.
86. Kivivuori, S. M., Anttila, R., Viinikka, L., Pesonen, K., and Siimes, M. A., Serum transferrin receptor for assessment of iron status in healthy prepubertal and early pubertal boys, *Pediatr. Res.*, 34, 297, 1993.
87. Cooper, M. J. and Zlotkin, S. H., Day-to day variation of transferrin receptor and ferritin in healthy men and women, *Am. J. Clin. Nutr.*, 64, 738, 1996.
88. Punnonen, K., Irjala, K., and Rajamaki, A., Iron-deficiency anemia is associated with concentrations of transferrin receptor in serum, *Clin. Chem.*, 40, 774, 1994.
89. Kuvibidila, S., Warrier, R. P., Ode, D., and Yu, L., Serum transferrin receptor concentrations in women with mild malnutrition, *Am. J. Clin. Nutr.*, 63, 596, 1996.
90. Yeung, G. S. and Zlotkin, S. H., Percentile estimates for transferrin receptors in normal infants 9-15 mo. of age, *Am. J. Clin. Nutr.*, 66, 342, 1997.
91. Viteri, F. E., The consequences of iron deficiency and anemia in pregnancy, in *Nutrient Regulation During Pregnancy, Lactation and Infant Growth*, Allen, L., King, J., and Lonnerdal, B., Eds., Plenum Press, New York, 1994, 127.
92. Fairweather-Tait, S., Iron, *Int. J. Vit. Nutr. Res.*, 63, 296, 1993.
93. Johnson, M. A., Iron: Nutrition monitoring and nutrition status, *J. Nutr.*, 120, 1486, 1990.
94. Baker, S. J. and Jacob, E., Iron, in *Tropical and Geographica Medicine*, Warren, K. S. and Mahmoud, A. A. F., Eds., McGraw-Hill, New York, 1984, 1045.
95. Cook, J. D., Skikne, B. S., Lynch, S. R., and Reusser, M. E., Estimates of iron sufficiency in the U.S. population, *Blood*, 68, 726, 1986.
96. Looker, A. C., Dallman, P. R., Carroll, M. D., Gunter, E. W., and Johnson, C. L., Prevalence of iron deficiency in the United States, *JAMA*, 277, 1997.
97. Simmons, W. K. and Gurney, J. M., Nutritional anemia in the English-speaking Caribbean and Suriname, *Am. J. Clin. Nutr.*, 35, 327, 1982.
98. Sayers, M. H., Iron, *Clinics in Laboratory Med.*, 1, 729, 1981.
99. Dallman, P. R., Iron deficiency: does it matter? *J. Int. Med.*, 226, 367, 1989.
100. Walter, T., deAndraca, I., Chadud, P., and Perales, C. G., Iron deficiency anemia: adverse effects on infant psychomotor development, *Pediatrics*, 84, 7, 1989.
101. Viteri, F. E. and Torun, B., Anaemia and physical work capacity, *Clinics in Haematology*, 3, 609, 1974.
102. Zhu, Y. I. and Haas, J. D., Iron depletion without anemia and physical performance in young women, *Am. J. Clin. Nutr.*, 66 334, 1997.
103. Li, R., Chen, X., Yan, H., Deurenberg, P., Garby, L., and Hautvast, J. G. A. J., Functional consequences of iron supplementation in iron-deficient female cotton mill workers in Beijing, China, *Am. J. Clin. Nutr.*, 59, 908, 1994.
104. Bates, C. J., Powers, H. J., and Thurnham, D. I., Vitamins, iron, and physical work, *Lancet*, 313, 1989.
105. Weaver, C. M. and Rajaram, S., Exercise and iron status, *J. Nutr.*, 122, 782, 1992.
106. Leibel, R. L., Pollitt, E., Kim, I., and Viteri, F., Studies regarding the impact of micronutrient status on behavior in man: iron deficiency as a model, *Am. J. Clin. Nutr.*, 35, 1211, 1982.
107. Pollitt, E., Saco-Pollitt, C., Leibel, R. L., and Viteri, F. E., Iron deficiency and behavioral development in infants and preschool children, *Am. J. Clin. Nutr.*, 43, 555, 1986.
108. Lozoff, B., Jimenez, E., and Wolf, A. W., Long-term developmental outcome of infants with iron deficiency, *N. Engl. J. Med.*, 325, 687, 1991.
109. Beard, J. L., Iron deficiency: assessment during pregnancy and its importance in pregnant adolescents, *Am. J. Clin. Nutr.*, 59, 502S, 1994.

110. Kaufer, M. and Casanueva, E., Relation of pregnancy serum ferritin levels to hemoglobin levels throughout pregnancy, *Eur. J. Clin. Nutr.*, 44, 709, 1990.

111. Dallman, P. R., Siimes, M. A., and Stekel, A., Iron deficiency in infancy and childhood, *Am. J. Clin. Nutr.*, 33, 86, 1980.

112. Bentley, D. P., Iron metabolism and anaemia in pregnancy, *Clinics in Haematology*, 14, 613, 1985.

113. Siimes, M. A., Iron requirement in low birthweight infants, *Acta Paediatr. Scan. Suppl.*, 296, 101, 1982.

114. Siimes, M. A. and Jarvenpaa, A.–L., Prevention of anemia and iron deficiency in very low-birth-weight infants, *J. Pediatr.*, 101, 277, 1982.

115. Scholl, T. O. and Hediger, M. L., Anemia and iron-deficiency anemia; compilation of data on pregnancy outcome, *Am. J. Clin. Nutr.*, 59, 492S, 1994.

116. Balan, V., Baldus, W., Fairbanks, V., Michels, V., Burritt, M., and Klee, G., Screening for hemochromatosis: a cost-effectiveness study based on 12,258 patients, *Gastroenterology*, 107, 453, 1994.

117. Gollan, J. L., Iron overload disease, *Alabama J. Med. Sci.*, 25, 40, 1988.

118. Gordeuk, V. R., Bacon, B. R., and Brittenham, G. M., Iron overload: causes and consequences, *Annu. Rev. Nutr.*, 7, 485, 1987.

119. Boyce, N., The value of screening for hemochromatosis, *Lab. News*, 23, 1, 1997.

120. Skikne, B. S. and Cook, J. D., Screening test for iron overload, *Am. J. Clin. Nutr.*, 46, 840, 1987.

121. Edwards, C. Q. and Kushner, J. P., Screening for hemochromatosis, *N. Engl. J. Med.*, 328, 1616, 1993.

122. Halliday, J. W., Inherited iron overload, *Acta Paediatr. Scand. Suppl.*, 361, 86, 1989.

123. Edwards, C. Q., Griffen, L. M., Drummond, C., Skolnick, M. H., and Kushner, J. P., Screening for hemochromatosis in healthy blood donors, *Ann. N.Y. Acad. Sci.*, 526, 258, 1988.

124. Bassett, M. L., Halliday, J. W., Bryant, S., Dent, O., and Powell, L. W., Screening for hemochromatosis, *Ann. N.Y. Acad. Sci.*, 526, 274, 1988.

125. Milman, N., Iron status markers in hereditary haemochromatosis: distinction between individuals being homozygous and heterozygous for the haemochromatosis allele, *Eur. J. Haematol.*, 47, 292, 1991.

126. Morrison, H. I., Semenciw, R. M., Mao, Y., and Wigle, D. T., Serum iron and risk of fatal acute myocardial infarction, *Epidemiology*, 5, 243, 1994.

127. Reunanen, A., Takkunen, H., Knekt, P., Seppanen, R., and Aromaa, A., Body iron stores, dietary iron intake and coronary heart disease mortality, *J. Int. Med.*, 238, 223, 1995.

128. Salonen, J. T., Nyyssonen, K., Korpela, H., Tuomilehto, J., Seppanen, R., and Salonen, R., High stored iron levels are associated with excess risk of myocardial infarction in Eastern Finnish men, *Circulation*, 86, 803, 1992.

129. Beard, J. L., Are we at risk for heart disease because of normal iron status, *Nutr. Revs.*, 51, 112, 1993.

130. Sempos, C. T., Looker, A. C., Gillum, R. F., and Makuc, D. M., Body stores and the risk of coronary heart disease, *N. Engl. J. Med.*, 330, 1119, 1994.

131. Prouex, W. R. and Weaver, C. M. Ironing out heart disease, *Nutr. Today*, 30, 16, 1995.

132. Ascherio, A., Willett, W. C., Rimm, E. B., Giovannucci, E. L., and Stampfer, M. J., Dietary iron intake and risk of coronary disease among men, *Circulation*, 89, 969, 1994.

133. Regnstrom, J., Tornvall, P., Kallner, A., Nilsson, J., and Hamsten, A., Stored iron levels and myocardial infarction at young age, *Atheroclerosis*, 106, 123, 1994.

134. Crawford, D. H. G., Powell, L. W., Halliday, J. W., and Leggett, B. A., Factors influencing disease expression in hemochromatosis, *Annu. Rev. Nutr.*, 16, 139, 1996.

135. Smith, J. L., Wickiser, A. A., Korth, L. L., Grandjean, A. C., and Schaefer, A. E., Nutritional status of an institutionalized aged population, *J. Am. Coll. Nutr.*, 3, 13, 1984.

136. Johnson, M. A., Fischer, J. G., Bowman, B. A., and Gunter, E. W., Iron nutriture in elderly individuals, *FASEB J.*, 8, 609, 1994.

137. Connor, J. R. and Beard, J. L., Dietary supplements in the elderly, *Nutr. Today*, 32, 102, 1997.

138. Ahluwalia, N., Lammi-Keefe, C. J., Bendel, R. B., Morse, E. E., Beard, J. L., and Haley, N. R., Iron deficiency and anemia of chronic disease in elderly women: a discriminant-analysis approach for differentiation, *Am. J. Clin. Nutr.*, 61, 590, 1995.

139. Mattila, K. S., Kuusela, V., Pelliniemi, T.–T., Rajamaki, A., Kaihola, H.–L., and Juva, K., Haematological laboratory findings in the elderly: influence of age and sex, *Scand. J. Clin. Lab. Invest.*, 46, 411, 1986.

140. Drabkin, D. L. and Austin, J. H., Spectrophotometric studies: spectrophotometric constants for common hemoglobin derivatives in human, dog, and rabbit blood, *J. Biol. Chem.*, 98, 719, 1932.

141. Langer, E. E., Haining, R. G., Labbe, R. F., Jacobs, P., Crossby, E. F., and Finch, C. A., Erythrocyte protoporphyrin, *Blood*, 40, 112, 1972.

142. Piomelli, S., A micromethod for free erythrocyte protoporphyrins: the FEP test, *J. Lab. Clin. Med.*, 81, 932, 1973.

143. Chisholm, J. J. and Brown, D. H., Micro-scale photofluorometric determination of 'free erythrocyte protoporphyrin' (protoporphyrin IX), *Clin. Chem.*, 21, 1669, 1975.

144. Piomelli, S., Brickman, A., and Carlos, E., Rapid diagnosis of iron deficiency by measurement of free erythrocyte porphyrins and hemoglobin: the FEP/hemoglobin ratio, *Pediatrics*, 57, 136, 1976.

145. Blumerg, W. E., Eisinger, J., Lamola, A. A., and Zuckerman, P., Zinc protoporphyrin level in blood determined by portable hematofluorometer: a screening device for lead poisoning, *J. Lab. Clin. Med.*, 89, 712, 1977.

146. Lamola, A. A., Eisinger, J., and Blumburg, W. E., Erythrocyte protoporphyrin/heme ratio by hematofluorometry, *Clin. Chem.*, 26, 677, 1980.

147. Labbe, R. F., Clinical utility of zinc protoporphyrin, *Clin. Chem.*, 38, 2167, 1992.

148. Schifman, R. B., Thomasson, J., and Evers, J., Red blood cell zinc protoporphyrin in pregnancy, *Am. J. Obstet. Gynecol.*, 157, 304, 1987.

149. Yip, R. and Dallman, P. R., Development changes in erythrocyte protoporphyrin: Roles of iron deficiency and lead toxicity, *J. Pediatrics*, 104, 710, 1984.

150. Mahaffey, K. R. and Annest, J. L., Association of erythrocyte protoporphyrin with blood lead level and iron status in the Second National Health and Nutrition Examination Survey, 1976–80, *Environmental Res.*, 41, 327, 1986.

151. Hastka, J., Lasserre, J.–J., Schwarzbeck, A., Strauch, M., and Hehlmann, R., Zinc protoporphyrin in anemia and chronic disorders, *Blood*, 81, 1200, 1993.

151a. Hastka, J., Lasserre, J. J., Schwarzbeck, A., Strauch, M., and Hehlmann, R., Washing erythrocytes to remove interference in measurement of zinc protoporphyrin by front-face hematology, *Clin. Chem.*, 38, 2184, 1992.

152. Bellotti, V., Bergamaschi, G., Caldera, D., Cazzola, M., Ciriello, M. M., Colotti, M. T., Dezza, L., Derie, G. M., and Quaglini, S., Clinical evaluation of erythrocyte zinc-protoporphyrin as a parameter of iron status, *Haematologica*, 64, 272, 1984.

153. Siegel, R. M. and LaGrone, D. H., The use of zinc protoporphyrin in screening young children for iron deficiency, *Clinical Pediatrics*, 33, 473, 1994.

154. Trundle, D. S., Erythrocyte zinc protoporphyrin, *Clin. Chem. News*, August, 8, 1984.

155. Trundle, D. S., Habel, D., and Bradley, H., Erythrocyte Zn PP in diagnosing iron depletion, *Laboratory Management*, July, 83, 1995.

156. Wharf, S. G., Fox, T. E., Fairweather-Tait, S. J., and Cook, J. D., Factors affecting iron stores in infants 4-18 months of age, *Eur. J. Clin. Nutr.*, 51, 504, 1997.

157. Cavill, I., Jacobs, A., and Worwood, M., Diagnostic methods for iron status, *Annu. Clin. Biochem.*, 23, 168, 1986.

158. Holyoake, T. L., Stott, D. J., McKay, P. J., Hendry, A., MacDonald, J. B., and Lucie, N. P., Use of plasma ferritin concentration to diagnose iron deficiency in elderly patients, *J. Clin. Pathol.*, 46, 857, 1993.

159. Painter, P., Clinical utility of serum ferritin measurements, *Clin. Lab. News.*, 21, 6, 1995.

160. Pootrakul, P., Skikne, B. S., and Cook, J. D., The use of capillary blood for measurements of circulating ferritin, *Am. J. Clin. Nutr.*, 37, 307, 1983.

161. Finch, C. A., Bellotti, V., Stray, S., Lipschitz, D. A., Cook, J. D., Pippard, M. J., and Huebers, H. A., Plasma ferritin determination as a diagnostic tool, *West. J. Med.*, 145, 657, 1986.

162. Craig, W., Iron status of vegetarians, *Am. J. Clin. Nutr.*, 59, 1233S, 1994.

163. Stoltzfus, R. J., Chwaya, H. M., Tielsch, J. M., Schulze, K. J., Albonico, M., and Saviali, L., Epidemiology of iron deficiency anemia in Zanzibari schoolchildren: the importance of hookworms, *Am. J. Clin. Nutr.*, 65, 153, 1997.

164. Reddy, M. and Cook, J. D., Assessment of dietary determinations of nonheme-iron absorption in humans and rats, *Am. J. Clin. Nutr.*, 54, 723, 1991.

165. Hunt, J. R., Mullen, L. M., Lykkem, G. I., Gallagher, S. K., and Nielsen, F. H., Ascorbic acid: effect on ongoing iron absorption and status in iron-depleted young women, *Am. J. Clin. Nutr.*, 51, 649, 1990.

166. Hallberg, L., Brune, M., and Rossander-Hulthen, L., Is there a physiological role of vitamin C in iron absorption, *Ann. N.Y. Acad. Sci.*, 498, 324, 1987.

167. Shaw, N.-S., Chin, C.-J., and Pan, W.-H., A vegetarian diet rich in soybean products compromises iron status in young students, *J. Nutr.*, 125, 212, 1995.

168. El Guindi, M., Skikne, B. S., Covell, A. M., and Cook, J. D., An immunoassay for human transferrin, *Am. J. Clin. Nutr.*, 47, 37, 1988.

169. Feraudi, M. and Mejia, L. A., Development and evaluation of a simplified method to collect blood samples to determine hemoglobin and hematocrit using chromatographic paper discs, *Am. J. Clin. Nutr.*, 45, 790, 1987.

170. *Scientific Table*, 7th edition, Diem, K. and Lentner, C., Eds., Ciba-Geigy Limited, Basle, Switzerland, 1970, 617.

171. Herbert, V., Jayctilleke, E., Shaw, S., Rosman, A. S., Giardina, P., Grady, R. W., Bowman, B., and Gunter, E. W., Serum ferritin iron, a new test, measures human body iron stores unconfounded by inflammation, *Stem Cells*, 15, 291, 1997.

172. McCammon, R. W., *Human Growth and Development*, Charles C. Thomas, Springfield, 1970, 224.

173. *Nutritional Anaemias*, World Health Organization Technical Report Series No. 405, World Health Organization, Geneva, Switzerland, 1968.

174. CDC Criteria for anemia in children and childbearing-aged women, *Morbidity Mortality Weekly Report (MMWR)*, 38/No. 22, 400, 1989.

175. Svanberg, B., Arvidson, B., Norrby, A., Rybo, G., and Solvell, L., Absorption of supplemental iron during pregnancy: a longitudinal study with repeated bone-marrow studies and absorption measurements, *Acta Obstet. Gynecol. Scand. Suppl.*, 48, 87, 1975.

176. Sjosteadt, T. E., Manner, P., Nummi, S., and Ekenved, G., Oral iron prophylaxis during pregnancy: a comparative study on different dosage regimens, *Acta Obstet. Gynecol. Scand. Suppl.*, 60, 3, 1977.

177. Puolakka, J., Janne, O., Pakarinen, A., Janvinen, A., and Vikko, R., Serum ferritin as a measure of iron stores during and after normal pregnancy with and without iron supplements, *Acta Obstet. Gynecol. Scand. Suppl.*, 95, 43, 1980.

178. Taylor, D. J., Mallen, C., McDougall, N., and Lind, T., Effect of iron supplementation on serum ferritin levels during and after pregnancy, *Br. J. Obstet. Gynecol.*, 89, 1011, 1982.

179. Hurtado, A., Morino, C., Delgado, E., Influence of anoxemia on the hemopoietic activity, *Arch. Int. Med.*, 75, 284, 1945.

180. *Bolivia Nutrition Survey*, A report by the Interdepartment Committee on Nutrition for National Defense, Washington D.C., June, 1964.

181. *Nutritional Evaluation of the Population of Central America and Panama*, Institute of Nutrition of Central America and Panama Nutrition Program, Centers for Disease Control, DHEW Publication No. (HSM)72-8120, Centers for Disease Control, Atlanta, GA, 1972.

182. O'Neal, R. M., Johnson, O. C., and Schaefer, A. E., Guidelines for classification and interpretation of group blood and urine data collected as part of the National Nutrition Survey, *Pediatr. Res.*, 4, 103, 1970.

183. Adams, P. C., Halliday, J. W., and Powell, L. W., Early diagnosis and treatment of hemochromatosis, *Adv. Int. Med.*, 34, 111, 1989.

184. Third Report on the World Nutrition Situation, Chapter 2, ACC/SCN Secretariat, C/O World Health Organization, Geneva, Switzerland, 1972, 19.

185. Seshadri, S., Nutritional anaemia in South Asia, in *Malnutrition in South Asia*, Gillespie, S., Ed., ROSA Publication No. 5, UNICEF Regional Office for South Asia, Kathmandu, 1997, 75.

186. Zhu, Y. I. and Haas, J. D., Response of serum transferrin receptor to iron supplementation in iron-depleted, nonanemic women, *Am. J. Clin. Nutr.*, 67, 271, 1998.
187. Hulthen, L., Lindstedt, G., Lundberg, P.–A., and Hallberg, L., Effect of a mild infection on serum ferritin concentrations — clinical and epidemiological implications, *Eur. J. Clinical Nutr.*, 52, 376, 1998.
188. Beard, J. L., Dawson, H., and Pinero, D. J., Iron metabolism: a comprehensive review, *Nutr. Rev.*, 54, 295, 1996.
189. Ahluwalia, N., Lonnerdal, B., Lorenz, S. G., and Allen, L. H., Spot ferritin assay for serum samples dried on filter paper, *Am. J. Clin. Nutr.*, 67, 88, 1998.
190. Hurtado, E. K., Classen, A. H., and Scott, K. G., Early childhood anemia and mild or moderate retardation, *Am. J. Clin. Nutr.*, 69, 115, 1999.
191. Virtanen, M. A., Viinkka, L. U., Virtanen, M. K. G., Svahn, J. C. E., Anttila, R. M., Krusius, T., Cook, J. D., Axelsson, I. E. M., Raiha, N. C. R., and Siimes, M. A., Higher concentrations of serum transferrin receptor in children than in adults, *Am. J. Clin. Nutr.*, 69, 252, 1999.

Iodine

Converting metric units to International System (SI) units:

Iodine

$\mu g/L \times 0.00793 = \mu mol/L$

$\mu mol/L \times 126.9 = \mu g/L$

atomic weight: 126.90

Thyroxine (T_4) (3,5,3'-5'-tetraiodothyronine)

molecular weight: 776.9

Iodothyronine (T_3) (3,5,3'-triiodothyronine)

molecular weight: 651.0

Creatinine

molecular weight: 113.12

Introduction

Iodine was the second element, iron being first, to be recognized as essential for health. Iodine was discovered in 1811 by Courtois during the production of gunpowder for Napolean.[5] Iodine is an integral part of the thyroid hormones triiodothyronine (T_3) and thyroxin (T_4). Thyroid hormones exert most, if not all, of their effects through the control of protein synthesis. They have a calorigenic effect, a cardiovascular effect, metabolic effect, and an inhibitory effect on the secretion of thyrotropin by the pituitary.

Most of thyroxine (T_4) and triiodothyronine (T_3) are transported in the plasma bound to carrier proteins. Thyroxine-binding protein is the major carrier of thyroid hormones with some bound also to thyroxine-binding prealbumin. Little free thyroxine is found in the plasma. The requirement for iodine is about 1 to 2 μg/kg body weight.

Seafood and seaweed are excellent sources of iodine. Use of iodized salt in the U.S. serves as an important source of iodine. In the United States approximately 10 to 12 g of iodized salt are consumed per person per day. Iodized salt contains 76 μg of iodine per gram.

Iodine Deficiency

Iodine deficiency is a common worldwide cause of endemic goiter and cretinism in children.[18,84,88] Globally, 5.7 million overt cretins exist.[94] When cretinism is observed in a population, a larger sector probably exists that is suffering from a subclinical iodine deficiency with some brain damage or loss of energy due to hypothyroidism.[41,42] The cretin child is dwarfed, mentally retarded, and inactive, with a pug and expressionless face and an enlarged tongue. Successful treatment requires diagnosis long before these obvious signs appear. In fact, iodine deficiency must be corrected before pregnancy to completely prevent fetal brain damage.[6,18,41,42] With the use of iodized salt, iodine deficiency is rarely observed in the United States.

Most European countries have some degree of endemic iodine deficiency disorder.[74-81] In Europe overall, more than 11% of the population suffered from goiter in 1993. Thus, more will be suffering from subclinical iodine deficiency.[21] Endemic goiter is particularly prevalent in many of the mountainous regions of Europe. Goiter prevalence is high in most South American countries, especially in the Andes mountain regions.[53] A high incidence also occurs in India, China, and Southeast Asia where a presence of up to 50% may be present.[6,18,23,25,57-67,73,90] Indonesia is a country with a high prevalence of iodine deficiency disorders (IDD).[89] Much of Africa has severe endemic goiter.[18,23,25,41,92,93] In 1990 it was estimated that about 211 million people in the less developed regions had endemic goiter.[18,23,25] Recent estimates indicate that 1.57 billion people worldwide are at risk of an iodine deficiency, with 655 million goitrous, and approximately 20 million suffering from varying degrees of mental retardation.[63,64,88]

Despite an iodization program in India, it is estimated that approximately 167 million people are exposed to the risk of iodine deficiency. Of these 54 million have goiter, 2.2 million are cretins, and 6.6 million have mild neurological disorders.[52]

It has been accepted that currently iodine deficiency is the single most cause of preventable mental defect in the world.[6,28,69] Unfortunately a simple field test does not exist to assess the prevalence of cerebral hypothyroidism in an iodine-deficient population. It has been suggested that the development of an instrument for measuring a subject's reaction times could be of use for assessing populations for iodine-deficiency disorders.[6] Iodine deficiency is most destructive on the brain. The deficiency results in the impairment of brain development during fetal life and early infancy at the time of maximum growth rate of the brain.[6,18,23,27,28]

Cretinism, the result of fetal hypothyroidism, has been described since antiquity.[6] The deficiency is associated with impaired fetal brain development, abnormal neurological signs, marked delay in growth and bone maturation, and with learning disabilities.[62,69] The prevention of cretinism requires the correction of an iodine deficiency before pregnancy or at the latest by the end of the second trimester of pregnancy.[6,56,65,66]

The term iodine-deficiency disorders (IDD) has been generally adopted to denote the spectrum of diverse effects in a population resulting from iodine deficiency that are preventable by correction of the iodine deficiency.[6,7] World Health Organization estimates that worldwide 20 million persons are suffering from varying degrees of iodine preventable brain damage.[19]

Laboratory Procedures

Various laboratory procedures are available to assess iodine deficiency, but many are not used nor necessary for establishing an iodine deficiency in a population.[24,48,53,55] These procedures are usually reserved for following small groups or patients with thyroid problems.[33-35] The procedures include measurement of serum thyroid hormone concentrations (T_3 and T_4), radioiodine uptake studies, thyroid stimulation hormones (TSH) assays, TRH responses and others.[50,53,55,91] These methods provide an indirect measure of iodine nutritional status. Biochemical hypothyroidism is indicative with a T_4 level of less than 38.6 nmol/L (3.0 µg/dL).[25]

Urine analyses for iodine usually employ automated equipment permitting the measurement of large numbers of samples possible.[12,26,40,82,85] Various methods for the determination of iodine utilize a chloric acid digestion of samples followed by the use of the ceric-arsenic catalytic system.[13-15,40,90] Iodine concentrations in urine have also been measured with a microplate adaptation and the use of the Sandell-Kolthoff reaction.[43] The results maybe expressed as the level of excretion per ml of urine or can be related to creatinine excretion, if creatinine levels are known.[36-41,43,45,83-85]

Recently, May et al.[90a] developed a simple, inexpensive, manual urinary iodine acid digestion method. The procedure was compared with the results obtained with five other methods performed in four different laboratories. A high correlation was obtained between all of the laboratories in the urinary iodine values reported.

Commercial radioimmunoassy kits and immunochemiluminometric assay methods are available that can be used with automated equipment to measure serum thyroxine (T_4) or thyroid stimulating hormone (TSH) levels.[33,91] Because of easier use and their better stability, TSH measurements are generally preferred. In infant neonatal hypothyroid screening programs,[29,31,32,91] these sensitive immunoassay procedures can be used to measure TSH or T_4 in blood samples obtained from infants and neonate with a heel stick. The specimens are placed on filter paper, dried, and analyzed.[41,45,46,51,56,91]

Immunometric assay procedures have been described for the measurement of thyrotropin and thyroglobulin in plasma, serum, or whole blood.[68] Dry blood spots on filter paper may also be used, which makes the procedure practical for use in remote field studies.[67,68,91] The assays have been evaluated in field studies carried out in Zimbabwe, India, Peru, Malaysia, Algeria and elsewhere.[91] Thyroglobulin measurements appear to be a more sensitive indicator of iodine deficiency than thyrotropin levels.[69] However, the results were obtained on children in areas with extreme iodine deficiency. Further studies on the use of these procedures in evaluating iodine deficiency in other population groups appear warranted.

From a study on iodine deficiency in Algeria, it was found that urinary iodine concentration was the most useful epidemiological indicator for assessing current iodine status, and thyroid volume and serum thyroglobulin levels as the best markers for assessing chronic effects.[73] Serum thyroxine (T_4) and thyroid stimulating hormone (TSH) levels and urinary iodine concentrations were used to evaluate iodine status in Zaire.[41] In northern Zaire, 25% of the neonates were found to suffer from hypothyroidism. Goiter prevalence in their mothers was over 75%.[41]

In a survey to evaluate the iodine status of Dutch adults, urinary iodine excretion was measured.[79] The results were expressed in three different ways: (1) urinary 24-hr iodide excretion, (2) iodide/creatinine ratio in 24-hr urine samples, and (3) 24-hr iodide excretion per kilogram of body weight. Iodide concentrations in the urine were measured by ion-pair reversed-phase HPLC with electrochemical detection.[82] The urinary creatinine concentrations were measured with a Technician Autoanalyzer procedure.[85] The survey population consisted of 824 adult subjects from Brielle, The Netherlands. The investigators concluded that urinary iodide excretion levels were useful for evaluating iodine status. It has been suggested, however, that excretion guidelines may need modification to reflect the effects of age and gender on iodine excretion.[79,80]

TABLE 97
World Health Organization Criteria for Urinary Iodine
Excretion

	Concentrations	
Iodine Excretion Status	**Conventional**	**SI Units**
1. Low Excretion		
Iodine/24-hr	100 µg	<0.78 µmol
Iodine/creatinine ratio	50 µg/gm	0.045 µmol/mmol
Iodine/kg body weight	2 µg/kg	<0.016 µmol/kg
2. Marginal Excretion		
Iodine/24-hr	50 µg	<0.39 µmol
Iodine/creatinine ratio	25 µg/gm	<0.022 µmol/mmol
Iodine/kg body weight	1 µg/kg	0.008 µmol/kg

From Reference 79.

TABLE 98
Guidelines for Urinary Iodine Levels for Children (ages 8–10 years)

Iodine Deficiency State	Iodine/Creatinine Ratio	Urinary Iodine (umol/L)
None	89	>0.79
Mild	45–89	0.40–0.79
Moderate	22–45	0.16–0.40
Severe	<22	<0.16

n = 396 children.
From Reference 43.

TABLE 99
Guidelines for Urinary Iodine Levels for Adults

Urinary Iodine	Deficient	Low	Acceptable	References
µg iodine/g creatinine	<25	25–49	>50	9, 24, 36, 53

Deficient State	µg/L Urine	µmol/L Urine	References
Mild	<100	<0.79	28–30, 69
Moderate	<50	<0.40	
Severe	<20	<0.16	

TABLE 100
Reference Laboratory Blood Values for Iodine Status

	Serum Analysis	
Iodine Status	**Thyroxine (T_4) µg/dL**	**Thyroid Stimulation Hormone mU/L**
A. Serum Biochemical Criteria For Children (1–7 years) [a]		
Euthyroid	≥6	≤10
Moderately hypothyroid	<6	<40
Severly hypothyroid	≤5	≥40
B. Serum Biochemical Criteria for Adults [b]		
Euthyroid (normal)	8 µg/dL	0.1– 5.0 mU/L
Hypothyroid	<6 µg/dL	>10 mU/L

[a] From Reference 41.
[b] From Reference 35.

Assessment of Iodine Nutritional Status

Estimating intakes and adequacy of dietary iodine is quite difficult.[14] Iodine content of foods varies widely as the iodine content of the soils on which they are grown. Soils of the Great Lakes region of the United States have a low iodine content. Water supplies contain iodine, but in variable amounts. Hence, dietary intake estimates of iodine can be inaccurate.

A more practical means of estimating iodine intake is the measurement of the urinary excretion of iodine.[10-12,14,36-40] However, this procedure has limitations.[43-45] Ideally a 24-hr urine collection should be used as the amount of iodine excreted in the urine may vary throughout a single day.[43] For an individual subject, a 24-hr collection is feasible although inconvenient. When large groups or populations are involved, it is necessary to resort to the use of random urine specimens, preferably collected fasting in the morning. The iodine excretion data are then expressed in terms of the amount of iodine excreted per gram of urinary creatinine.[12,36-39] When applied to a population, the procedure permits an overall characterization of the iodine status of the population. This has been demonstrated in surveys of populations with iodine deficiency problems.[8,9,11,16,17,73,74,77-81,89]

Daily urinary excretion of iodine closely reflects iodine intake. Expressing urinary iodine concentrations in terms of urinary creatinine concentration has been questioned when applied to areas where large inter- and intraindividual variations in urinary creatinine excretion exist.[43-45] However, urinary iodine concentrations remains a useful and valuable measure for assessing current iodine status in a population.[43,45,89] It has been suggested that the reliability of the procedure could be substantially improved by measuring the iodine concentrations in two or more casual urine samples from the same subject, taken on consecutive days.[43] Various procedures are available for the determination of iodine present in urine samples.[11-15,39,40,43] Use of automated or semi-automated procedures permit the rapid analysis of large numbers of sample.[12,15,43,86,87]

Iodine Excretion Guidelines

Values used for defining "low" and "deficient" are somewhat arbitrary but with usage have proven reasonable and justified. In the United States, the overall median iodine excretion was in the area of 250 µg per gram of creatinine.[8,9] A "low" urinary excretion level has been considered 50 µg or less of iodine per gram of creatinine, while "deficient" has been considered less than 25 µg of iodine per gram of creatinine excreted.[12,14,36,37]

Urinary iodine concentrations of <0.79 µmol /L (100 µg/L) are considered mildly deficient, <0.40 µmol/L (<50 µg/L) moderately deficient, while urinary iodine concentrations of <0.16 µmol/L (20 µg/L) are classified as severely iodine deficient.[8,9,43,69]

Surveys

Evidence of an iodine deficiency may be obtained from physical examination that reveal the presence of an enlarged thyroid and cretinism.[2,7,24,35,41,42,53] The extent of the problem can be pursed with the application of laboratory measurements. Dietary information on the intake of iodine can be useful but often is unreliable. More often, daily iodine excretion measurements are performed. Ideally, 24-hr urinary collections are preferred.[79] However, such collections are subject to a large error and are not practical for use in large surveys.[10] Hence, random urine collections are used and the iodine present related to the creatinine present in the sample (e.g., μg iodine per gram of creatinine).[12,36-38,43,54,55] Iodine excretions of less than 50 μg per gram of creatinine are considered an indication of an iodine deficiency.[24,36] Others consider a mean iodine excretion value below 60 μg per gram of creatinine to be of concern, with a level of only 40 μg per gram of creatinine considered serious.[23]

A urinary excretion of 100 μg/24 hr in adolescent boys and girls appeared to be indicative of an inadequate intake of iodine as experienced in Czechoslovakia where goiter persists.[70,71] In Switzerland, where iodine deficiency has been eliminated by iodization of salt, the urinary excretion of iodine was found to be 150 μg/day.[78]

The excretion of iodine per gram of creatinine is greater in females than in males because of the lower excretion of creatinine due to the relatively smaller muscle mass of females.[10] Thus Frey et al.[10] (Figure 56) found the mean 24-hr excretion of iodine in a group of adult

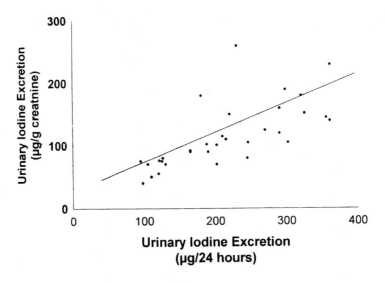

FIGURE 56

Relationship of urinary iodine excretion in 24 hr samples to the urinary excretion of iodine per gram of creatinine in a random afternoon sample (adult males). (Adapted from Frey, Rosenlund, and Torgersen.[10])

Norwegian males to be 216 ± 14 μg, while in an adult female group the mean iodine excretion was 165 ± 18 μg. However, when expressed on the basis of per kilogram of body weight, the iodine excretion for the two sexes was almost equal. An average iodine excretion of 2.7 μg/kg was observed in the women and 2.8 μg/kg in the men.[10] A close correlation was found between the mean total 24-hour iodine excretion and the mean excretion of iodine per gram of creatinine in an afternoon specimen.[10]

Radioiodine uptake methods are used in thyroid patient care and diagnostic needs, but rarely applied to iodine nutritional assessment or nutrition survey work.[47-50] Detailed descriptions of radioisotope methods and other procedures available for investigating thyroid diseases are summarized elsewhere.[50]

Pregnancy

Urine excretion of iodine remains essentially constant throughout pregnancy.[1] However, because of the increased rate of creatinine excretion during pregnancy, 24-hr urine collections should be used. Increases were observed during pregnancy in the plasma levels of thyroxine binding globulin, total thyroxine (T_4) and triiodothyronine.[1] Because of the major changes in iodine metabolism during pregnancy, the evaluation of iodine nutritional status is difficult during this period.

Goitrogens

Goitrogens occur naturally in certain foods and may cause goiter. Numerous goitrogens have been identified in cabbage, broccoli, turnips, cauliflower, and other members of the *Brassica* family.[3] Usually their presence in the average diet appears to be of little consequence. Additional iodine in the diet normally prevents their effects. In populations with a high intake of cassava, the thiocyanate present may act as a goitrogen and impair the uptake of iodine by the thyroid gland.[3,49,53,66]

Toxicity

High intakes of iodine may induce goiter because organification of iodine is blocked when the plasma concentration of iodine exceeds 15 to 25 µg/ml.[2,4] This has been documented in the Japanese, who have a high intake of iodine in seaweed, which is high in iodine. An intake in adults between 50 and 1000 µg/day of iodine is considered safe.

Hashimoto's thyroiditis and iodine-induced thyrotoxicosis (jodbasedow) are possible results of excess iodine intake.[2] Although other factors are involved, including genetic and immunologic.[2] Adverse effects of excess iodine may require information on the urinary iodine excretion, thyroid autoantibodies, and family history of thyroid disorders.

Iodine toxicity has not been considered a significant clinical or public health problem in the United States.[4] But with the current lower intake of iodine in the diet, an increase in goiter may occur. Monitoring of urinary iodine excretion as utilized in the Ten-State Nutrition Survey may be desired in the future.[8,9] Although widespread iodine deficiency goiter was not observed in this survey, an overall goiter prevalence of 3.1% was found.[8,9]

Excessive intakes of iodine are highly unlikely in the United States, but has been observed in some Japanese inhabitants living in coastal areas and have a high intake of seaweed. Their diets may provide a daily intake of iodine in excess of 50 mg. Excessive intakes of iodine can be monitored by the determination of urinary iodine levels. Prolonged excessive intakes of iodine may lead to thyrotoxicosis. An intake of 2000 µg of iodine is considered excessive and potentially harmful.

Summary

One of the major world nutritional problems is iodine deficiency. The presence of cretinism and goiter in a population is an indication of iodine deficiency. Iodine nutritional status may be assessed by the determination of iodine excretion in the urine. For this 24-hr collections or random urine samples may be used. For population studies, the collection of casual urine samples is more practical and feasible. The iodine levels are expressed as micrograms per 100 ml/L of urine or as micrograms per gram of creatinine present in the same urine sample.

An indirect measure of iodine nutritional status can be obtained through the determination of serum levels of thyroxine (T_4) or thyroid stimulating hormone. Convenient commercial radioimmunoassay kit methods are available for this purpose. Performing the two measurements can generally provide laboratory confirmation of a diagnosis of either hyperthroidism or hypothyroidism.

References

1. *Laboratory Indices of Nutritional Status in Pregnancy*, National Research Council - National Academy of Sciences, Washington D.C., 1978.
2. Talbot, J. M., Fisher, K. D., and Carr, C. J., *A Review of the Effects of Dietary Iodine on Certain Thyroid Disorders*, Life Sciences Research Office, Federation of American Societies for Experimental Biology, Bethesda, MD, 1976.
3. Van Etten, C. H., Goitrogens, in *Toxic Constituents of Plant Foods*, Liener, I. E., Ed., Academic Press, New York, 1969, 103.
4. Talbot, J. M., Fisher, K. D., and Carr, C. J., A *Review of the Significance of Untoward Reaction to Iodine in Foods*, Life Sciences Research Office, Federation of American Societies for Experimental Biology, Bethesda, MD, 1974.
5. Chapman, E. M., The history of the discovery of iodine and its many uses, *Alabama J. Med. Science*, 24, 216, 1987.
6. Hetzel, B. S., Historical development of the concepts of the brain-thyroid relationship, in *The Damaged Brain of Iodine Deficiency*, Stanbury, J. B., Ed., Cognizant Communications, New York, 1994, 1.
7. Hetzel, B. S., The iodine deficiency disorders (IDD) and their eradication, *Lancet*, 2, 1126, 1983.
8. Trowbridge, F. L., Hand, K. A., and Nichaman, M. Z., Findings relating to goiter and iodine in the Ten-State Nutrition Survey, Bethesda, MD, *Am. J. Clin. Nutr.*, 28, 712, 1975.
9. Ten-State Nutrition Survey IV-Biochemical, Iodine, U.S. Department of Health, Education, and Welfare, Washington D.C., DHEW Publication No (HSM) 72-8132, IV, chap. 7.
10. Frey, H. M. M., Rosenlund, B., and Torgersen, T. P., Value of single urine specimens in estimation of 24-hour urine iodine excretion, *Acta Endocrinologica*, 72, 287, 1973.
11. Mantel, M., Improved method for the determination of iodine in urine, *Clin. Chem. Acta*, 33, 39, 1971.
12. Garry, P. J., Lashley, D. W., and Owen, G. M., Automated measurement of urinary iodine, *Clin. Chem.*, 19, 950, 1973.
13. Zak, B., Willard, H. H., Myers, G. B., and Boyle, A. J., Choric acid method for determination of protein-bound iodine, *Anal. Chem.*, 24, 1345, 1952.
14. Benotti, J. and Benotti, N., Protein-bound and total iodine-Zak method modified in *Manual for Nutrition Surveys*, 2nd edition, Interdepartmental Committee on Nutrition for National Defense, Washington D.C., 1963, 155.

15. Benotti, J. and Benotti, N., Protein-bound iodine, total iodine, and butanol-extractable iodine by partial automation, *Clin. Chem.*, 9, 408, 1963.

16. Follis, R. H. Jr., Vanprapa, K., and Damrongsaki, D., Studies on iodine nutrition in Thailand, *J. Nutr.*, 76, 159, 1962.

17. Stanbury, J. B., Iodine metabolism and physiological aspects of endemic goitre, *Bull World Health Org.*, 18, 201, 1958.

18. Matovinovic, J., Endemic goiter and cretinism at the dawn of the third millenium, *Annu. Rev. Nutr.*, 3, 341, 1983.

19. World Health Organization, Report to 43rd World Health Assembly, Geneva, Switzerland, 1990.

20. Hetzel, B. S., Potter, B. J., and Dulberg, E. M., The iodine deficiency disorders: Nature, pathogenesis and epidemiology, *World Rev. Nutr. Diet.*, 62, 59, 1990.

21. *Regional Nutrition Programme Advisory Group*, Copenhagen, 28-30 August 1995, Nutrition Unit, World Health Organization, Copenhagen, 1995.

22. Kelly, F. C. and Snedden, W. W., Prevalence and geographical distribution of endemic goitre, in *Endemic Goitre*, WHO Monograph Series No. 44, World Health Organization, Geneva, Switzerland, 1960, 27.

23. Stanbury, J. B. and Matovinovic, J., Iodine, endemic goiter, and endemic cretinism, in *Tropical and Geographic Medicine*, Warren, K. S. and Mahmoud, A. A. F., Eds., McGraw-Hill Book Company, New York, 1984, 1064.

24. *Manual For Nutrition Surveys*, 2nd edition, Interdepartmental Committee on Nutrition for National Defense, National Institutes of Health, Bethesda, MD, 1963.

25. Clugston, G. A. and Hetzel, B. S., Iodine, in *Modern Nutrition in Health and Disease*, 8th edition, Volume 1, Shils, M. E., Olson, J. A., and Shike, M., Eds., Lea & Febiger, Philadelphia, 1994, 252.

26. *The Prevention and Control of Iodine Deficiency Disorders*, Hetzel, B. S., Dunn, J. T., and Stanbury, J. B., Eds., Elsevier, 1987.

27. Halpern, J.-P., The neuromotor deficit in endemic cretinism and its implications for the pathogenesis of the disorder, in *The Damaged Brain of Iodine Deficiency*, Stanbury, J. B., Ed., Cognizant Communications Corp., New York, 1994, 15.

28. Dunn, J. T., Societal implications of iodine deficiency and the value of its prevention, in *The Damaged Brain of Iodine Deficiency*, Stanbury, J. B., Ed., Cognizant Communications Corp., New York, 1994, 309.

29. Dunn, J. T. and van der Haar, F., A practical guide to the correction of iodine deficiency, International Council for Control of Iodine Deficiency Disorders, The Netherlands, 1990.

30. WHO/UNICEF/ICCIDD, Use of Indicators for Assessment and Monitoring IDD Programs, Geneva, Switzerland, 1992.

31. Barden, H. S. and Kessel, R., The costs and benefits of screening for congenital hypothyroidism in Wisconsin, *Soc. Biol.*, 31, 185, 1985.

32. Dagenais, D. L., Courville, L., and Dagenais, M. G., A cost-benefit analysis of the Quebec network of genetic medicine, *Canada Soc. Sci. Med.*, 20, 601, 1985.

33. Hay, I. D. and Klee, G. G., Tests of thyroid function, in *Medicine for the Practicing Physician*, 4th edition, Hurst, J. W., Ed., Appleton & Lange, Stamford, 1996, 590.

34. Gardner, D. F., Hyperthyroidism, in *Medicine for the Practicing Physician*, 4th edition, Hurst, J. W., Ed., Appleton & Lange, Stamford, 1996, 593.

35. Wilber, J. F., Hypothyroidism, *in Medicine for the Practicing Physician*, 4th edition, Hurst, J. W., Ed., Appleton & Lange, Stamford, 1996, 599.

36. O'Neal, R. M., Johnson, O. C., and Schaefer, A. E., Guidelines for classification and interpretation of group blood and urine data collected as part of the National Nutrition Survey, *Pediat. Res.*, 4, 103, 1970.

37. Jolin, T. and Excobar Del Rey, R., Evaluation of iodine/creatinine ratios of casual samples as indices of daily urinary iodine output during field studies, *J. Clin. Endocrinology Metab.*, 25, 540, 1965.

38. Plough, I. C. and Consolazio, C. F., The use of casual urine specimens in the evaluation of the excretion rates of thiamine, riboflavin and N'-methylinidotinamide, *J. Nutr.*, 69, 365, 1959.

39. Mantel, M., Improved method for the determination of iodine in urine, *Clin. Chem. Acta*, 33, 39, 1971.

40. Benotti, J., Benotti, N., Pino, S., and Gardyna, H., Determination of total iodine in urine, stool, diets, and tissue, *Clin. Chem.*, 19, 932, 1973.

41. Vanderpas, J. and Thilly, C. H., Endemic neonatal, infantile, and juvenile hypothyroidism in Ubangi, Northern Zaire: clinical consequences and prevention, in *The Damaged Brain of Iodine Deficiency*, Stanbury, J. B., Ed., Cognizant Communications Corp., New York, 1994, 209.

42. Connolly, K. J. and Pharoah, P. O. D., Subclinical effects of iodine deficiency: problems of assessment, in *The Damaged Brain of Iodine Deficiency*, Stanbury, J. B., Ed., Cognizant Communications Corp., New York, 1994, 27.

43. Furnee, C. A., van der Haar, F., West, C. E., and Hautvast, J. G. A. J., A critical appraisal of goiter assessment and the ratio of urinary iodine to creatinine for evaluating iodine status, *Am. J. Clin. Nutr.*, 59, 1415, 1994.

44. Greenblatt, D. J., Ransil, B. J., Harmatz, J. S., Smith T. W., Duhme, D. W., and Kochweser, J., Variability of 24-hour urinary creatinine excretion by normal subjects, *J. Clin. Pharmacol*, 16, 321, 1976.

45. Bourdoux, F., Seghus, P., and Mafuta, M. et al, Biochemical and statistical methods, in Nutritional Factors Involved in the Goitrogenic Action of Cassava, Delange, F., Iteke, F. B., and Ermans, A. M., Eds., International Development Research Center (IDRC), Ottawa, Canada, 1982, 51.

46. Larsen, P. R. and Browkin, K., Thyroxine immunoassay using filter paper blood samples for screening neonates for hypothyroidism, *Pediatr. Res.*, 9, 604, 1975.

47. Rall, J. E., Recent advances in the diagnosis of the diseases of the thyroid, *Clin. Chem. Acta*, 25, 339, 1969.

48. Lucis, O. J., Cummings, G. T., Matthews, S., and Burry, C., Laboratory observations of assays of serum thyroxine and protein-bound iodine, *J. Nucl. Med.*, 10, 160, 1969.

49. Delange, F. and Ermans, A. M., Role of a dietary goitrogen in the etiology of endemic goiter on Idjwi Island, *Am. J. Nutr.*, 24, 1354, 1971.

50. *Tietz Textbook of Clinical Chemistry*, 2nd edition, Burtis, C. A. and Ashwood, E. R., Eds., W. B. Saunders, Orlando, FL, 1994.

51. Maberly, G., Iodine deficiency disorders: contemporary scientific issues and international programmatic approaches, *J. Nutr.*, 124, 1473S, 1994.

52. Ranganathan, S. and Reddy, V., Human requirements of iodine and safe use of iodized salt, *Nutrition News*, Vol. 16, No. 1, National Institute of Nutrition, Hyderabad, India, 1995.

53. Hetzel, B. S. and Dunn, J. T., The iodine deficiency disorders: their nature and prevention, *Annu. Rev. Nutr.*, 9, 21, 1989.

54. Bourdoux, P. P., Measurement of iodine in the assessment of iodine deficiency, *Iodine Deficiency Disorder Newsletter*, 4, 8, 1988.

55. Bourdoux, P., Thilly, C., Delange, F., and Ermans, A. M., A new look at old concepts in laboratory evaluation of endemic goiter, in *Towards the Eradication of Endemic Goiter, Cretinism, and Iodine Deficiency*, Dunn, J. T., Pretell, E. A., Daza, C. H., Viteri, F. E., Eds., Pan. American Health and Organization, Washington D.C., 1986, 115.

56. Larsen, P. R., Merker, A., and Parlow, A. F., Immunoassay of human thyroid stimulating hormone used in dried blood samples, *J. Clin. Endocrinol. Metab.*, 42, 987, 1976.

57. Djokomoeljanto, R., Iodine deficiency in Indonesia: reassessment of its control program, in *Human Nutrition Better Nutrition Better Life*, Tanphaichitr, V., Dahlan, W., Suphakarn, V., and Valyasevi, A., Eds., Aksornsmai Press, Bangkok, 1984, 318.

58. Kochupillai, N., Godbole, M. M., Pandav, C. S., Karmarkar, M. G., Vasuki, K., and Ahuja, M. M. S., Thyroid status among newborns from iodine deficient environments in India, in *Human Nutrition Better Nutrition Better Life*, Tanphaichitr, V., Dahlan, W., Suphakarn, V., and Valyasevi, A., Eds., Aksornsmai Press, Bangkok, 1984, 329.

59. Hetzel, B. S., Overview on control of iodine deficiency in Southeast Asia, in *Human Nutrition Better Nutrition Better Life*, Tanphaichitr, V., Dahlan, W., Suphakorn, V., and Valyasevi, A., Eds., Aksornsmai Press, Bangkok, 1984, 307.

60. Suwanik, R., Pleehachinda, R., Boonamsiri, V., Tuntawiroon, M., and Pattanachak, C., Endemic goiter and endemic cretins in Thailand: a review of experiences with experiments of its control, in *Human Nutrition Better Nutrition Better Life*, Tanphaichitr, V., Dahlan, W., Suphakarn, V., and Valyasevi, A., Eds, Aksornsmai Press, Bangkok, 1984, 325.

61. Ma T., Lu, T. Z., Tan, Y. B., Chen, B. Z., and Zhu, X. Y., Control of iodine deficiency disorders in China, in *Human Nutrition Better Nutrition Better Life*, Tanphaichitr, V., Dahlan, W., Suphakarn, V., and Valyasevi, A., Eds., Aksornsmai Press, Bangkok, 1984, 313.

62. Tiwari, B. D., Godbole, M. M., Chauopadhyay, N., Mandal, A., and Mithal, A., Learning disabilities and poor motivation to achieve due to prolonged iodine deficiency, *Am. J. Clin. Nutr.*, 63, 782, 1996.

63. Yusuf, H. K. M., Quazi, S., Islan, M. N., Hoque, T., Rahman, K. M., Mohiduzzaman, M., Nahar, B., Rakman, M. M., Khan, M. A., Shakidullah, M., Baquer, M., and Pandav, C. S., Current status of iodine-deficiency disorders in Bangladesh, *Lancet*, 343, 1367, 1994.

64. Global prevalence of iodine deficiency disorders: micronutrient deficiency information system (MDIS) Working Paper No. 1, WHO/UNICEF/ICCIDD, Geneva, Switzerland, 1993, 5.

65. Xue-Yi, C., Xin-Min, J., Zhi-Hong, D., Rakeman, M. D., Ming-Li, Z., O'Donnell, K., Tai, M., Amette, K., Delong, N., and DeLong, G. R., Timing of vulnerability of the brain to iodine deficiency in endemic cretinism, *N. Engl. J. Med.*, 331, 1739, 1994.

66. Topliss, D. J., Iodine-deficiency disorders, *Med. J. Australia*, 150, 669, 1989.

67. Khin-Maung-Naing, Cho-Nwe-Oo, Tin-Tin-Oo, and Thane-Toe, A study on the aetiology of endemic goitre in lowland Burma, *Eur. J. Clin. Nutr.*, 43, 693, 1989.

68. Missler, U., Gutekunst, R., and Wood, W. G., Thyroglobulin is a more sensitive indicator of iodine deficiency then thyrotropin: development and evaluation of dry blood spot assays for thyrotropin and thyroglobulin in iodine-deficient geographical areas, *Eur. J. Clin. Chem. Clin. Biochem.*, 32, 137, 1994.

69. Dunn, J. T., Iodine supplementation and the prevention of cretinism, *Ann. NY Acad. Sci.*, 678, 158, 1993.

70. Tajtakova, M., Hancinova, D., Langer, P., Tajtak, J., Folder, O., Malinovsky, E., and Varga, J., Thyroid volume of East Slovakian adolescents determined by ultrasound 40 years after the introduction of iodized salt, *Klin. Wochenschr.*, 66, 749, 1988.

71. Tajtakova, M., Hancinova, D., Langer, P., Tajtak, J., Malinovsky, E., and Varga, J., Thyroid volume by ultrasound in boys and girls 6–12 years of age under marginal iodine deficiency as related to the age of puberty, *Klin. Wochenschr.*, 68, 503, 1990.

72. Benmiloud, M., Chaouki, M. L., Gutekunst, R., Teichert, H.-M., Wood, W. G., and Dunn, J. T., Oral iodized oil for correcting iodine deficiency: Optimal dosing and outcome indicator selection, *J. Clin. Endocrinol. Metab.*, 79, 20, 1994.

73. Pang, X.-P., Ouyang, A., Su, T.-S., and Hershmann, J. M., Thyroid function of subjects with goitre and cretinism in an endemic goitre area of rural China after use of iodized salt, *Acta Endocriologica* (Copenhagen), 118, 444, 1988.

74. Goitre and iodine deficiency in Europe, Report of the Subcommittee for the Study of Endemic Goitre and Iodine Deficiency of the European Thyroid Association, *Lancet*, 1289, 1985.

75. Delang, F., Heidemann, P., Bourdoux, P., Larsson, A., Vigneri, R., Klett, M., Beckus, C., and Stubbe, P., Regional variations of iodine nutrition and thyroid function during the neonatal period in Europe, *Biol. Neonate*, 49, 322, 1986.

76. Pedersen, K. M., Borlum, K. G., Knudsen, P. R., Hansen, E. -S., Johannesen, P. L., and Laurberg, P., Urinary iodine excretion is low and serum thyroglobulin high in pregnant women in parts of Dennmark, *Acta Obstet. Gynecol. Scand.*, 67, 413, 1988.

77. Delange, F. and Burgi, H., Iodine deficiency disorders, in *Eur. Bull. World Health Organization*, 67, 317, 1989.

78. Burgi, H., Supersaxo, Z., and Selz, B., Iodine deficiency diseases in Switzerland one hundred years after Theodor Kocher's survey: a historical review with some new goitre prevalence data, *Acta Endocrinologica*, 123, 577, 1990.

79. Brug, J., Lowik, M. R. H., van Binsbergen, J. J., Odink, J., Egger, R. J., and Wedel, M., Indicators of iodine status among adults, *Annu. Nutr. Metab.*, 36, 129, 1992.

80. Nohr, S. B., Laurberg, P., Borlum, K.-G., Pederson, K. M., Johannesen, P. L., Damm, P., Fuglsang, E., and Johansen, A., Iodine deficiency in pregnancy in Dennmark, *Acta Obstet. Gynecol. Scand.*, 72, 350, 1993.

81. Aghini-Lombardi, F., Pinchers, A., Antonangeli, L., Rago, T., Fenzi, G. F., Nanni, P., and Vitti, P., Iodized salt prophylaxis of endemic goiter: an experience in Toscano (Italy), *Acta Endocrinologica*, 129, 497, 1993.

82. Odink, J., Bogoards, J. J. P., Sandman, H., Egger, R. J., Arkesteyn, G.A., and de Jong, P., Excretion of iodine in 24-h urine as determined by ion-pair reversed-phase liquid chromatography with electrochemical detection, *J. Chromatogr.*, 431, 309, 1988.

83. Siedel, J., Mollering, H., and Ziegenhorn, J., Sensitive color reagent for the enzymatic determination of creatinine, *Clin. Chem.*, 30, 968, 1984.

84. Follis, R. H. Jr., Patterns of urinary iodine excretion in goitrous and nongoitrous areas, *Am. J. Clin. Nutr.*, 14, 253, 1964.

85. Auto-Analyzer Method File N-56, Technicon Corp., Tarrytown, NY.

86. Rendl, J., Seybold, S., and Barner, W., Urinary iodine determination by paired-ion reversed-phase HPLC with electrochemical detection, *Clin. Chem.*, 40, 908, 1994.

87. Tsuda, K., Namba, H., Norura, T. et al., Automated measurement of urinary iodine with use of ultraviolet irradiation, *Clin. Chem.*, 41, 581, 1995.

88. Dunn, J. T., Extensive personal experience, Seven deadly sins in confronting endemic iodine deficiency, and how to avoid them, *J. Clin. Endocrinol. Metab.*, 81, 1332, 1996.

89. Pardede, L. V. H., Hardjowasito, W., Gross, R., Dillon, D. H. S., Totoprajogo, O. S., Yosoprawoto, M., Waskito, L, and Untoro, J., Urinary iodine excretion is the most appropriate outcome indicator for iodine deficiency at field conditions at District Level, *J. Nutr.*, 128, 1122, 1998.

90. Zargar, A. H., Shah, J. A., Mir, M. M., Laway, B. A., Prevalence of goiter in school children in Kashmir Valley, India, *Am. J. Clin. Nutr.*, 62, 1020, 1995.

90a. May, S. L., May, W. A., Bourdoux, P. P., Pino, S., Sullivan, K. M., and Maberly, G. F., Validation of a single manual urinary iodine method for estimating the prevalence of iodine-deficiency with other methods, *Am. J. Clin. Nutr.*, 65, 1441, 1997.

91. Sullivan, K. M., May, W., Nordenberg, D., Houston, R., and Maberly, G. F., Use of thyroid stimulating hormone testing in newborns to identify iodine deficiency, *J. Nutr.*, 127, 55, 1997.

92. Todd, C. H. and Dunn, J. T., Intermittent oral administration of potassium iodide solution for the correction of iodine deficiency, *Am. J. Clin. Nutr.*, 67, 1279, 1998.

93. Alnwick, D., Weekly iodine supplements work, *Am. J. Clin. Nutr.*, 67, 1103, 1998.

94. Malnutrition in South Asia, A regional profile, Gillespie, S., Ed., Rosa Publication No. 5, UNICEF, Regional Office of South Asia, Kathmanda, Nepal, November, 1997.

95. Third Report on the World Nutrition Situation, Chapter 2, ACC/SCN Secretariat, C/O World Health Organization, Geneva, Switzerland, December, 1997, 19.

Zinc

Converting metric units International System (SI) units:

μmol/L × 0.0654 = μg/mL

μg/mL × 15.3 = μmol/L

atomic weight: 65.4

History of Zinc Essentiality

In 1934, zinc was reported to be essential for the rat.[20] Over twenty years later, zinc was found to prevent and treat parakeratosis in swine.[21] In 1963 in Iran, the essentiality of zinc in the human was demonstrated in the classical report of Prasad and associates.[22] This was followed by the recognition of zinc deficiency in Egypt.[83] The early history of zinc deficiency in the human has been the subject of several reviews.[23,24,34,39,50,51,82] In subsequent years, the literature on zinc deficiency in the human has become extensive (Table 101).[29,34,35,52]

Occurrence of Zinc Deficiency

The occurrence of zinc deficiency is more widespread and prevalent than originally considered.[132,133] Countries with recognized zinc deficiency include Iran, Egypt, Turkey, Portugal, Morocco, Mexico, Canada, and Yugoslavia.[82,105,109] Populations subsisting mainly on cereal proteins are more likely to have a zinc deficiency. It is estimated that 30% of Chinese children are zinc deficient.[81,84] Children in the United States have been observed to have zinc deficiency.[29,31-33] Zinc deficiency may occur in subjects with non-insulin-dependent diabetes.[150,151] Early total parenteral nutrition preparations were devoid of zinc and zinc deficiencies were observed with their use.[35] Some patients with malabsorption syndromes have been reported to develop a zinc deficiency.[29] Acrodermatitis enteropathica, which results in a severe skin and intestinal disorder is due to a metabolic error that produces zinc malabsorption.[35,39,40] Chronic use of diuretics may result in low plasma levels of zinc.[27,108] A conditioned zinc deficiency may be caused by a number of factors as summarized by Sandstead.[108] Serum zinc levels in males appear to be age-related. Serum zinc levels rise from about 80 μg/dL at age 3 to 8 years to 95 μg/dL at age 18 years and then fall off at age 45 years and returns again to levels of 80 μg/dL. An age-related variation in serum zinc levels was not noted in females.[16,24] Serum zinc levels did not differ between blacks and whites.[16] Obese males and females have serum zinc concentrations that were 24 to 34% lower than non-obese subjects.[143] Zinc deficiency is often noted in patients with homozygous sickle disease.[94-96]

TABLE 101
Some Literature Values for Guidance in the Evaluation of Zinc Status

	Serum Zinc (μmol/L)	Reference (Year)
1. Infants and Children		
Age		142 (1987)
0–5 d (*n* = 27)	9.9–21.4	
1–5 yr (*n* = 77)	10.3–18.1	
6–9 yr (*n* = 44)	11.8–16.4	
10–14 yr (*n* = 36; males)	11.6–15.4	
10–14 yr (*n* = 23; females)	12.1–18.0	
15–19 yr (*n* = 55; males)	9.8 –17.9	
15–19 yr (*n* = 31; females)	9.2 –15.4	
2. Preschool Children (Canada)		
Serum zinc		142 (1987)
Male and females (*n* = 74)	17.0 ± 2.0 μmol/L	
3. Adults		
Serum zinc		19 (1982)
Men military personnel (*n* = 2,029)	17.9 ± 6.4 μmol/L	
Women military personnel (*n* = 386)	16.2 ± 0.3 μmol/L	
4. Elderly (70–85 yr)		
Plasma zinc (*n* = 24)	11.0 μmol/L	135 (1984)
Serum zinc (*n* = 53)	13.0 μmol/L	137 (1988)
5. Pregnancy		
Non-pregnant (*n* = 28)	14.0 μmol/L	66 (1981)
2nd trimester (*n* = 60)	9.8 ± 1.2 μmol/L	
3rd trimester (*n* = 50)	9.8 ± 1.2 μmol/L	
Non-pregnant (*n* = 17)	12.2 ± 2.1 μmol/L	138 (1984)
1st trimester (*n* = 34)	11.9 ± 1.7 μmol/L	
2nd trimester (*n* = 39)	9.7 ± 1.3 μmol/L	
3rd trimester (*n* = 15)	8.7 ± 1.6 μmol/L	
Non-pregnant (*n* = 61)	13.9 μmol/L	69 (1986)
1st trimester (*n* = 36)	10.6 μmol/L	
2nd trimester (*n* = 31)	8.9 μmol/L	
3rd trimester (*n* = 42)	9.2 μmol/L	
Non-pregnant (*n* = 14)	14.3 ± 1.1 μmol/L	74 (1988)
2nd trimester (*n* = 84)	11.5 ± 2.7 μmol/L	
3rd trimester (*n* = 84)	10.8 ± 7.0 μmol/L	
6. U.S. Navy Trainees (Male)		
Plasma zinc (*n* = 270)	13.4 ± 0.2 μmol/L	144 (1989)
Urine zinc (*n* = 270)	11.1 ± 0.3 μmol/L	
7. Hair zinc		
(a) Adults (*n* = 96)	2.25–3.93 μmol/L	52 (1981); 136 (1979); 142 (1987; 143 (1988)
	127–257 μg/g	
(b) Males (*n* = 62)	103 ± 35 μg/g	
Females (*n* = 44)	129 ± 34 μg/g	

Sickle cell patients have lower serum zinc concentrations.[106,146a] Their serum levels of retinol-binding protein and alkaline phosphatase, two zinc dependent proteins, were also lower than normal.[95]

Zinc Essentiality and Functions

Zinc is involved in a large array of metabolic actions in the body. As examples, zinc is involved in acid-base balance, amino acid metabolism, protein synthesis, zinc-finger proteins, nucleic acid synthesis, folate availability, vision, immune system, reproduction, and the development and functioning of the nervous system.[24,29,36-41,46,49,82]

With the broad range of zinc participation in metabolic processes, it is only to be expected that a zinc deficiency can lead to a variety of physiological and development impairments.[24,29,75,82,101,102] Thus, a zinc deficiency has been associated with ezematous scaling, psoriasiform rash, growth restriction, hypogonadism, delayed puberty, slow wound healing, hypogeusia, photophobia, acrodermatitis, abnormal dark adaptation, impaired taste and smell, anorexia, and mental aberrations.[24,40,82]

More than 200 enzymes are zinc dependent, including carbonic anhydrase, alcohol dehydrogenase, alkaline phosphatase, RNA polymerase, DNA polymerase, nucleoside phosphorylase, protein kinase C, Cu/Zn superoxide dismutalse, and pteroylpoly-glutamate hydrolase. Numerous reviews exist that provide details regarding the essentiality of zinc.[36-39,44,45,75,78,108,122]

Diet and Zinc Sources and Intakes

Zinc is ubiquitous and thus it is rarely lacking in the food intake; however, all cereals contain phytate and fiber which binds zinc, forming an unabsorbable complex. The zinc contained in animal protein is readily available. Hence, zinc present in vegetarian diets has less bioavailability then the zinc in non-vegetarian diets. In contrast to earlier reports, folate supplements do not interfere with the utilization or intestinal absorption of zinc.[103,104,107] Food sources of zinc are meat, liver, eggs, and seafoods, especially oysters.[1] Milk, cheese, and some grain products can be a significant source of zinc.[1]

Dietary intake data indicate that a substantial number of the U.S. population consume considerably less than the Recommended Daily Allowance for zinc. Reports indicate that women consume up to 39% less zinc than the recommended zinc allowance of 15 mg per day.[16,42] Children consumed only 77% of their recommended zinc intake. This would suggest that the potential for a zinc deficiency may exist in some U.S. populations. Zinc deficiency has been described in infants and children, particularly during treatment of malnutrition.[33,34,57,82,110]

Elderly subjects have been reported to have a high incidence of a mild zinc deficiency.[85,96,111,137,139] Plasma zinc concentrations fall somewhat in the elderly.[85] Impaired cellular immune function was found in mildly zinc-deficient elderly and in patients with sickle cell anemia.[96]

Zinc Nutritional Assessment

General

Evaluation of zinc status has been handicapped by the lack of sensitive and specific methods to assess zinc nutrition.[75,117,121] Despite the participation of zinc in many metabolic functions, specific and sensitive methods to assess zinc nutritional status are not available.[52,75,121] However, the measurement of zinc concentrations in serum or plasma have been commonly used to evaluate zinc status, recognizing the values may be influenced by infection, stress, pregnancy, exercise, aging, meal eating and other physiological factors.[17,76,77,79,88,119,121,147,149] Laboratories often consider plasma zinc concentrations greater than 10.8 µmol/L (0.75 µg/ml) as an acceptable level.

Sample Collection for Zinc Analyses

Numerous factors are known to affect serum or plasma zinc concentrations.[16,17,35,75,76,147] For example, trace element free blood collecting tubes are required to minimize zinc contamination. Without their use, plasma zinc concentrations may be artifactily elevated by 20 to 25%. Heparin, but not EDTA, may be used as an anticoagulant. Similarly, falsely high zinc concentrations will occur when whole blood samples are held at room temperature for more than one hour before separating plasma or serum from the erythrocytes.[17,75] Blood samples should be processed immediately or refrigerated until separation.[17,75] Fasting plasma or serum samples should be obtained as food intake may increase zinc levels.[75,77] Hemolysis must be avoided as the concentration of zinc in erythrocytes is about ten-fold higher than that of plasma or serum.[122]

Plasma and serum zinc concentrations are highly correlated with plasma and serum albumin concentrations (Table 102). Over 80% of the zinc present in plasma is bound to albumin. Consequently, in hypoalbuminemia, plasma zinc concentrations may be low in the absence of dietary deficiency of zinc.[41] Plasma zinc levels may be influenced also by infection, stress, age, use of oral contraceptive agents, and pregnancy.[16,41,147] Patients with Down syndrome often have low serum levels of zinc.[43] Even the time of day when the blood samples were obtained can influence the level of zinc present in the plasma.[16,42] Numerous other factors may affect the zinc concentration in various tissues and urine.[19,134]

TABLE 102
Quick Reference Guide For Interpretation
of Plasma Zinc Concentrations

	µg/mL	µmol/L
Undesirable	<0.75	<11.5
Low/Borderline	0.75–0.85	11.5–13.0
Acceptable/Desirable	0.85–1.25	13.0–19.0
Elevated	>1.50	>23.0

Atomic Absorption Spectrometry

Atomic absorption spectrometry is the procedure commonly used to measure zinc concentrations in biological specimens.[146] Before the development of atomic absorption spectrometry, zinc was commonly measured by methods based on the dithizone colormetric procedure.[145] The atomic absorption spectrometry procedure is simple, sensitive, fast and accurate.[52,122-124] Certified zinc controls are available (e.g., Bio-Rad, Anaheim, CA 92806; National Institutes of Science and Technology, Gaithersburg, MA, 20889). In 1985, Smith et al.[124] provided an extensive listing from the literature of normal serum and plasma zinc concentrations. Earlier values have been summarized by Halsted et al.,[34] Johnson and Sauberlich,[19] Versieck and Cornelis,[134] and Jacob.[52] Since 1968, all of the analyses were performed by atomic absorption spectrometry. In general, mean plasma and serum zinc concentration range from 12.5 to 19.0 µmol/L (0.82 to 1.24 µg/mL). These authors have provided a careful evaluation of procedures for sample collecting, sample handling, sample preparation, analytical methodologies for measurement of zinc in plasma.[124] Plasma zinc concentrations below 10.7 µmol/L (70 µg/dL) have been considered to be at risk for zinc deficiency.[16,42,105,125] Procedures for analyzing zinc levels in neutrophils, lymphocytes, plasma, and erythrocytes have also been described in detail by Prasad[125] and others.[121,126,148]

Angiotensin-Converting Enzyme and Zinc Status

Angiotensin-converting enzyme (ACE) is a zinc metalloenzyme which converts angiotensin I to angiotensin II. Zinc deficient rats and humans were reported to have lowered serum activities of serum angiotensin-converting enzyme.[90,91,97] The activity in serum could be restored by the *in vitro* addition of zinc. Subsequently plasma angiotensin-converting enzyme activity and its *in vitro* zinc stimulation of the enzyme were investigated as a method to assess zinc nutrition in the human.[92,93] However, the procedure proved to be too insensitive to serve as an indicator of zinc status in the human.[93]

Plasma Alkaline Phosphatase and Plasma 5-Nucleotidase

The activity of the zinc-dependent plasma enzyme 5'-nucleotidase appears responsive to acute changes in zinc intake.[111,150,151] Thus, the activity of the enzyme fell promptly within 15 days in adults receiving a moderately low zinc diet (3.97 mg/d).[111] Normal values were restored within 6 days of zinc repletion. The measurement warrants further study as a possible functional test for zinc deficiency, such as in diabetics.[150,151] It must be recognized that certain conditions, such as liver disease, may give rise to elevated 5'-nucleotidase activities.

Plasma alkaline phosphatase (actually a group of enzymes) (E.C.3.1.3.1), also zinc dependent, did not respond to changes in zinc intake.[111] Other reports have also indicated that plasma alkaline phosphatase activity measurements lacked sensitivity and specficity.[113] Both plasma alkaline phosphatase activity and plasma 5'-nucleotidase activity can be readily measured spectrophotometrically with the use of commercial assay kits (e.g., Sigma Chemicals, St. Louis, MO). The measurement of alkaline phosphatase activity in neutrophils has been used for the diagnosis of zinc deficiency.[30,65] Lymphocyte 5'-nucleotidase activities also fall in the human with a mild zinc deficiency.[112] However, the isolation of the lymphocytes and the conduct of the assay can be tedious.

Thymulin

Thymulin is a thymus-specific hormone found in serum that requires the presence of zinc for its biological activity.[27,28] Mild zinc deficiency results in a decrease in serum thymulin activity. The decrease in activity may be reversed by the *in vitro* addition of zinc.[27] The assay of serum thymulin activity, with and without the *in vitro* addition of zinc, holds promise as a sensitive functional procedure for evaluating even a mild zinc deficiency.[24]

Zinc Assessment and Blood Components

Leucocytes and Zinc Levels

To obtain information on the body zinc status, blood leucocyte zinc concentrations have been measured.[70,71,121] Because of methodological problems, the measurement has received only limited use; however, with the current availability of rapid and simplified techniques to isolate leucocytes, this zinc assessment procedure should see increased use. Leucocyte zinc concentrations appear to be more sensitive than serum zinc concentrations in reflecting zinc status.[113]

Lymphocytes Zinc Levels

The results obtained in a controlled human zinc deficiency study indicated that zinc concentrations in lymphocytes, granulocytes, and platelets may provide a sensitive criterion for diagnosing a mild deficiency of zinc.[25,122] These peripheral blood cells have a high turnover rate and consequently appear to be more sensitive to a zinc deficit. The zinc content of these cells may be measured by flameless atomic absorption spectrometry.[26]

Erythrocyte Measurements

Because of the long half-life of erythrocytes, erythrocyte zinc concentrations do not represent acute or recent changes in zinc intakes. Consequently, erythrocyte zinc concentrations cannot be considered a reliable indicator of acute zinc deficiencies but may be useful as an indicator of a chronic zinc deficiency.[73]

    Erythrocyte metallothionein measurements have also been investigated as to usefulness in the evaluation of zinc status. The sensitivity of the procedure is uncertain, but reports indicate that it may reflect long-term or severe zinc depletion.[111,113-115]

    Erythrocyte carbonic anhydrase activity also lacks sensitivity as only a modest reduction in activity occurs with a severe zinc deficiency.

Zinc Clearance Tests

Body zinc clearance tests have been applied to children for the detection of marginal zinc deficiency.[89] Zinc clearance from the serum was followed over a period of two hours following an injection of zinc sulfate. Although the procedure may have merit, only 11 Japanese boys were studied. The investigators concluded "that body zinc kinetics studies will reveal some cases of marginal zinc deficiency."[89]

    Occasionally zinc loading tests have been used to evaluate zinc status.[48,118,129] However, the procedure is time-consuming, lacks sensitivity, and requires several timed blood collections. The procedure appears unreliable as an index of zinc status.[129]

Hair Zinc Concentration

Hair zinc analyses have been used as a measure of zinc status.[34,52,127,128] The results have been difficult to interpret and in general considered unreliable.[52,66,117,129] Severe zinc deficiency may result in normal zinc concentrations probably due to severely diminished growth of hair during deficiency.[50] Standards for evaluating hair zinc levels have not been established. Hair zinc levels below 100 μg/g of hair have been considered indicative of inadequate zinc nutrition.[40] Other reports suggest that a zinc level of less than 70 μg/g is a marker of zinc deficiency.[54]

Urine Zinc Levels

Low intakes of zinc result in reduced zinc urinary excretion.[72,73,130,141] Excretions of less than 3 μmol/d (<200 μg/d) of zinc have been considered low.[72,73] However, the measurement of urinary zinc excretions has received little use in the assessment of zinc status. A 24-hr urinary excretion of zinc has not been considered a reliable indicator of zinc status.

Zinc Status and the Second National Health and Nutrition Examination Survey

During the Second National Health and Nutrition Examination Survey, 1976–1980 (NHANES-II),[16,42,148] serum zinc values were obtained on 14,770 U.S. persons 3 to 74 years old. Zinc was measured by flame atomic absorption spectroscopy.

Serum zinc values were influenced by sample collection conditions. Serum zinc values collected on persons in the morning after an overnight fast were significantly higher than those obtained in the afternoon or from non-fasting subjects. Serum zinc values for males were relatively low during childhood, increased during adolescence and peaked in early childhood.[16,42] Older adults and elderly had lower serum zinc values. Pregnant women had lower serum zinc values than did non-pregnant women. Women who used oral contraceptive agents had lower serum zinc values than nonuser women.[16,19,42] In the Second National Health and Nutrition Examination Survey, a serum zinc level of 70 μg/dL or lower was considered low.[16,42] The survey observed that low serum zinc values occurred in less than 2% of the U.S. males and in less than 3% in the U.S. women. However, it was concluded that serum zinc values were not definitive for the assessment of zinc nutritional status.[16,42] Mean serum zinc concentrations for oral contraceptive users was 81.5 μg/dL; for nonusers, 84.9 μg/dL; and for males (20 to 44 years), 93.0 μg/dL.[16,42]

Pregnancy and Zinc Status

The observation that low serum zinc concentrations during pregnancy correlated with increased risks to the infant, maternal morbidity, abnormal deliveries, and infant cogenital malformations, stimulated interest in means of providing adequate zinc nutrition and in the assessment of zinc status.[62,64,65,75,80]

During pregnancy, plasma and serum zinc concentrations fall from the tenth week of gestation and onwards.[61,63-65,68,74,86,87,134] During late pregnancy serum zinc levels of 50 to 60 μg/dL are observed.[53,54,66,67,75] Serum zinc concentrations equal to or below 53.2 μg/dL were considered to indicate a low zinc status.[67] Zinc levels of <10 μmol/L (0.65 μg/ml) have also been considered low.[58] The gradual decline in serum zinc levels during pregnancy has been considered physiological for the normal women. However, only part of the decline can be related to an increase in blood volume and a decline in serum albumin level during pregnancy.[61,75]

With this regard, the concentrations of zinc in leucocytes were observed to be lower in mothers who had a small gestational age babies compared with mothers who produced normal babies.[62] Adequate zinc nutrition has been shown to lower the incidence of complication of pregnancy as in the prevention of premature births particularly in pregnant adolescents.[55,56,58,59,63,75,79] Zinc supplements in women with relatively low plasma zinc concentrations in early pregnancy was associated with greater infant head circumferences and birth weight.[79] Low maternal plasma and leucocyte zinc concentrations have been considered predictors of pregnancy complications and abnormal labor.[58-60,67,75,79] Failure of infants and toddlers to thrive may be associated with a mild zinc deficiency.[57]

Erythrocyte zinc concentrations may increase in late pregnancy. Approximately 80% of the zinc in erythrocytes is bound to carbonic anhydrase. An increased synthesis of this enzyme may account for the higher erythrocyte zinc concentrations observed.[68,69]

Toxicity

Zinc toxicity, although rare, may occur.[8] Zinc toxicity has been reported in patients receiving prolonged oral zinc therapy or total parenteral nutrition. The use of prolonged zinc supplements of more than 30 mg per day should be considered only with medical supervision. Excess zinc intake may block copper absorption and lead to a copper deficiency state.[14] Excess intakes of zinc are reflected in elevated levels of zinc in the plasma or red blood cells and in lowered laboratory indices of copper status.[2] Pharmacological amounts of zinc are used in the treatment of patients with Wilson's disease.[4-7] Wilson's disease was effectively treated with a regimen of 25 mg 3 times daily of elemental zinc.[9] Although normal zinc status is important for normal immune function, excessive intakes of zinc have been reported to impair certain immune responses in adult men.[10,13]

Other reports regarding potential toxic effects of excess intake of zinc have been recently summarized.[15] Zinc intakes of 30 mg per day were considered to be safe with no known adverse effects.[12] However, an intake of 60 mg per day of zinc produced a decrease in erythrocyte Cu/Zn superoxide dismutase activity,[11] indicating an adverse effect on copper status.

Summary

Plasma or serum zinc concentrations are easily measured in the laboratory by atomic absorption spectrometry. Low plasma zinc concentrations are usually caused by a dietary zinc deficiency. Leucocyte zinc analyses and lymphocyte 5'-nucleotidase activities may be more sensitive and specific indicators of zinc status than plasma zinc values, but the current procedures are more tedious to perform. With careful interpretation, plasma zinc concentrations remain the best way to evaluate zinc status in the human. Plasma or serum zinc concentrations 10.7 μmol/L (0.70 μg/mL) are considered low. Plasma zinc concentrations from 10.7 μmol/L to 13.0 μmol/L (0.70 to 0.85 μg/mL) have been considered to indicate a marginal zinc status (Tables 101 and 102).

References

1. Pennington, J. A. T. and Schoen, S. A., Contributions of food groups to estimated intakes of nutritional elements: results from the FDA total diet studies, 1982–1991, *Int. J. Vit. Nutr. Res.*, 66, 342, 1996.
2. Sandstead, H. H., Requirements and toxicity of essential trace elements, *Am. J. Clin. Nutr.*, 61, 621S, 1995.
3. Prasad, A., Brewer, G., Schoomaker, E., and Rabbani, P., Hyporupremia induced by zinc therapy in adults, *JAMA*, 240, 2166, 1978.
4. Hoogenroad, T. and Van den Hammer, C., 3 years of continuous oral zinc therapy in 4 patients with Wilson's disease, *Acta Neurol. Scand.*, 67, 356, 1983.
5. Brewer, G., Hill, G., Prasad, A., Cossack, Z., and Rabbani, P., Oral zinc therapy for Wilson's disease, *Annu. Int. Med.*, 99, 314, 1983.

6. Brewer, G., Hill, G., Nostrani, T., Sams, J., Wells, J., and Prasad, A., Treatment of Wilson's disease with zinc. III. Prevention of reaccumulation of hepatic copper, *J. Lab. Clin. Med.*, 109, 526, 1987.

7. Brewer, G. and Yusbasiyan, G., Wilson's disease, *Medicine*, 71, 139, 1992.

8. Calesnick, B. and Dinan, A. M., Zinc deficiency and zinc toxicity, AFP: Clinical *Pharmacology*, 37, 267, 1988.

9. Brewer, G. J., Yuzbasiyan-Gurkan, V., Johnson, V., Dick, R. D., and Wang, Y., Treatment of Wilson's disease with zinc XII: dose regimen requirements, *Am. J. Med. Sci.*, 305, 199, 1993.

10. Chandra, R. K., Excessive intake of zinc impairs immune responses, *J. Am. Med. Assoc.*, 252, 1443, 1984.

11. Yadrick, M. K., Kenney, M. A., and Winterfeldt, E. A., Iron, copper, and zinc status: response to supplementation with zinc or zinc and iron in adult females, *Am. J. Clin. Nutr.*, 49, 145, 1989.

12. Cantilli, R., Abernathy, C. O., and Donohue, J. M., Derivation of the reference dose for zinc, in *Risk Assessment of Essential Elements*, Mertz, W., Abernathy, C. O., and Olin, S. S., Ed., ILSI Press, Washington D.C., 1994, 113.

13. Greger, J. L., Zinc: overview from deficiency to toxicity, in *Risk Assessment of Essential Elements*, Mertz, W., Abernathy, C. O., and Olin, S. S., Ed., ILSI Press, Washington D.C., 1994, 91.

14. Fischer, P. W. F., Giroux, A., and L'Abbe, A. R., Effect of zinc supplementation on copper status in adult man, *Am. J. Clin. Nutr.*, 40, 743, 1984.

15. Hathcock, J. N., *Vitamin and Mineral Safety*, Council for Responsible Nutrition, Washington D.C., 1997.

16. Pilch, S. M. and Senti, F. R., Assessment of the zinc nutritional status of the U.S. population based on data collected in the Second National Health and Nutrition Examination Survey, 1976–1980, Federation of American Societies for Experimental Biology, Bethesda, MD, 1984.

17. Tamura, T., Johnston, K. E., Freeberg, L. E., Perkins, L. L., and Golderberg, R. L., Refrigeration of blood samples prior to separation is essential for the accurate determination of plasma or serum zinc concentrations, *Biol. Trace Element Res.*, 41, 165, 1994.

18. Solomons, N. W., On the assessment of zinc and copper nutrition in man, *Am. J. Clin. Nutr.*, 32, 856, 1979.

19. Johnson, H. L. and Sauberlich, H. E., Trace element analysis in biological samples, in *Clinical, Biochemical, and Nutritional Aspects of Trace Elements*, Prasad, A. S., Ed., Alan R. Liss, Inc., New York, 1982, 405.

20. Todd, W. R., Elvehijem, C. A., and Hart, E. B., Zinc nutrition of the rat, *Am. J. Physiol.*, 107, 146, 1934.

21. Tucker, H. E. and Salmon, W. D., Parakeratosis or zinc deficiency disease in pigs, *Proc. Soc. Exp. Biol. Med.*, 88, 613, 1955.

22. Prasad, A. S., Schalert, A. R., Miale, A. Jr., Farid, Z., and Sandstead, H. H., Zinc and iron deficiencies in male subjects with dwarfism and hypogonadism but without ancylostomiasis and schistomiasis or severe anemia, *Am. J. Clin. Nutr.*, 12, 437, 1963.

23. Prasad, A. S., Metabolism of zinc and its deficiency in human subjects, in Zinc Metabolism, Prasad, A. S., Ed., Charles W. Thomas, Springfield, IL, 1966, 250.

24. Prasad, A. S., Discovery of human zinc deficiency and studies in an experimental human model, *Am. J. Clin. Nutr.*, 53, 403, 1991.

25. Prasad, A. S., Rabbani, P., Abbasi, A., Bowersox, F., and Fox, M. R. S., Experimental zinc deficiency in humans, *Annu. Int. Med.*, 89, 483, 1978.

26. Wang, H., Prasad, A. S., and DuMouchelle, E., Zinc in platelets, lymphocytes, and granulocytes by flameless atomic absorption spectrophotometry, *J. Micronutrient Anal.*, 5, 181, 1989.

27. Prasad, A. S., Meftah, S., Abdallah, J., Kaplan, J., Brewer, G. J., Bach, J. F., and Dardenne, M., Serum thymulin in human zinc deficiency, *J. Clin. Invest.*, 82, 1202, 1988.

28. Dardenne, M., Pleau, J. M., Nabarra, B., Lefrancier, P., Derrun, M., Choay, J., and Bach, J. F., Contribution of zinc and other metals to the biological activity of the serum thymic factor, *Proc. Natl. Acad. Sci. U.S.A.*, 79, 5370, 1982.

29. Prasad, A. S., Clinical, biochemical and nutritional spectrum of zinc deficiency in human subjects: an update, *Nutr. Rev.*, 41, 197, 1983.

30. Prasad, A. S., Abbasi, A. A., Rabbani, P., and DuMouchelle, E., Effect of zinc supplementation on serum testosterone level in adult male sickle cell anemia subjects, *Am. J. Hematol.*, 10, 119, 1981.
31. Walravens, P. A. and Hambidge, K. M., Nutritional zinc deficiency in infants and children, in *Zinc Metabolism: Current Aspects in Health and Disease*, Brewer, G. J., and Prasad, A. S., Eds., Alan R. Liss, New York, 1977, 61.
32. Hambidge, K. M., Walravens, P. A., Brown, R. M., Webster, J., White, S., Anthony, M., and Roth, M. L., Zinc nutrition of preschool children in the Denver Head Start Program, *Am. J. Clin. Nutr.*, 29, 734, 1976.
33. Walravens, P. A., Krebs, N. F., and Hambidge, K. M., Linear growth of low income preschool children receiving a zinc supplement, *Am. J. Clin. Nutr.*, 38, 195, 1983.
34. Halsted, J. A., Smith, J. C. Jr., and Irwin, M. I., A compectus of research on zinc requirements of man, *J. Nutr.*, 104, 345, 1974.
35. Solomons, N. W., Recent progress in zinc nutrition research, *Nutrition Update*, 1, 123, 1983.
36. Chester, J. K., Trace element-gene interactions, *Nutr. Rev.*, 50, 217, 1992.
37. Hambidge, K. M., Casey, C. E., and Krebs, N. F., Zinc, in *Trace Elements in Human and Animal Nutrition*, 5th Edition, Vol. 2, Mertz, W., Ed., Academic Press, Orlando, 1986, 1.
38. Chesters, J. K., Biochemistry of zinc in cell division and tissue growth, in Zinc in Human Biology, Mills, C. F., Ed., ILSI, London, 1989, 109.
39. Prasad, A. S., Nutritional zinc today, *Nutrition Today*, March/April, 4, 1981.
40. King, J. C. and Keen, C. L., Zinc, in *Modern Nutrition in Health and Disease*, Shils, M. E., Olson, J. A. and Shike, M., Eds., Lea & Febiger, Philadelphia, 1994, 214.
41. Myrvik, Q. N., Immunology and nutrition, in *Modern Nutrition in Health and Disease*, Shils, M. E., Olson, J. A., and Shike, M., Eds., Lea & Febiger, Phildelphia, 1994, 623.
42. Pilch, S. M. and Senti, F. R., Analysis of zinc data from the Second National Health and Nutrition Examination Survey (NHANES-II), *J. Nutr.*, 115, 1393, 1985.
43. Bjorksten, B., Back, O., Gustavson, K. H., Hallmans, G., Hagglof, B., and Tarnvik, A., Zinc and immune function in Down's Syndrome, *Acta Paediatr. Scand.*, 69, 183, 1980.
44. Vallee, B. L. and Galdes, A., The metallobiochemistry of zinc enzymes, *Adv. Enzymol.*, 56, 282, 1984.
45. Wu, F. Y.-H. and Wu, C.-W., Zinc in DNA replication and transcription, *Annu. Rev. Nutr.*, 7, 251, 1987.
46. Golub, M. S., Keen, C. L., Gershwin, M. E., and Hendrickx, A. G., Developmental zinc deficiency and behavior, *J. Nutr.*, 125, 2263S, 1995.
47. Walravens, P. A., Zinc nutrition in infants and children, in *Clinical, Biochemical, and Nutritional Aspects of Trace Elements*, Prasad, A. S., Ed., Alan R. Liss, Inc., New York, 1982, 129.
48. Solomons, N. W., Jacobs, R. A., Pineda, O., and Viteri, F., Studies on the bioavailability of zinc in man II, Absorption of zinc from organic and inorganic sources, *J. Lab. Clin. Med.*, 94, 335, 1979.
49. Smith, J. C. Jr., Interrelationship of zinc and vitamin A metabolism in animal and human nutrition: a review, in *Clinical, Biochemical, and Nutritional Aspects of Trace Elements*, Prasad, A. S., Ed., Alan R. Liss, Inc., New York, 1982, 239.
50. Prasad, A. S., Nutritional metabolic role of zinc, *Fed. Proc.*, 26, 172, 1967.
51. Prasad, A. S., Zinc deficiency syndrome in man: A historical review, *Intr. Rev. Neurobiology*, (Supplement 1), Academic Press, New York, 1972, 1.
52. Jacob, R. A., Zinc and copper, *Clinics in Laboratory Medicine*, Vol. 1, W. B. Saunders, Philadelphia, 1981, 743.
53. Hambidge, K. M. and Droegemueller, W., Changes in plasma and hair concentrations of zinc, copper, chromium, and manganese during pregnancy, *Obstet. Gynecol.*, 44, 666, 1974.
54. Hambidge, K. M. and Mauer, A. M., Trace elements, in *Laboratory Indices of Nutritional Status in Pregnancy*, Food and Nutrition Board, National Academy of Sciences, Washington D.C., 1978, 157.
55. Cherry, F. F., Sandstead, H. H., Rajas, P., Johnson, L. K., Batson, H. K., and Wang, X. B., Adolescent pregnancy associations among body weight, zinc nutriture, and pregnancy outcome, *Am. J. Clin. Nutr.*, 50, 945, 1989.

56. Neggers, V. H., Cutter, G. R., Acton, R. T., Alvarez, J. O., Bonner, J. L., Golderberg, R. J., Go, R. C., and Roseman, J. M., A positive association between maternal serum zinc concentrations and birth weight, *Am. J. Clin. Nutr.*, 51, 678, 1990.

57. Walravens, P. A., Hambidge, K. M., and Koepfer, D. M., Zinc supplementation in infants with a nutritional pattern of failure to thrive: a double-bind, controlled study, *Pediatrics*, 83, 532, 1989.

58. Jameson, S., Zinc status in pregnancy: the effect of zinc therapy on perinatal mortality, prematurity, and placental ablation, *Ann. NY Acad. Sci.*, 678, 178, 1993.

59. Lazebnik, N., Kuhnert, B. R., Kuhnert, P. M., and Thompson, K. L., Zinc status, pregnancy complications, and labor abnormalities, *Am. J. Obstet. Gynecol.*, 158, 161, 1988.

60. Wells, J. L., James, D. K., Luxton, R., and Pennock, C. A., Maternal leucyte zinc deficiency at start of third trimester as a predictor of fetal growth retardation, *Br. Med. J.*, 294, 1054, 1987.

61. Breskin, M. W., Worthington-Roberts, B. S., Knopp, R. H., Brown, Z., Plovie, B., Mottet, N. K., and Mills, J. L., First trimester serum zinc concentrations in human pregnancy, *Am. J. Clin. Nutr.*, 38, 943, 1983.

62. Meadows, N. J., Smith, M. F., Keeling, P. W. N., Ruse, W., Day, J., Scopes, J. W., and Thompson, R. P. H., Zinc and small babies, *Lancet*, 11, 1135, 1981.

63. Kynast, G. and Saling, E., The relevance of zinc in pregnancy, *J. Perinat. Med.*, 8, 171, 1980.

64. Metcoff, J., Costiloe, J. P., Crosby, W., Bentle, L., Seshachalam, D., Sandstead, H. H., Bodwell, C. E., Weaver, F., and McClaim, P., Maternal nutrition and fetal outcome, *Am. J. Clin. Nutr.*, 34, 708, 1981.

65. Hambidge, K. M., Krebs, N. F., Jacobs, M. A., Favier, A., Guyette, L., and Inkle, D. M., Zinc nutritional status during pregnancy: a longitudinal study, *Am. J. Clin. Nutr.*, 37, 429, 1983.

66. Vir, S. C., Love, A. H. G., and Thompson, W., Zinc concentration in hair and serum of pregnant women in Belfast, *Am. J. Clin. Nutr.*, 34, 2800, 1981.

67. Hunt, I. F., Murphy, N. J., Cleaver, A. E., Faraji, B., Swendseid, M. E., Coulson, A. H., Clark, V. A., Laine, N., Davis, C. A., and Smith, J. C. Jr., Zinc supplementation during pregnancy: zinc concentration of serum and hair from low-income women of Mexican descent, *Am. J. Clin. Nutr.*, 37, 572, 1983.

68. Swanson, C. A. and King, J. C., Zinc and pregnancy outcome, *Am. J. Clin. Nutr.*, 46, 763, 1987.

69. Qvist, I., Abdulla, M., Jagirstad, M., and Svensson, S., Iron, zinc, and folate status during pregnancy and two months after delivery, *Acta Obstet. Gynecol. Scand.*, 65, 15, 1986.

70. Jones, R. B., Keeling, P. W. N., Hilton, P. J., and Thompson, R. P., The relationship between leucocyte and muscle zinc in health and disease, *Clin. Sci.*, 60, 237, 1981.

71. Patrick, J. and Dervich, C., Leukocyte zinc in the assessment of zinc status, *CRC Crit. Rev. Clin. Lab. Sci.*, 20, 95, 1984.

72. Hess, F. M., King, J. C., and Margen, S., Zinc excretion in young women on low zinc intake and oral contraceptive agents, *J. Nutr.*, 107, 1610, 1977.

73. Baer, M. T. and King, J. C., Tissue levels and zinc excretion during experimental zinc depletion in young men, *Am. J. Clin. Nutr.*, 39, 556, 1984.

74. Argemi, J., Serrano, J., Gutievez, M. C., Ruiz, M. S., and Gil, A., Serum zinc binding capacity in pregnant women, *Annu. Nutr. Metab.*, 32, 121, 1988.

75. Tamura, T. and Goldenberg, R. L., Zinc nutriture and pregnancy, *Nutr. Res.*, 16, 139, 1995.

76. English, J. L. and Hambidge, K. M., Plasma and serum zinc concentrations: Effects of time between collection and separation, *Clin. Chim. Acta*, 175, 211, 1988.

77. King, J. C., Hambidge, K. M., Wescott, J. L., Kern, D. L., and Marshall, G., Daily variation in plasma zinc concentrations in women fed meals at six-hour intervals, *J. Nutr.*, 124, 508, 1994.

78. Vallee, B. L. and Falchuk, K. H., The biochemical basis of zinc physiology, *Physiol. Rev.*, 73, 79, 1993.

79. Goldenberg, R. L., Tamura, T., Neggers, Y., Copper, R. L., Johnston, K. E., DuBard, M. B., and Hauth, J. C., The effect of zinc supplementation on pregnancy outcome, *JAMA*, 274, 463, 1995.

80. McMichael, A. J., Dreosti, I. E., and Gibson, G. T., Maternal zinc status and pregnancy outcome: A prospective study, in *Clinical Applications of Recent Advances in Zinc Metabolism*, Prasad, A. S., Dreosti, I. E., and Hetzel, B. S., Eds., Alan R. Liss, New York, 1982, 53.

81. Penland, J. G., Sandstead, H. H., Alcock, N. W., Xue-Cun, C., Jue-Sheng, L., Jia-Jiu, Y., and Faji, Z., Cognitive and psychomotor effects of zinc supplementation of urban Chinese children, *FASEB J.*, 10, A290, 1996.

82. Prasad, A. S., Clinical manifestations of zinc deficiency, *Annu. Rev. Nutr.*, 5, 341, 1985.

83. Sandstead, H. H., Prasad, A. S., Schulert, A. R., Farid, Z., Miale, A. Jr., Bassilly, S., and Darby, W. J., Human zinc deficiency, endocrine manifestations and response to treatment, *Am. J. Clin. Nutr.*, 20, 422, 1967.

84. Xue-Cun, C., Tai-An, Y., Jin-Sheng, H., Qiu-Yan, M., Zhi-Min, H., and Li-Xiang, L., Low levels of zinc in hair and blood, pica, anorexia, and poor growth in Chinese preschool children, *Am. J. Clin. Nutr.*, 42, 694, 1985.

85. Sandstead, H. H., Henriksen, L. K., Greger, J. L., Prasad, A. S., and Good, R. A., Zinc nutriture in the elderly in relation to taste acuity, immune response, and wound healing, *Am. J. Clin. Nutr.*, 36, 1046, 1982.

86. Apgar, J., Zinc and reproduction, *Annu. Rev. Nutr.*, 5, 43, 1985.

87. Apgar, J., Zinc and reproduction, An update, *J. Nutr. Biochem.*, 3, 266, 1992.

88. King, J. C., Assessment of zinc status, *J. Nutr.*, 120, 1474, 1990.

89. Nakamura, T., Nishiyama, S., Futagoishi-Suginokara, Y., Matsuda, I., and Higashi, A., Mild to moderate zinc deficiency in short children: Effect of zinc supplementation on linear growth velocity, *J. Pediatr.*, 123, 65, 1993.

90. Reeves, P. G. and O'Dell, B. L., An experimental study of the effect of zinc on the activity of angiotension converting enzyme in serum, *Clin. Chem.*, 31, 581, 1985.

91. Tamura, T., Freeberg, L. E., Johnston, K. E., and Keen, C. L., *In vitro* zinc stimulation of angiotensin-converting enzyme activities in various tissues of zinc-deficient rats, *Nutr. Res.*, 14, 919, 1994.

92. Tamura, T., Johanning, G. L., Goldenberg, R. L., Johnston, K. E., and DuBard, M. B., Effect of angiotensin-converting enzyme gene polymophism on pregnancy outcome, enzyme activity, and zinc concentration, *Obstet. Gynecol.*, 88, 497, 1996.

93. Tamura, T., Goldenberg, R. L., Johnston, K. E., Freeberg, L. E., DuBard, M. B., and Thomas, E. A., *In vitro* zinc stimulation of angiotensin-converting enzyme activities in human plasma, *J. Nutr. Biochem.*, 7, 55, 1996.

94. Phebus, C. K., Maciak, B. J., Gloninger, M. F., and Paul, H. S., Zinc status of children with sickle cell disease: relationship to poor growth, *Am. J. Hematol.*, 29, 67, 1988.

95. Prasad, A. S., Ortega, J., Brewer, G. H., Oberleas, D., and Schoomaker, E. B., Trace elements in sickle cell disease, *JAMA*, 235, 2396, 1976.

96. Kaplan, J., Hess, J. W., and Prasad, A. S., Impaired interleukin-2 production in the elderly: association with mild zinc deficiency, *J. Trace Elements in Experimental Med.*, 1, 3, 1988.

97. Bakan, N., Bakan, E., Suerdem, M., and Yigitoglu, M. R., Serum zinc and angiotensin-converting enzyme levels in patients with lung cancer, *Bio Factors*, 1, 177, 1988.

98. Walravens, P. A. and Hambidge, K. M., Growth of infants fed a zinc supplemented formula, *Am. J. Clin. Nutr.*, 29, 1114, 1976.

99. Hambidge, K. M., Walravens, P. A., Casey, C. E., Brown, R. M., and Bender, C., Plasma zinc concentrations of breast-fed infants, *J. Pediatr.*, 94, 607, 1979.

100. Golden, B. E. and Golden, M. H. N., Plasma zinc, rate of weight gain, and the energy cost of tissue deposition in children recovering from severe malnutrition on cow's mild or soya protein based formula, *Am. J. Clin. Nutr.*, 34, 892, 1981.

101. Okade, A., Zinc in clinical surgery - a research review, *Japanese J. Surg.*, 20, 635, 1990.

102. Morrison, S. A., Russell, R. M., Carney, E. A., and Oakes, E. V., Zinc deficiency: a cause of abnormal dark adaptation in cirrhotics, *Am. J. Clin. Nutr.*, 31, 276, 1978.

103. Butterworth, C. E., Hatch, K., Cole, P., Sauberlich, H. E., Tamura, T., Cornwell, P., and Soon, S.–J., Zinc concentration in plasma and erythrocytes of subjects receiving folic acid supplementation, *Am. J. Clin. Nutr.*, 47, 484, 1988.

104. Keating, J. N., Wade, L., Stokstad, E. L. R., and King, J. C., Folic acid: effect on zinc absorption in humans and in the rat, *Am. J. Clin. Nutr.*, 46, 835, 1987.

105. Rosado, J. L., Sopez, P., Munoz, E., Martinez, H., and Allen, L. H., Zinc supplementation reduced mortality, but neither zinc nor iron supplementation affected growth or body composition of Mexican preschoolers, *Am. J. Clin. Nutr.*, 61, 13, 1997.

106. Reed, J. O., Redding-Lallinger, R., and Orringer, E. P., Nutrition and sickle cell disease, *Am. J. Hematol.*, 24, 441, 1987.

107. Kauwell, G. P. A., Bailey, L. B., Gregory, J. F. III, Bowling, D. W., and Cousins, R. J., Zinc status is not adversely affected by folic acid supplementation and zinc intake does not impair folate utilization in human subjects, *J. Nutr.*, 125, 66, 1995.

108. Sandstead, H. H., Requirement of zinc in human subjects, *J. Am. Coll. Nutr.*, 4, 73, 1985.

109. Gibson, R. S., Smit Vanderkooy, P. D., MacDonald, A. C., Goldman, A., Ryan, B. A., and Berry, M., A growth-limiting, mild zinc-deficiency syndrome in some Southern Ontario boys with low height percentiles, *Am. J. Clin. Nutr.*, 49, 1266, 1989.

110. Schlesinger, L., Arevalo, M., Arredondo, S., Diaz, M., Lonnerdal, B., and Stekal, A., Effect of a zinc-fortified formula on immunocompetence and growth of malnourished infants, *Am. J. Clin. Nutr.*, 56, 49, 1992.

111. Bales, C. W., DiSilvestro, R. A., Curie, K. L., Plaisted, C. S., Joung, H., Galanos, A. N., and Lin, P.–H., Marginal zinc deficiency in older adults: responsiveness of zinc status indicators, *J. Am. Coll. Nutr.*, 13, 455, 1994.

112. Meftah, S., Prasad, A. S., Lee, D. Y., and Brewer, G. J., Ecto 5′ nucleotidase (5′N T) as a sensitive inductor of human zinc deficiency, *J. Lab. Clin. Med.*, 118, 306, 1991.

113. Thompson, R. P., Assessment of zinc status, *Proc. Nutr. Soc.*, 50,19, 1991.

114. Grider, A., Bailey, L. B., and Cousins, R. J., Erythrocyte metallothionein as an index of zinc status in humans, *Proc. Natl. Acad. Sci.*, 87, 1259, 1990.

115. Thomas, E. A., Bailey, L. B., Kauwell, G. A., Lee, D.–Y., and Cousins, R. J., Erythrocyte metallothionein response to dietary zinc in humans, *J. Nutr.*, 122, 2408, 1992.

116. Boosalis, M. G., Evans, G. W., and McClain, C. J., Impaired handling of orally administered zinc in pancreatic insufficiency, *Am. J. Clin. Nutr.*, 37, 268, 1983.

117. Sauberlich, H. E., Methods for the assessment of nutritional status, in *Nutritional Aspects of Aging*, Volume I, Chen, L. H., Ed., CRC Press, Boca Raton, FL, 1987, 131.

118. Sullivan, J. F., Jetton, M. M., and Burch, R. E., A zinc tolerance test, *J. Lab. Clin. Med.*, 93, 485, 1979.

119. Brasad, A. S., Oberleas, D., and Halsted, J. A., Determination of zinc in biological fluids by atomic absorption spectrophotometry in normal and cirrhotic subjects, *J. Lab. Clin. Med.*, 66, 508, 1965.

120. Markowitz, M. E., Rosen, J. F., and Mizruchi, M., Circadian variations in serum zinc (Zn) concentrations: correlation with blood ionized calcium, serum total calcium and phosphate in humans, *Am. J. Clin. Nutr.*, 41, 689, 1985.

121. Aggett, P. J. and Favier, A., Zinc, *Int. J. Vit. Nutr. Res.*, 63, 301, 1993.

122. Whitehouse, R. C., Prasad, A. S., Rabbani, P. I., and Cossack, Z. T., Zinc in plasma, neutrophils, lymphocytes and erythrocytes as determined by flameless atomic absorption spectrometry, *Clin. Chem.*, 28, 475, 1982.

123. Smith, J. C. Jr., Butrimovitz, G. P., and Purdy, W. C., Direct measurement of zinc in plasma by atomic absorption spectroscopy, *Clin. Chem.*, 25, 1487, 1979.

124. Smith, J. C., Holbrook, J. T., and Danford, D. E., Analysis and evaluation of zinc and copper in human plasma and serum, *J. Am. Colleg. Nutr.*, 4, 627, 1985.

125. Prasad, A. S., Laboratory diagnosis of zinc deficiency, *J. Am. Colleg. Nutr.*, 4, 591, 1985.

126. Goode, H. F., Kelleher, J., and Walker, B. E., Zinc concentrations in pure populations of peripheral blood neutrophils, lymphocytes and monocytes, *Annu. Clin. Biochem.*, 26, 89, 1989.

127. Buckley, R. A., Chem, H. C. A., and Dreosti, I. E., Radioisotopic studies concerning the efficacy of standard washing procedures for the cleansing of hair before zinc analyses, *Am. J. Clin. Nutr.*, 40, 840, 1984.

128. Friel, J. K. and Ngyuen, C. D., Dry- and wet-washing techniques compared in analyses for zinc, copper, manganese, and iron in hair, *Clin. Chem.*, 32, 739, 1986.

129. Fickel, J. F., Freeland-Graves, J. H., and Roby, M. J., Zinc tolerance tests in zinc deficient and zinc supplemented diets, *Am. J. Clin. Nutr.*, 43, 47, 1986.

130. Taylor, C. M., Bacon, J. R., Aggett, P. J., and Bremner, I., Homeostatic regulation of zinc absorption and endogenous losses of zinc-deprived men, *Am. J. Clin. Nutr.*, 53, 755, 1991.
131. Gunter, E. W., Turner, W. E., Neese, J W., and Bayse, D. D., Laboratory procedures used by the Clinical Division, Center for Disease Control for the Second Health and Nutrition Examination Survey (HANES-II) 1976-1980, Centers for Disease Control, Atlanta.
132. Hambidge, K. M., Zinc deficiency in young children, *Am. J. Clin. Nutr.*, 65, 160, 1997.
133. Gibson, R. S., Zinc nutrition in developing countries, *Nutr. Res. Rev.*, 7, 151, 1994.
134. Versieck, J. and Cornelis, R., *Trace Elements in Human Plasma or Serum*, CRC Press, Boca Raton, FL, 1989.
135. Bunker, V., Hinks, L. J., Lawson, M. S., and Clayton, B. E., Assessment of zinc and copper status of healthy elderly people using metabolic balance studies and measurement of leucocyte concentrations, *Am. J. Clin. Nutr.*, 40, 1096, 1984.
136. McKenzie, J. M., Content of zinc in serum, urine, hair, and toenails of New Zealand adults, *Am. J. Clin. Nutr.*, 32, 570, 1979.
137. Swanson, C. A., Mansourian, R., Diven, H., and Rapin, C. –H., Zinc status of healthy elderly adults: response to supplementation, *Am. J. Clin. Nutr.*, 48, 343, 1988.
138. Zimmerman, A. W., Dunham, B. S., Nochimson, D. J., Kaplan, B. M., Clive, J. M., and Kunkel, S. L., Zinc transport in pregnancy, *Am. J. Ostet. Gynecol.*, 149, 523, 1984.
139. Smith, J. C. Jr. and Hsu, J. M., Trace elements in aging research: emphasis on zinc, copper, chromium, and selenium, in *Nutritional Approaches to Aging Research*, Moment, G. B., Ed., CRC Press, Boca Raton, FL, 1982, 120.
140. Lockitch, G., Halstead, A. C., Wadsworth, L., Quigley, G., Reston, L., and Jacobson, B., Age- and sex-specific pediatric reference intervals and correlations for zinc, copper, selenium, iron, vitamins A and E, and related proteins, *Clin. Chem.*, 34, 1625, 1988.
141. Johnson, P. E., Hunt, C. D., Milne, D. B., and Mullen, L. K., Homeostatic control of zinc metabolism in men: zinc excretion and balance in men fed diets low in zinc, *Am. J. Clin. Nutr.*, 57, 557, 1993.
142. Vanderkooy, P. D. S., and Gibson, R. S., Food consumption patterns of Canadian preschool children in relation to zinc and growth status, *Am. J. Clin. Nutr.*, 45, 609, 1987.
143. Chen, M.–D., Lin, P.–Y., Lin, W.–H., and Cheng, V., Zinc in hair and serum of obese individuals in Taiwan, *Am. J. Clin. Nutr.*, 48, 1307, 1988.
144. Singh, A., Day, B. A., DeBolt, J. E., Trostmann, U. H., Bernier, L. L., and Deuster, P. A., Magnesium, zinc, and copper status of U.S. Navy SEAL trainees, *Am. J. Clin. Nutr.*, 49, 695, 1989.
145. Hoch, F. L. and Vallee, B. L., Precipitation by trichloroacetic acid as a simplification in the determination of zinc in blood and its components, *J. Biol. Chem.*, 181, 295, 1949.
146. Falchuk, K. H., Hilt, K. L., and Vallee, B. L., Determination of zinc in biological samples by atomic absorption spectrometry, *Methods Enzymol.*, 158, 422, 1988.
146a. Prasad, A. S., Malnutrition in sickle cell disease patients, *Am. J. Clin. Nutr.*, 66, 423, 1997.
147. Brown, E. H., Effect of infections on plasma zinc concentration and implications for zinc status assessment in low-income countries, *Am. J. Clin. Nutr.*, 68, 425S, 1998.
148. Gunter, E. W., Turner, W. E., Neese, J. W., and Bayse, D. D., Laboratory procedures used by the Clinical Chemistry Division, Centers for Disease Control for the Second Health and Nutrition Examination Survey (HANES-II), Atlanta, 1981.
149. Bahl, R., Bhandari, N., Hambidge, K. M., and Bhan, M. K., Plasma zinc as a predictor of diarrheal and respiratory morbidity in children in an urban slum setting, *Am. J. Clin. Nutr.*, 68, 414S, 1998.
150. Blostein-Fujii, A., DiSilvestro, R. A., Frid, D., Katz, C., and Malarkey, W., Short-term zinc supplementation in women with non-insulin-dependent diabetes mellitus: effects on plasma 5'-nuleotidase activities, insulin-like growth factor I concentrations, and lipoprotein oxidation rates *in vitro*, *Am. J. Clin. Nutr.*, 66, 639, 1997.
151. Sandstead, H. H. and Egger, N. G., Is zinc nutriture a problem in persons with diabetes mellitus, *Am. J. Clin. Nutr.*, 66, 681, 1997.

Copper

Converting metric units to International System (SI) units:

μmol/L × 0.0635 = μg/mL

μg/mL × 15.7 = μmol/L

atomic weight: 63.55

Although the nutrition essentiality of copper was established in animal studies in the 1920s and 1930s,[6] many years passed before copper was accepted as an essential nutrient for the human.[7-10,23]

The essentiality of copper was settled with the discovery in 1962 of Menkes disease, a rare genetic disease, which responds to copper therapy.[35] The features of copper deficiency are now recognized to incluce hypocupremia normocytic or megaloblastic anemia, neutropenia, and osteoporosis.[10,18,19,26,50,59,60,63] Other manifestations of a copper deficiency are depigmentation of the hair and skin, kinky hair, lethargy, neurological disturbances, and abnormalities of connective tissue with skeletal abnormalites.[60,63] Impaired cross-linking of elastin and collagen occurs which results in premature rupture of membranes leading to death.

Subsequently, copper deficiency due to an inadequate intake of copper has been reported.[9,10,30-33,42,60] This has occurred in premature infants fed for an extensive period solely a modified cow's milk formula. A copper deficiency was considered to exist in malnurished Peruvian and Chilean children.[20,21] Numerous reports exist on copper deficiency in subjects on total parenteral nutrition.[9,25-28] Hypocupremia has been observed in other diseased conditions, including kwashiorkor, tropical and nontropical sprue, and the nephrotic syndrome.[7,42,55,59,74]

Excessive intakes of zinc or iron can induce a copper deficiency.[10-13] Zinc supplements have been used to treat sickle cell anemia patients. However, excessive amounts or prolonged use of zinc may cause a copper deficiency by interfering with the intestinal absorption of copper.[29] Evidence exists of an association of copper deficiency in the human with the development of cardiovascular disease has been proposed.[1,2,43,84]

Legumes, liver, nuts, whole-grain breads and cereals, shrimp and oysters are good sources of copper with 30 to 40% of the copper in the diet absorbed.[58,59,63]

Metabolism

Copper participates in the functions of a number of enzymes. The functions of these enzymes explain many of the clinical signs associated with a copper deficiency. Some of the important copper-dependent enzymes are:[10,53,59,82]

Superoxidase dismutase (EC 1.15.1.1) (free radical detoxification)

Lysyl oxidase (EC 1.4.3.13) (cross-linking of elastin and collagen)

Ceruloplasmin (EC 1.16.3.1) (copper transport; oxidase activity)

Tyrosinase (EC 1.14.18.1) (melanin production)

Cytochrome C oxidase (EC 1.9.3.1) (electron-transport system)

Dopamine-β-hydroxylase (EC 1.14.17.1) (catecholamine formation)

S-adenosylhomocysteine hydrolase (sulfur amino acid metabolism and copper metabolism)

Assessment of Copper Nutritional Status

General

Copper deficiency is uncommon in the human and when it occurs it is usually associated with other modifying conditions. They include infection, inflammation, pregnancy, hepatitis, cirrhosis, estrogen therapy, cancer, and protein energy deficiency.[10,35] Copper nutritional status has been evaluated by plasma or serum copper levels.[10,15,22,23,40,88]

Serum or plasma copper concentrations may be measured by colorimetric methods or by atomic absorption spectroscopy, inductively coupled plasma emission spectroscopy, and other procedures.[40,41,54,57,61] Plasma copper is easily quantitated by flame atomic absorption spectroscopy.[61,65,72] For analysis, plasma or serum required only a dilution with water. Standard reference materials for copper analyses are available from the National Institute of Standards and Technology, Gaithersburg, MD. Hypocupremia has been considered to exist with serum copper concentrations of <0.75 µg/mL (11.8 µmol/L).[83]

As functional measurements, serum ceruloplasmin levels and Cu/Zn superoxide dismutase activities in erythrocytes are used. Other static measurements used to assess copper status in the human include levels of copper in whole blood, erythrocytes, leukocytes, hair, and urine.[14-17,56,57,66,88] Urinary measurements of hydroxylysine have been investigated as a functional measurement of copper status.[88]

Of the measurements available to assess copper status, plasma or serum copper and serum ceruloplasmin levels, and erythrocyte Cu/Zn superoxide dismutase levels are the easiest to perform and most widely used.[63,85,88]

Ceruloplasmin (Ferroxidase I)

Ceruloplasmin (EC 1.16.3.1) contains six atoms of copper per molecule and accounts for over 90% of the copper present in plasma. Ceruloplasmin may be measured immunologically or by its oxidase activity. Plasma ceruloplasmin may be determined by radial immunodiffusion with commercial assay kits available (Behring Diagnostics, Somerville, NJ). It can also be determined enzymatically based on the ceruloplasmin p-phyenylenediamine oxidase activity.[39] Measurement of ceruloplasmin based on its oxidase activity may be preferred over immunological methods because of its great sensitivity to a copper deficiency.

Plasma measurements of copper are essentially a measurement of ceruloplasmin. Hence, copper status may be evaluated by the measurement of either plasma copper concentrations or by the measurement of ceruloplasmin. In a controlled study, volunteer young men were fed low copper-containing diets (0.38 mg/day) for a period of 66 days.[78,87] Over this period of time, serum copper concentrations fell significantly as well as a reduction in ceruloplasmin activity and in ceruloplasmin concentrations. With severe copper deficiency, serum (plasma) levels of ceruloplasmin and of copper fall to levels that are 30% of normal levels.[33] At birth, infants have low concentrations of serum copper due to the delayed synthesis of ceruloplasmin by the body.[7] By six to eighteen months of age, serum ceruloplasmin concentrations and serum copper concentrations have reached levels equal to or above adults.[49,51,62,64]

Plasma concentrations of copper and ceruloplasmin may be altered by a number of factors that must be considered in evaluation of copper status.[54,73,74] This includes the effects of infection, estrogen, age, sex differences, and pregnancy.[10,37,55,57] Women have higher plasma copper levels and ceruloplasmin levels than men.[45-47] The use of oral contraceptive agents may increase the plasma copper concentrations above those of non-users.[34,37,47] Plasma copper levels are higher in the elderly than those of younger populations.[48,56]

Serum Concentrations of Copper in Military Personnel[34]

Sex	Number	Copper	
		µg/dL	µmol/L
Men	2033	107 ± 23	16.8 ± 3.6
Women			
All	386	129 ± 33	20.3 ± 5.2
OCA users	31	188 ± 55	29.6 ± 8.6
Non-users	355	124 ± 25	19.5 ± 3.9

Cu/Zn Superoxide Dismutase

Approximately 60% of the copper found in red blood cells is present as Cu/Zn superoxide dismutase.[10,14,62] However, superoxide dismutase is produced at the time of erythrocyte formation, and therefore has a slow turnover rate corresponding to the life of the erythrocyte. Consequently, red blood cell copper levels and red cell Cu/Zn superoxide dismutase levels or activity can serve as a measure of long-term copper nutrition. White blood cells have a shorter turnover rate and also contain superoxide dismutase. Their use could provide information on more recent copper intake and status.

Superoxide dismutase (SOD) (EC 1.15.1.1) represent a group of metalloenzymes that catalyze the dismutation of superoxide anion radicals (O_2^-) to oxygen and hydrogen peroxide. The types of superoxide dismutase that exist include:

Cu/Zn superoxide dismutase (cytoplasm)

Manganese superoxide dismutase (mitochondria)

Iron superoxide dismutase (cytosol)

Extracellular superoxide dismutase (extracellular fluids)

Commercial kits are available for the measurement of Cu/Zn superoxide dismutase in human serum, plasma, and urine. For this purpose, an enzyme-linked immunosorbent assay (ELISA) is available from ENDOGEN, Inc., Cambridge, MA. Another kit provides for a spectrophotometric assay of superoxide dismutase activity (Cabiochem-Novabiochem Corp., San Diego, CA). The assay is independent of the type of superoxide dismutase present and may be used with plasma or red blood cells. It has application in identifying patients with Downs syndrome. Serum and urine levels of Cu/Zn superoxide dismutase are elevated in these patients.[5] Normally the serum levels of Cu/Zn superoxide dismutase are very low and have not been useful for assessing copper status. Other methods have been used to measure red cell superoxide dismutase activity.[69]

Cytochrome C Oxidase (EC 1.9.3.1):

Cytochrome-C oxidase activity in platelets and mononucleated leukocytes is sensitive to copper nutrition.[38] However, the wide subject-to-subject variability encountered has made the usefulness of this index of copper status uncertain.[37-39] Red blood cell Cu/Zn superoxide dismutase and platelet cytochrome-C activity measurements and plasma immunoreactive ceruloplasmin determinations probably provide a better measure of metabolically active copper than either plasma copper concentration or plasma ceruloplasmin activity alone.[37]

An interesting study was conducted with 12 postmenopausal women fed for 105 days a diet low in copper.[68] During this period, plasma copper and plasma ceruloplasmin did not change. However, during this period, erythrocyte superoxide dismutase activity was reduced (3450 to 2600 U/g hemoglobin) as well as platelet cytochrome C oxidase activity and platelet copper concentrations.

This would indicate that measurement of erythrocyte superoxide dismutase activity and platelet cytochrome C oxidase activity would be more sensitive indicators of copper status than plasma copper concentrations or plasma ceruloplasmin concentrations. Guides for use in the interpretation of the results will require further development before general use can be expected. Other studies have also reported that erythrocyte superoxide dismutase measurements were a more sensitive indicators of copper status than were serum copper or serum ceruloplasmin concentrations.[17,36-38,40,70,71,85]

Other Measures

The copper containing enzyme, lysyloxidase, is reduced in activity with a marked deficiency of copper. Deficiency of this enzyme results in impaired collagen metabolism that is reflected in an increased urinary excretion of hydroxylysine. Quantitation of hydroxylysine may serve as a functional indicator of copper status.

Several other measures have been investigated but have not been considered useful or reliable.[86] They include copper concentrations in urine, sweat, saliva, and hair.[10,14,17,26,67] Hair has been reported to contain copper at levels of 15 to 16 µg/g[44] or higher.[66] Full-term infants had copper concentrations of 16.5 µg/g.[52]

Wilson's Disease

In Wilson's disease, a rare genetic disorder, copper accumulates excessively in the liver and tissues.[35,59] These patients usually have increased serum copper concentrations and low ceruloplasmin levels.[7,35] Chelation therapy with D-penicillamine is effective in its treatment. The effectiveness can be followed by plasma copper and ceruloplasmin measurements.

Copper Toxicity

An intake of 0.5 mg per day of copper per kilogram of body weight has been considered safe by FAO/WHO.[24,76] A dietary intake of this magnitude would be highly unlikely in the United States.[25,43] Copper intake of 10 to 15 mg can result in metallic taste, diarrhea and vomitting.[23,35] Severe copper intakes may result in intravascular hemolysis, jaundice, renal failure, vascular collapse and death. Most instances of copper toxicity have been related to environmental exposure, including accidental ingestion of copper (usually copper sulfate by children), water and foods prepared or stored in copper vessels, industrial exposures to copper, and iatrogenic causes (e.g., intrauterine contraceptive devices and hemodialysis).[35,59]

The Food and Nutrition Board of the U.S. National Research Council considers in their Recommended Dietary Allowances that a copper intake of 0.4 to 0.6 mg/d is safe for infants 0 to 0.5 y age and of 1.5 to 3.0 mg/d for adults.[75]

Summary

Erythrocyte Cu/Zn superoxide dismutase measurements can serve as an index of long-term copper status. As an alternative, assessment of copper status may be made by the determination of serum concentrations of copper or of serum ceruloplasmin, and ceruloplasmin activity. These measurements may provide information as to current or more recent copper intakes and status. Interpretation of the analytical findings requires consideration of factors that influence the conditions of the subject, including age, gender, pregnancy, and nutrition. With further study, platelet cytochrome C oxidase activity measurements may prove to be a sensitive index of copper status. Serum copper concentrations of >0.75 μg/mL (>11.8 μmol/L) are considered acceptable (Table 103).

TABLE 103
Some Literature Values for Guidance in Evaluation of Copper Status

Subject and Determination	Value	Reference
1. Infants		
Serum copper (μmol/L)		
0–5 day (*n* = 27)	1.4–7.2	64
1–5 yr (*n* = 77)	12.6–23.6	64
10–14 yr (M, *n* = 36)	12.6–19.0	64
10–14 yr (F, *n* = 23)	12.9–18.9	64
Serum copper (μmol/L)		
5 day	7.1 ± 1	62
1 month	9.9 ± 2	62
6–12 months	17.4 ± 3	62
2. Infants (Finland)		
Plasma copper (μmol/L)		
0 month (*n* = 198)	4.57 ± 0.16	41
6 months (*n* = 182)	15.28 ± 0.31	41
12 months (*n* = 190)	19.67 ± 0.31	41
Plasma cerulplasmin concentration		
(immunodiffusion) (μmol/L)		
0 month (*n* = 198)	0.90 ± 0.07	41
6 months (*n* = 192)	2.54 ± 0.07	41
12 months (*n* = 191)	3.21 ± 0.07	41
3. Adults		
Serum/plasma copper (μmol/L)		
Adolescent females		
White 14–16 yr (*n* = 30)	18.2 ± 1	73
Black 14–16 yr (*n* = 26)	19.0 ± 1	73
Women (63 ± 8.8 yr) (*n* = 12)		
Plasma copper	17.2 ± 2.2	68
Plasma ceruloplasmin		
Enzyme assay	453 ± 16 mg/L	68
Radioimmunoassy	367 ± 45 mg/L	68
Erythrocytes		
Superoxide dismutase	3450 ± 485 U/g Hb	68
Platelets		
Cytochrome C oxidase	1660 ± 290 U/g protein	68

TABLE 103 (continued)
Some Literature Values for Guidance in Evaluation of Copper Status

Subject and Determination	Value	Reference
4. Adult Women		
20–29 yr (*n* = 10)		
Plasma copper	15.9 ± 4.2 µmol/L	46
Plasma ceruloplasmin		
Radioimmunodiffusion assay	330 ± 61 mg/L	46
Enzyme assay	502 ± 128 mg/L	46
Superoxide dismutase	2839 ± 464 U/g Hb	46
Age 50–59 years (*n* = 12)		
Plasma copper	17.2 ± 2.8 µmol/L	46
Plasma ceruloplasmin		
Radioimmunodiffusion assay	370 ± 77 mg/L	46
Enzyme assay	517 ± 85 mg/L	46
Superoxide dismutase	3360 ± 823 U/g Hb	46
5. Young Men (n = 11)		
Plasma copper	14.8 ± 0.3 µmol/L	78
Plasma ceruloplasmin concentration	302 ± 6.0 mg/L	78
Plasma ceruloplasmin activity	79.1 ± 2.1 U/L	78
6. Adults (Northern Ireland)		
Plasma copper (µmol/L)		
Males (*n* = 1142)	17.9 ± 3.3	47
Females (*n* = 1034) (not pregnant or using OCA)	20.1 ± 3.9	47
7. Adults (Belgium)		
Serum copper (µmol/L)		
Males (*n* = 25)	16.2 ± 2.8	54
Females (*n* = 21)	17.7 ± 4.5	54
8. Adults		
Plasma copper (µmol/L)		
Men (*n* = 55) (overall range)	8.8–175	37
Women		
None OCA users (*n* = 65)	10.7–26.6	37
OCA users (*n* = 21)	15.7–31.5	37

(continues)

TABLE 103 (continued)
Some Literature Values for Guidance in Evaluation of Copper Status

Subject and Determination	Value	Reference
9. Serum Copper (μg/mL)		
Men		
18–60 yr (*n* = 244)	0.75–1.50 μg/mL	45
> 60 yr (*n* = 29)	1.0–1.55 μg/mL	45
Women		
18 yr and over (*n* = 83)	1.05–1.85 μg/mL	45
10. Adults		
Plasma or serum		
Ceruloplasmin	51–176 U/L	24
Ceruloplasmin	94–116 U/L	70
Ceruloplasmin	180–400 mg/L	60, 79
Erythrocytes		
Cu/Zn Superoxide dismutase (mg/g)	0.471 ± 0.067	74
Copper (μmol/L)	4.8–20.8	14
Copper (μmol/L)	17.3	62
Whole Blood		
Copper (μmol/L)	13–22	15
Copper (μmol/L)	13.5	65
11. Elderly		
Elderly women (Canada)		
Serum copper (μmol/L)		
70.3 yr (mean) (*n* = 90)	19.1 ± 4.5	77
Elderly (United Kingdom)		
Plasma copper (μmol/L)		
Female patients (*n* = 15; 71–93 yr)	20.03 ± 3.78	48
Controls (*n* = 11; 30–44 yr)	15.64 ± 1.35	48
Elderly (United Kingdom) (*n* = 24)		
Male and female (69–85 yr)		
Plasma copper (μmol/L)	19.4	56, 57
Plasma ceruloplasmin (mg/L)	330	56, 57
Whole blood copper (μmol/L)	13.4	56, 57

References

1. Klevay, L. M., Coronary heart disease: zinc/copper hypothesis, *Am. J. Clin. Nutr.*, 28, 764, 1975.
2. Klevay, L. M., Copper and ischemic heart disease, *Biolog. Trace Element Res.*, 5, 245, 1983.
3. Nebot, C., Moutrt, M., Huet, P., Xu, J. Z., Yadan, J. C., Chavdiere, J., Spectrophotometric assay of superoxide dismutase activity based on the activated autooxidation of a tetracyclic catechol, *Anal. Biochem.*, 214, 442, 1993.
4. Robberecht, W., Sapp, P., Viaene, M. K., Rosen, D., McKenna-Yasek, D., Haines, J., Horvitz, R., Theys, P., and Brown, R. J., Cu/Zn superoxide dismutase activity in familial and sporadic amyotrophic lateral sclerosis, *J. Neurochem.*, 62, 384, 1994.
5. Porstmann, T., Wietschke, R., Cobet, G., Larenz, K., Grunow, R., John, S., Ballmann, R., Stamminger, G., and von Bachr, R., Immunochemical quantification of Cu/Zn superoxide dismutase in prenatal diagnosis of Down's Syndrome, *Hum. Genet.*, 85, 362, 1990.
6. Elvehjem, C. A., The biological significance of copper and its relation to iron metabolism, *Physiol. Rev.*, 15, 471, 1935.
7. Carturight, G. E. and Wintrobe, M. M., The question of copper deficiency in man, *Am. J. Clin. Nutr.*, 15, 94, 1964.
8. Underwood, E. J., Copper, in *Trace Elements in Human and Animal Nutrition*, 4th edition, Academic Press, New York, 1977, 56.
9. William, D. M., Copper deficiency in humans, *Semin. Hematology*, 20, 118, 1983.
10. Danks, D. M., Copper deficiency in humans, *Annu. Res. Nutr.*, 8, 235, 1988.
11. Barclay, S. M., Aggett, P. J., Lloyd, D. J., and Duffy, P., Reduced erythrocyte superoxide dismutase activity in low birth weight infants given iron supplements, *Pediatr. Res.*, 29, 297, 1991.
12. Fisher, P. W. F., Giroux, A., and L'Abbe, M. R., Effect of zinc supplementation on copper status in adult men, *Am. J. Clin. Nutr.*, 40, 743, 1984.
13. Yadrick, M. K., Kenney, M. A., and Winterfeldt, E. A., Iron, copper, and zinc status: response to supplementation with zinc or zinc and iron in adult females, *Am. J. Clin. Nutr.*, 49, 145, 1989.
14. Delves, H. T., Assessment of trace element status, *Clin. Endocrinol. Metab.*, 14, 725, 1985.
15. Iyengar, G. V., *Elemental Analysis of Biological Systems*, Vol. 1, CRC Press, Boca Raton, FL, 1989, 155.
16. Bunker, V. W., Hinks, L. J., Stansfeld, M. F., Lawson, M. S., and Clayton, B. E., Metabolic balance studies for zinc and copper in housebound elderly people and the relationship between zinc balance and leukocyte zinc concentrations, *Am. J. Clin. Nutr.*, 46, 353, 1987.
17. Turnlund, J. R., Keen, C. L., and Smith, R. G., Copper status and urinary and salivary copper in young men at three levels of dietary copper, *Am. J. Clin. Nutr.*, 51, 658, 1990.
18. Menkes, J. H., Alter, M., Steigledger, G. K., Weakly, D. R., and Sung, J. H., A sex-linked recessive disorder with retardation in growth, peculiar hair, and focal cerebral and cerebellar degeneration, *Pediatrics*, 29, 764, 1962.
19. Danks, D. M., Stevens, B. J., Campbell, P. E., Gillespie, J. M., Walker-Smith, J., Blomfield, J., Turner, B., Menkes' kinky-hair syndrome, *Lancet*, 1, 1100, 1972.
20. Cardano, A., Baertl, J. M., and Graham, G. G., Copper deficiency in infancy, *Pediatrics*, 34, 324, 1964.
21. Castillo-Duran, C. and Uauy, R., Copper deficiency impairs growth of infants recovering from malnutrition, *Am. J. Clin. Nutr.*, 47, 710, 1988.
22. Solomons, N. W., On the assessment of zinc and copper nutriture in man, *Am. J. Clin. Nutr.*, 32, 856, 1979.
23. Mason, K. E., A conspectus of research on copper metabolism and requirements, *J. Nutr.*, 109, 1979, 1979.
24. FAO/WHO (Food and Agriculture Organization/World Health Organization), *Evaluation of Food Additives*, WHO Technical Report Series No 462, World Health Organization, Geneva, Switzerland, 1971.

25. Cordano, A., The role played by copper in the physiopathology and nutrition of the infant and the child, *Annu. Nestle*, 33, 1, 1974.
26. Dunlap, W. M., Jamrs, G. W. III, and Hume, D. M., Anemia and neutropenia caused by copper deficiency, *Annu. Int. Med.*, 80, 470, 1974.
27. Heller, R. M., Kirchner, S. G., O'Neill, J. A., Hough, A. J., Howard, L., Krame, S. S., and Green, H. L., Skeletal changes of copper deficiency in infants receiving prolonged total parenteral nutrition, *J. Pediatr.*, 92, 947, 1978.
28. Karpil, J. T. and Peden, V. H., Copper deficiency in long-term parenteral nutrition, *J. Pediatr.*, 80, 32,1972.
29. Prasad, A. S., Brewer, G. J., Schoomaker, E. B., and Rabbani, P., Hypocupremia induced by Zinc therapy in adults, *J. Am. Med. Assoc.*, 240, 2166, 1978.
30. AL-Rashid, R. A. and Spangler, J., Neonatal copper deficiency, *N. Engl. J. Med.*, 285, 841, 1971.
31. Ashkenozi, A., Levin, S., Djaldetti, M., Fishel, E., and Benvenisti, D., The syndrome of neonatal copper deficiency, *Pediatrics*, 52, 525, 1973.
32. Sutton, A. M., Harvie, A., Cockburn, F., Farquharson, J., and Logan, R. W., Copper deficiency in the preterm infant of very low birthweight: four cases and a reference range for plasma copper, *Arch. Dis. Child.*, 60, 644, 1985.
33. Manser, J. I., Crawford, C. S., Tyrala, E. E., Brodsky, N. L., and Grover, W. D., Serum copper concentrations in sick and well preterm infants, *J. Pediatr.*, 97, 795, 1980.
34. Johnson, H. L. and Sauberlich, H. E., Trace element analysis in biological samples, in *Clinical, Biochemical, and Nutritional Aspects of Trace Elements*, Prasad, A. S., Ed., Alan R. Liss, Inc., New York, 1982, 405.
35. Williams, D. M., Clinical significance of copper deficiency and toxicity in the world population, in *Clinical, Biochemical and Nutritional Aspects of Trace Elements*, Prasad, A. S., Ed., Alan R. Liss, Inc., New York, 1982, 277.
36. Klevay, L. M., Inman, L., Johnson, L. A. K., Lawler, M., Mahalko, J. R., Milne, D. R., Lukaski, H. C., Bolonchuk, W., and Sandstead, H. H., Increased cholesterol in plasma in a young man during experimental copper depletion, *Metabolism*, 33, 1112, 1984.
37. Milne, D. B. and Johnson, P. E., Assessment of copper status: effect of age and gender on reference ranges in healthy adults, *Clin. Chem.*, 39, 883, 1993.
38. Milne, D. B., Klevay, L. M., and Hunt, J. R., Effects of ascorbic acid supplements and a diet marginal in copper on indices of copper nutriture in women, *Nutr., Res.*, 8, 865, 1988.
39. Prohaska, J. R. and Wells, W. W., Copper deficiency in developing rat brain: a possible model for Menkes' steely-hair disease, *J. Neurochem.*, 23, 91, 1974.
40. Milne, D. B., Assessment of copper nutritional status, *Clin. Chem.*, 40, 1479, 1994.
41. Salmenpera, L., Sumes, M. A., Nanto, V., and Perheetupa, J., Copper supplementation: failure to increase plasma copper and ceruloplasmin concentrations in healthy infants, *Am. J. Clin. Nutr.*, 50, 843, 1989.
42. Castillo-Duran, C., Fisberg, M., Valenzuela, A., Egana, J. I., and Usey, R., Controlled trial of copper supplementation during recovery from marasmus, *Am. J. Clin. Nutr.*, 37, 898, 1983.
43. Klevay, L. M., The role of copper, zinc, and other chemical elements on ischemic heart disease, in *Metabolism of Trace Elements in Man*, Vol. 1, Renmert, O. W., and Chan, W. -Y., Ed., CRC Press, Boca Raton, FL, 1984, 129.
44. Gibson, R. S., Anderson, B. M., and Sabry, J. H., The trace metal status of a group of post-menopausal vegetarians, *J. Am. Diet. Assoc.*, 82, 246, 1983.
45. Schreurs, W. H. P., Kloss, J. A., Muys, T., and Haesen, J. P., Serum copper levels in relation to sex and age, *Int. J. Vit. Nutr. Res.*, 52, 68, 1981.
46. Johnson, P. E., Milne, D. B., and Lykken, G. I., Effects of age and sex on copper absorption, biological half-life, and status in humans, *Am. J. Clin. Nutr.*, 56, 917, 1992.
47. McMaster, D., McCrum, E., Patterson, C. C., McF Kerr, M., O'Reilly, D., Evans, A. E., and Love, A. H. G., Serum copper and zinc in random samples of the population of Northern Ireland, *Am. J. Clin. Nutr.*, 56, 440, 1992.
48. Field, H. P., Whitley, A. J., Srimivason, T. R., Walker, B. E., and Kelleher, J., Plasma and leucocyte zinc concentrations and their response to zinc supplementation in an elderly population, *Int. J. Vit. Nutr. Res.*, 57, 311, 1987.

49. Salmenpera, L., Perheentupa, J., Pakarinen, P., and Sumes, M. A., Cu nutrition in infants during prolonged exclusive breast-feeding: low intake but rising serum concentrations of Cu and ceruloplasmin, *Am. J. Clin. Nutr.*, 43, 251, 1986.

50. Walranens, P. A., Nutritional importance of copper and zinc in neonates and infants, *Clin. Chem.*, 26, 185, 1980.

51. Perlaman, M., Chan, W.-Y., Ramadan, T. Z., McCaffree, M. A., and Rennert, O. M., Serum copper and ceruloplasmin in pre-term infants: prospective study, *J. Am. College Nutr.*, 1, 155, 1982.

52. Friel, J. K., Gibson, R. S., Balassa, R., and Watts, J. L., A comparison of the zinc, copper and manganese status of very low birth weight pre-term and full-term infants during the first twelve months, *Acta Paediatr. Scand.*, 73, 596, 1984.

53. Sorenson, J. T. J., Soderberg, L. S. F., and Chang, L. W., Radiation protection and radiation recovery with essential metallaelement chelates, *Proc. Soc. Expt. Biol. Med.*, 210, 191, 1995.

54. Versieck, J., Barbier, F., Speecke, A., and Hoste, J., Manganese, copper, and zinc concentrations in serum and packed blood cells during acute hepatitis, chronic hepatitis, and posthepatitic cirrhosis, *Clin. Chem.*, 20, 1141, 1974.

55. Brown, K. H., Lanata, C. F., Yuen, M. L., Peerson, J. M., and Butron, B., Potential magnitude of the missclassification of a population's trace element status due to infection: example from a survey of young Peruvian children, *Am. J. Clin. Nutr.*, 58, 549, 1993.

56. Bunke, V. W., Hinks, L. T., Lawson, M. S., and Clayton, B. E., Assessment of zinc and copper status of healthy elderly people using metabolic balance studies and measurement of leucocyte concentrations, *Am. J. Clin. Nutr.*, 40, 1096, 1984.

57. Bunker, V. W. and Clayton, B. E., Research review: studies in the nutrition of elderly people with particular reference to essential trace elements, *Age and Aging*, 18, 422, 1989.

58. Lonnerdal, B., Bioavailability of copper, *Am. J. Clin. Nutr.*, 63, 821S, 1996.

59. Linder, M. C. and Hazegh-Azam, M., Copper biochemistry and molecular biology, *Am. J. Clin. Nutr.*, 63, 797S, 1996.

60. Olivares, O. and Uauy, R., Copper as an essential nutrient, *Am. J. Clin. Nutr.*, 63, 791S, 1996.

61. Sunderman, F. W. Jr., Atomic absorption spectrometry of trace metals in clinical pathology, *Human Pathology*, 4, 549, 1973.

62. Shaw, J. C. L., Trace elements in the fetus and young infants. II. Copper, manganese, selenium, and chromium, *Am. J. Dis. Child.*, 134, 74, 1980.

63. Salomons, N. W., Biochemical, metabolic, and clinical role of copper in human nutrition, *J. Am. College Nutr.*, 4, 83, 1985.

64. Lockitch, G., Halstead, A. C., Wadsworth, L., Quigley, G., Reston, L., and Jacobson, B., Age- and sex-specific pediatric reference intervals and correlations for zinc, copper, selenium, iron, vitamins A and E, and related proteins, *Clin. Chem.*, 34, 1625, 1988.

65. Liska, S. K., Kerkay, J., and Pearson, K. H., Determination of copper in whole blood, plasma and serum using Zeeman effect atomic absorption spectroscopy, *Clin. Chim. Acta*, 150, 11, 1985.

66. Vuori, E., Salmela, S., Akerblom, H. K., Vukari, J., Uhari, M., Suoninen, P., Pietikainen, M., Pesonen, E., Lahde, P. L., and Dahl, M., Atherosclerosis precursors in Finnish children and adolescents. III. Serum and hair copper and zinc concentrations, *Acta Paediatr. Scand. Suppl.*, 318, 205, 1985.

67. Deeming, S. B. and Webir, C. W., Hair analysis of trace minerals in human subjects as influenced by age, sex, and contraceptive drugs, *Am. J. Clin. Nutr.*, 31, 1175, 1978.

68. Milne, D. B. and Nielsen, F. H., Effect of a diet low in copper on copper-status indicators in postmenopausal women, *Am. J. Clin. Nutr.*, 63, 358, 1996.

69. Winterbourne, C. C., Hawkins, R. E., Brian, M., and Carrell, R. W., The estimation of red cell superoxide dismutase activity, *J. Lab. Clin. Med.*, 85, 337, 1975.

70. Reiser, S., Smith, J. C. Jr., Mertz, W., Holbrooks, J. T., Scholfield, D. J., Powell, A. S., Canfield, W. K., and Canary, J. J., Indices of copper status in humans consuming a typical American diet containing either fructose or starch, *Am. J. Clin. Nutr.*, 42, 242, 1985.

71. Milne, D. B., Johnson, P. E., Klevay, L. M., and Sandstead, H. H., Effect of copper intake on balance, absorption, and status indices of copper in men, *Nutr. Res.*, 10, 975, 1990.

72. Evenson, M. A., Measurement of copper in biological samples by flame or electrothermal atomic spectrometry, *Meth. Enzymol.*, 158, 351, 1988.

73. Sloane, B. A., Gibbons, C. C., and Hegsted, M., Evaluation of zinc and copper nutritional status and effects upon growth of southern adolescent females, *Am. J. Clin. Nutr.*, 42, 235, 1985.

74. Turnlund, J. R., Copper nutrition, bioavailability and the influence of dietary factors, *J. Am. Dietet. Assoc.*, 88, 303, 1988.

75. National Research Council, Food and Nutrition Board, *Recommended Dietary Allowances*, 10th ed., National Academy Press, Washington D.C., 1989, 224.

76. Olivares, M. and Uauy, R., Limits of metabolic tolerance to copper and biological basis for present recommendations and regulations, *Am. J. Clin. Nutr.*, 63, 846S, 1996.

77. Gibson, R. S., Martinez, O. B., and MacDonald, A. C., The zinc, copper, and selenium status of a selected sample of Canadian elderly women, *J. Gerontology*, 40, 296, 1985.

78. Kelley, D. S., Daudeu, P. A., Taylor, P. C., Mackey, B. E., and Turnlund, J. R., Effects of low-copper diets on human immune response, *Am. J. Clin. Nutr.*, 62, 412, 1995.

79. Hankiewiez, V. J. and Sevecek, E., Untersuchungen uber den kupfer und zeruloplasmingehalt bei frauen wahrend der schwangerschaft und bei solchen mit gewissen gynokologischen krankheiten, *Zentralbl. Gynaekol.*, 96, 905, 1975.

80. Hambidge, K. M. and Maner, A. M., Trace elements, in *Laboratory Indices of Nutritional Status in Pregnancy*, National Research Council, National Academy of Sciences, Washington D.C., 1978, 157.

81. Turnlund, J. R., Scott, K. C., Peiffer, G. L., Jang, A. M., Keyes, W. R., Keen, C. L., and Saknashi, T. M., Copper status of young men consuming a low-copper diet, *Am. J. Clin. Nutr.*, 65, 72, 1997.

82. Bethin, K. E., Petrovic, N., and Ettinger, M. J., Identification of a major hepatic copper binding protein as S-adenosylhomocysteine hydrolase, *J. Biol. Chem.*, 270, 20698, 1994.

83. Rodriguez, M. C. N., Henriquez, M. S., Turon, A. F. M., Nova, F. J., Diaz, J. G., and Leon, P. B., Trace elements in chronic alcoholism, *Trace Element Med.*, 3, 164, 1986.

84. Medeiros, D. M. and Wildman, R. E. C., New findings on a unified perspective of copper restriction and cardiomyopathy, *Proc. Soc. Expt. Biol. Med.*, 215, 299, 1997.

85. Milne, D. B., Copper intake and assessment of copper status, *Am. J. Clin. Nutr.*, 67, 1041S, 1998.

86. Prohaska, J. R., Tamura, T., Percy, A. K., and Turnlund, J. R., *In vitro* copper stimulation of plasma peptidylglyine alpha-amidating monooxygenase in Menkes disease variant with occipital horns, *Pediatric Res.*, 42, 862, 1997.

87. Turnlund, J. R., Keyes, W. R., Peiffer, G. L., and Scott, K. C., Copper absorption, excretion, and retention by young men consuming low dietary copper determined by using the stable isotope ^{65}Cu, *Am. J. Clin. Nutr.*, 67, 1219, 1998.

88. Arnaud, J., Copper, *Int. J. Vit. Nutr. Res.*, 63, 308, 1993.

Selenium

Converting metric units to International System (SI) units:

μmol/L x 0.079 = μg/mL

μg/mL x 12.7 = μmol/L

atomic weight: 78.96

Introduction

Studies on selenium nutrition before 1970 have been summarized in a document of the National Academy of Sciences[1] which was revised in 1983. Early interests in selenium were related to its toxic effects when in the 1930s the element was shown to cause "alkali disease" and "blind staggers" that occurred in livestock in South Dakota, Wyoming, and other areas of Western United States.[1-4]

The concept that selenium had an essential role in nutrition was not considered until the reports in 1957 demonstrated that selenium prevented the occurrence of liver necrosis in rats[5,6] and exudative diathesis in chicks.[7-9] Shortly thereafter, selenium was found to prevent white muscle disease in calves and lambs.[10,11]

The importance of selenium in human nutrition was established with the recognition of its association with two diseases that occur in China: Keshan disease and Kaschin-Beck disease.[19-22,33,41,124] Selenium supplementation has been highly successful in controlling these two diseases.[24,69,124] Keshan disease is an endemic cardiomyopathy that affects primarily children and young women.[21,42] Kaschin-Beck disease is an endemic osteoarthritic condition that occurs during preadolescent and adolescent years.[23] The selenium content of the soil is very low in the areas of China where these diseases occur. Selenium levels in blood and hair are low.[124,128,129]

Selenium deficiency has been reported in patients on total parenteral nutrition.[17,20,43-45,108,109,134] In one instance, the patient suffered from muscle weakness and loss of ability to walk.[17,20] Selenium supplementation corrected the condition. Patients with Crohn's disease appear to be at risk of developing a selenium deficiency.[119] Selenium concentrations in plasma and erythrocytes may be depressed in HIV-positive patients, in AIDS patients, and in alcoholics.[136-138]

Dietary Sources of Selenium

Most meats, poultry, sea foods, baked products and cereal grains are good sources of selenium (15 to 60 μg/100 g edible portion).[56] Most vegetables, legumes, and fruits are relatively low in selenium content. Interesting, Brazil nuts contain an astonishing high concentration of selenium (2960 µg/100 g edible portion).[56420]

Determination of Selenium

Fluorometric Procedure

Versieck and Cornelis have succinctly described the various analytical techniques that are used to assay trace elements in plasma or serum.[46] However, many of the procedures described are not applicable for the measurement of the low levels of selenium present in biological materials.

Olson et al.[50] has summarized the various methods that have been used before 1973 for the determination of selenium in biological materials. The methods noted include (a) colorimetry, (b) spectrophotometry, (c) fluorometry, (d) atomic absorption spectrophotometry, (e) gas chromatography, (f) neutron activation analysis, and (g) X-ray fluoroescence analyses.

Before 1980, most selenium analyses were based upon spectrophoto-fluorometric procedures.[27,50,75,82,95] Following wet ashing of the sample, the selenium is reacted with a fluorescing agent to form a fluorescent complex that is then extracted. Both 3,3'-diaminobenzidine (DAB) and 2,3-diaminophthalene (DAN) have been used for this purpose. DAN has received the greater use because it was more sensitive, accurate, easier to use, and permitted automation.[35-37,51,52,82] Fluorometry and atomic absorption spectrometry remain the commonly used procedure to measure selenium in biological materials.[91,95] Gas chromatography/mass spectrometry methods have received some use.[95,96]

Modifications of the fluorometric procedure of Watkinson[37,51,52] are commonly used to measure selenium in whole blood, serum, erythrocytes, and urine.[81] The procedure requires digestion of the sample to remove organic material followed by reacting with 2,3-diaminonaphthaline. The selenium complex is then extracted into decahydronaphthalene (Decalin), followed by fluorometric measurement of the complex with an excitation wavelength of 369 nm and an emission wavelength of 525 nm. The procedure has been modified to provide for an automated determination of selenium[37,52] as well as for a single-test tube method.[36,55] The single tube fluorometric method for the determination of selenium in biological specimens, as described by Koh and Benson,[76] is very sensitive, reliable, and applicable to the analysis of large numbers of samples.

Various modifications have been reported on improvements in the fluorometric determination of selenium in biological materials.[46,50-52,75,81,82,84] Patterson et al.[81] simplified the sample digestion step required for fluorometric measurements of selenium. The procedure was considered acceptable as judged by comparison of the fluorometric obtained values on blood, serum, and urine with those obtained by hydride-generation atomic absorption spectrometry.

Atomic Absorption Spectrometry

For laboratories that possess the necessary equipment, graphite furance atomic absorption spectrometry and hydride generation atomic absorption spectrometry provide a sensitive and convenient means for measuring selenium in blood samples.[46,50,85,89,94,95,101,103] A tedious aspect of selenium analysis with fluorometric methods has been the requirement of sample digestion to remove the organic material present in the samples. Commonly nitric and perchloric acids are used. Hydride generation atomic absorption spectrometry measurements of selenium in serum requires a careful digestion of the sample.[74,85,99,104] This can be avoided with the use of atomic absorption spectrometry with Zeeman background correction.[61,80,91]

McMaster et al.[80] have described an automated system for measuring glutathione peroxidase activities and selenium concentrations in serum and whole blood that requires no sample treatment other than sample dilution. The system consisted of a centrifugal analyzer and an atomic absorption spectrophotometer with Zeeman background correction. The procedure permitted the measurement of the four parameters on at least 35 subjects per day and was applicable to epidemiological surveys.[80] Only a total of 500 μL of whole blood was required to perform the four analyses.

As with all trace element analytical procedures, the avoidance of contamination is essential.[46,97] Even the contamination of samples may negate results. Hence, selenium analyses of hair and finger nails are generally not reliable due to contamination such as from the selenium often present in shampoos.[79] However, information on selenium content of toenails has been obtained in several studies.[114-117]

Other Analytical Procedures

Various other procedures have been used for the determination of selenium in biological samples, such as by proton-induced X-ray emission.[38,39] This procedure is rather complex and requires special equipment. Similarly neutron activation analysis, mass spectrometry, and other nonroutine methods have seen limited use because of the requirement for expensive equipment, time needed to perform the analyses, and high technician expertise.[95,96,98]

Glutathione Peroxidase

Glutathione peroxidase (EC 1.11.1.9) functions in the following general reaction:

$$ROOH + 2\,GSH \xrightarrow{\text{glutathione peroxidase}} ROH + GSSG + H_2O$$

Erythrocyte glutathione peroxidase activity has been considered a functional index of long-term selenium status.[125] One unit has been defined as one μmol NADPH oxidized per minute. Erythrocyte selenium levels may also indicate long-term selenium status. Plasma concentrations of selenium have been considered the most sensitive index of short-term changes in selenium status. Measurement of selenium concentrations in platelets have also been suggested for assessing selenium status.[72]

When a selenium deficient subject was supplemented with selenium, a rapid increase occurred in the plasma glutathione peroxidase activity.[107] This was followed after a 4 to 6 week lag period with an increase in the erythrocyte glutathione peroxidase activity.[107] Apparently selenium can only be incorporated in newly formed erythrocytes.[107] Erythrocyte glutathione peroxidase has a half-life of 30 days while serum selenium concentrations have a half-life of one day.[108]

Glutathione peroxidase contains four selenocysteine residues and catalyzes the reduction of organic hydroperoxides. Erythrocyte and serum glutathione peroxidase forms differ funtionally and structurally and, hence, technically should be measured separately.

For time-saving reasons, whole blood samples rather than erythrocyte preparations are often used for glutathione peroxidase activity assays. The enzyme-linked procedure of the method of Paglia and Valentine[77] has been commonly used for the assay of erythrocyte glutathione peroxidase. The procedure has received several modifications.[61,79,105,123]

All of the glutathione peroxidase activity in human plasma appears attributable to a plasma-specific glutathione peroxidase (pl-GSHPx; p-GSHPx).[141,142] Glutathione peroxidase activity in the red blood cells is attributable to a different glutathione peroxidase; namely, cellular glutathione peroxidase (c-GSPHx; RBC-GSHPx).[141,143] Several enzyme-linked immunoassay (ELISA) kits are available to measure the plasma-specific glutathione peroxidase activity in plasma. The immunoassay is performed with the use of 96-well plates and a microplate-reader to measure absorbance at 405-nm wavelength. Blood samples should be obtained with the use of heparin as the anticoagulant. Assay kits are available from R & D Systems, Minneapolis, MN, and from Calbiochem-Novabiochem Corporation, San Diego, CA.

A radioimmunoassay has also been described for measuring glutathione peroxidase protein in human serum.[92,93] Only 10 μL of serum was required for the assay. The glutathione peroxidase protein levels correlated strongly with glutathione peroxidase activity ($r = 0.94$) and correlated somewhat less with serum selenium concentrations ($r = 0.64$). The glutathione peroxidase protein in serum was stable for at least 10 months when held at −20°C.

Whole blood glutathione peroxidase activity correlated with erythrocyte selenium concentrations.[61,129] Glutathione peroxidase activity increased with increasing concentrations of selenium in whole blood or erythrocytes until a level of 100 ng/mL of selenium in the whole blood was reached or a level of 140 ng/mL of selenium in the erythrocytes was reached.[47] At this level, the blood glutathione peroxidase activity plateaued. This concentration of erythrocyte selenium and the associated blood glutathione peroxidase activity can serve as guidelines for selenium nutritional status. In another study, plasma glutathione peroxidase activities correlated with both plasma selenium concentrations and with whole blood selenium concentrations in both children and men.[129]

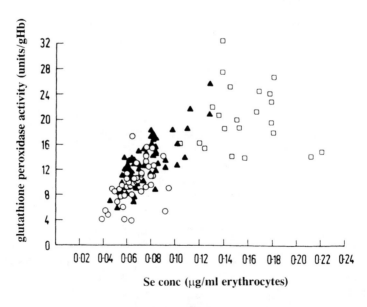

FIGURE 57

Relationship between selenium concentration of erythrocytes and glutathione peroxidase activity of whole blood from human subjects.[32,47] (With permission.)

The use of plasma and erythrocyte glutathione peroxidase activity measurements for assessing selenium status have been summarized by a number of investigators.[27,34,48,73,111,123]

The activity of glutathione peroxidase in serum is stable for at least six weeks when stored at −20°C.[80] Glutathione peroxidase activity in whole blood was less stable with evidence of deterioration occurring within 2 weeks of storage.[80]

Platelet Glutathione Peroxidase

Measuring platelet glutathione peroxidase activity has been suggested as a means of evaluating selenium status.[48,105] Platelet glutathione peroxidase activity reflects the dietary intake of selenium. Platelets have been reported to contain 782 ± 127 ng of selenium per gram of platelets.[102]

Alfthan et al.[105] reported that the mean dietary intake of selenium in Finland was 100 µg/d. It was estimated that the plasma selenium concentration needed to achieve maximal platelet glutathione peroxidase activity was 1.25 to 1.45 µmol/L. With the 100 µg/d intake of selenium in Finnland, glutathione peroxidase activity was saturated in the plasma and erythrocytes and almost saturated in the platelets. Approximately 50% of the dietary intake of selenium was excreted in the urine. The mean urinary selenium excretion was 0.72 µmol/d (57 µg/d) with a range of 0.50 to 1.22 µmol/d (40 to 97 µg/d). Information from this report can be useful in evaluating selenium nutritional status.

Assessment of Selenium Status

Since 1960, a vast number of studies have been reported on the determination, metabolism, functions, and requirements of selenium by the human. These studies have provided the basis for methods used in the evaluation of selenium status in the human. Many of these efforts have been summarized in a number of excellent publications and reviews.[12-16,31,32,49,54,95,121,122,125,126,133,135]

A number of selenoproteins have been recognized to exist reflecting various roles for selenium.[12,15,17,49,131] For example, type I iodothyronine 5′-deiodinase (EC 3.8.1.4) contains selenium and participates in the conversion of thyroxine to triiodothyronine.[15,40,132] Cellular glutathione peroxidase (EC 1.11.1.9) was the first selenium dependent enzyme found.[19] Measurement of the enzyme activity of this enzyme has been used extensively to evaluate selenium nutritional status.[61] Subsequently extracellular glutathione peroxidase was observed.[18] Selenium nutritional status can be followed also by measuring the activity of this enzyme in plasma.[61]

However, much of the selenium in plasma is present in selenoprotein P.[120] Approximately 44% of the selenium in plasma has been shown to be present as selenoprotein P. Glutathione peroxidase accounted for 12% of the plasma selenium.[120] A radioimmunoassay has been developed to measure plasma levels of selenoprotein P.[120] Selenoprotein P concentrations correlated with plasma selenium concentrations.[120] With further development into an assay kit it could serve as another means for evaluating selenium nutritional status in the human.

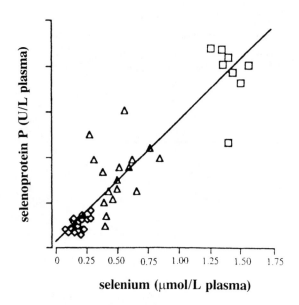

FIGURE 58

Comparison of selenoprotein P concentrations in plasma with plasma selenium concentrations in Chinese subjects (men 17 years and older). (Hill et al.[120] With permission.)

When selenium supplementation was withdrawn from patients on total parenteral nutrition, platelet glutathione peroxidase activity was significantly decreased within one week, while plasma glutathione peroxidase activity and plasma selenium levels were significantly decreased by three weeks.[110] Erythrocytes showed no changes in selenium indices during this period. These changes were promptly reversed with reintroduction of selenium supplementation. These results would indicate that platelet glutathione peroxidase activity could be a sensitive index for evaluating selenium status.[111] A disadvantage is the time required to prepare the platelets and the greater blood sample volume required.[78] However, the measurement has received application. As an example, healthy adults and blood donors in England had a mean serum selenium concentration of 92 μg/L. Serum selenium concentrations and platelet glutathione peroxidase activities indicated that a substantial number of the subjects had a low selenium nutritional status.[112]

Serum or plasma selenium concentrations may be a more sensitive indicator of selenium status than whole blood selenium concentrations. Plasma selenium concentrations can provide an index of short-term selenium status as plasma selenium levels respond more quickly to changes in selenium intakes or supplements.[27] Red blood cells or whole blood selenium concentrations can provide information on the long-term selenium status.

Blood selenium levels reflect the dietary intake of selenium.[32] Populations living in areas with low soil levels of selenium commonly have lower than normal plasma selenium concentrations. Plasma concentrations of selenium averaged 1.51 μmol/L in subjects living in Ohio where the soil selenium levels are low.[28,29] Low serum selenium concentrations are observed in Finland, China, and New Zealand populations where the soils are very low in selenium.[30-32,124] Selenium intake has been shown to be a predictor of tissue selenium concentration.[106] Selenium intake was found to be strongly correlated with the selenium concentration in serum, whole blood, and toenails.[88]

Urine analyses for selenium have been of limited use in evaluating selenium status.[100,105] In population studies urine selenium analyses can provide a qualitative assessment of selenium status and intake.[27] Selenium has been measured in urine with the use of fluorometric procedures that require only 400 µL of sample.[84] The mean selenium urinary excretion of a group of Canadian men was 124.5 ± 76.0 µg per day.[84] Other balance studies indicate that approximately 50% of the selenium intake is excreted in the urine.[105]

Infants and Children

In general, children have lower plasma or serum selenium concentrations than adults.[46,65-68,118,119,125] However, these concentrations may vary according to dietary selenium intake for a given area that may reflect soil selenium levels.[27,32] Serum levels of preterm and term infants have been reported to be low (0.81 to 0.93 µmol/L) when compared to adolescents and adults (1.83 µmol/L).[91,106]

During pregnancy, whole blood and erythrocyte selenium concentrations declined.[125] Plasma and erythrocyte glutathione peroxidase activities also decreased after the 20th week of pregnancy. The results indicate an increased requirement for selenium in pregnant women.[125]

Elderly

The effects of aging on selenium status appear variable. Earlier reports indicated that aging *per se* had only a minimal effect on selenium status.[70,71] The effects observed related largely to decreased food intake. Nevertheless, healthy elderly subjects (>65 yr) had significantly lower levels of selenium in plasma and whole blood when compared with younger subjects.[71] Institutionalized elderly had even lower selenium levels. However, erythrocyte glutathione peroxidase activities were the same for all groups.

In another report aging was associated with a progressive decrease in selenium status and serum selenium levels. The decrease was considered to be independent of changes in their dietary intake of selenium.[74] Serum selenium concentrations of 1.18 ± 0.19 µmol/L in the 20 to 39 year age group fell to 0.9 ± 0.19 µmol/L in the group 75 years of age and above.[74] In general, these concentrations would indicate an acceptable selenium status. Similar effects of aging on reducing serum selenium concentrations have been reported by other investigators.[86-88] In a few reports, these changes were not observed.[70,90]

Adults

In the United States, Canada, and Japan, serum selenium concentrations usually range between 100 to 200 µg/L (1.26 to 2.53 µmol/L). The serum selenium concentrations of European countries are somewhat less ranging from 50 to 110 µg/L (0.63 to 1.39 µmol/L). The mean serum selenium concentration for samples collected from adults in 10 different countries was 79.8 µg/L (1.0 µmol/L).[124] Variations were noted in the serum selenium concentration of people from different parts of Europe (Greece: 63 ± 14 µg/L vs. England: 109 ± 14 µg/L).[79,126,127]

Although various methods have been used to measure selenium in biological materials in comparisons of the methods, comparable results are generally obtained.[82,89,94,95,97,103] This has been enhanced by the use of standard references materials (SMR) available from the National Institute of Standards and Technology, Gaithersburg, MD.

However, such reference materials are not available for glutathione peroxidase measurements. Furthermore, no standardized method has been adopted for the measurement of glutathione peroxidase activity, although procedures based on the coupled assay of Paglia and Valentine[77] are often used. Thus, many laboratories express their results in the following manner: one unit of enzyme activity is defined as micromoles of NADPH oxidized per minute (25°C), and results expressed as units per gram of hemoglobin or per liter of plasma. Otherwise, comparison of results between laboratories can be difficult.

Since glutathione peroxidase is the major known metabolically functional form of selenium, its measurement may be more informative than measurements of selenium for evaluating selenium nutritional status. Thus, a need to use standardized methods is necessary in order to compare values between laboratories.

Toxicity

Although selenium is essential for human health, it is also a very toxic element.[1,2,12,18,25,26,32,83,121,128,130] For selenium, the range between an essential level and a toxic level is narrow. Selenium toxicity results in loss of hair and nails, accompanied by lesions of the skin and changes in the nervous system.[25] Toxic signs of selenium excess were observed in subjects with blood selenium levels of 13.3 μmol/L and above.[26] For the human, a selenium intake of up to 500 μg/day has been considered tolerable.[130] However, other studies indicate that the maximum tolerable selenium level in humans could be in the range of 1000 to 1500 μg/day.[130]

Urinary selenium measurements are probably a better indicator of selenium toxicity than blood selenium determinations. To avoid selenium toxicity, an acceptable urinary level of selenium should fall below 100 μg/L.[53]

Summary

Selenium nutritional status may be assessed by determining the selenium concentrations and the glutathione peroxidase enzyme activities in plasma, erythrocytes, and whole blood. Plasma or serum selenium concentrations can serve as an indicator of recent selenium intakes while erythrocyte concentrations can serve as indicators of long-term selenium intakes reflecting the 120-day lifespace of the erythrocytes.[113] Glutathione peroxidase measurements provide an indication of selenium functional status.

Fluorometry and graphite-furnace atomic absorption spectrometry are commonly used to measure selenium concentrations in whole blood and blood components. Glutathione peroxidase activities can be readily determined in erythrocytes, plasma, and platelets with the use of standardized methods. As a general guide, plasma or serum concentrations of 100 μg/L and above represent selenium nutritional adequacy (Tables 104 to 107).

TABLE 104

Some Literature Reference Values for Selenium Parameters for U.S. Populations (Additional reference values have been summarized elsewhere)[35,46,96]

Selenium Concentrations in Blood and Blood Components		
Source	Selenium Concentration (μmol/L)	Reference
U.S.A. (Plasma)		
Preterm infants (*n* = 20)	0.81 ± 0.19	91
Term infants (*n* = 20)	0.96 ± 0.12	
1–5 years (*n* = 20)	1.52 ± 0.15	
6–9 years (*n* = 20)	1.64 ± 0.19	
>10 years (*n* = 20)	1.83 ± 0.26	
U.S.A. (Seleniferous Area)		
Men and Women	Women (*n* = 20) Men (*n* = 24)	88
Serum (μmol/L)	2.17 ± 0.49 2.04 ± 0.27	
Whole Blood (μmol/L)	3.32 ± 1.03 3.14 ± 0.51	
Urine (μmol/d)	1.28 ± 0.95 1.77 ± 1.05	
Adult Men (*n* = 12)		115
Serum (μmol/L)	1.53 ± 0.03	

Population Group (Adults)	**ng/mg Hb**	**μg /ml Whole Blood**	**123**
South Dakota (*n* = 21)	2.78 ± 0.97	0.397 ± 0.129	128
Oregon (*n* = 23)	1.46 ± 0.20	0.202 ± 0.250	
New Zealand (*n* = 34)	0.45 ± 0.8	0.059 ± 0.011	

U.S.A.

Group	Serum Selenium Mean Values (μg/mL)	Reference
Age		98
< 55 yr (*n* = 43)	0.135	
> 55 yr (*n* = 68)	0.136	
Race		98
Black (*n* = 49)	0.132	
White (*n* = 60)	0.139	
Sex		98
Female (*n* = 51)	0.134	
Male (*n* = 60)	0.137	
Adults (*n* = 16)	0.112	97
Men (*n* = 27)	0.136 ± 4	28
Women (*n* = 27)	0.133 ± 4	

TABLE 105
Some Literature Selenium Values Reported From Several Countries

Selenium Concentrations in Blood and Blood Components		
Source	**Selenium Concentrations**	**Reference**
Northwest England		112
(low selenium area) (n = 275)		
Adults		
Serum selenium (μmol/L)	1.16	
Poland		140
Women (n = 49)		
Plasma (μmol/L)	0.70 ± 0.12	
Red cells (μmol/L)	1.48 ± 0.22	
Northern Ireland	**Men** (n = 48) **Women** (n = 52)	80
Serum (μmol/L)	1.08 ± 0.22 0.98 ± 0.19	
Whole blood (μmol/L)	1.15 ± 0.22 1.15 ± 0.20	
England	**Men and Women** (means)	71
Selenium	< 65 yr > 65 yr	
Plasma (μmol/L)	1.20 1.03	
Whole blood (μmol/L)	1.37 1.23	
Red cells (μmol/L)	1.60 1.49	
Platelets (nmol/g protein)	27.6 26.6	
	Selenium (μg/dL)	
China	Plasma Whole blood	129
Boys (n = 22)		
Dechany	1.3 ± 0.5 1.8 ± 1.0	
Mianning	4.0 ± 1.1 4.7 ± 0.9	
Beijing	11.9 ± 1.2 12.6 ± 0.7	
Men (n = 22)		
Dechany	1.6 ± 0.4 2.2 ± 0.7	
Mianning	4.2 ± 1.1 5.3 ± 0.69	
Beijing	11.1 ± 1.1 12.7 ± 1.5	
Low Se area (n = 40)	2.7 ± 0.9	25
Adequate Se area (n = 1745)	9.5 ± 0.9	
High Se area (n = 72)	320 (30–750)	118
France		
Boys and Girls (n = 186)	**Serum Selenium (μmol/L)**	
3–16 yr	0.85 ± 0.33	

TABLE 106
Literature Values For Glutathione Peroxidase Activity

Source	Activity	Reference
Finland (15 men)		105
Plasma (U/L)	358 ± 46	
Red cells (U/g Hb)	9.4 ± 1.3	
Platelets (U/g protein)	185 ± 28	
Northern Ireland		80
Serum		
Men (*n* = 48) (U/L)	248 ± 50	
Women (*n* = 52) (U/L)	217 ± 46	
England		71
Red cells (U/g Hb)	24.1	
Platelets (U/g protein)	133	
Northwest England (Low Se area)		112
Adults (*n* = 275)		
Platelets (U/g protein)	2.51	
Poland		140
Women (n = 49)		
Plasma (U/L)	369.9 ± 81.4	
Red cells (U/g Hb)	33.0 ± 17.5	

TABLE 107
Selenium Concentration in Toenails and Hair

Source	Concentration	References
U.S.A.		
Toenails (μmol/kg)	10.4 ± 1.5	114
Toenails (mg/kg)	0.823 ± 0.197	114
Toenails (μmol/kg)	13.2 ± 1.1	115
U.S.A. (residing in seleniferous area)		
Toenails (μmol/kg)		
Women (*n* = 20)	15.7 ± 3.7	88
Men (*n* = 24)	14.8 ± 2.5	
Finland (*n* = 166)		
Toenails (mg/kg)	0.47 ± 0.09	116
China		
Hair selenium (μg/g)		25
Low selenium area	0.16 ± 0.04	
Adequate selenium area	0.36 ± 0.17	
High selenium area	32.2 (4.1–100)	

References

1. National Research Council, *Selenium in Nutrition*, National Academy of Sciences, Washington D.C., 1971 (Revised in 1981).
2. Moxon, A. L. and Rhian, M., Selenium poisoning, *Physiol. Rev.*, 23, 305, 1943.
3. Shrift, A., Biological activities of selenium compounds, *Bot. Rev.*, 24, 550, 1958.
4. Rosenfeld, I. and Beath, O. A., *Selenium: Geobotany, Biochemistry, Toxicity and Nutrition*, Academic Press, New York, 1964.
5. Schwarz, K. and Foltz, C. M., Selenium as an integral part of Factor 3 against dietary necrotic liver degeneration, *J. Am. Chem. Soc.*, 79, 3292, 1957.
6. Schwarz, K., The nutritional significance of selenium — A symposium, *Fed. Proc.*, 20, 665, 1961.
7. Patterson, E. L., Milstrey, R., and Stokstad, E. L. R., Effect of selenium in preventing exudative diathesis in chicks, *Proc. Soc. Exp. Biol. Med.*, 95, 617, 1957.
8. Scott, M. L., Bieri, J. G., Briggs, G. M., and Schwarz, K., Prevention of exudative diathesis by factor 3 in chicks on vitamin E-deficient torula yeast diets, *Poultry Sci.*, 36, 1155, 1957 (Abstract).
9. Stokstad, E. L. R., Patterson, E. L., and Milstrey, R., Factors which prevent exudative diathesis in chicks on torula yeast diets, *Poultry Sci.*, 36, 1160, 1957.
10. Muth, O. H., Oldfield, J. E., Remmert, L. F., and Schubert, J. R., Effects of selenium and vitamin E white on muscle disease, *Science*, 128, 1090, 1958.
11. Hogue, D. E., Proctor, J. F., Warner, R. G., and Loosli, J. K., Relation of selenium, vitamin E and an unidentified factor to muscular dystrophy (stiff-lamb or white muscle disease) in the lamb, *J. Anim. Sci.*, 21, 25, 1962.
12. Sunde, R. A., Molecular biology of selenoproteins, *Annu. Rev. Nutr.*, 10, 451, 1990.
13. Burk, R. F., Molecular biology of selenium with implications for its metabolism, *FASEB J.*, 5, 2274, 1991.
14. Levander, O. A., Scientific rationale for the 1989 recommended dietary allowance for selenium, *J. Am. Diet. Assoc.*, 91, 1572, 1991.
15. Burk, R. F. and Hill, K. E., Regulation of selenoproteins, *Annu. Rev. Nutr.*, 13, 65, 1993.
16. *Selenium in Biology and Medicine*, Burk, R. F., Ed., Springer Verlag, New York, 1994.
17. Thomson, C. D., Clinical consequences and assessment of low selenium status, *NZ Med. J.*, 104, 376, 1991.
18. Takahashi, K. and Cohen, H. J., Selenium-dependent glutathione peroxidase protein and activity: immunological investigations on cellular and plasma enzymes, *Blood*, 68, 640, 1986.
19. Rotruck, J. T., Pope, A. L., Ganther, H. E., Swanson, A. B., Hafeman, D., and Hoekstra, W. G., Selenium: biochemical role as a component of glutathione peroxidase, *Science*, 179, 588, 1973.
20. Van Rij, A. M., Thomson, C. D., McKenzie, J. M., and Robinson, M. F., Selenium deficiency in total parenteral nutrition, *Am. J. Clin. Nutr.*, 32, 2076, 1979.
21. Keshan Disease Research Group of the Chinese Academy of Science, Observations on effect of sodium selenium in prevention of Keshan disease, *Chin. Med. J.*, 92, 471, 1979.
22. Levander, O. A., and Burk, R. F., Selenium, in *Modern Nutrition in Health and Disease*, Volume 1, 8th edition, Shils, M. E., Olson, J. A., and Shike, M., Eds., Lea & Febiger, Philadelphia, PA, 1994.
23. Mo, D., Pathology and selenium deficiency in Kashin-Beck disease, in *Selenium in Biology and Medicine*, Combs, G. F. Jr., Spallholz, J. E., Levander, O. A., and Oldfield, J. E., Eds., Van Nostrand Reinhold, New York, 1987, 924.
24. Yang, G., Ge, K., Chen, J., and Chen, X. S., Selenium-related endemic diseases and the daily selenium requirement, *World Rev. Nutr. Diet.*, 55, 98, 1988.
25. Yang, G., Wang, S., Zhou, R., and Sun, S., Endemic selenium intoxication of humans in China, *Am. J. Clin. Nutr.*, 37, 872, 1983.
26. Yang, G., Yin, S., Zhou, R., Gu, L., Yan, B., Liu, Y., Studies of safe maximal daily dietary Se-intake in a seleniferous area in China, *J. Trace Elem. Electrolytes Hlth. Dis.*, 3, 123, 1989.
27. Thomson, C. D. and Robinson, M. F., Selenium in human health and disease with emphasis on those aspects peculiar to New Zealand, *Am. J. Clin. Nutr.*, 33, 303, 1980.

28. Snook, J. T., Palmquist, D. L., Moxon, A. L., Cantor, A. A., and Vivian, V. M., Selenium status of a rural (predominantly Amish) Community living in a low-selenium area, *Am. J. Clin. Nutr.*, 38, 620,1983.

29. Levander, O. A. and Morris, V. C., Dietary selenium levels needed to maintain balance in North American adults consuming self-selected diets, *Am. J. Clin. Nutr.*, 39, 809, 1984.

30. Robinson, M. F., Selenium in human nutrition in New Zealand, *Nutr. Rev.*, 47, 99, 1989.

31. Levander, O. A., Selenium: Biochemical actions, interactions, and some human health implications, in *Clinical, Biochemical, and Nutritional Aspects of Trace Elements*, Prasad, A. S., Ed., Alan R. Liss, New York, 1982, 345.

32. Robinson, M. F., Clinical effects of selenium deficiency and excess, in *Clinical, Biochemical, and Nutritional Aspects of Trace Elements*, Prasad, A. S., Ed., Alan R. Liss, New York, 1982, 325.

33. Keshan Disease Research Group of the Chinese Academy of Science, Epidemiologic studies on the etiologic relationship of selenium and Keshan disease, *Chinese Med. J.*, 92, 477, 1979.

34. Burk, R. F., Selenium in nutrition, *World Rev. Nutr. Diet*, 30, 88, 1978.

35. Johnson, H. L. and Sauberlich, H. E., Trace element analysis in biological samples, in *Clinical, Biochemical, and Nutritional Aspects of Trace Elements*, Prasad, A. S., Ed., Alan R. Liss, New York, 1982, 405.

36. Spallholz, J. E., Collins, G. F., and Schwarz, K., A single-test-tube method for the fluorimetric microdetermination of selenium, *Bioinorg. Chem.*, 9, 453, 1978.

37. Brown, M. W. and Watkinson, J. H., An automated fluorometric method for the determination of nanogram quantities of selenium, *Annu. Chim. Acta*, 89, 29, 1979.

38. Simonoff, M., Hamon, C., Moretto, P., Llabador, Y., and Simonoff, G., High sensibility Pixe determination of selenium in food and biological samples using a preconcentration technique, *Nucl. Instrum. Methods Phys. Res.*, B31, 442, 1988.

39. Delmas-Beauvieux, M.-C., Peuchant, E., Couchouron, A., Constans, J., Sergeant, C., Simonoff, M., Pellegrin, J.-L., Leng, B., Contri, C., and Clerc, M., The enzymatic antioxidant system in blood and glutathione status in human immunodeficiency virus (HIV)-infected patients: effects of supplementation with selenium or β-carotene, *Am. J. Clin. Nutr.*, 64, 101, 1996.

40. Arthur, J. R., Nicol, F., and Beckett, G. J., Hepatic iodothyronine 5′-deiodinase, The role of selenium, *Biochemi. J.*, 272, 537, 1990.

41. Levander, O. A., Ager, A. L. Jr., and Beck, M. A., Vitamin E and selenium: contrasting and interacting nutritional derterminants of host resistance to parasitic and viral infections, *Proc. Nutr. Soc.*, 54, 475, 1995.

42. Yang, F. Y., Lin, Z. H., Xing, J. R., Li, S. G., Yang, J., San, S., and Wu, L. Y., Se deficiency is a necessary but no sufficient factor required for the pathogenesis of Keshan disease, *J. Clin. Biochem. Nutr.*, 16, 101, 1994.

43. Johnson, R. A., Baker, S. S., and Fallon, J. T., An accidental case of cardiomyopathy and selenium deficiency, *N. Engl. J. Med.*, 304, 1210, 1981.

44. Waston, R. D., Cannon, R. A., Kurland, G. S., Cox, K. L., and Frates, R. C., Selenium responsive myositis during prolonged home parenteral nutrition in cystic fibrosis, *JPEN*, 9, 58, 1985.

45. Brown, M. R., Cohen, H. J., Lyones, J. M., Curtis, T. W., Thunberg, B., Cochran, W. H., and Klish, W. J., Proximal muscle weakness and selenium deficiency associated with long-term parenteral nutrition, *Am. J. Clin. Nutr.*, 43, 549, 1986.

46. Versieck, J. and Cornelis, R., *Trace Elements in Human Plasma or Serum*, CRC Press, Boca Raton, FL, 1989.

47. Rea, H. M., Thomson, C. D., Campbell, D. R., and Robinson, N. J., Relation between erythrocyte selenium concentrations and glutathione peroxidase (EC 1.11.1.9) activities of New Zealand residents and visitors to New Zealand, *Br. J. Nutr.*, 42, 201, 1979.

48. Thomson, C. D., Steven, S. M., van Rij, A. M., Wade, C. R., and Robinson, M. F., Selenium and vitamin E supplementation: activities of glutathione peroxidase in human tissues, *Am. J. Clin. Nutr.*, 48, 316, 1988.

49. Burk, R. F., Recent developments in trace element metabolism and function: newer roles for selenium in nutrition, *J. Nutr.*, 119, 1051, 1989.

50. Olson, O. E., Palmer, I. S., and Whitehead, E. I., Determination of selenium in biological materials, *Meth. Biochem. Anal.*, 21, 39, 1973.

51. Watkinson, J. H., Fluorometric determination of selenium in biological material with 2,3-diaminonaphthalene, *Anal. Chem. Acta*, 38, 92, 1966.
52. Watkinson, J. H., Semi-automated fluorometric determination of nanogram quantities of selenium in biological material, *Anal. Chem. Acta*, 105, 319, 1979.
53. Glover, J. R., Selenium in human urine: a tentative maximum allowable concentration for industrial and rural populations, *Annu. Occup. Hyg.*, 10, 3, 1967.
54. Combs, G. F. Jr. and Combs, S. B., The nutritional biochemistry of selenium, *Annu. Rev. Nutr.*, 4, 257, 1984.
55. Alfthan, G., A micromethod for the determination of selenium in tissues and biological fluids by single-test-tube fluorimetry, *Anal. Chim. Acta*, 165, 189, 1984.
56. Provisional Table on the Selenium Content of Foods, Human Nutrition Information Service, United States Department of Agriculture, Beltsville, MD, 1992, Document HNIS/PT-109.
57. Kahn, H. L., Peterson, G. E., and Shallis, J. E., Atomic absorption microsampling with the sampling boat technique, *Atomic Absorption Newsletter*, 7, 35, 1968.
58. Kerber, J. D. and Fernandez, F. J., Determination of trace metals in aqueous solution with the Delves sampling cup technique, *Atomic Absorption Newsletter*, 10, 78, 1971.
59. Baird, R. B., Pourian, S., and Gabrilian, S. M., Determination of trace elements of selenium in wastewater by carbon rod atomization, *Anal. Chem. Acta*, 44, 1887, 1972.
60. Carnick, G. R., Manning, D. C., and Stavin, W., Determination of selenium in biological materials with platform furnace atomicabsorption spectroscopy and Zeeman background correction, *Analyst*, 108, 1297, 1983.
61. Pleban, P. A., Munyani, A., and Beachum, J., Determination of selenium concentration and glutathione peroxidase activity in plasma and erythrocytes, *Clin. Chem.*, 28, 311, 1982.
62. Schmid, P. J. and Royer, J. L., Submicrogram determination of arsenic, selenium, antimony, bismuth by atomic absorption utilizing sodium borahydride reduction, *Anal. Letters*, 6, 17, 1973.
63. Clinton, O. E., Determination of selenium in blood and plant material by hydride generation and atomic absorption spectroscopy, *Analyst*, 102, 187, 1977.
64. Inhat, M., Selenium in food: evaluation of atomic absorption spectrometric techniques involving hydrogen selenide generation and carbon-furnace atomization, *J. Assoc. Off. Anal. Chem.*, 59, 911, 1976.
65. Westermarck, T., Raunu, P., Kirjarinta, M., and Lappalainen, L., Selenium content of whole blood and serum in adults and children of different ages from different parts of Finland, *Acta Pharmacol. Toxicol.*, 40, 465, 1977.
66. Lombeck, L., Kasperek, K., Harbisch, H. D., Feinendegen, L. E., and Bremer, H. J., The selenium state of healthy children, *Eur. J. Pediatr.*, 125, 81, 1977.
67. Verlinden, M., van Sprundel, M., Van der Auwera, J. C., and Eylenbosch, W. J., The selenium status of Belgian population groups. II. Newborne, children, and the aged, *Biol. Trace Element Res.*, 5, 103, 1983.
68. Lombeck, I., The evaluation of selenium state in children, *J. Inherit. Metab. Dis.*, 6 (Suppl. 1), 83, 1983.
69. Keshan Disease Research Group, Observation on effect of sodium selenite in prevention of Keshan disease, *Chin. Med. J.*, 92, 471, 1979.
70. Lane, H. W., Warren, D. C., Taylor, B. J., and Stool, E., Blood selenium and glutathione peroxidase levels and dietary selenium of free-living and institutionalized elderly subjects, *Proc. Soc. Expt. Biol. Med.*, 173, 87, 1983.
71. Campbell, D., Bunker, V. W., Thomas, A. J., and Clayton, B. E., Selenium and vitamin E status of healthy and institutionalized elderly subjects: analysis of plasma, erythrocytes and platelets, *Br. J. Nutr.*, 62, 221, 1989.
72. Neve, J., Vertongen, F., and Molle, L., Selenium deficiency, *Clinics in Endocrinology and Metabolism*, 14, 629, 1985.
73. Beutler, E., Glutathionine peroxidase (GSH-Px), in *A Manual of Biochemical Methods*, 2nd edition, Grune and Stratton, New York, 1979, 71.
74. Olivieri, O., Stanzial, A. M., Girelli, D., Trevison, M. T., Guarini, P., Terzi, M., Caffi, S., Fontana, F., Casaril, M., Ferrari, S., and Corrocher, R., Selenium status, fatty acids, vitamins A and E, and aging: the Nove Study, *Am. J. Clin. Nutr.*, 60, 510, 1994.

75. Olson, O. E., Palmer, I. S., and Cary, E. E., Modification of the official fluorometric method for selenium in plants, *JAOAC*, 58, 117, 1975.

76. Koh, T. -S. and Benson, T. H., Critical reappraisal of fluorometric method for determination of selenium in biological materials, *JAOAC*, 66, 918, 1983.

77. Paglia, D. E. and Valentine, W. N., Studies on quantitative and qualitative characterization of erythrocyte glutathione peroxidase, *J. Lab. Clin. Med.*, 70, 158, 1979.

78. Levander, O. A., DeLoach, D. P., Morris, V. C., and Moser, P. B., Platelet glutathione peroxidase as an index of selenium status in rats, *J. Nutr.*, 113, 55, 1983.

79. Dube, P., Chutsch, M., and Krauser, C., Trace elements-evaluation of environmental exposure and medical diagnosis, in *Trace Elements in Human Health and Disease*, World Health Organization, Regional Office for Europe, Cophenhagen, 1987.

80. McMaster, D., Bell, N., Anderson, P., and Love, A. H. G., Automated measurement of two indicators of human selenium status, and applicability to population studies, *Clin. Chem.*, 36, 211, 1990.

81. Petterson, J., Hansson, L., Ornemark, U., and Olin, A., Fluorimetry of selenium in body fluids after digestion with nitric acid, magnesium nitrate hexahydrate, and hydrochloric acid, *Clin. Chem.*, 34, 1908, 1988.

82. Tamari, Y., Ohmori, S., and Hiraki, K., Fluorometry of nanogram amounts of selenium in biological samples, *Clin. Chem.*, 32, 1464, 1986.

83. Wilber, C. G., Toxicology of selenium: a review, *Clin. Toxicol.*, 17, 171, 1980.

84. Lalonde, L., Jean, Y., Roberts, K. D., Chapdelaine, A., and Bleau, G., Fluorometry of selenium in serum and urine, *Clin. Chem.*, 28, 172, 1982.

85. Neve, J., Methods in determination of selenium states, *J. Trace Elem. Electrolytes Hlth. Dis.*, 5, 1, 1991.

86. Bunker, V. W., Lawson, M. S., Stanfield, M. F., and Clayton, B. E., Selenium balance studies in apparently healthy and house-bound elderly people eating self-selected diets, *Br. J. Nutr.*, 59, 45, 1988.

87. Lockitch, G., Selenium: clinical significance and analytical concepts, *Crit. Rev. Clin. Lab. Sci.*, 27, 483, 1989.

88. Swanson, C. A., Longnecker, M. P., Veillon, C., Howe, S. M., Levander, O. A., Taylor, P. R., McAdam, P. A., Brown, C. C., Stampfer, M. J., and Willett, W. C., Selenium intake, age, gender, and smoking in relation to indices of selenium status of adults residing in a seleniferous area, *Am. J. Clin. Nutr.*, 52, 858, 1990.

89. Dillon, L. J., Hilderbrand, D. C., and Groon, K. S., Flameless atomic absorption determination of selenium in human blood, *Atomic Spectroscopy*, 3, 5, 1982.

90. McAdam, P. A., Smith, D. K., Feldman, E. B., and Hames, C., Effect of age, sex, and race on selenium status of healthy residents of Augusta, GA, *Biol. Trace, Elem. Res.*, 6, 3, 1984.

91. Jacobson, B. E., and Lockitch, G., Direct determination of selenium in serum by graphite-furnace atomic absorption spectrometry with deuterium background: correction and a reduced palladium modifier, Age specific ranges, *Clin. Chem.*, 34, 709, 1988.

92. Huang, W. and Akesson, B., Radioimmunoassay of glutathione peroxidase in human serum, *Clin. Chim. Acta*, 219, 139, 1993.

93. Takahashi, K., Newburger, P. E., and Cohen, H. J., Glutathione peroxidase protein: absence in selenium deficiency states and correlation with enzyme activity, *J. Clin. Invest.*, 77, 402, 1986.

94. Oster, O. and Prellivitz, W., A methodological comparison of hydride and carbon furnace atomic absorption spectroscopy for the determination of selenium in serum, *Clin. Chim. Acta*, 124, 277, 1982.

95. Lewis, S. A., Determination of selenium in biological matrices, *Meth. Enzymol.*, 158, 391, 1988.

96. Ducros, V. and Favier, A., Gass chromatographic-mass spectrometric method for the determination of selenium in biological samples, *J. Chromatogr.*, 583, 35, 1992.

97. Ericson, S. P., McHalsky, M. L., Rabinow, B. E., Kronholm, K. G., Areco, C. S., Weltzer, J. A., and Ayd, S. W., Sampling and analysis techniques for monitoring serum for trace elements, *Clin. Chem.*, 32, 1350, 1986.

98. Willett, W. C., Polk, B. F., Morris, J. S., Stampfer, M. J., Pressel, S., Rosner, B., Taylor, J. O., Schneider, K., and Hames, C. G., Prediagnostic serum selenium and risk of cancer, *Lancet*, 1, 130, 1983.

99. Tam, G. K. H. and Lacroix, G., Dry ashing, hydride generation atomic absorption spectrometric determination of arsenic and selenium in foods, *J. Assoc. Off. Anal. Chem.*, 65, 647, 1982.

100. Geahchan, A. and Chambon, P., Fluorametry of selenium in urine, *Clin. Chem.*, 26, 1272, 1980.

101. Tulley, R. T. and Lehmann, H. P., Flameless atomic absorption spectrophotometry of selenium in whole blood, *Clin. Chem.*, 28, 1448, 1982.

102. Kasperek, K., Iyengar, G. V., Kiem, J., Borberg, H., and Emil, L., Elemental composition of platelets. III. Determination of Ag, Au, Cd, Co, Sc, Mo, Rb, Sb, and Se in normal human platelets by neutron activation analysis, *Clin. Chem.*, 25, 711, 1979.

103. Morisi, G., Patriarca, M., and Menotti, A., Improved determination of selenium by Zeeman atomic absorption spectrometry, *Clin. Chem.*, 34, 127, 1988.

104. Reamer, D. C. and Veillon, C., Preparation of biological materials for determination of selenium by hydride generation - atomic absorption spectrometry, *Anal. Chem.*, 53, 1192, 1981.

105. Alfthan, G., Aro, A., Arvilommi, H., and Huttunen, J. K., Selenium metabolism and platelet glutathione peroxidase activity in healthy Finnish men: effects of selenium yeast, selenite, and selenate, *Am. J. Clin. Nutr.*, 53, 120, 1991.

106. Smith, A. M., Chen, L. W., and Thomas, M. R., Selenate fortification improves selenium status of term infants fed soy formula, *Am. J. Clin. Nutr.*, 61, 44, 1995.

107. Cohen, H. J., Chovaniec, M. E., Mistretta, D., and Baker, S. S., Selenium repletion and glutathione peroxidase - differential effects on plasma and red blood cell enzyme activity, *Am. J. Clin. Nutr.*, 41, 735, 1985.

108. Vandepas, J. B., Dumont, J. E., Contempre, B., and Diplock, A. T, Iodine and selenium deficiency in northern Zaire, *Am. J. Clin. Nutr.*, 52, 1087, 1990.

109. Vinton, N. E., Dahlstrom, K. A., Strobel, C. T., and Ament, M. E., Macrocytosis and pseudoalbinism: manifestations of selenium deficiency, *J. Pediatr.*, 111, 711, 1987.

110. Sando, K., Hoki, M., Nezu, R., Takagi, Y., and Okada, A., Platelet glutathione peroxidase activity in long-term total parenteral nutrition with and without selenium supplementation, *JPEN*, 16, 54, 1992.

111. Levander, O. A., Considerations on the assessment of selenium status, *Federation Proc.*, 44, 2579, 1985.

112. Pearson, D. J., Day, J. P., Suarez-Mendez, V. J., Miller, P. F., Owen, S., and Woodcock, A., Human selenium status and glutathione peroxidase activity in north-west England, *Eur. J. Clin. Nutr.*, 44, 277, 1990.

113. Cohen, H. J., Chovaniec, M. E., Mistretta, D., and Baker, S. S., Selenium repletion and glutathione peroxidase - differential effects on plasma and red blood cell enzyme activity, *Am. J. Clin. Nutr.*, 41, 735, 1985.

114. Hunter, D. J., Morris, J. S., Stampfer, M. J., Colditz, G. A., Speizer, F. E., and Willett, W. C., A prospective study of selenium status and breast cancer risk, *JAMA*, 264, 1128, 1990.

115. Longnecker, M. P., Stampfer, M. J., Morris, J. S., Spate, V., Baskett, C., Mason, M., and Willett, W. C., A 1-y trial of the effect of high-selenium bread on selenium concentrations in blood and toenails, *Am. J. Clin. Nutr.*, 57, 408, 1993.

116. Ovaskainen, M.-L., Virtamo, J., Alfthan, G., Haukka, J., Pietinen, P., Taylor, P. R., and Huttunen, J. K., Toenail selenium as an indicator of selenium intake among middle-aged men in an area with low soil selenium, *Am. J. Clin. Nutr.*, 57, 662, 1993.

117. Morris, J. S., Stampfer, M. J., and Willett, W., Dietary selenium in humans, Toenails as an indicator, *Biolog. Trace Element Res.*, 5, 529, 1983.

118. Malvy, D. J.-M., Arnaud, J., Burtschy, B., Richard, M.-J., Favier, A., Houot, O., and Amedee-Manesme, O., Reference values for serum zinc and selenium of French healthy children, *Eur. J. Epidemiol.*, 9, 155, 1993.

119. Rannem, T., Ladefoged, K., Hylander, E., Hegnhoj, J., and Jarnum, S., Selenium status in patients with Crohn's disease, *Am. J. Clin. Nutr.*, 56, 933, 1992.

120. Hill, K. E., Xia, Y., Akesson, B., Boeglin, M. E., and Burk, R. F., Selenoprotein P concentration in plasma is an index of selenium status in selenium deficient and selenium supplemented Chinese subjects, *J. Nutr.*, 126, 138, 1996.

121. Bedwal, R. S., Nair, N., Sharma, M. P., and Mathur, R. S., Selenium - its biological perspectives, *Medical Hypothesis*, 41, 150, 1993.

122. Lavander, O. A., Recent developments in selenium nutrition, *Nutrition Update*, 1, 147, 1983.

123. Whanger, P. D., Beilstein, M. A., Thomson, C. D., Robinson, M. F., and Howe, M., Blood selenium and glutathione peroxidase activity of populations in New Zealand, Oregon, and South Dakota, *FASEB J.*, 2, 2996, 1988.

124. Chen, X., Yang, G., Chen, J., Chen, X., Wen, Z., and Ge, K., Studies on the relations of selenium and Keshan disease, *Biolog. Trace Element Res.*, 2, 91, 1980.

125. Litov, R. E. and Combs, G. F. Jr., Selenium in pediatric nutrition, *Pediatrics*, 87, 339, 1991.

126. Neve, J., Physiological and nutritional importance of selenium, *Experientia*, 47, 187, 1991.

127. Thorling, E. B. and Overvad, K., Selenium status in Denmark, A comparison with 16 sites in Europe, *Trace Elements in Human Health and Diesease*, World Health Organization Regional Office For Europe, Copenhagen, 1987.

128. Whanger, P. D., A country with both selenium deficiency and toxicity: some thoughts and impressions, *J. Nutr.*, 119, 1236, 1989.

129. Xia, Y., Hill, K. E., and Burk, R. F., Biochemical studies of a selenium-deficient population in China: measurement of selenium, glutathione peroxidase and other oxidant defense indices in blood, *J. Nutr.*, 119, 1318, 1989.

130. Kaller, L. D. and Exon, J. H., The two faces of selenium-deficiency and toxicity - are similar in animals and man, *Can. J. Vet. Res.*, 50, 297, 1986.

131. Ursini, F., Maiorino, M., and Gregolin, C., The selenoenzyme phospholipid hydroperoxidase glutathione peroxidase, *Biochem. Biophys. Acta*, 839, 62, 1985.

132. Arthur, J. R., The role of selenium in thyroid hormone metabolism, *Can. J. Physiol. Pharmacol.*, 69, 1648, 1991.

133. Freake, H. C., Molecular biological approaches to studying trace minerals: why should clinicians care, *J. Am. College Nutr.*, 12, 294, 1993.

134. Kien, C. L. and Ganther, H. E., Manifestations of chronic selenium deficiency in a child receiving total parenteral nutrition, *Am. J. Clin. Nutr.*, 37, 319, 1983.

135. Bettger, W. J., Zinc and selenium, site-specific versus general oxidation, *Can. J. Physiol. Pharmacol.*, 71, 721, 1993.

136. Dworkin, B. M., Selenium deficiency in HIV infection and the acquired immunodeficiency syndrome (AIDS), *Chemico-Biological Interactions*, 91, 181, 1994.

137. Dworkin, B., Rosenthal, W. S., Jankowski, R. H., Gordon, G. G., and Haldea, D., Low blood selenium levels in alcoholics with and without advanced liver disease, Correlations with clinical and nutritional status, *Digest. Dis. Sciences*, 30, 838, 1985.

138. Dutta, S. K., Miller, P. A., Greenberg, L. B., and Levander, O. A., Selenium and acute alcoholism, *Am. J. Clin. Nutr.*, 38, 713, 1983.

139. Baker, S. S., Lerman, R. H., Krey, S. H., Crocker, K. S., Hirsh, E. F., and Cohen, H., Selenium deficiency with total parenteral nutrition: reversal of biochemical and functional abnormalities by selenium supplementation: a case report, *Am. J. Clin. Nutr.*, 38, 769, 1983.

140. Zachara, B. A., Wardak, C., Didkowski, W., Maciag, A., and Marchaluk, E., Changes in blood selenium and glutathione concentrations and glutathione peroxidase activity in human pregnancy, *Gynocol. Obstet. Invest.*, 35, 12, 1993.

141. Avissar, N., Semmon, J. R., Palmer, I. S., and Cohen, H. J., Partial sequence of human plasma glutathione peroxidase and immunologic indentification of milk glutathione peroxidase as the plasma enzyme, *J. Nutr.*, 121, 1243, 1991.

142. Maddipati, K. R., Gasparski, C., and Marnett, L. J., Characterization of the hydroperoxide-reducing activity of human plasma, *Arch. Biochem. Biophys.*, 254, 9, 1987.

143. Takahoshi, K., Avissar, N., Whitin, J., and Cohen, H. J., Purification and characterization of human plasma glutathione peroxidase: a selenoglycoprotein distinct from known cellular enzyme, *Arch. Biochem. Biophys.*, 256, 677, 1987.

144. Tyrala, E. E., Borschel, M. W., and Jacobs, J. R., Selenate fortification of infant formulas improved the selenium status of preterm infants, *Am. J. Clin. Nutr.*, 64, 860, 1996.

Manganese

Converting metric units to International System (SI) units:

ng/mL × 18.2 = nmol/L

nmol/L × 0.0549 = ng/mL

atomic weight: 54.938

Manganese metabolism, requirement, and roles in health and disease were extensively reviewed in 1994.[4,41] The essentiality of manganese has been regularly demonstrated in animal species, but comparable evidence for needs of manganese by the human is very limited.[1-4] A study conducted in 1973 involved one male subject fed a purified diet that provided about 0.35 mg per day of manganese.[5] Over a period of 17 weeks on the diet, his serum manganese concentration fell 55%. He developed dermatitis, hair changes, gastrointestinal symptoms, and weight loss. These symptoms disappeared with manganese supplementation. No measurements were made for manganese concentrations in blood, serum, or other fluids, which may support the existence of a manganese deficiency.

Manganese-dependent enzymes are involved in many areas of metabolism, which includes manganese-dependent superoxide dismutase, pyruvate carboxylase, arginase, glycosyl synthetase, glycosyltransferases, and galactose transferase.[20,30] In animals a manganese deficiency is reflected in impaired growth, skeletal defects, neurological problems, and loss of reproductive capacity. Although manganese participates in numerous enzymatic systems, their measurement has not served as the basis for a functional assessment of manganese nutritional status.[20,30]

Average dietary intake of manganese by adults range from 2.6 to 3.0 mg manganese per day.[24] The RDA considers an intake of 2.0 to 5.0 mg per day of manganese adequate for the adult human.[33] The manganese requirement for adult human may not always be attained as suggested by balance studies and from manganese supplement studies.[1-3,23,24] Although manganese supplements usually increase the serum manganese concentrations, the changes were not sufficient to be used as an indicator of nutritional status of manganese.[23,24] Under conditions where a severely depleted manganese condition was induced by feeding young men a manganese-deficient diet, urinary excretion of manganese was reduced.[3] The few studies conducted to date on manganese metabolism have not established any useful indicators of manganese nutritional status. Several laboratories have reported manganese levels in hair samples.[20,29,34] A wide range of values have been reported suggesting that manganese analyses of hair may be of little assessment value (e.g., 0.18 to 5.46 nmol/g).[20] In a carefully conducted study with 15 subjects, hair was reported to contain 0.26 ± 0.05 micrograms of manganese per gram dry weight.[29] Similar levels of manganese were reported for hair from 1-year-old infants.[34]

As more is known about the manganese-dependent enzymes, functional tests for the assessment of manganese nutritional status may evolve. In this respect, the manganese-depended superoxide dismutase (EC 1.15.1.1.) has been investigated.[37,38] Lymphocyte manganese-dependent superoxide dismutase activity was studied in adult women over a period of 124 days.[23,25] The experimental group received 15 mg of manganese per day. The supplement produced a significant increase in serum manganese concentrations and in lymphocyte manganese-dependent superoxide dismutase activity.[23]

The investigators suggested that lymphocyte manganese-dependent superoxide dismutase activity along with serum manganese concentrations would be useful in monitoring toxicological exposure to manganese.[23] Studies on subjects known to be deficient in manganese will be required to determine whether lymphocyte manganese-dependent superoxide dismutase activity may serve as a functional assessment of manganese deficiency. Lymphocyte manganese-dependent superoxide dismutase activity of eleven healthy women was 1.74 ± 0.14 k U/g protein.[23]

Manganese concentrations of mononuclear blood cells may have potential use as an indicator of manganese nutritional status.[40] Mononuclear blood cell manganese levels fell in 25 patients maintained on total parenteral nutrition, while the manganese levels in whole blood and plasma remained unchanged.[40]

Manganese-dependent superoxide dismutase levels have been measured in serum from human subjects with the use of sensitive ELISA kits (enzyme-linked immunosorbent assay) (Ube Industries ltd., Tokyo; Endogen Inc., Boston, MA)[37,38] The mean serum levels of manganese-dependent superoxide dismutase of healthy male and female subjects were 99.8 ± 24.8 and 88.8 ± 20.8 ng/mL, respectively.[37] The subjects consisted of 207 females and 194 males. Of note, hemolysis of erythrocytes did not effect the serum manganese-dependent superoxide dismutase levels. In contrast, copper-zinc dependent superoxide dismutase levels are influenced by hemolysis as erythrocytes are high in this enzyme.[37,38] Although serum manganese-dependent superoxide levels were markedly increased in patients with acute myocardial infection and with malignant diseases, it remains to be studied whether low levels of the enzyme would occur with a manganese deficiency.

Determination of Manganese

Sample contamination is a serious problem in analyses for manganese. Extreme care must be employed in order to obtain reliable and reproducible values.[7,8,14,19,21,39] Serum levels of manganese can be accurately measured with the use of graphite furnace atomic absorption spectrometry and employing background correction.[7-10,14,15,36] Less than 200 µL of serum or plasma are required. Radiochemical neutron activation analysis has also been successfully applied to serum or plasma.[7,8] Several review articles summarize some of the factors and problems associated with the determination of manganese in biological materials.[20,21] The use of reference materials is essential and are available from the U.S. National Institute of Standards and Technology, Gaithersburg, MD. Other reference materials have been successfully used.[20,21,28] The accompanying tables provides reference values from published documents as to the manganese levels in various biological samples. Because of earlier methodological problems, emphasis has been placed on values reported since 1984 (Tables 108 and 109).

Toxicity of Manganese

Dietary intakes of 8 to 9 mg of manganese per day produced no known toxic effects in the human.[6] Manganese toxicity has been observed only in workers exposed to high levels of manganese in the dust or fumes in the air.[41]

TABLE 108

Literature Values For Manganese Concentrations in Human Biological Samples

Sample	Manganese Values for Normal Human Subjects		References	Year
	Concentration			
	μg/L	nmol/L		
Serum/Plasma				
Males (*n* = 25)	0.59 ± 0.12	10.7 ± 2.2	8, 13,17	1974
Females (*n* = 21)	0.55 ± 0.14	10.0 ± 2.5	8,13,17	1974
Adults (*n* = 9)	0.58 (0.36–0.96)	10.6 (6.6–17.5)	15	1981
Adults (*n* = 46)	0.57 ± 0.13	10.3 ± 2.3	11,12	1986
Men & Women (*n* = 16)	0.57 ± 0.18	10.3 ± 3.3	14	1986
Males (*n* = 20)	1.30 (0.90–1.70)	23.7 (16.4–30.9)	22	1994
Females (*n* = 19)	1.23 (0.90–2.20)	22.4 (16.4–40.0)	22	1994
Women (*n* = 11)	0.95 ± 0.11	17.3 ± 2.0	23	1992
Men (*n* = 19)	0.63 ± 0.15	11.4 ± 2.7	21	1991
Women (*n* = 12)	0.53 ± 0.18	9.7 ± 3.3	21	1991
Men (*n* = 10)	1.06 ± 0.05	19.3 ± 1	24	1990
Adults (*n* = 48)	0.88 ± 0.11	16 ± 2	27	1990
Packed Red Cells				
Adults (*n* = 46)	15.0 ± 4.9	273 ± 89	12	1986
Males (*n* =25)	13.6 ± 3.2	248 ± 58	13	1974
Females (*n* = 21)	16.9 ± 6.0	308 ± 109	13	1974
Adults (*n* = 48)	16.6 ± 1.2	302 ± 22	27	1990
Whole Blood				
Adults (*n* = 48)	10.9 ± 10.9	198 ± 11	27	1990
Adults (*n* = 31)	11.2 ± 4.6	204 ± 84	40	1994
Males (*n* = 19)	9.0 (7.5–11.3)	164 (136–206)	22	1994
Women (*n* = 19)	9.7 (7.0–13.7)	177 (127–249)	22	1994
Children (*n* = 42)	8.5 (7.7–9.4)	155 (140–172)	31	1989
0-12 mon. (*n* = 44)	16.9 ± 0.58	308 ± 10.6	32	1985
13 mon.-17 yr. (*n* = 76)	14.4 ± 0.40	262 ± 25	32	1985
Pregnancy				
Whole Blood (*n* = 20)				
Trimester:				
I	7.4 (4.3–14.7)	135 (79–268)	36	1993
II	9.4 (6.0–22.4)	171 (109–408)	36	1993
III	13.1 (7.3–21.0)	238 (133–383)	36	1992
Blood Components				
Platelets (*n* = 48)	0.054 ± 0.021 nmol/10⁹ cells		27	1990
Mononuclear cells	8.84 ± 4.18 ng/10⁸ cells		40	1990
Leukocytes				
Mononucleated	6.75 ± 2.48 nmol/10⁹ cells		27	1990
Polynucleated	6.53 ± 2.42 nmol/10⁹ cells		27	1990
Human Milk (*n* = 8)				
1st month	6.6 ± 4.7	120 ± 86	26	1984
3rd month	3.5 ± 1.4	64 ± 25	26	1984
1st month (*n* = 11)	4.1 ± 1.6	75 ± 29	18	1985
Urine				
Adult Men (*n* = 10)	7.0 ± 0.5 nmol Mn/g creatinine		24	1990
Adult Women (*n* = 11)	10.6 ± 1.9 nmol Mn/d		23	1992

n = number of subjects studied.

TABLE 109
Manganese-Dependent Superoxide Dismutase Levels in the Human

Sample	Concentration (ng/mL)	References	Year
Serum			
Adult males (n = 194)	99.8 ± 24.8	37	1990
Adult females (n = 204)	88.8 ± 20.8	37	1990
Males and females (n = 28)	102.6 ± 3.7	38	1991
Lymphocytes			
Women (47)	1.85 ± 0.16 U/g protein	23	1992

n = number of subjects studied.

Summary

Further studies may establish if changes in manganese-dependent dismutase (Mn SOD) activity values may serve as means of monitoring manganese exposure in the human. Further studies are also needed to determine whether low manganese concentrations in blood, serum or erythrocytes may serve to evaluate manganese nutritional status. Similarly, low lymphocyte manganese-dependent superoxide dismutase activity may prove useful in assessing manganese status. Analyses for manganese require recognition of contamination problems and the need for suitable analytical equipment and reference standards. At present, no established method is available for assessing manganese nutritional status in the human.

References

1. Freeland-Graves, J. H., Bales, C. W., and Behmardi, F., Manganese requirements of humans, in *Nutritional Bioavailability of Manganese*, Kies, C., Eds., American Chemical Society, Washington D.C., 1987.
2. Freeland-Graves, J. H., Behamardi, F., Bales, C. W., Dougherty, V., Lin, P.-H., Crosby, J. B., and Trickett, P. C., Metabolic balance of manganese in young men consuming diets containing five levels of dietary manganese, *J. Nutr.*, 118, 764, 1988.
3. Friedman, B. J., Freedland-Graves, J. H., Bales, C. W., Behmardi, R. L., Shorey-Kutschke, R. L., Willis, R. A., Crosby, J. B., Trickett, P. C., and Houston, S. D., Manganese balance and clinical observations in young men fed a manganese-deficient diet, *J. Nutr.*, 117, 133, 1987.
4. Manganese in Health and Disease, Klimis-Tavantzis, D. J., Eds., CRC Press, Boca Raton, FL, 1994.
5. Doisy, E. A. Jr., Effects of deficiency in manganese upon plasma levels of clotting proteins and cholesterol in man, in *Trace Element Metabolism in Animals*. II. Hoekstra, W. G., Suttie, J. W., Ganther, H. E., and Mertz, W., Eds., University Park Press, Baltimore, MD, 1974, 668.
6. WHO (World Health Organization), Trace elements in human nutrition, Report of a WHO Expert Committee, *WHO Technical Report Series No. 532*, World Health Organization, Geneva, Switzerland, 1973.
7. Versiek, J. and Cornelis, R., *Trace Elements in Plasma or Serum*, CRC Press, Boca Raton, FL, 1989.
8. Versiek, J., Barbier, F., Speecke, A., and Hoste, J., Normal manganese concentrations in human serum, *Acta Endocrinol.*, 76, 783, 1974.

9. Tsalev, D. L. and Zaprianov, Z.K., *Atomic Absorption Spectrometry in Occupational and Environmental Health Practice*, Vols. I and II, CRC Press, Boca Raton, FL, 1983.

10. Welz, B., *Atomic Absorption Spectrometry*, 2nd edition,Verlag Chemie, Deerfield Beach, FL, 1985.

11. Wallaeys, B., Cornelis, R., Meer, L., and Lameire, N., Trace elements in patients with renal insufficiency on continuous ambulatory peritoneal dialysis, *Acta Pharmacol. Toxicol.*, 59 (Suppl. 7), 435, 1986.

12. Wallaeys, B., Cornelis, R., and Lameire, N., Trace elements in serum, packed cells, and dialysate of CAPD patients, *Kidney Int.*, 30, 599, 1986.

13. Versieck, J., Barbier, F., Speecke, A., and Hoste, J., Manganese, copper, and zinc concentrations in serum and packed blood cells during acute hepatitis, chronic hepatitis, and posthepatic cirrhosis, *Clin. Chem.*, 20, 1141, 1974.

14. Ericson, S. P., McHalsky, M. L, Rabinow, B. E., Kronholm, K. G., Arceo, C. S., Weltzier, J. A., and Ayd, S. W., Sampling and analysis techniques for monitoring serum for trace elements, *Clin. Chem.*, 32, 1350, 1986.

15. Halls, D. J. and Fell, G. S., Determination of manganese in serum and urine by electrothermal atomic absorption spectrometry, *Anal. Chim. Acta.*, 129, 205, 1981.

16. McLeod, B. F. and Robinson, M. F., Dietary intake of manganese by New Zealand infants during the first six months of life, *Br. J. Nutr.*, 27, 229, 1972.

17. Versieck, J. and Cornelis, R., Normal levels of trace elements in human blood plasma or serum, *Anal. Chim. Acta*, 116, 217, 1980.

18. Casey, C. E., Hambidge, K. M., and Neville, M., Studies in human lactation: zinc, copper, manganese, and chromium in human milk in the first month of lactation, *Am. J. Clin. Nutr.*, 41, 1193, 1985.

19. Versieck, J., Trace element analysis — a plea for accuracy, *Trace Element Med.*, 1, 1, 1984.

20. Baruthio, F., Guillard, O., Arnaud, J., Pierre, F., and Zawislak, R., Determination of manganese in biological materials by electrothermal atomic absorption spectrometry: a review, *Clin. Chem.*, 34, 227, 1988.

21. Neve, J. and Leclercq, N., Factors affecting determinations of manganese in serum by atomic absorption spectrometry, *Clin. Chem.*, 37, 723, 1991.

22. Finley, J. W., Johnson, P. E., and Johnson, L. K., Sex affects manganese absorption and retention by humans from a diet adequate in manganese, *Am. J. Clin. Nutr.*, 60, 949, 1994.

23. Davis, C. D. and Greger, J. L., Longitudinal changes of manganese-dependent superoxide dismutase and other indexes of manganese and iron status in women, *Am. J. Clin. Nutr.*, 55, 747, 1992.

24. Greger, J. L., Davis, C. D., Suttie, J.W., and Lyle, B. J., Intake, serum concentrations, and urinary excretion of manganese by adult males, *Am. J. Clin. Nutr.*, 51, 457, 1990.

25. Marklund, S. and Marklund, G., Involvement of the superoxide anion in the autoxidation of pyrogallol and a convenient assay for superoxide dismutase, *Eur. J. Biochem.*, 47, 469, 1974.

26. Stastny, D, Vogel, R. D., and Picciano, M. F., Manganese intake and serum manganese concentrations of human milk-fed and formula-fed infants, *Am. J. Clin. Nutr.*, 39, 872, 1984.

27. Milne, D. B., Sims, R. L., and Ralson, N. V. C., Manganese content of the cellular components of blood, *Clin. Chem.*, 36, 450, 1990.

28. Versieck, J., Vanballenberghe, L., DeKessel, A., Certification of a second-generation biological reference material (freeze-dried human serum) for trace element determinations, *Anal. Chim. Acta*, 204, 63, 1988.

29. Guillard, O., Brugier, J. C., Piriou, A., Menard, M., Gombert, J., and Reiss, D. Improved determination of manganese in hair by use of a mini-autoclave and flameless atomic absorption spectrometry with Zeeman background correction: an evaluation in unexposed subjects, *Clin. Chem.*, 30, 1642, 1984.

30. Sorenson, J. R. J., Soderberg, L. S. F., and Chang, L. W., Radiation protection and radiation recovery with essential metalloelement chelates, *Proc. Soc. Expt. Biol. Med.*, 210, 191, 1995.

31. Hall, A. J., Margetts, B. M., Barker, D. J. P., Walsh, H. P. J., Redfern, T. R., Taylor, J. F., Dangerfield, P., Delves, H. T., and Shuttler, I. L., Low blood manganese levels in Liverpool children with Perthes' disease, *Paediatr. Perinat. Epidemiol.*, 3, 131,1989.

32. Dupont, C. L. and Tanaka, Y., Blood manganese levels in children with convulsion disorders, *Biochem. Med.*, 33, 246, 1985.

33. National Research Council, *Recommended Dietary Allowance*, National Academy of Sciences, 10th edition, Washington D.C., 1989.

34. Friel, J. K., Gibson, R. S., Balassa, R., and Watts, J. L., A comparison of the zinc, copper, and manganese status of very low birth pre-term and full-term infants during the first twelve months, *Acta Paediatr. Scand.*, 73, 596, 1984.

35. Johnson, H. L. and Sauberlich, H. E., Trace element analyses in biological samples, in *Clinical, Biochemical, and Nutritional Aspects of Trace Elements*, Prasad, A. S., Ed., Alan Liss, Inc., New York, 1982, 405.

36. Tholin, K., Palm, R., Hallmans, G., and Sandetrom, B., Manganese status during pregnancy, *Ann. N.Y. Acad. Sci.*, 678, 359, 1993.

37. Kawaguchi, T., Suzuki, K., Matsuda, Y., Nishiura, T., Uda, T., Ono, M., Sekiya, C., Ishikawa, M., Iino, S., Endo, Y., and Taniguchi, N., Serum-manganese-superoxide dismutase: normal values and increased levels in patients with acute myocardial infraction and several malignant diseases determined by an enzyme-linked immunosorbent assay using a monoclonal antibody, *J. Immunol. Meth.*, 127, 249, 1990.

38. Ohno, H., Matsuura, N., Ishikawa, M., Sato, Y., Endo, Y., and Taniguchi, N., Serum manganese-superoxide dismutase in patients with diabetes mellitus and thyroid-dysfunction as judged by an ELISA, *Horm. Metab. Res.*, 23, 449, 1991.

39. Allain, P., Mauras, Y., and Grangeray, C., The determination of acid precipitation for manganese determination in human whole blood, *Annu. Clin. Biochem.*, 24, 518, 1987.

40. Matsuda, A., Kimura, M., Takeda, T., Katsoka, M., Sato, M., and Itokawa, Y., Changes in manganese content of mononuclear blood cells in patients receiving total parenteral nutrition, *Clin. Chem.*, 40, 829, 1994.

41. Greger, J. L. and Malecki, E. A., Manganese: how do we know our limits? *Nutrition Today*, 32, 116, 1997.

Chromium

Converting metric units to International System (SI) units:

ng/mL × 19.306 = nmol/L

nmol/L × 0.052 = ng/mL

atomic weight: 51.996

Chromium is an essential trace mineral.[3,5,12] Evidence for this has been summarized in a number of reviews.[12,15-18,28,37,39] In the human, a deficiency of chromium may result in increased plasma LDL-cholesterol levels, impaired glucose and amino acid utilization, and peripheral neuropathy.[2,6-8,16-18] The use of trivalent chromium has been effective in the treatment of pronounced chromium deficiency.[2,4,9] Subsequently, other studies have reported that mild diabetics and other individuals with hypoglycemia or impaired glucose tolerance respond to chromium administration.[1,9,12,28,31,32]

Dietary studies of adult subjects in the U.S. indicate that their chromium intakes are below the minimum safe and adequate chromium intake (50 to 200 µg/day) suggested by the RDA.[4,14,21] Hence, there has been a need for laboratory procedures that may determine whether or not an inadequate chromium nutritional status exists.

At present, there is no satisfactory test to diagnose a chromium deficiency. Since glucose intolerance can result from a chromium deficiency, an improved response in glucose tolerance to chromium treatment has been used as an indicator of chromium deficiency.[15] For such a response test, 5 g or 10 g/day of brewer's yeast (a rich source of chromium) or 200 µg/day of trivalent chromium (Cr Cl$_3$) have been used.[27,31]

Blood and urine chromium measurements have been conducted as a possible means of identifying a chromium deficiency. However, these measurements have been difficult to perform.[24,26,35,36] Only a limited number of laboratories have the specialized techniques to conduct accurate chromium measurements. Consequently, the measurements have had only a limited ability to identify a nutritional deficit of chromium in the human. Only 200 µL of serum is required for a chromium analysis.[36]

Schemaier et al. determined chromium in whole blood serum by Zeeman electrothermal atomic absorption spectrophotometer.[24] They found the mean chromium levels in whole blood and serum from apparently healthy individuals to be 0.371 µg/L (n = 37) for whole blood and 0.130 µg/L (n = 19) for serum. Anderson et al. determined the serum concentration of chromium in adult males (n = 48) and females (n = 28) by graphite furnace atomic absorption.[10] A chromium level of 0.13 ± 0.02 µg/L of serum was found. No differences were noted between males and females.

A group of Canadian men (n = 52) were found to have serum chromium concentrations of 0.15 µg/L (range 0.12 to 0.20).[29] Plasma chromium levels of healthy elderly individuals were not different from those of young adults.[30] The average concentration of chromium in human milk has been reported to be 0.27 ± 0.10 ng/mL.[34]

Urinary excretion of chromium has not been established as a means of evaluating chromium nutritional status.[4,10,13,19,22] The average daily urinary excretion of chromium for adult males and females was the same (0.19 ± 0.01 µg). Urinary chromium did not appear to be a useful indicator of chromium nutritional status, but maybe a useful indicator of chromium intake.[13] In general, the daily urinary chromium excretion was relatively constant regardless of intake.[4,13] Earlier studies with less reliable procedures reported considerably higher 24-hour urinary chromium excretion levels by normal subjects (e.g., 0.8 to 150 µg/day).[13]

Determination of Chromium

Serum chromium can be determined by electrothermal or graphite furnace atomic absorption.[10,11,20,24,26,33,35] Extreme care must be employed to avoid contamination.[11,20,24,25,35] Even blood collecting tubes must be established as free of chromium.[24] Consequently early observations are unreliable with elevated and variable levels of serum or plasma chromium reported.[10,11,12,20] Levels reported before 1980 must be regarded with suspect and probably should not be accepted.[12] With a recognition of contamination problems, the availability of improved analytical methods, and the use of certified quality controls, reliable chromium analyses of serum and urine are now possible.[18,20,35] Certified standard reference materials (SRM) are available from the National Institute of Standards and Technology, Gaithersburg, MD (Table 110).

TABLE 110
Reference Values For Chromium Concentrations

	Chromium Values For Normal Human Subjects			
	Concentrations			
Sample	µg/L	nmol/L	References	Year
Serum/Plasma				
Males (*n* = 48)	0.13 ± 0.02	2.50 ± 0.38	13	1985
Females (*n* = 28)	0.13 ± 0.02	2.50 ± 0.38	13	1985
Adults (*n* = 19)	0.13 ± 0.08	2.50 ± 1.54	24	1985
Elderly (*n* = 23)	0.27 ± 0.08	5.19 ± 1.54	27	1985
Adults (*n* = 16)	0.19 ± 0.07	3.65 ± 1.35	36	1986
Men (*n* = 52)	0.15 (0.12–0.20)	2.89 (2.31–3.85)	29	1987
Human Milk				
(*n* = 9)	0.27 ± 0.10	5.19 ± 1.92	34	1985
Urine				
Females (*n* = 15)	0.20 ± 0.03	3.85 ± 0.58	13	1983
Males (*n* = 27)	0.17 ± 0.02	3.27 ± 0.38	13	1983
Adults (*n* = 32)	0.19 ± 0.01	3.65 ± 0.19	4	1985

n = is the number of subjects studied.

Toxicity of Chromium

Trivalent chromium, the form present in diets, is considered safe with no harmful effects recognized.[2] Rats fed diets containing 100 mg/kg of chromium demonstrated no toxicity.[1] Absorbed chromium is readily excreted in the urine.[4] However, the safety of long-term use of chromium supplements has been questioned and may need further study.[23,38]

Summary

Satisfactory measurements to evaluate chromium nutritional status are not available. Serum, plasma, and urine concentrations of chromium have been studied, often in conjunction with glucose loads, but the results are difficult to interpret and apply to the assessments of chromium status. Analyses for chromium require the recognition of contamination problems and the need for suitable analytical equipment and reference standards.

References

1. IPCS (International Programme on Chemical Safety), Chromium, *Environmental Health Criteria*, 61, World Health Organization, Geneva, Switzerland, 1988.
2. Glinsmann, W. H. and Mertz, W., Effect of trivalent chromium on glucose tolerance, *Metabolism*, 15, 510, 1966.
3. Mertz, W., Chromium occurrence and function in biological systems, *Physiol. Rev.*, 49, 163, 1969.
4. Anderson R. A. and Kozlovsky, A. D., Chromium intake, absorption, and excretion of subjects consuming self-selected diets, *Am. J. Clin. Nutr.*, 41, 1177, 1985.
5. Schroeder, H. A., Chromium deficiency in rats: a syndrome simulating diabetes mellitus with retarded growth, *J. Nutr.*, 88, 439, 1966.
6. Jeejeebhoy, K. N., Chu, R. C., Marlis, E. B., Greenberg, G. R., and Bruce-Robertson, A., Chromium deficiency, glucose intolerance and neuropathy reversed by chromium supplementation in a patient receiving long-term total parental nutrition. *Am. J. Clin. Nutr.*, 30, 531, 1977.
7. Freund, H., Atamian, S., and Fischer, J. E., Chromium deficiency during total parental nutrition, *J. Am. Med. Assoc.*, 241, 496, 1979.
8. Brown, R. O., Forloines-Lynn, S., Cross, R. E., and Heizer, W. D., Chromium deficiency after long-term total parental nutrition, *Dig. Dis. Sci.*, 31, 661, 1986.
9. Anderson, R. A., Polansky, M. M., Bryden, N. A., Roginski, E. E., Mertz, W., and Glinsmann, W. H., Chromium supplementation of human subjects: effects on glucose, insulin and lipid variables, *Metabolism*, 32, 894, 1983.
10. Anderson, R. A., Bryden, N. A., and Polansky, M. M., Serum chromium of human subjects: effect of chromium supplementation and glucose, *Am. J. Clin. Nutr.*, 41, 571, 1985.
11. Veillon, C., Patterson, K. Y., and Bryden, N. A., Determination of chromium in human serum by electrothermal atomic absorption spectrometry, *Am. Clin. Acta*, 164, 67, 1984.
12. Mertz, W., Chromium in human nutrition: a review, *J. Nutr.*, 123, 626, 1993.
13. Anderson, R. A., Polansky, M. M., Bryden, N. A., Patterson, K. Y., Veillon, C., and Glinsmann, W. H., Effects of chromium supplementation on urinary Cr excretion of human subjects and correlation of Cr excretion with selected clinical parameters, *J. Nutr.*, 113, 276, 1983.
14. National Research Council, *Recommended Dietary Allowances*, 10th edition, National Academy of Sciences, Washington D.C., 1989.
15. Clinical Nutrition Cases, Is chromuim essential for humans, *Nutr. Rev.*, 46, 17, 1988.
16. Wallach, S., Clinical and biochemical aspects of chromium deficiency, *J. Am. Coll. Nutr.*, 4, 107, 1985.
17. Borel, J. S. and Anderson, R. A., Chromium, *Biochemistry of the Essential Ultratrace Elements*, Chapter 8, Frieden, E., Ed., Plenum Publications, New York, 1984, 175.
18. Anderson, R. A., Chromium metabolism and its role in disease processes in man, *Clin. Physiol. Biochem.*, 4, 31, 1986.
19. Veillon, C., Patterson, K. Y., and Bryden, N. A., Direct determination of chromium in human urine by electrothermal atomic absorption spectrometry, *Anal. Chim. Acta*, 136, 233, 1982.

20. Versieck, J. and Cornelis, R., *Trace Elements in Human Plasma or Serum*, CRC Press, Boca Raton, FL, 1989.

21. Anderson, R. A., Bryden, N. A., and Polansky, M. M., Dietary chromium intake: freely chosen diets, institutional diets, and individual foods, *Biol. Trace Element Res.*, 32, 117, 1992.

22. Anderson, R. A., Polansky, M. M., Bryden, N. A., Roginski, E. E., Patterson, K. K., Veillon, C., and Glinsmann, W., Urinary chromium excretion of human subjects: effects of chromium supplementation and glucose loading, *Am. J. Clin. Nutr.*, 36, 1184, 1982.

23. Stearns, D. M., Belbruno, J. J., and Wetterhahn, K. E., A prediction of chromium (III) accumulation in humans from chromium dietary supplements, *FASEB J.*, 9, 1650, 1995.

24. Schermaier, A. J., O'Connor, L. H., and Pearson, K. H., Semi-automated determination of chromium in whole blood and serum by Zeeman electrothermal atom is absorption spectrophotometry, *Clin. Chim. Acta.*, 152, 123, 1985.

25. Versieck, J. and Cornelis, R., Normal levels of trace metals in human plasma or serum. *Anal. Chim. Acta*, 116, 217, 1980.

26. Veillon, C., Analytical chemistry of chromium. *Sci. Total Environ.*, 86, 65, 1989.

27. Offenbacher, E. G., Rinko, C. J., and Pi-Sunyer, F. X., The effects of inorganic chromium and brewer's yeast on glucose tolerance, plasma lipids, and plasma chromium in elderly subjects, *Am. J. Clin. Nutr.*, 42, 454, 1985.

28. Anderson, R. A., Essentiality of chromium in humans. *Sci. Total Environment*, 86, 75, 1989.

29. Randall, J. A. and Gibson, R. S., Serum and urine chromium as indices of chromium status in tannery workers, *Proc. Soc. Extl. Bio. Med.*, 185, 16, 1987.

30. Offenbacher, E. G., Chromium in the elderly, *Biol. Trace Element Res.*, 32, 123, 1992.

31. Anderson, R. A., Polansky, M. M., Bryden, N. A., Bhathena, S. J., and Canary, J. J., Effects of supplemental chromium on patients with symptoms of reactive hypoglycemia, *Metabolism*, 36, 351, 1987.

32. Martinez, O. B., MacDonald, A. C., Gibson, R. S., and Bourne, D., Dietary chromium and effect of chromium supplementation on glucose tolerance of elderly Canadian women, *Nutr. Res.*, 5, 609, 1985.

33. Granadaillo, V. A., Parra de Machado, L., and Romero, R. A., Determination of total chromium in whole blood, blood components, bone, and urine by fast furnace program electrothermal atomization AAS and using neither analyte information nor background correction, *Anal. Chem.*, 66, 3624, 1994.

34. Casey, C. E., Hambidge, K. M., and Neville, M. C., Studies in human lactation: zinc, copper, manganese and chromium in human milk in the first month of lactation, *Am. J. Clin. Nutr.*, 41, 1193, 1985.

35. Christensen, J. M., Holst, E., Bonde, J. P., and Knudsen, L., Determination of chromium in blood and serum: evaluation of quality control procedures and estimation of reference values in Dutch subjects, *Sci. Total Environment*, 132, 11, 1993.

36. Ericson, S. P., McHalsky, M. L. Rabinow, B. E., Kronholm, K. G., Arceo, C. S., Weltzer, J. A., and Ayd, S. W., Sampling and analysis techniques for monitoring serum for trace elements, *Clin. Chem.*, 32, 1350, 1986.

37. Offenbacher, E. G. and Pi-Sunyer, F. X., Chromium in human nutrition, *Annu. Rev. Nutr.*, 8, 543, 1988.

38. Lukaski, H. C., Bolonchuk, W. W., Siders, W. A., and Milne, D. B., Chromium supplementation and resistance training: effects on body composition, strength, and trace element status of men, *Am. J. Clin. Nutr.*, 63, 954, 1996.

39. Nielsen, F., Controversial chromium, *Nutrition Today*, 31, 226, 1996.

Molybdenum

Converting metric units to International System (SI) units:

ng/mL × 10.42 = nmol/L

nmol/L × 0.0959 = ng/mL

atomic weight: 95.94

Molybdenum is an essential nutrient for animals, but its importance in human health has been uncertain, since a molybdenum deficiency in the human has seldom been recognized.[1-3] Nevertheless, molybdenum is a component of the metalloenzymes aldehyde oxidase, xanthine oxidase, and sulfite oxidase. These enzymes also contain iron.[1-3,5-7,22-25]

Xanthine oxidase (EC 1.2.1.37) is required for the terminal oxidation of purines for the formation uric acid; aldehyde oxidase (EC 1.2.3.1) acts on a wide spectrum of compounds, including aldehydes; and sulfite oxidase (EC 1.8.2.1) is necessary for the metabolism of sulfur to sulfate to enable its excretion. Absence of the sulfite oxidase is lethal, while the absences of xanthine oxidase and aldehyde oxidase are relatively benign.[26]

Human investigations on molybdenum deficiency and metabolism have been difficult to conduct because of the inability to formulate diets with a low content of the element along with its apparent low daily requirement.[13] However, subsequent studies have established molybdenum as an essential trace element for the human.[1-3,10]

For example, prolonged use of total parenteral nutrition in a patient with an acquired short bowel syndrome developed clinical symptoms that were associated with laboratory findings that included hypouricemia, hypouricosuria, hypermethioninemia, and exceedingly low excretion of inorganic sulfate in the urine.[1-3,10] Molybdate treatment improved the clinical condition, suggesting a diet-induced molybdenum deficiency.[10] Subsequently a number of patients with a genetic deficiency of molybdenum-containing enzymes has established the essentiality of molybdenum for the human.[1,2,5] The condition is usually the result of a deficiency in the molybdenum cofactors.[17-19,22-25] At least 47 patients have been identified with molybdenum cofactor deficiency.[26]

Determination of Molybdenum

Reports on the molybdenum levels in serum and other biological specimens are limited.[4,8,9] Molybdenum measurements are performed with the use of atomic absorption spectrophotometry and atomic emission spectrometry.[4] These procedures provide for the sensitivity required to measure the low levels of molybdenum present in biological samples. Earlier reported values for molybdenum are open to question because of unreliable analytical methods and contamination problems.[9] The failure to use quality controls and certified reference standards further complicated the interpretation of these studies.

Molybdenum is conserved at low intakes but is rapidly excreted in the urine when the intake is high.[13,14] Urinary levels of molybdenum could possibly serve as an indicator of low as well as high intakes of molybdenum.[14,15] Table 111 lists some published reference values for molybdenum levels in plasma, serum, and human milk.

TABLE 111
Reference Values For Molybdenum Concentrations

Molybdenum Values For Normal Human Subjects				
	Concentrations			
Sample	µg/L	nmol/L	References	Year
Serum (n = 24)	0.8 ± 0.2	8.34 ± 2.1	4	1986
Serum (n = 30)	0.58 ± 0.21	6.04 ± 2.19	9	1979
(no difference between men and women)	0.28–1.17	2.92–2.19		
Plasma (n = 7)	0.59 ± 0.23	6.15 ± 2.40	8	1979
Human Milk (n = 13)				
Day 1 (n = 13)	15.0 ± 6.1	156.3 ± 63.6	16	1987
Day 30 (n = 13)	1–2	10–20	16	1987
Day 5 (n = 6)	10.2 ± 3.7	106.2 ± 38.5	21	1988
Day 30 (n = 6)	2.6 ± 2.2	27.1 ± 22.9	21	1988

Molybdenum Cofactor Deficiency

Molybdenum cofactor deficiency as associated with an inborn error of metabolism would appear not to be associated with a dietary deficiency of molybdenum. Subjects placed on low molybdenum (22 µg/day) diets for over 100 days exhibited no clinical symptoms of a deficiency other than the urinary excretion of molybdenum fell.[14] Of interest, in the metabolism of molybdenum cofactor urothione is produced and excreted in the urine.[26] Molybdenum cofactor deficient patients excrete little if any urothione.[25,26] Normal subjects excrete from 50 to 600 ng/mg creatinine.[26] Whether a dietary deficiency of molybdenum would relate to the urinary excretion levels of urothione remains to be investigated. Urothione can be measured by HPLC chromatography.[26]

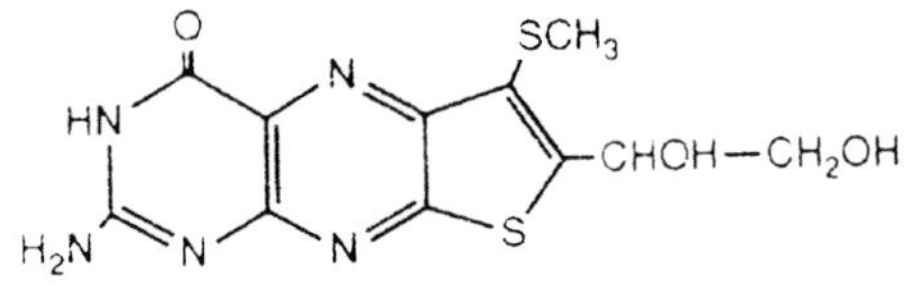

FIGURE 59
Structure of urothione.

Although measurement of the products or substrates of the molybdenum requiring enzyme in the blood or urine may be useful in diagnosing these rare genetic disorders (inborn error of metabolism), their use in the recognition of a dietary deficiency of molybdenum remains unknown.

In a study with premature infants, a significant correlation was observed for urine molybdenum levels and molybdenum intakes as well as for plasma molybdenum levels and uric acid excretion.[20]

Toxicity

In high amounts, molybdenum is toxic (e.g., >100 mg/kg food).[1,27] This was observed early in cattle grazing on pastures growing on high molybdenum soils. This involved an antagonism of molybdenum to copper since supplements of copper are usually beneficial.[1,27] In the human, high dietary intakes of molybdenum have been associated with soils high in molybdenum and may relate to the high incidence of gout observed in these areas.[1,27] Blood levels of molybdenum as high as 170 ng/mL have been reported in subjects from these regions. Surveys indicate that in the United States the daily intake of molybdenum normally ranges between 50 and 350 µg (0.52–3.65 µmol).[11-13] Dietary intakes between 22 and 1500 µg/d by adult men were considered safe.[13]

Summary

Although molybdenum has been established as an essential nutrient, the occurrence of a deficiency of the element is highly unlikely in view of its normal abundance in the diet.

No established method is available for the assessment of a molybdenum nutritional status, but several possibilities exist for investigation.

The measurement of molybdenum is difficult to perform and requires extremely careful laboratory techniques to avoid contamination. In addition, the use of quality controls and certified reference materials is essential in order to obtain reliable results.[28]

References

1. Rajagopalan, K. V., Molybenum: an essential trace element in human nutrition, *Annu. Rev. Nutr.*, 8, 401, 1988.
2. Rajagopalan, K. V., Molybdenum: an essential element, *Nutr. Rev.*, 45, 321, 1987.
3. Anonymous, Molybdenum deficiency in TPN, *Nutr. Rev.*, 45, 337, 1987.
4. Ericson, S. P., McHalsky, M. L., Rabinow, B. E., Kronholm, K. G., Areco, C. S., Weltzer, J. A, and Ayd, S. W., Sampling and analysis techniques for monitoring serum for trace elements, *Clin. Chem.*, 32, 1350, 1986.
5. Nielsen, F. H., Ultratrace elements, in *Modern Nutrition in Health and Disease*, Shils, M. E., Olsen, J. A., and Shike, M., Eds., 8th edition, Lea and Febiger, Philadelphia, 1994, 269.
6. Richert, D. A. and Westerfield, W. W., Isolation and identification of the xanthine oxidase cofactor as molybdenum, *J. Biol. Chem.*, 203, 915, 1953.
7. DeRenzo, E. C., Kaleita, E., Heytler, P. G., Oleson, J. J., Hutchings, B. L., and Williams, J. H., Identification of the xanthine oxidase factor as molybdenum, *Arch. Biochem. Biophys.*, 45, 247, 1953.
8. Kasperek, K., Lyenar, G. V., Kiem, J., Borberg, H., and Fernendegen, L. E., Elemental composition of Platelets, Part III, Determination of Ag, Au, Cd, Co, Cr, Cs, Mo, Rb, Sb, and Se in normal human platelets by neutron activation analysis, *Clin. Chem.*, 25, 711, 1979.
9. Versieck, J., Hoste, J., Barbier, F., Vanballenberghe, L., deRudder, J., and Cornelis, R., Determination of molybdenum in human serum be neutron activation analyses, *Clin. Chim. Acta*, 87, 135, 1978.

10. Abumrad, N. N., Schneider, A. J., Steel, D., and Rogers, L. S., Amino acid intolerance during prolonged total parenteral nutrition reversed by molybdate therapy, *Am. J. Clin. Nutr.*, 34, 2551, 1981.

11. Tsongas, T. A., Meglen, R. R., Walravens, P. A., and Chappell, W. R., Molybdenum in the diet: an estimate of average daily intake of the United States, *Am. J. Clin. Nutr.*, 33, 1103, 1980.

12. Pennington, J. A. T. and Jones, J. W., Molybdenum, nickel, cobalt, vanadium, and strontium in total diets, *J. Am. Diet. Assoc.*, 87, 1644, 1987.

13. Turnlund, J. R., Keyes, W. R., and Peiffer, G. L., Molybdenum absorption, excretion, and retention studied with stable isotopes in young men at five dietary intakes of dietary molybdenum, *Am. J. Clin. Nutr.*, 62, 790, 1995.

14. Turnland, J. R., Keyes, W. R., Peiffer, G. L., and Chiang, G., Molybdenum absorption, excretion, and retention studied with stable isotopes in young men during depletion and repletion, *Am. J. Clin. Nutr.*, 61, 1102, 1995.

15. Thompson, K. H. and Turnlund, J. R., Kinetic model of molybdenum metabolism developed from dual stable isotope excretion in men consuming a low molybdenum diet, *J. Nutr.*, 126, 963, 1996.

16. Casey, C. E. and Neville, M. C., Studies in human lactation. III. Molybdenum and nickel in human milk during the first month of lactation, *Am. J. Clin. Nutr.*, 45, 921, 1987.

17. Johnson, J. L., Wuebbens, M. M., Mandell, R., and Shih, V. E., Molybdenum cofactor biosynthesis in humans, *J. Clin. Invest.*, 83, 897, 1989.

18. Bakker, H. D., Abeling, N. G. G. M., ten Houten, R., van den Blij, J. F., Overweg-Plandsoen, W. C. G., Wanders, R. J. A., and van Genmjs, A. H., Molybdenum cofactor deficiency can mimic postanoxic encephalopathy, *J. Inher. Metab. Dis.*, 16, 900, 1993.

19. Arnold, G. L., Greene, C. L., Stout, J. P., and Goodman, S. I., Molybdenum cofactor deficiency, *J. Pediatr.*, 123, 595, 1993.

20. Bougle, D., Foucault, D., Voirin, J., Bureau, F., and Duhamel, J. F., Molybdenum in the premature infant, *Biol. Neonate*, 59, 201, 1991.

21. Bougle, D., Bureau, F., Faucault, P., Duhamel, J. F., Muller, G., and Drosdowsky, M., Molybdenum content of term and preterm human milk during the first 2 months of lactation, *Am. J. Clin. Nutr.*, 48, 652, 1988.

22. Roth, A., Nogues, C., Monnet, J. P., Ogier, H., and Saudubray, J. M., Anatomo-pathological findings in a case of combined deficiency of sulfite oxidase and xanthine oxidase with a defect of molybdenum cofactors, *Virchows Archiw (Pathol. Anat.)*, 405, 379, 1985.

23. Gray, R. G. F., Green, A., Basu, S. N., Constantine, G., Condie, R. G., Dorche, C., Vianey-Liaud, C., and Desjacques, P., Antenatal diagnosis of molybdenum cofactor deficiency, *Am. J. Ostet. Gynecol.*, 163, 1203, 1990.

24. Johnson, J. L., Waud, W. R., Rajagopalan, K. V., Duran, M., Beemer, F. A., and Wadman, S. K., Inborn errors of molybdenum metabolism: combined deficiencies of sulfite oxidase and xanthine dehydrogenase in a patient lacking the molybdenum cofactor, *Proc. Natl. Acad. Sci. USA*, 77, 3715, 1980.

25. Johnson, J. L., Wuebbens, M. M., Mandell, R., and Shih, V. E., Molybdenum cofactor deficiency in a patient previously characterized as deficient in sulfite oxidase, *Biochem. Med. Metab. Biol.*, 40, 86, 1988.

26. Johnson, J. L., Rajagopalan, K. V., and Wadman, S. K., Human molybdenum cofactor deficiency, in *Chemistry and Biology of Pteridines and Folates*, Plenum Press, New York, 1993, 373.

27. Mills, C. F. and Davis, G. K., Molybdenum, in *Trace Elements in Human and Animal Nutrition*, Vol. 1, 5th edition, Mertz, W., Ed., Academic Press, Orlando, FL, 1987, 429.

28. Environmental Health: *Trace Elements In Human Health and Disease*, Grandjean, P., Ed., Series No. 26, World Health Organization, Copenhagen, Denmark, 1987.

Arsenic, Boron, Fluorine, Nickel, Silicon, Tin, Vanadium, and Sulfur

Several reviews have considered the essentiality and physiological importance of ultratrace elements (e.g., bromine, cadmium, lead, lithium).[9-13,16-19] From these reviews it is apparent that considerably more information is required to establish their essentiality, functions, interactions, and level of requirement. Undoubtedly some of the ultratrace elements will prove to have nutritional significance with important roles in human nutrition. Not until then will there be a need for assessing their nutritional status in the human.

Arsenic
atomic weight: 74.92

The essentiality of arsenic has been demonstrated for several animal species, including rats, chicks, and goats.[12,13,17,18] Evidence suggests that arsenic may participate in the metabolism of arginine, methionine, and zinc.[13,17,18] Growth and reproduction may be impaired. An essentiality of arsenic for the human has not been established.

Boron
atomic weight: 10.81

Rat studies indicate that boron may be beneficial for optimal calcium metabolism, and therefore, for optimal bone formation.[3,9,10,12,19] Human investigations also suggest an involvement of boron in calcium and magnesium metabolism.[9,15]

Fluorine
atomic weight: 19.00

Fluorine has not been demonstrated to be an essential nutrient for the human or animals.[13] However, it participates in the prevention of tooth decay and in the formation of fluoroapetite and in the enhancement of bone density.[2,21]

Nickel
atomic weight: 58.69

The essentiality of nickel has been reported for the chick, rat and other animals, but its importance in human health has not been well established.[4,11] Nickel levels in the serum of 11 non-pregnant women was reported as 122 ± 25 µg/L (range: 9 to 301 µg/L).[6,7,11] This level is higher than values reported by others (3 to 60 µg/L).[6] Nickel metabolism has been investigated in the human with oral use of isotope ^{62}Ni.[20]

Silicon
atomic weight: 28.09

Silicon appears to be an essential element for the chick and rat, but a corresponding need for the human has not been established.[1,5] Controlled human studies on silicon deprivation remain to be conducted.

Tin
atomic weight: 118.7

Although tin was reported to be essential for the rat, these observations have not been confirmed. If tin proves to be essential for the human, the requirement would be small. The levels of tin in the diet probably precludes the likelihood of a deficiency occurring.

Vanadium
atomic weight: 50.94

Vanadium is considered essential for chicks and rats.[8,14] Specific biological functions of vanadium are unclear, but it may be involved in lipid metabolism and in bone development.

Sulfur
atomic weight: 32.06

The majority of the sulfur present in the body exists as the sulfur-containing amino acids; methionine, cystine, cysteine, and homocystine. These compounds serve to provide the sulfur needed for the formation of other sulfur-containing compounds. Inorganic sulfates and sulfides represent only a small fraction of the total sulfur in the body. Aside from the dietary needs for methionine, biotin and thiamin represent the only other dietary requirement for sulfur. Other sulfur-containing biological components, including the semi-essential taurine, are synthesized by the body.

References

1. Carlisle, E. M., A silicon requirement for normal skull formation in chicks, *J. Nutr.*, 110, 352, 1980.
2. Richmond, V. L., Thirty years of fluoridation: a review, *Am. J. Clin. Nutr.*, 41, 129, 1985.
3. Meachan, S. L., Taper, L. J., and Volpe, S. L., Effect of boron supplementation on blood and urinary calcium, magnesium, and phosphorus, and urinary boron in athletic and sedentary women, *Am. J. Clin. Nutr.*, 61, 341, 1995.
4. Schnegg, A. and Kirchgessner, M., Changes in hemoglobin content, erythrocyte count and hematocrit in nickel deficiency, *Nutr. Metab.*, 19, 268, 1975.
5. Carlisle, E. M., Silicon, *Nutr. Rev.*, 33, 257, 1975.
6. Anonymous, Transient hypernickelemia following delivery, *Nutr. Revs.*, 42, 157, 1984.
7. Rubanyi, G., Birtalan, I., Grergely A., and Kovach, A. G. B., Serum nickel concentrations in women during pregnancy, during parturition, and post partum, *Am. J. Obstet. Gynecol.*, 143, 167, 1982.
8. Uthus, E. O. and Nielsen, F. H., Effect of vanadium, iodine and their interaction on growth, blood variables, liver trace elements and thyroid status indices in rats, *Magnesium Trace Elem.*, 9, 219, 1990.
9. Nielsen, F. H., Trace and ultratrace elements in health and disease, *Comprehensive Therapy*, 17, 20, 1991.
10. Nielsen, F. H., New essential trace elements for the lifesciences, *Biological Trace Element Res.*, 26-27, 599, 1990.
11. Nielsen, F. H., Nickel, in *Trace Elements In Human And Animal Nutrition*, Vol. 1, 5th edition, Mertz, W., Ed., Academic Press, San Diego, CA, 1987, 245.
12. Nielsen, F. H., Nutritional significance of the ultratrace elements, *Nutr. Revs.*, 46, 337, 1988.
13. Nielsen, F. H., Ultratrace elements in nutrition, *Annu. Rev. Nutr.*, 4, 21, 1984.
14. Nielsen, F. H., Vanadium, *Trace Elements In Human and Animal Nutrition*, Vol. 1, 5th edition, Mertz, W., Ed., Academic Press, San Diego, CA, 1987, 275.
15. Nielsen, F. H., Hunt, C. D., Mullen, L. M., and Hunt, J. R., Effect of dietary boron on mineral, estrogen, and testosterone metabolism in postmenopausal women, *FASEB J.*, 1, 394, 1987.
16. Nielsen, F. H., Possible future implications of nickel, arsenic, silicon, vanadium, and other ultratrace elements in human nutrition, in *Clinical, Biochemical, and Nutritional Aspects of Trace Elements*, Prasad, A. S., Ed., Alan R. Liss, New York, 1982, 379.
17. Nielsen, F. H., Possible future implications of ultratrace elements in human health and disease, in *Essential and Toxic Trace Elements in Human Health and Disease*, Prasad, A. S., Ed., *Current Topics in Nutrition and Disease*, Vol. 18, Alan R. Liss, New York, 1988, 277.
18. Nielsen, F. H., Ultratrace minerals, in *Modern Nutrition in Health and Disease*, Shils, M. E., Olson, J. A., and Shike, M., Eds., 8th edition, Vol. 1, Lea & Febiger, Philadelphia, 1994, 269.
19. Mertz, W., Essential trace metals: New definitions based on new paradigm, *Nutr. Rev.*, 51, 287, 1993.
20. Patriarca, M., Lyon, T. D. B., and Fell, G. S., Nickel metabolism in humans investigated with an oral stable isotope, *Am. J. Clin. Nutr.*, 66, 616, 1997.
21. Raiten, D. J., Talbot, J. M., and Waters, J. H., Assessment of nutrient requirements for infant formulas, *J. Nutr.*, 128, 2059S, 1998.

Section IV

Protein-Energy Malnutrition

Protein-Energy Malnutrition

Introduction

History has recorded many famines. The food shortages resulting from famines cause weight loss, wasting, and death from starvation in the affected population. In the early 1930s, a condition termed "kwashiorkor" was described by Cicely Williams, while working in Ghana.[16] Kwashiorkor means the "disease of the displaced child."[16]

In developing countries four major deficiency diseases occur; namely, protein-energy malnutrition, vitamin A deficiency, nutritional anemias, and iodine deficiency. The deficiencies will most likely effect newborns, weanlings, and women of reproductive age.[96]

Protein-energy malnutrition is generally the result of inadequate intake or utilization of food, particularly of energy and protein. Protein-energy malnutrition of children may be classified as (a) low height-for-age (stunting) or (b) low weight-for-height (wasting).[19,97] The values are compared in relation to reference data from healthy populations. It is estimated that up to one-third of childhood deaths occurring between 6 and 60 months of age in developing countries may be attributable to protein-energy malnutrition.[96]

The World Health Organization has indicated that at least 500 million children in the world suffer from protein-energy malnutrition.[3,179] Protein-energy malnutrition is mainly caused by inadequate food intake. A deficiency of energy is more important and more frequent than protein deficiency.[17,38-40] Kwashiorkor is often regarded as the result of protein deficiency while nutritional marasmus is the result of an energy deficiency. Nutritional marasmus is associated with severe wasting, while kwashiorkor is characterized by exhibiting edema.[18,19] Waterlow suggested that acute malnutrition be termed **wasting** and that chronic malnutrition be termed **stunting**, while a combined condition of acute and chronic malnutrition be considered wasting and stunting (Table 112).[1-3,14,19]

TABLE 112
Simplified Classification of Protein-Energy Malnutrition

Condition	Body Weight as % of Standard	Edema	Deficit in Weight for Height
Underweight child	80–60	0	Minimal
Nutritional dwarfing	<60	0	Minimal
Kwashiorkor	80–60	+	++
Marasmus	<60	0	++
Marasmic kwashiorkor	<60	+	++

From FAO and WHO report (1971).[148]
 + = mild
++ = markedly deficient

The most common form of malnutrition occurring in the hospital setting is that of protein-energy malnutrition.[130-138] Protein-energy malnutrition affects about 50% of patients hospitalized for 2 or more weeks on general medical and surgical wards in U.S. hospitals. Disconcerting is that patients with evidence of malnutrition have significantly longer average hospital stays, higher mortality rates, and a greater frequency of surgical complications.

Clinical Protein-Energy Malnutrition

Kwashiorkor patients usually have a well-nourished appearance;[1-4,92] however, they have a tendency to develop edema, pressure sores, easily pluckable hair, and anergy on immune skin testing. Marasmus usually presents a starved appearance with diminished skinfold thickness. Protein undernutrition with adequate energy intake, as occurs in the kwashiorkor child, leads to a severe and potentially lethal form of fatty liver.[4,92] Untreated, the majority of the children result in death. When both dietary intakes of protein and energy are inadequate, growth may be severely restricted, but the fatty liver condition does not occur.[1-4] Kwashiorkor cases usually responds quickly to treatment, while the response to treatment in maramus patients may be slower.[2,3] Protein-energy malnutrition has been considered in detail by Waterlow.[1] A number of reviews on protein-energy malnutrition are available for indepth considerations.[2-6,43,44,48,49,61-67,80,92]

Anthropometric Parameters

Severe forms of protein-energy malnutrition can be diagnosed relatively easily from their clinical manifestation.[3,14] Milder forms of protein-energy malnutrition are more difficult to clinically diagnose. Anthropometric procedures as well as bioclinical measurements have been useful for this purpose although their limitations in sensitivity and specificity are recognized. The most commonly used anthropometric measurements for assessing child growth and nutritional status are weight-for-height, height-for-age, weight-for-age, mid-upper-arm circumference, and triceps skin-fold thickness.[2,3,40,105,111,112,122,123]

Anthropometry methods are noninvasive, inexpensive, universally applicable, and can reflect nutritional and health status.[2,3,40,105] Reference standards and guides have been developed by the World Health Organization, National Center for Health Statistics, and the National Health and Nutrition Examination Surveys.[2,3,20,21,105,112-121] References have been developed for various age groups, including newborns, infants, children, adolescents, and adults.[105,111-121]

Other measurements can provide detailed information on body composition and may indirectly provide an assessment of protein status. Most of these measurements entail special equipment or facilities that are not routinely available. Hence, these procedures are commonly limited to research applications. Some of these methods include bioimpedance analysis, dual-energy X-ray absorptiometry (DXA), isotope dilution, magnetic resonance imaging, and underwater weighing (Table 113).[106-110]

Biochemical Assessment of Protein-Energy Malnutrition

Biochemical procedures have the potential of providing the most objective and quantitative assessment of protein and energy status. Anthropometric, clinical, and dietary data can aid in the evaluation. Although a number of biochemical evaluation procedures are available, no single test can be considered as an ideal and reliable indicator of protein status.[143,176] Some of these biochemical procedures will be briefly considered in this section.

TABLE 113
Height and Weight Ranges
for Men and Women

Height*	Weight in Pounds**
4'10"	91–119
4'11"	94–124
5'0"	97–128
5'1"	101–132
5'2"	104–137
5'3"	107–141
5'4"	111–146
5'5"	114–150
5'6"	118–155
5'7"	121–160
5'8"	125–164
5'9"	129–169
5'10"	132–174
5'11"	136–179
6'0"	140–184
6'1"	144–189
6'2"	148–195
6'3"	152–200
6'4"	156–205
6'5"	160–211
6'6"	164–216

* without shoes
** without clothes
Derived from National Research
Council (1989) for adults.[178]

Serum Total Protein (Tables 114 and 115)

Although total serum protein levels have been commonly measured in nutrition surveys, the results themselves appear to be of little value as a sensitive and specific index for estimating protein intake or protein nutritional status.[173] In general, changes in serum proteins have been difficult to evaluate despite the voluminous literature on the subject. Often total serum protein levels are elevated in population groups living in the tropical and subtropical areas even in the presence of inadequate protein intakes.[164] These elevated serum protein levels appear to be largely due to environmental effects rather than of ethnic origin.

TABLE 114
Normal Plasma Protein Concentrations as Suggested by Feldman[124]

Protein	Turnover Rate (T½ days)	Normal Range
Albumin	18	35–54 g/L
Transferrin	8	2.0–4.0 g/L
Prealbumin (transthyretin)	2	230–430 mg/L
Retinol-binding protein	0.5	30–70 mg/L

TABLE 115
Plasma Protein Concentrations in Elderly Chinese Age 60–75 years

Protein	Men	Women
Total protein (g/L)	78 ± 5.1 (161)	78.0 ± 4.8 (240)
Albumin (g/L)	42.8 ± 3.4 (156)	42.8 ± 3.1 (238)
Prealbumin (transthyretin) (mg/L)	358 ± 136.0 (154)	382.9 ± 152.3 (212)
Retinol-binding protein (mg/L)	70.5 ± 20.2 (155)	72.2 ± 19.4 (230)
Transferrin (g/L)	2.58 ± 0.75 (150)	2.41 ± 0.5 (228)

Values in parenthesis = number of subjects studied.
Adapted from Woo et al., *Europ. J. Clin. Nutr.*, 42, 903, 1988.

Serum Albumin

In the past, the measurements of plasma albumin was the method of choice for monitoring a subjects' protein status.[100] However, albumin measurements have not been helpful in following the response of protein changes to protein intervention. The plasma level of albumin does not reflect immediate changes in protein levels because of the long turn-over rate of albumin (18 days).

For example, the effect of total parenteral nutrition on the plasma proteins of protein-depleted patients was investigated by Carpentier et al.[104] They found that after five days of total parenteral nutrition the initially depressed transthyritin (prealbumin) and retinol-binding protein concentrations had returned to the normal range. A moderate rise occurred in the plasma transferrin concentration, while the albumin concentration had not significantly increased.

Nevertheless, low serum albumin levels are often associated with various medical conditions. The 18-day turnover rate of serum albumin is rather long and hence, it is not a good measure of protein-energy malnutrition.[49,65,66,104,127] However, serum albumin is easy to measure and is routinely available in most clinical laboratories. Serum albumin may be quantified by the bromcreosol green method[101,102] or by the bromcreosol purple procedure.[102,103]

Plasma Amino Acids

Plasma amino acid levels have been extensively studied in both the malnourished and normal infants.[61,62] Of the plasma amino acids studied, valine concentrations had some correlation with protein-energy malnutrition.[91] The usefulness of this marker in evaluating protein-energy status may be limited because plasma amino acids and proteins can change rapidly by sepsis, stress, or by marked changes in the quantity or balance of protein and energy in the diet.

Plasma amino acid levels exhibit also a circadian rhythm. Fasting plasma samples are necessary for analyses. Levels vary widely between subjects and the results are calculated as essential: non-essential amino acid ratios. Results suggest that the ratios may be useful in detecting extremes of protein-energy malnutrition.[93] The amino acid ratio precedure requires the separation and measurement of the following amino acids.[149-153]

$$\text{Amino acid ratio (NE:E)} = \frac{\text{Glycine + serine + glutamine + taurine}}{\text{Isoleucine + leucine + valine + methionine}}$$

Saunders et al.[94] have noted that the amino acid profile of a protein-energy malnourished child appears to reflect the immediately preceding dietary protein intake and may not necessarily be useful in assessing nutritional status. In general, the essential amino acid levels are reduced, and the non-essential amino acid levels are elevated in children suffering from protein deficiency.

Following the ingestion of protein, plasma amino acid concentrations rise, but within a short time, they return to the relatively constant level observed in the fasting state.[95] In severe protein depletion, characteristic changes in blood amino acid concentrations do occur and persist. However, before the plasma amino acid changes become evident, clinical conditions can already be recognized. Consequently, plasma amino acid changes are not a suitable or sensitive indicator of the onset of malnutrition.[95]

Plasma Alkaline Ribonuclease Activity

Plasma alkaline ribonuclease activity (EC 3.1.4.2.2) is increased with impaired protein status.[53-60] Hence, its measurement has been studied as to its usefulness as an indicator of protein nutritional status.[54] Scott[59] has described a method for the determination of alkaline ribonuclease activity in serum. The enzyme is comparatively easy to measure and requires only a small quantity of serum or plasma. Malnourished infants and children had initially high enzyme activity. The high enzyme activity returned to normal within 2 to 4 weeks. The time required was related to the level and quality of protein used in the rehabilitation.[54] A change in plasma alkaline ribonuclease activity may be noted within one week after change in nutrition support.[54] Scott et al.[54] suggest that the greatest potential use of the assay may be in monitoring the response of malnourished patients to dietary changes. Serum alkaline ribonuclease activity was reported to be higher in chronic alcoholics than normal controls.[60] This may suggest that some overall protein malnutrition exists in chronic alcoholics.

Insulin-Like Growth Factor I (IGF-I, Somatomedin C)

Insulin-like growth factor I is universally lowered in the serum of subjects with protein-energy malnutrition.[126] Its restoration is dependent upon the provision of adequate protein rather than of energy. In contrast, the restoration of serum prealbumin levels is more dependent upon energy intake than protein.[44]

The half-life of IGF-I is 12 to 15 hours.[126] Low serum IGF-I levels of chronically malnourished subjects can be normalized by adequate nutrition, but it may require 9 to 29 days. A number of conditions, aside from malnutrition, may decrease serum IGF-I concentrations. Some of the conditions are anorexia nervosa, inflammatory bowel disease, celiac disease, HIV-1 infection, and fasting.[126] Measurements of serum levels of IGF-I hold promise as an index of nutritional status. In addition, the measurement could serve as a marker to follow the response of a patient to nutrient support.[126,129,130]

IGF-I measurement were reported to be more sensitive and specific than measurement of albumin, prealbumin, transferrin or retinol-binding protein.[126] Furthermore it was reported that IGF-I values were more informative than anthropometric measurements (e.g., triceps skinfold thickness and mid-upper-arm circumference.[126,128]

Insulin-like growth factor I (IGF-I; Somatomedin C) can be easily measured in serum with the use of commercially available radioimmunoassay kits (DiaSorin, Stillwater, MN). A sample size of 200 μL is utilized. Since the assay requires the use of ^{125}I, a gamma counter is required for reading the samples. Quality controls are provided with the assay kits.

Plasma Transferrin

Plasma transferrin metabolism was altered in children with severe protein-energy malnutrition.[41] Only a fair correlation was observed between plasma transferrin and indices of wasting. The investigator concluded that transferrin concentration was not a very good indicator of protein nutritional status.[41] Plasma transferrin has a turnover rate of 8 to 9 days.[43,44]

Commercial assay kits are available for measuring serum levels of transferrin (e.g., The Binding Site, Inc., San Diego, CA; DiaSorin, Stillwater, MN).

3-Methylhistidine

During the breakdown of muscle protein in the process of protein turnover, 3-methylhistidine is formed and excreted quantitatively in the urine. Urinary excretion of 3-methylhistidine is decreased in protein-energy malnutrition in adults and children.[50,51] Excretion of 3-methylhistidine increases again with protein and energy treatment. These findings indicated that a qualitative and quantitative relationship may exist between 3-methylhistidine excretion and protein-energy malnutrition.

The urinary excretion of 3-methylhistine has been studied as a marker for protein-energy malnutrition status.[50,51] Although applicable in healthy subjects, the method was not useful in evaluating protein-energy malnutrition patients because of variable 3-methylhistidine turnover rates.[42,50,52] Plasma methylhistidine levels have been used to follow changes in muscle protein catabolism with protein therapy, particularly with total parenteral nutrition.

Plasma Retinol-Binding Protein

Plasma retinol binding protein has a turnover rate of 4 to 24 hours.[43-45] With its short half-life, plasma retinol-binding protein measurements have been used to evaluate protein-energy deprivation and to follow the response to nutritional therapy.[45,48,177] Plasma concentrations of retinol, retinol-binding protein, and prealbumin (transthyretin) are reduced in protein-energy malnourished subjects.[177] The availability of commercial kits permit the measurement of plasma retinol-binding protein easily and quickly on a few microliters of sample (Calbiochem-Behring Corp., San Diego, CA; The Binding Site, San Diego, CA).

Plasma Transthyretin (Prealbumin; Thyroxine-Binding Prealbumin)

Transthyretin (prealbumin) is present in the plasma complexed with retinol-binding protein.[98] These proteins have a rapid turnover, with a half-life of 2 to 3 days.[44] When energy and/or protein intake is below normal, plasma concentrations of transthyretin will decrease quickly, within 3 to 4 days.[98] Interpretation of plasma transthyretin findings requires careful consideration in view of factors that may influence protein synthesis, such as inflammatory responses, certain liver disorders, renal disease, and iron status.[26,44,48,98]

In neonatal infants, serum transthyretin concentrations provided a rapid, accurate, and convenient means to monitor protein-energy adequacy and response to dietary changes.[125] In general, plasma concentrations of transthyretin (prealbumin) appear to be a very sensitive parameter for indicating the efficiency of a nutritional therapy.[48] Failure of plasma transthyretin levels to return to a normal concentration may portend a poor prognosis.[99,136]

Commercial turbidimetric and radial immunodiffusion (RID) assay kits are available for measuring serum levels of transthyretin (prealbumin) and of transferrin (e.g., The Binding Site, Inc., San Diego, CA; DiaSorin, Stillwater, MN). The assay kits are convenient, sensitive, stable, and easy to use, have a small sample requirement, and are reliable. Control materials are supplied with the kits. Reading of the RID plates require the use of a jewelers' eye-piece or an electronic radial immunodiffusion plate reader.

Guidelines for Serum Transthyretin Concentrations (mg/dL)

Normal	Marginally Deficient	Deficient	Elevated
20–40	10–17	<10	>40

Nitrogen Balance

Adequacy of protein intake may be determined by nitrogen balance measurement. The determination is expressed as follows:

$$\text{Nitrogen balance} = \frac{\text{protein intake as g/day}}{6.25} - \left(\begin{array}{c} \text{urinary urea N/day} \\ + \text{ 3 or 4 as fecal losses} \end{array} \right)$$

A positive nitrogen balance is indicative of nitrogen retention and net protein synthesis. A negative nitrogen balance indicates inadequate protein intake resulting in net protein catabolism. Nitrogen balance studies are relatively expensive to conduct and often prone to errors.[48] Nitrogen balance studies are of limited use as an indicator of nutritional status.

Urinary Creatinine – Height Index

The relationship of milligrams of creatinine excreted per unit of time per centimeter of body height has been used in evaluating protein nutritional status in chidren and other age groups.[138,139,145,146]

$$\text{creatinine–height index (CHI)} = \frac{\text{creatinine excretion by subject (mg/24 hr)}}{\text{creatinine excretion by normal child of same height}}$$
$$\text{(mg/24 hr)}$$

Although 24-hr urine collections are preferred, shorter collection periods have been used at the expense of precision.[139-142] Expressing creatinine excretion in terms of height is preferred over that of per kilogram of body weight since variations in adipose tissues do not effect the former.[139-142] Moreover, knowledge as to the exact age of the child is not essential since the CHI norms are based only on the expected creatinine excretion of normal children of the height of the malnourished child. The creatinine-height index agreed closely with the potassium-height index as an indirect measure of the relative mass and the degree of protein depletion and repletion in malnourished children.[139,141,144] Suggested norms for use in comparing creatinine excretion in children in reference to height have been published.[139-141] Limitations in the use of the urinary creatinine-height index have been reviewed (Figures 60 and 61).[140-143]

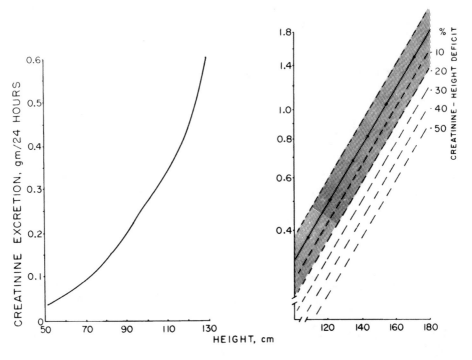

FIGURE 60
Relationship between urinary creatinine excretion (g/24 hr) and height (cm) for children (Adapted from Viteri et al.[139,141] and Mendez and Buskirk[140]).

Although the requirement for carefully timed urine collections limits its field use, the measurement could be of value in assessing the recovery of malnourished children as well as in the detection of marginal protein-calorie malnutrition.[138,139,142] More recently a creatinine arm index was proposed as an alternative for the creatinine-height index. The objective was to provide a more age-independent index for nutritional assessment applicable to adults and elderly.[147] The index requires further evaluation as to its reliability and usefulness.

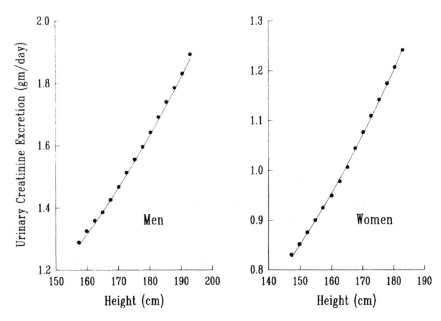

FIGURE 61

Relationship between urinary creatinine excretion (g/24 hr) and height (cm) for adult men and women. (Derived from Blackburn et al.)[67]

Fasting Urinary Urea-Creatinine Ratio

Since urea is the principal end product of protein metabolism in the human, the use of nitrogen to creatinine ratios and urea to creatinine ratios have been proposed for evaluating dietary protein intakes.[163-166]

$$\text{urea−creatinine ratio} = \frac{\text{mg urea nitrogen/ml urine}}{\text{mg creatinine/ml urine}}$$

Under laboratory conditions, an increase or a decrease in the level of protein intake is paralleled by marked changes in the urinary urea/creatinine ratio. When the technique has been applied in the field variable results have been reported.[166,167] Since 24-hr urine collections are difficult to obtain from children, especially in field nutrition studies, random urine samples have been commonly employed, recognizing their limitations.[166] The recommended procedure for collecting the fasting random urine sample is to discard the first urine void in the morning and collect the second. Urea-creatinine ratio values must be interpreted with general caution as creatinine excretion is related to age, sex, diet, muscle mass, and other factors. Clearly defined guidelines are not available. Nevertheless, the urea-creatinine ratio can be useful if it is recognized that it is primarily a measure of dietary rather than of nutritional status. The ratio is a reflection of the recent dietary intake and does not indicate the actual protein nutriture of an individual.[166,168] However, the ratio, when applied to population groups, may provide a general evaluation of the quantity of protein ingested.

Urinary Hydroxyproline Index

Hydroxyproline, a product of collagen metabolism, is excreted in reduced amounts by malnourished and protein-depleted children.[61,62,154-156] From these observations, the hydroxyproline index was proposed.[156,157]

$$\text{urinary hydroxyproline index} = \frac{\mu M \text{ hydroxyproline/ml urine}}{\mu M \text{ creatinine/ml urine/kg body wt.}}$$

$$= \frac{\mu M \text{ hydroxyproline/ml urine} \times \text{kg body wt.}}{\mu M \text{ creatinine/ml urine}}$$

Most reliable results are obtained when 24-hr urine collections are employed. In studies with children, 24-hr urine collections are not practical. However, expressing the urinary hydroxyproline excretion values in terms of creatinine excretion has permitted the use of random urine samples.[155,157,158] To avoid falsely high hydroxyproline excretions due to dietary ingestion of the amino acid, fasting morning urine collections are recommended. When the hydroxyproline excretions are expressed in terms of creatinine excretion, differences between adult males and females are eliminated. The age of the subject is, however, a major factor in the interpretation of urinary hydroxyproline levels.[155,158] This is because the rate of hydroxyproline excretion in normal children decreases with increasing age, as the rate of growth drops,[159] while that of creatinine excretion increases.[158]

The highest absolute hydroxyproline excretion of any group of normal subjects is seen in the rapidly growing adolescent (11 to 16 years).[160] Between ages 16 and 24 years, there is a gradual reduction in hydroxyproline excretion. The large variation in hydroxyproline excretion between normal individuals limits the use of the measurement to young children where the index appears to have virtue in the assessment of growth rate. For this age group, Whitehead and others[154,155,157,158,161] have found the urinary hydroxyproline index to be a useful biochemical test for evaluating nutritional status. However, the hydroxyproline index does not diagnose whether the growth retardation is due to protein and/or energy malnutrition or to certain other disease conditions.[162]

Pediatric Protein-Energy Malnutrition

Pediatric kwashiorkor disorders occur in children shortly after weaning from breast feeding.[1-4,6] The child commonly shows growth retardation, maintains subcutaneous adipose tissue, lethargy, fatigue, anemia, and hepatomegaly.[4,25] Skin lesions that resemble those of pellagra are often present on the feet, legs, and face. Hair is often depigmented and easily plucked. These skin lesions have been described in detail by McLaren.[27] Hypoalbuminemia usually exists that progresses to edema. The critical pathologic conditions are fatty liver and atrophy of the skeletal muscles.[4] These subjects usually respond favorably by providing an adequate intake of protein and energy.[5]

Malnutrition results in reduced physical activity and work output, decreased resistance to infection, and impaired cognitive performance.[1-3,6,7,22-24] Malnutrition (PEM), reflected in an underweight population, has a prevalence of about 50% in South Asia.[8,9] In South East Asia, 32% of the children were underweight. Similarly, 30% of the children of the

Sub-Saharan region of Africa were underweight. In 1995, worldwide over 150 million children, age 0 to 60 months, were underweight.[8] Most children with kwashiorkor or marasmius will die within the year; many die with diarrhea.[14] The prevalence of protein-energy malnutrition for children under 4 years of age has been reported as 66% for Bangladesh; 51% for Indonesia; 52% for Pakistan; 61% for India; 34% for Philippines; 26% for Thailand; and 14% for Singapore.[9,10]

Evaluation of cases of edematous protein-energy malnutrition reported in North America has provided clear evidence that protein deficiency is an essential prerequisite for kwashiorkor and marasmic kwashiorkor to develop.[36] A low ratio of protein to energy leads to hypoalbuminemia and the consequent edema.

From a study of 29 infants with edematous protein-energy malnutrition, Rossouw[37] reported the following clinical and laboratory findings:

Entity	Number of Infants
Edema	29 of 29
Skin changes	20 of 25
Hair changes	17 of 21
Hypoalbuminemia (<35 g/L)	28 of 28
Anemia (hemoglobin <110 g/L)	20 of 26
Low serum urea (<1.8 mmol/L)	14 of 23

Studies conducted in 1969 on preschool Navajo Indian children revealed cases of kwashiorkor and marasmus.[12,13] Out of 616 children admitted to the hospital, 15 cases of kwashiorkor and 29 cases of marasmus were observed. Within 4 years with the use of infant and child-feeding programs, marasmus essentially disappeared and kwashiorkor was reduced by 50%.[13]

Adult Protein-Energy Malnutrition

Chronic energy malnutrition probably occurs in adults in the regions with high childhood protein-energy malnutrition, but little information is available as to the extent.[11] However, a survey in India in 1996 found nearly 50% of the adults suffered from chronic energy deficiency as indicated by their body mass index.[15] Nearly 9% of the children exhibited severe malnutrition and 1 to 3% had clinical signs of kwashiorkor/marasmus.

Adult protein-energy malnutrition during famines may appear as kwashiorkor or a kwashiorkor-like condition exhibiting edema.[180] Marasmus in adults may be associated with diverse conditions, including chronic infection such as AIDS or severe tuberculosis, anorexia, malignant neoplasmas, and some forms of malabsorption.

Protein-Energy Malnutrition in Geriatric Populations

Studies in nursing home populations have found protein-energy malnutrition to be a common problem.[81,82] In one study, based on anthropometric and biomedical measurements, 52% of the individuals were considered malnourished.[81] Of the patients ($n = 227$), 24% were hypoalbuminemic, 19% were of a kwashiorkor-marasmus mix, and 9% were marasmus. In addition, 28% of the patients were anergic and 76% were anemic. Other investigations of geriatric patients have commonly observed protein-energy undernutrition.[80,82-88] Low serum albumin concentrations are often encountered.[181] Serum albumin concentrations of less than 38 g/L are associated with increased morbidity, mortality, and disability in the elderly.[86,89] Serum albumin concentrations were positively associated with total muscle mass in men and women.[86]

The First National Health and Nutrition Examination Survey included 4,728 individuals aged 55 to 74 yrs.[88] Hypoalbuminemia was defined as <35 g/L (1.2% of the subjects) or as ≤38 g/L (7.9% of the subjects).[88] Hypoalbuminemia is commonly considered a marker of protein-energy undernutrition. However, as noted elsewhere, hypoalbuminemia may be associated also with liver and renal disease, infection, inflammation, trauma, and surgical stress.[90]

Hemodialysis and Protein-Energy Malnutrition

Protein-energy malnutrition has been associated with hemodialysis patients.[30-36] A causitive role has been ascribed to an inadequacy of nourishment before dialysis and in the early stage of regular dialysis.[31] Hemodialysis patients with protein-energy malnutrition were found to have lower serum prealbumin and plasma leucine concentrations. Analysis of essential amino acids and prealbumin concentration may serve to follow the protein nutritional status of hemodialysis patients.[31,32]

Hakin and Levin have reviewed studies on malnutrition in hemodialysis patients.[30] They have summarized some of the biochemical measurements that may assist in identifying protein-energy malnutrition in hemodialysis patients as follows:[33]

Indices	Deficient Level
1. Serum albumin	<4.0 g/dL
2. Serum transferrin	<200 mg/dL
3. Prealbumin	<29 mg/dL
4. Serum IGF-1 concentration	<300 µg/L
5. Serum cholesterol	<150 mg/dL

Hair Changes with Protein-Energy Malnutrition

Changes in hair morphology have also been proposed as indices for assessing early protein-energy malnutrition in children.[174,175] It has long been recognized that children suffering from protein-energy malnutrition have change in the texture, color, and pluckability of their hair.[169]

Similar changes have been produced in experimentally protein-deprived adults.[174,175] To quantitate the changes in hair pluckability, a calibrated mechanical instrument, named a trichotillometer, was devised by Krumdieck.[28,29] The instrument determines the force required to epilate individual hairs. The instrument was applied to adult hospitalized patients and to a group of Nigerians. Trichotillometry requires little skill and is quick and inexpensive. The results supported the view that the ease of hair pluckability was related to kwashiorkor (protein depletion) rather than to energy depletion.[29]

Immunocompetence

Immune competence may be reduced in the subject with protein malnutrition due to a failure of protein synthesis.[80] Immune deficiency leads to increased susceptibility to infection, and an elevated mortality. Chandra has studied extensively the use of immunocompetence as a functional index of nutritional status and vulnerability to disease.[75-79] He noted that "assessment of immunocompetence by currently available methods in conjunction with other methods of nutritional assessment can identify individuals who are most in need of appropriate nutritional support and thus provide crucial prognostic information in terms of risk of disease, duration of hospitalization, and chances of survival."[78] The competence may be evaluated with the use of various skin test antigens.[68-79] Skin test antigens commonly used include Candida, mumps, Trichophyton, streptokinase-streptodornase, tuberculosis antigen, and Proteus.[69-71,73] A test kit that contains seven different antigens has been manufactured by the Merieux Institute, Lyon, France, and distributed by Merieux Institute, Miami, FL.[69] The use of seven antigens provided a more reliable identification of malnourished patients than when a lower number of antigens were used in the test.[69]

However, depressed cellular immunity may be due to factors other than protein malnutrition. Other nutritional factors, such as vitamin A and zinc may be involved, as well as non-nutritional factors including burns, trauma, infections, liver disease, renal disease, and neoplasmas.[78,79]

Summary (Table 116)

The major functional consequences of protein-energy malnutrition are reduction in muscle mass and ultimate body size, decreased work capacity and physical activity, and immunosuppression with the attendant increased risk of infections and death. Studies estimate that up to one-third of the childhood deaths occurring between 6 and 60 months of age in developing countries may be related to protein-energy malnutrition.[96]

No single biochemical procedure that can satisfactorily evaluate protein and energy malnutrition in early or sub-clinical states is available. The severe forms of malnutrition, kwashiorkor and marasmus, are clinically recognizable. Anthropometric measurements such as weight, height, skinfold, arm circumference, and age, can be extremely useful in the diagnosis of these forms of malnutrition.

A growing number of laboratory procedures are available for evaluating protein-energy malnutrition. Some of the older procedures used included serum total protein, serum albumin, plasma amino acids, nitrogen balance, urinary creatinine-height index, 3-methylhistidine, urea-creatinine ratio, urinary hyproxyproline index, and plasma alkaline ribonuclease activity.

More recently, the assessment of protein-energy status has involved the measurements of plasma concentrations of transthyritin (formerly known as prealbumin), transferrin, retinol-binding protein, and IGF-I. Plasma albumin is routinely measured, although it lacks the sensitivity desired for evaluating protein-energy malnutrition. Plasma transthyretin measurements are a more sensitive indicator of protein-energy malnutrition and its use should be considered for identifying and following patients with possible malnutrition.

TABLE 116

Suggested Guidelines for the Interpretation of Biochemical Indices Used in Evaluating Protein and Energy Deficiencies

	Less thanAcceptable (at Risk)			
Measurement or Index	Deficient (High Risk)	Low (Medium Risk)	Acceptable (Low Risk)	References
1. Serum protein (g/dL)				169–171
0–11 months		<5.0	≥5.0	
1–5 years		<5.5	≥5.5	
6–17 years		<6.0	≥6.0	
Adults	<6.0	6.0–6.4	≥6.5	
Pregnant, 2nd and 3rd trimester	<5.5	5.5–5.9	≥6.0	
2. Serum albumin (g/d/l)				161, 169–172
0–11 months		<2.5	≥2.5	
1–5 years	(<2.8)	<3.0	≥3.0	
6–17 years	(<2.8)	<3.5	≥3.5	
Adults	<2.8	2.8–3.4	≥3.5	
Pregnant, 1st trimester	<3.0	3.0–3.9	≥4.0	
Pregnant, 2nd and 3rd trimester	<3.0	3.0–3.4	≥3.5	
3. Nonessential/essential amino acid ratio (NE/E)[a]				
All ages	>3.0	2.0–3.0	<2.0	150–152, 161, 173
4. Hydroxyproline index 3 mon. to 10 yrs of age	<1.0	1.0–2.0	>2.0	154, 156, 157, 160, 161, 173
5. Creatinine Height Index 3 months to 17 yrs	<0.5	0.5–0.9	>0.9	139–141, 146
6. Urea/creatinine Ratio	<6.0	6.0–12.0	>12.0	164, 166, 173

[a] Value depends upon the analytical method employed and the procedure used to calculate the ratio.

The use of several biochemical measurements carefully interpreted can, when used in conjunction with clinical and anthropometric assessments, provide a reasonable evaluation of protein and energy nutritional status.

References

1. Waterlow, J. C., *Protein Energy Malnutrition*, Edward Arnold Publication, London, 1992.
2. Torun, B. and Chew, F., Protein-energy malnutrition, in *Modern Nutrition in Health and Disease*, 8th Edition, Shils, M. E., Olson, J. A., and Shike, M., Eds., Lea & Febiger, Philadelphia, 1994, 950.
3. Latham, M. C., Protein-energy malnutrition, in *Present Knowledge in Nutrition*, 6th Edition, Brown, M. L., Ed., International Life Science Institute, Nutrition Foundation, Washington D.C., 1990, 39.
4. Rudman, D. and Feller, A. G., Liver disease, in *Present Knowledge in Nutrition*, 6th Edition, Brown, M. L., Ed., International Life Sciences Institute, Nutrition Foundation, Washington D.C., 1990, 385.
5. Klein, S., Kinney, J., Jujeebhoy, K., Apers, D., Hellerstein, M., Murray, M., and Twomey, P., Nutrition support in clinical practice: Review of published data and recommendations for future research directions. *Am. J. Clin. Nutr.*, 66, 683, 1997.
6. Torun, B. and Viteri, F. E., Protein-energy malnutrition, in *Tropical and Geographic Medicine*, Warren, K. S. and Mahmoud, A. A. F., Eds., McGraw-Hill, New York, 1984.
7. Scrimshaw, N. S., Consequences of hunger for individuals and societies, *Federation Proc.*, 45, 2421, 1986.

8. UN ACC Sub-committee on Nutrition, *SCN NEWS*, No. 14, July 1997, UN Development Programme, One United Nation Plaza, New York.
9. United Nations Update on the Nutrition Situation: 1996, ACC/SCN Secretariat, % World Health Organization, Geneva, 27, Switzerland.
10. Heywood, P. F. and Marks, G. C., Nutrition and Health in South-East Asia, *Med. J. Australia*, 159, 133, 1993.
11. James, W. P. T., Ferro-Luzzi, A., and Waterlow, J. C., Definition of chronic energy deficiency in adults, Report of a working party of the International Dietary Energy Consultancy Group, *Eur. J. Clin. Nutr.*, 42, 969, 1988.
12. Van Duzen, J., Carter, J., Secondi, J., and Federspial, C., Protein and caloric malnutrition among preschool Navajo Indian children, *Am. J. Clin. Nutr.*, 22, 1362, 1969.
13. Van Duzen, J., Carter, J. P., and Vander Zwagg, R., Protein and calorie among preschool Navajo Indian children, a follow-up, *Am. J. Clin. Nutr.*, 29, 657, 1976.
14. Latham, M. C., Protein-energy malnutrition – its epidemiology and control, *JEPTO*, 10, 169, 1990.
15. Bhaskaram, P., Malnutrition – A critical determinant of progressive forms of tuberculosis, *Nutrition News*, National Institute of Nutrition, Hyderabad, India, 17, 1, 1996.
16. Williams, C. D., A nutritional disease of childhood associated with a maze diet, *Arch. Dis. Child.*, 8, 423, 1933.
17. McLaren, D. S., The great protein fiasco, *Lancet*, ii, 93, 1974.
18. Waterlow, J. C., Kwashiorkor revisited: the pathogenesis of oedema in kwashiorkor and its significance, *Trans. Roy. Soc. Trop. Med. Hyg.*, 78, 436, 1984.
19. Waterlow, J. C., Classification and definition of protein-caloric malnutrition, *Br. Med. J.*, 3, 566, 1972.
20. United States Dept. of Health, Education and Welfare (DHEW): NCHS Growth Curves for Children from birth to 18 years, Publication PHS 78-1650, Hyattsville, DHEW, 1970.
21. WHO: Measuring Change in Nutritional Status, Geneva, Switzerland, World Health Organization, 1983.
22. Chandra, R. K., Nutrition, immunity and infection: present knowledge and future directions, *Lancet*, I, 688, 1983.
23. Beisel, W. R., Metabolic effect of infection, *Prog. Food Nutr. Sci.*, 8, 43, 1984.
24. Chandra, R. K., Nutritional regulation of immunity and infection: from epidemiology to clinical practice, *J. Ped. Gastroent. and Nutr.*, 5, 844, 1985.
25. Gomez, F., Galvan, R. R., Cravioto, J., and Frenk, S., Malnutrition in infancy and childhood, with special reference to kwashiorkor, *Adv. Pediatrics*, 7, 131, 1995.
26. Hedlund, J. U., Hansson, L. O., and Ortqvist, A. B., Hypoalbuminemia in hospitalized patients with community-acquired pneumonia, *Arch. Int. Med.*, 155, 1438, 1995.
27. McLaren, D. S., Skin in protein energy malnutrition, *Arch. Dermatol.*, 123, 1674, 1987.
28. Chase, E. S., Weinsier, R. L., Laven, G. T., and Krumdieck, C. L., Trichotillometry: the quantitation of hair pluckability as a method of nutritional assessment, *Am. J. Clin. Nutr.*, 34, 2280, 1981.
29. Smelser, D. N., Smelser, N. B., Krumdieck, C. L., Schreeder, M. T., and Laven, G. T., Field use of hair epilation force in nutrition status assessment, *Am. J. Clin. Nutr.*, 35, 342, 1982.
30. Hakim, R. M. and Levin, N., Malnutrition in hemodialysis patients, *Am. J. Kidney Dis.*, 21, 125, 1993.
31. Marckmann, P., Nutritional status of patients on hemodialysis and peritoneal dialysis, *Clin. Nephrology*, 29, 75, 1988.
32. Oksa, H., Ahonen, K., Pasternack, A., and Marnela, K.–M., Malnutrition in hemodialysis patients, *Scand. J. Urol. Nephrol.*, 25, 157, 1991.
33. Bansal, V. K., Pickering, J., Ing, T. S., Ventuna, L. L., and Hano, J. E., Protein-caloric malnutrition and cutaneous energy in hemodialysis maintained patients, *Am. J. Clin. Nutr.*, 33, 1608, 1980.
34. Kluthe, R., Nutritional management of patients treated with dialysis with special reference to RDT patients, *Acta Chir. Scand.*, 498, 102, 1980.
35. Thurberg, B. J., Swamy, A. P., and Cestero, R. V. M., Cross-sectional and longitudinal nutritional measurements in maintenance hemodialysis patients, *Am. J. Clin. Nutr.*, 34, 2005, 1981.

36. Wolfson, M., Strong, C. J., Minuturn, D., Gray, D. K., and Kopple, J. D., Nutritional status and lymphocyte function in maintenance hemodialysis patients, *Am. J. Clin. Nutr.*, 39, 547, 1984.
37. Rossouw, J. E., Kwashiorkor in North America, *Am. J. Clin. Nutr.*, 49, 588, 1989.
38. Gopalan, C., The contribution of nutrition research to the control of undernutrition: The Indian experience, *Annu. Rev. Nutr.*, 12, 1, 1992.
39. Srikantia, S. G., Protein caloric malnutrition in Indian children, *Indian J. Med. Res.*, 57, 36, 1969.
40. Heymsfield, S. B., Tighe, A., and Wang, Z.–M., Nutritional assessment by anthropometric and biochemical methods, in *Modern Nutrition in Health and Disease*, 8th Edition, Shils, M. E., Olson, J. A., and Shike, M., Eds., Lea & Febiger, Philadelphia, 1994, 812.
41. Morlese, J. F., Forrester, T., Del Rosario, M., Frazer, M., and Jahoor, F., Transferrin kinetics are altered in children with severe protein-energy malnutrition, *J. Nutr.*, 127, 1469, 1997.
42. Lukaski, H. and Mendez, J., Relationship between fat-free weight and urinary 3-methylhistidine excretion in man, *Metabolism*, 29, 758, 1980.
43. Young, V. R., Marchini, J. S., and Cortiella, J., Assessment of protein nutritional status, *J. Nutr.*, 120, 1296, 1990.
44. Benjamin, D. R., Laboratory tests and nutritional assessment, Protein-energy status, *Pediatr. Clin. North Amer.*, 36, 139, 1989.
45. Sachs, E. and Bernstein, L. H., Protein markers of nutritional status as related to sex and age, *Clin. Chem.*, 32, 339, 1986.
46. Ingenbleek, Y., van der Schrieck, H. G., de Nayer, P., and de Visscher, M., The role of retinol-binding protein in protein-calorie malnutrition, *Metabolism*, 24, 633, 1975.
47. Ingenbleek, Y., van der Schrieck, H. G., de Nayer, P., and de Visscher, M., Albumin, transferrin and the thyroxine-binding prealbumin/retinol-binding protein (TBPA-RBP) complex in assessment of malnutrition, *Clin. Chim. Acta*, 63, 61, 1975.
48. Carpentier, Y. A., Barthel, J., and Bruyns, J., Plasma protein concentration in nutritional assessment, *Proc. Nutr. Soc.*, 41, 405, 1982.
49. Golden, M. H. N., Transport proteins as indices of protein status, *Am. J. Clin. Nutr.*, 35, 1159, 1982.
50. Nagabhushan, V. S. and Rao, B. S. N., Studies on 3-methylhistidine metabolism in children with protein-energy malnutrition, *Am. J. Clin. Nutr.*, 31, 1322, 1978.
51. Munro, H. N. and Young, V. R., Urinary excretion of N′-methylhistidine (3-methylhistidine): a tool to study metabolic responses in relation to nutrient and hormonal status in health and disease in man, *Am. J. Clin. Nutr.*, 31, 1608, 1978.
52. Heymsfield, S. B., McManus, C., Stevens, V., and Smith, J., Muscle mass: reliable indicator of protein-energy malnutrition severity and outcome, *Am. J. Clin. Nutr.*, 35, 1192, 1982.
53. Scott, P. H., Berger, H. M., and Kenward, C. et al., Plasma alkaline ribonuclease and nitrogen retention in low birthweight infants, *Br. J. Nutr.*, 40, 459, 1978.
54. Scott, P. H., Berger, H. M., and Wharton, B. A., A critical assessment of plasma alkaline ribonuclease as an indicator of protein nutritional status in infancy, *Annu. Clin. Biochem.*, 21, 357, 1984.
55. Albanese, A. A., Orto, L. A., and Zavattaro, D. N. et al., Protein metabolic significance of blood ribonuclease levels in man, *Nutr. Rept. Int.*, 4, 151, 1971.
56. Sigulem, D. M., Brasel, J. A., and Valesco, E. G. et al., Plasma and urine ribonuclease as a measure of nutritional status in children, *Am. J. Clin. Nutr.*, 26, 793, 1973.
57. Prabhavathi, P., Mohanran, M., and Reddy, V., Ribonuclease activity in plasma and leucocytes of malnourished children, *Clin. Chim. Acta*, 79, 591, 1977.
58. Reddy, V., Mohanran, M., and Prabhavathi, P., Alkaline ribonuclease activity in plasma and leucocytes of malnourished women, *Nutr. Metab.*, 22, 357, 1978.
59. Scott, P. H., A method for the determination of alkaline ribonuclease (E.C. 3.1.4.22) activity in human serum, *Anal. Biochem.*, 100, 233, 1979.
60. Duane, P. and Peters, T. J., Nutritional status in alcoholics with and without chronic skeletal muscle myopathy, *Alcohol & Alcoholism*, 23, 271, 1988.
61. Copper, A. and Heird, W. C., Nutritional assessment of the infant, in *Parenteral Nutrition in the Infant Patient*, Filer, L. J. and Leathem, W. D., Eds., Abbott Laboratories, North Chicago, IL, 1983, 13.

62. Copper, A. and Heird, W. C., Nutritional assessment of the pediatric patient including the low birth weight infant, *Am. J. Clin. Nutr.*, 35, 1132, 1982.
63. Georgieff, M. K. and Sasanow, S. R., Nutritional assessment of the neonate, *Clinics in Perimatology*, 13, 73, 1986.
64. Nadeau, L., Forest, J.–C., Masson, M., Morrissette, I., Lariviere, F., and Michele, C., Biochemical markers in the assessment of protein-calorie malnutrition in premature neonates, *Clin. Chem.*, 32, 1269, 1986.
65. Blazey, M. E., Brewer, E. M., Hudson, M. A., and Wilson, M. F., Nutritional assessment of protein status, *Dimensions of Critical Care Nursing*, 5, 328, 1986.
66. Grant, J., Custer, P., and Thurlow, J., Current techniques of nutritional assessment, *Surg. Clin. North Am.*, 61, 437, 1981.
67. Blackburn, G. L., Bistrian, B. R., Maini, B. S., Schlamm, H. T., and Smith, M. F., Nutritional and metabolic assessment of the hospitalized patient, *J. Parenteral and Enteral Nutr.*, 1, 11, 1977.
68. Stinnett, J. D., Protein-caloric malnutrition and host defense, in *Nutrition and the Immune Response*, CRC Press, Boca Raton, FL, 1983, 111.
69. Linn, B. S., Delayed hypersensitivity skin testing in nutritional assessment, *Am. Surgeon*, 53, 628, 1987.
70. Sauberlich, H. E., Implications of nutritional status on human biochemistry, physiology, and health, *Clin. Biochem.*, 17, 132, 1984.
71. Cunningham-Rundles, S., Effects of nutritional status on immunological functions, *Am. J. Clin. Nutr.*, 35, 1202, 1982.
72. Parent, G., Chevalier, P., Zalles, L., Sevilla, R., Bustos, M., Dhenin, J. M., and Jambon, B., *In vitro* lymphocyte-differentiating effects of thymulin (Zn-FTS) on lymphocyte subpopulations of severely malnourished children, *Am. J. Clin. Nutr.*, 60, 274, 1994.
73. Fakhir, S., Ahmad, P., Faridi, M. M. A., and Rattan, A., Cell-mediated immune responses in malnourished host, *J. Tropical Pediatrics*, 35, 175, 1989.
74. Bhaskaram, P., Nutrition-immunization interactions and relevance to child health, *Nutrition News*, 17, 1, 1996.
75. Chandra, R. K., Immunocompetence as a functional index of nutritional status, *Br. Medical Bulletin*, 37, 89, 1981.
76. Chandra, R. K. and Kumari, S., Nutrition and immunity: an overview, *J. Nutr.*, 124, 1433S, 1994.
77. Chandra, R. K., Chandra, S., and Gupta, S., Antibody affinity and immune complexes after immunization with tetanus toxoid in protein-energy malnutrition, *Am. J. Clin. Nutr.*, 40, 131, 1984.
78. Puri, S. and Chandra, R. K., Nutritional regulation of host resistance and predictive value of immunologic tests in assessment of outcome, *Pediatric Clinics North Am.*, 32, 499, 1985.
79. Chandra, R. K., 1990 McCollum Award Lecture, Nutrition and immunity: lessons from past and new insights into the future, *Am. J. Clin. Nutr.*, 53, 1087, 1991.
80. Haider, M. and Haider, S. Q., Assessment of protein-calorie malnutrition, *Clin. Chem.*, (Review) 30, 1286, 1984.
81. Pinchcofsky-Devin, G. D. and Kaminski, M. V. Jr., Incidence of protein-calorie malnutrition in the nursing home population, *J. Am. Coll. Nutr.*, 6, 109, 1987.
82. Sullivan, D. H. and Carter, W. J., Insulin-like growth factor I as an indicator of protein-energy undernutrition among metabolically stable hospitalized elderly, *J. Am. Coll. Nutr.*, 13, 184, 1994.
83. Sullivan, D. H. and Walls, R. C., Impact of nutritional status on morbidity in a population of geriatric rehabilitation patients, *J. Am. Geriatr. Soc.*, 42, 471, 1994.
84. McClave, S. A., Mitoraj, T. E., Thielmeier, K. A., and Greenburg, R. A., Differentiating subtypes (hypalbuminemic vs marasmic) of protein-calorie malnutrition: incidence and clinical significance in a University hospital setting, *J. Parent. Enter. Nutr.*, 18, 337, 1992.
85. Sullivan, D. H., Patch, G. A., Walls, R. C., and Lipschitz, D. A., Impact of nutrition status on morbidity and mortality in a select population of geriatric rehabilitation patients, *Am. J. Clin. Nutr.*, 51, 749, 1990.
86. Baumgartner, R. N., Koehler, K. M., Romero, L., and Garry, P. J., Serum albumin is associated with skeletal muscle in elderly men and women, *Am. J. Clin. Nutr.*, 64, 552, 1996.

87. Sullivan, D. H., Risk factors for early hospital readmission in a select population of geriatric rehabilitation patients: the significance of nutritional status, *J. Am. Geriatr. Soc.*, 40, 798, 1992.

88. Reuben, D. B., Moore, A. A., Damesyn, M., Keller, E., Harrison, G. G., and Greendale, G. A., Correlates of hypoalbuminemia in community-dwelling older persons, *Am. J. Clin. Nutr.*, 66, 38, 1997.

89. Corti, M.–C., Guralnik, J. M., Salive, M. E., and Sorkin, J. D., Serum albumin level and physical disability as predictors of mortality in older persons, *JAMA*, 272, 1036, 1994.

90. Rothschild, M. A., Oratz, M., and Schreiber, S., Serum albumin, *Hepatology*, 8, 385, 1988.

91. Young, G. A. and Hill, G. L., Evaluation of protein-energy malnutrition in surgical patients from plasma valine and other amino acids, proteins, and anthropometric measurements, *Am. J. Clin. Nutr.*, 34, 166, 1981.

92. McLaren, D. S., A fresh look at protein-energy malnutrition in the hospitalized patient, *Nutrition*, 4, 1, 1988.

93. Stegink, L. D. and Baker, G. L., Serum amino acid levels of Northern Alaskan Eskimo infants and children, *Am. J. Clin. Nutr.*, 23, 1642, 1970.

94. Sauders, S. J., Truswell, A. S., Barbezat, G. O., Wittman, W., and Hansen, J. D. L., Plasma free amino acid pattern in protein-calorie malnutrition, *Lancet*, 2, 795, 1967.

95. Harper, A. E., Plasma amino acid concentrations in relation to evaluation of nutritional status, in *Nutritional Assessment – Present Status, Future Directions and Prospects*, Report of the second Ross conference on Medical Research, Ross Laboratories, Columbus, 1981, 29.

96. Brown, K. H. and Solomons, N. W., Nutritional problems of developing countries, *Infectious Disease Clinics of North Am.*, 5, 297, 1991.

97. Waterlow, J. C., Note on the assessment and classification of protein-energy malnutrition in children, *Lancet*, 2, 87, 1973.

98. Ingenbleek, Y. and Young V., Transthyretin (prealbumin) in health and disease: nutritional implications, *Annu. Rev. Nutr.*, 14, 495, 1994.

99. Fulop, T., Herrmann, F., and Rapil, C. H., Prognostic role of serum albumin and prealbumin levels in elderly patients at admission to a geriatric hospital, *Arch. Gerontol. Geriatr.*, 12, 31, 1991.

100. Herrmann, F. R., Safran, C., Levkoff, S. E., and Minaker, K. L., Serum albumin level on admission as a predictor of death, length of stay and readmission, *Arch. Int. Med.*, 152, 125, 1992.

101. Doumas, E. T., Watson, W. A., and Biggs, H. G., Albumin standards and the measurement of serum albumin with bromcresol green, *Clin. Chim. Acta*, 31, 87, 1971.

102. Frederichsen P. and Kierulf, P., A more accurate dye-binding method for the routine determination of serum albumin, *Clin. Chem.*, 25, 1180, 1979.

103. Pinnel, A. E. and Northam, B. E., New automated dye-binding method for serum albumin determination with bromcresol purple, *Clin. Chem.*, 24, 80, 1978.

104. Carpentier, J. B. S. and Bruyns, J., Plasma protein concentration in nutritional assessment, *Proc. Nutr. Soc.*, 41, 405, 1982.

105. de Onis, M. and Habicht, J. –P., Anthropometric reference data for international use: recommendation from a World Health Organization Expert Committee, *Am. J. Clin. Nutr.*, 64, 650, 1996.

106. Heymsfield, S. B., Wang, Z., Baumgarter, R. N., and Ross, R., Human body composition: advances in models and methods, *Annu. Rev. Nutr.*, 17, 527, 1997.

107. Fogelholm, M. and van Marken Lichtenbelt, W., Comparison of body composition methods: a literature analysis (Review), *Eur. J. Clin. Nutr.*, 51, 495, 1997.

108. Khaled, M. A., McCutcheon, M. J., Reddy, S., Pearman, P. L., Hunter, G. R., and Weinsier, R. L., Electrical impedance in assessing human body composition: the BIA method, *Am. J. Clin. Nutr.*, 47, 789, 1988.

109. Kuczarski, R. J., Fanelli, M. T., and Koch, G. G., Ultrasonic assessment of body composition in obese adults: overcoming the limitations of the skinfold caliper, *Am. J. Clin. Nutr.*, 45, 717, 1987.

110. Van Loan, M. and Mayclin, P., A new TOBEC instrument and procedure for the assessment of body composition: use of Fourier coefficients to predict lean body mass and total body water, *Am. J. Clin. Nutr.*, 45, 131, 1987.

111. Robbins, G. E. and Trowbridge, F. L., Anthropometric techniques and their application, in *Nutrition Assessment*, Simko, M. D., Cowell, C., and Gilbride, J. A., Eds., Aspen Systems Corp., Rockville, 1984, 69.

112. Roche, A. F., Guo, S., Baumgastner, R. N., Chumlea, W. C., Ryan, A. S., and Kuzmarski, R. J., Reference data for weight, stature, and weight/stature in Mexican Americans from Hispanic Health and Nutrition Examination Survey (HHANES 1982-1984), *Am. J. Clin. Nutr.*, 51, 917S, 1990.

113. Najjar, M. F. and Rowland, M., Anthropometric reference data and prevalence of overweight, United States, 1976-1980, Washington D.C.: US Government Printing Office, 1987 (Vital and health statistics, Series 11, No. 238, [DHEW Publication (PHS) 87-16885]).

114. Frisancho, A. R., New standards of weight and body composition by frame size and height for assessment of nutritional status of adults and the elderly, *Am. J. Clin. Nutr.*, 40, 808, 1984.

115. Geissler, C. A. and Miller, D. S., Problem with the use of "weight for height" tables, *J. Nutr.*, 115, 1546, 1985.

116. Rao, K. V. and Rao, N. P., Association of growth status and the incidence of nutrition deficiency signs, *Am. J. Clin. Nutr.*, 28, 209, 1975.

117. Bishop, C. W., Bowen, P. E., and Ritshey, S. J., Norms for nutritional assessment of American adults by upper arm anthropometry, *Am. J. Clin. Nutr.*, 34, 2530, 1981.

118. WHO, Physical status: the use and interpretation of anthropometry, Report of a WHO Expert Committee, World Health Organ. Tech. Report, Series 1995, 854.

119. Waterlow, J. C., Buzina, R., Keller, W., Lane, J. M., Nichaman, M. Z., and Tanner, J. M., The presentation and use of height and weight data for comparing nutritional status of groups of children under age of 10 years, Bull. World Health Organ., 55, 489, 1977.

120. WHO, Measuring change in nutritional status, Geneva, Switzerland: World Health Organization, 1983.

121. WHO Working Group, Use and interpretation of anthropometric indicators of nutritional status, Bull. World Health Organ., 64, 929, 1986.

122. Velzeboer, M. F., Selwyn, B. J., Sargent, F., Pollitt, E., and Delgado, H., Evaluation of arm circumference as a public health index of protein energy malnutrition in early childhood, *J. Trop. Pediatr.*, 29, 135, 1983.

123. Ball, T. M. and Pust, R. E., Arm circumference vs. arm circumference/head circumference ratio in the assessment of malnutrition in rural Malawian children, *J. Tropical Pediatr.*, 39, 298, 1993.

124. Feldman, E. B., *Essentials of Clinical Nutrition*, F. A. Davis, Philadelphia, 1988, 72.

125. Thomas, M. R., Massoudi, M., Byrne, J., Mitchell, M. A., Eggert, L. D., and Chan, G. M., Evaluation of transthyretin as a monitor of protein-energy intake in preterm and sick neonatal infants, *J. Parenteral Enteral Nutr.*, 12, 162, 1988.

126. Thissen, J.–P., Ketelslegers, J.–M., and Underwood, L. E., Nutritional regulation of the insulin-like growth factors, *Endocrine Revs.*, 15, 80, 1994.

127. Klein, S., The myth of serum albumin as a measure of nutritional status, *Gastroenterology*, 99, 1845, 1990.

128. Unterman, T. G., Vazquez, R. M., Sla, A. J., Martyn, P. A., and Phillips, L. S., Nutrition and somatomedin, XIII, Usefulness of somatomedin-C in nutritional assessment, *Am. J. Med.*, 78, 228, 1985.

129. Clemmons, D. R., Underwood, L. E., Dickerson, R. N., Brown, R. O., Hak, L. J., MacPhee, R. D., and Heizer, W. D., Use of plasma somatomedin-C/insulin-like growth factor-I measurements to monitor the response to nutritional repletion in malnourished patients, *Am. J. Clin. Nutr.*, 41, 191, 1985.

130. Powers, D. A., Franse, V. L., Brown, R. O., Hinson, A., and Cowan, G. S. M. Jr., Serum fibronectin and somatomedin-C as nutritional markers in adults receiving total parenteral nutrition, *Clin. Pharmcol.*, 7, 889, 1988.

131. Heimburger, D. C. and Weinsier, R. L., Hospital-associated malnutrition, in *Medicine for the Practicing Physician*, Hurst, J. W., Ed., 4th Edition, Appleton & Lange, Stamford, 1996, 128.

132. Coats, K. G., Morgan, S. L., Bartolucci, A. A., and Weinsier, R. L., Hospital-associated malnutrition: a re-evaluation 12 years later, *J. Am. Diet. Assoc.*, 92, 27, 1993.

133. Weinsier, R. L. and Morgan, S. L., *Fundamentals of Clinical Nutrition*, Mosby, St. Louis, 1993.

134. Weinsier, R. L., Bacon, J. A., and Butterworth, C. E. Jr., Hospital-associated malnutrition, *Alabama J. Med. Sci.*, 19, 402, 1982.

135. Friedmann, J. M., Jensen, G. C., Smiciklas-Wright, H., and McCamish, M. A., Predicting early nonelective hospital readmission in nutritionally compromised older adults, *Am. J. Clin. Nutr.*, 65, 1714, 1997.

136. Boles, J. M., Garre, M. A., Youinou, P. Y., Mialon, P., Menez, J. F., Jouquan, J., Miossec, P. J., Pennec, Y., and Le Menn, G., Nutritional status in intensive care patients: evaluation in 84 unselected patients, *Critical Care Med.*, 11, 87, 1993.

137. Bakerman, S. and Strausbach, P. H., Malnutrition: the laboratory and the clinic, *Laboratory Management*, 1984, 13.

138. Mitchell, C. O. and Lipschitz, D. A., The effect of age and sex on the routinely used measurements to assess the nutritional status of hospitalized patients, *Am. J. Clin. Nutr.*, 36, 340, 1982.

139. Viteri, F. E. and Alvarado, J., The creatinine height index: its use in the estimation of the degree of protein depletion and repletion in protein calorie malnourished children, *Pediatrics*, 46, 696, 1970.

140. Mendez, J. and Buskirk, E. R., Creatinine-height index, *Am. J. Clin. Nutr.*, 24, 385, 1971.

141. Viteri, F. E., Alvarado, J., and Alleyne, G. A. O., Reply to Drs. Mendez and Buskirk, *Am. J. Clin. Nutr.*, 24, 386, 1971.

142. Viteri, F. E., Creatinine-height index in malnourished children, *Nutr. Rev.*, 30, 24, 1972.

143. Anon., Creatinine-height index in malnourished children, *Nutr. Rev.*, 29, 134, 1971.

144. Alleyne, G. A. O., Viteri, F., and Alvarado, J., Indices of body composition in infantile malnutrition: total body potassium and urinary creatinine, *Am. J. Clin. Nutr.*, 23, 875, 1970.

145. Standard, K. L., Wills, V. G., and Waterlow, J. C., Indirect indicators of muscle mass in malnourished infants, *Am. J. Clin. Nutr.*, 7, 271, 1959.

146. Arroyave, G. and Wilson, D., Urinary excretion of creatinine of children under different nutritional conditions, *Am. J. Clin. Nutr.*, 9, 170, 1961.

147. Van Hoeyweghen, R. J., De Leeuw, I. H., Vandewoude, M. F. J., Creatinine arm index as alternative for creatinine height index, *Am. J. Clin. Nutr.*, 56, 611, 1992.

148. Joint FAO/WHP Expert Committee on Nutrition, Eighth Report, FAO nutrition meetings report series No. 49, Food and Agriculture Organization, Rome, 1971.

149. Whitehead, R. G., Rapid determination of some plasma amino acids in subclinical kwashiorkor, *Lancet*, 1, 250, 1964.

150. Whitehead, R. G. and Dean, R. F. A., Serum amino acids in kwashiorkor, II, An abbreviated method of estimation and its application, *Am. J. Clin. Nutr.*, 14, 320, 1964.

151. Simmons, W. K., The plasma amino acid ratio as an indicator of the protein nutrition status: A review of recent work, *Bull. W.H.O.*, 42, 480, 1970.

152. Whitehead, R. G. and Dean, R. F. A., Serum amino acids in kwashiorkor, I, Relationship to clinical condition, *Am. J. Clin. Nutr.*, 14, 313, 1964.

153. Saunders, S. J., Truswell, A. S., and Hansen, J. D. L., Plasma free amino acid pattern in protein-calorie malnutrition, *Lancet*, 2, 795, 1967.

154. Katz, St. I., The amino acid ratio and hydroxyproline creatinine index in marginal protein-calorie malnutrition, *Trop. Georgr. Med.*, 22, 389, 1970.

155. Howells, G. R., Wharton, B. A., and McCance, R. A., Value of hydroxypyroline indices in malnutrition, *Lancet*, 1, 1082, 1967.

156. Whitehead, R. G., Urinary excretion of hydroxyproline in kwashiorkor, *Lancet*, 1, 203, 1966.

157. Whitehead, R., Hydroxyproline creatinine ratio as an index of nutritional status and rate growth, *Lancet*, 2, 567, 1965.

158. McLaren, D. S., Loshkajian, H., and Kanawati, A. A., Urinary creatinine and hydroxyproline in relation to childhood malnutrition, *Br. J. Nutr.*, 24, 641, 1970.

159. Allison, D. J., Walker, A., and Smith, Q. T., Urinary hydroxyproline: creatinine ratio of normal humans at various ages, *Clin. Chim. Acta*, 14, 729, 1966.

160. Crowne, R. S., Wharton, B. A., and McCance, R. A., Hydroxyproline indices and hydroxyproline/creatinine ratios in older children, *Lancet*, 1, 395, 1969.

161. Whitehead, R. G., Biochemical tests in differential diagnosis of protein and calories deficiencies, *Arch. Dis. Child.*, 42, 479, 1967.
162. LeRoy, E. C., The technique and significance of hydroxyproline measurement in man, *Adv. Clin. Chem.*, 10, 213, 1967.
163. Assessment of protein nutritional status, A committee report, *Am. J. Clin. Nutr.*, 23, 807, 1970.
164. Arroyave, G., The estimation of relative nutrient intake and nutritional status by biochemical methods: proteins, *Am. J. Clin. Nutr.*, 11, 447, 1962.
165. Powell, R. C., Plough, I. C., and Baker, E. M. III, The use of nitrogen to creatinine ratios in random urine specimens to estimate dietary protein, *J. Nutr.*, 73, 47, 1961.
166. Simmons, W. K., Urinary urea nitrogen/creatinine ratio as indicator of recent protein intake in field studies, *Am. J. Clin. Nutr.*, 25, 539, 1972.
167. Dugdale, A. E. and Edkins, E., Urinary urea/creatinine ratio in healthy and malnourished children, *Lancet*, 1, 1062, 1964.
168. Arroyave, G. and Lee, M., Variation in urinary excretion of urea and N′-methylnicotinamide during the day comparison with fasting levels, *Arch. Latinoam. Nutr.*, 16, 125, 1966.
169. Manual for Nutrition Surveys, 2nd Ed., Interdepartmental Committee on Nutrition for National Defense, Superintendent of Documents, U.S. Government Printing Office, Washington D.C., 1963.
170. Oberman, J. W., Gregory, K. O., Burke, F. G., Ross, S., and Rice, E. C., Electrophoretic analysis of serum proteins in infants and children, I, Normal values from birth to adolescence, *N. Engl. J. Med.*, 255, 743, 1956.
171. O′Neal, R. M., Johnson, O. C., and Schaefer, A. E., Guidelines for classification and interpretation of group blood and urine data collected as part of the National Nutrition Survey, *Pediatr. Res.*, 4, 103, 1970.
172. Whitehead, R. G., Frood, J. D. L., and Poskitt, E. M. E., Value of serum-albumin measurements in nutritional surveys: A reappraisal, *Lancet*, 2, 287, 1971.
173. Simmons, W. K. and Bohdal, M., Assessment of some biochemical parameters related to protein-calorie nutrition in children, *Bull. WHO*, 42, 897, 1970.
174. Bradfield, R. B. and Margen, S., Morphological changes in human scalp hair during protein deprivation, *Science*, 157, 438, 1970.
175. Bradfield, R. B., Protein deprivation: comparative response of hair roots, serum protein, and urinary nitrogen, *Am. J. Clin. Nutr.*, 24, 405, 1971.
176. Millward, D. J., Methods for assessing protein nutriture in individuals and populations, in *Group of Europeans Nutritionist: Nutritional Status Assessment for Individuals and Population Groups*, Fidanza, F., Ed., Perugia, 1986, 109.
177. Large, S., Neal, G., Glover, J., Thanangkul, O., and Olson, R.E., The early changes in retinol-binding protein and prealbumin concentrations in plasma of protein-energy malnourished children after treatment with retinol and improved diet, *Br. J. Nutr.*, 43, 393, 1980.
178. NIDDK, Proposed dietary guideline emphasizes weight maintenance, Weight-Control Information Network (WIN Notes), National Institutes of Health, Washington D.C., Fall, 1995.
179. Third Report on the World Nutrition Situation, Chapter 2, ACC/SCCN Secretariat, C/O World Health Organization, Geneva, Switzerland, December, 1997, 19.
180. Collins, S., Myatt, M., and Golden, B., Dietary treatment of severe malnutrition in adults, *Am. J. Clin. Nutr.*, 68, 193, 1998.
181. Lesourd, B. M., Nutrition and immunity in the elderly: modification of immune responses with nutritional treatments, *Am. J. Clin. Nutr.*, 66, 478S, 1997.

Section V

Essential Fatty Acids Deficiencies

Essential Fatty Acids Deficiencies

Linoleic Acid

molecular weight: 280.4

Linolenic Acid

molecular weight: 278.4

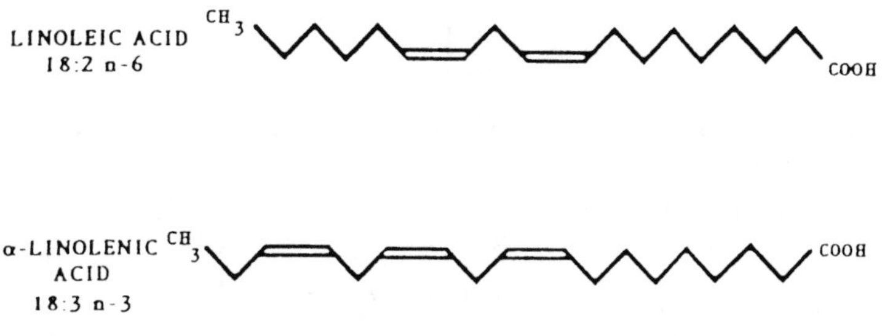

FIGURE 62
Structure of linoleic acid and α-linolenic acid.

History

The essentiality of linoleic acid for the rat was demonstrated by Burr and Burr[1,2] in 1925. However, the essentiality for the human was not established until 1958 by Wiesen, Hansen, and Adam.[3,4] The essential fatty acids came into the fore with the introduction of fat-free total parenteral nutrition (TPN) in 1969 by Dudrick et al.[7] for the treatment of seriously ill patients.

Dermatological changes were observed in patients on the fat-free TPN preparation for only 3 weeks,[6] however, biochemical evidence of an essential fatty acid deficiency exists long before the development of the scaly dermatitis.[5,6] Besides the dermatitis, a human essential fatty acid deficiency may result in impaired growth in children, fatty liver, abnormal platelet function, delayed wound healing, neurological abnormalities and impaired resistance to infection.[5,7,10,12] Several reviews are available that consider the roles of the essential fatty acids in health and disease.[11-22,33,34,47,55,60,62,63]

Dietary Sources of Essential Fatty Acids

Hepburn et al.[56] complied extensive tables on the content of α-linolenic acid (omega-3) in common food items and seafood products. They have also provided the contents of eicosapentaenoic acid (20:5 ω3) and docosahexaenoic acid (22:6 ω3) in a large number of seafood products. Cold water fish are a common source in the diet of 20:5 ω3 and 22:6 ω3 fatty acids. Alpha-linolenic acid (18:3 ω3) is provided mainly by vegetable oils. Rapeseed oil (canola) contains 11%; soybean oil, 6.8%; walnut oil, 10%; wheat germ oil, 7%; butter, 1.5%; and margarine, 2.8%.

Linoleic acid (18:2 ω6) content is quite high in most vegetable oils: safflower oil contains 77%; sunflower oil, 69%; corn oil, 61%; soybean oil; 54%; peanut oil, 33%; canola oil, 22%; olive oil, 8%; margarine, 17%; lard, 11%; chicken fat, 21%; beef fat, 3%; and butterfat, 2%. Hunter[57] has provided additional information on the dietary intakes of α-linolenic acid by United States and Canadian populations. Blackcurrent seed oil, borage oil, and primrose oil can serve as sources of γ-linolenic acid.[60]

Metabolism of Linolenic Acid and Linoleic Acid

Linoleic and linolenic acids are considered essential and must be obtained from the diet.[8-11,51,60,62] An essential fatty acid (EFA) deficiency status in the human can be categorized into three stages:[6] (1) biochemical essential fatty acid depletion, (2) biochemical essential fatty acid deficiency, and (3) clinical essential fatty acid deficiency. These stages can be established by the determination of the essential fatty composition of the total serum lipids.[6,9]

The essentiality of linoleic acid and α-linolenic acid, relates to their ability to incorporate into lipids and to serve as precursors in the biosynthesis of eicosanoids. Linoleic acid serves as a precursor of arachidonic acid which is metabolized to prostaglandins, leukotrienes, and thromboxand.[18-20]

The following is a simplified outline of the metabolic pathways of linoleic acid and linolenic acid in the body.

Metabolism of Linoleic Acid (*n*-6) and α-Linolenic Acid (*n*-3) (abbreviated)

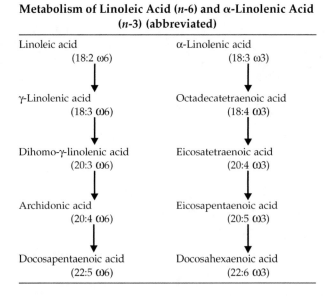

Deficiency of Linoleic Acid and Linolenic Acid

Occurrence of Deficiency

Dietary deficiency of linolenic acid (18:3 ω-3) and linoleic acid (18:2 ω-6) during development has been shown to result in lower levels of 20:4 ω-6 and 22:6 ω-3 in the central nervous system.[17,19,22] These changes have been associated with altered learning behavior and visual function.[17,19,22-25] Thus, the synthesis of 20:4 ω-6 and of 22:6 ω-3 depends upon a dietary intake of 18:2 ω-6 and of 18:3 ω-3, respectively.[19,22]

A deficiency in linoleic acid and arachidonic acid is often associated with protein-energy malnutrition in children,[27] infants,[46] and malnourished elderly patients.[35,36] Cutaneous hypersensitivity is impaired in these groups. Essential fatty acids deficiency may be a contributing factor in this immunodeficiency state.[35,36]

Altered essential fatty acid metabolism has been reported in some boys with attention-deficient hyperactivity disorder.[28] Fatty acid deficiency has also been implicated in the nutrition of premature infants.[47-51,58] Infants at birth have low essential fatty acid levels and, hence, are more prone to an essential fatty acids deficiency.[58] The onset of an essential fatty acid deficiency can be rapid and its incidence is high in low-birth weight-infants.[47,50]

Vegetarian subjects have lower serum levels of docosahexaenoic acid than omnivores.[21,26] Patients with severe fat malabsorption diseases have been observed with biochemical signs of an essential fatty acid deficiency.[52] Some evidence suggests that the use of essential fatty acids may have benefits in reducing cardiovascular risk.[41-43]

Total Parenteral Nutrition

Since the initial report of Dudrick et al.,[7] numerous reports have appeared on essential fatty acid deficiencies occurring in patients sustained on fat-free TPN preparations.[5,6,11,19,39,61] Patients on total parenteral nutrition (TPN) now receive supplements of vitamins and trace minerals. Lipids providing essential fatty acids are usually given as either a separate infusion or mixed with other TPN components. Intralipid preparation (KabiVitram, Inc., Alameda, CA) is commonly used for this purpose.[53]

Linolenic Acid Deficiency

For some time, linoleic acid was the only fatty acid definitely known to be essential to man.[10,17] The first case of linolenic acid deficiency was reported by Holman et al.[10,17] in 1982 while studying a 6-year-old girl on a linolenic acid-poor parenteral formula. The girl developed paresthesia, blurred vision, and difficulties in walking. The condition corrected with the feeding of a α-linolenic acid rich diet.[10] Subsequently, other investigators have reported on the essentiality of α-linolenic acid.[11,12,17,36,37,42,43]

Assessment of Essential Fatty Acid Deficiency

In the absence of dietary linoleic acid, the endogenous oleic acid (18:1 ω-9) is elongated and desaturated to form 5,8,11-eicosatrienoic acid (5,8,11–20:3 ω-9). This unusual fatty acid is referred to as the Mead acid.[54] Measurement of this acid can serve as an indicator of an essential fatty acid deficiency state. Normally only trace amounts of this fatty acid are found in the plasma.[9] An essential fatty acid depletion is associated with a decrease in plasma linoleate and arachidonate percentages.[47]

Holman introduced the use of the triene/tetraene ratio (20:3 ω-9/20:4 ω-6) as a criterion for identifying an essential fatty acid deficiency.[4,14,30-32] A deficiency is characterized by an increase in the 5,8,11-eicosatrienoate/arachidonate (triene/tetraene) ratio. A ratio greater than 0.4 has been considered abnormal, indicating an essential fatty acid deficiency.[9,45] The ratio is less than 0.2 in normal subjects.[4,14,31,32,35] The triene/tetraene ratio is a sensitive diagnostic index of essential fatty acid deficiencies which were considered to be associated only with total paranteral nutrition.[39,40] However, with the use of the triene/tetraene ratio as an index of essential fatty acid status, essential fatty acid deficiency was found to occur in other conditions. Included are patients with fat malabsorption, elderly subjects with peripherol vascular disease, and kwashiorkor.[27]

Methods

Fatty acid are usually analyzed by gas-liquid chromatography procedures[14,19,28,29] and by capillary gas chromatography-mass spectrometry.[38] Blood samples require extraction and purification, followed by derivatization. Separation and identification of the individual fatty acids is performed by gas chromatography.[14,32,45,47,52,59]

Summary

Linoleic acid and alpha-linolenic acid are considered the essential fatty acids. The occurrence of essential fatty acid deficiency associated with total parenteral nutrition has been alleviated with the use of commercial clinical nutrition preparations that provide the essential fatty acids. However, occasionally an essential fatty deficiency may occur due to other circumstances. Essential fatty acid deficiency can be biochemically diagnosed by determining the level of certain unsaturated fatty acids in serum or plasma. When linoleic acid is deficient in the diet, serum levels of linoleic and arachidonic acids fall and the level of the trienoic acid, 5,8,11-eicosatrienoic, is increased. The ratio of 5,8,11-eicosatrienoic acid and arachidonic acid (20:4 ω-6) levels in serum lipids can provide an index of essential fatty acid status in the human. In normal subjects the triene/tetraene ratio for serum is below 0.4.

References

1. Holman, R. T. and George O. Burr and the discovery of essential fatty acids, *J. Nutr.*, 118, 535, 1988.
2. Burr, G. O. and Burr, M. M., New deficiency disease produced by rigid exclusion of fat from the diet, *J. Biol. Chem.*, 82, 345, 1929.

3. Wiese, H. F., Hansen, A. E., and Adam, D. J. D., Essential fatty acids in infant nutrition: I. Linoleic acid requirements in terms of serum di- tri- and tetraenoic acid levels, *J. Nutr.*, 66, 345, 1958.

4. Hansen, A. E., Wiese, H. F., Boelsche, A. N., Haggard, M. E., Adam, D. J. D., and Davis, H., Role of linoleic acid in infant nutrition, Clinical and chemical study of 428 infants fed on milk mixtures varying in kind and amount of fat, *Pediatrics*, 31 (Suppl. 1, Part 2), 171, 1963.

5. Caldwell, M. D., Human essential fatty acid deficiency: a review, in *Fat Emulsions in Parenteral Nutrition*, Meng, H. C., Wilmore, D. W., Eds., American Medical Association, Chicago, 1976, 24.

6. Tanphaichitr, V., Fat in parenteral nutrition, in *Human Nutrition: Better Nutrition Better Life*, Tanphaichitr, V., Dahlan, W., Suphakarn, V., and Valyasevi, A., Eds., Aksornsmai Press, Bangkok, Thailand, 1984, 160.

7. Dudrick, S. J., Wilmore, D. W., Vas, H. M., and Rhoads, J. E., Long-term total parenteral nutrition with growth, development, and positive nitrogen balance, *Surgery*, 64, 134, 1969.

8. Mead, J. F., Nutrients with special functions: essential fatty acids, in *Nutrition and the Adult: Macronutrients*, Alfin-Slater, R. B. and Kritchevsky, D., Eds., Plenum Press, 1980, 213.

9. Holman, R. T., Function and biologic activities of essential fatty acids in man, in *Fat Emulsions in Parenteral Nutrition*, Meng, H. C., and Wilmore, D. W., Eds., American Medical Association, Chicago, 1976, 5.

10. Holman, R. T., Johnson, S. B., and Hatch, T. F., A case of human linolenic acid deficiency involving neurological abnormalities, *Am. J. Clin. Nutr.*, 35, 617, 1982.

11. Bjerve, K. S., Lovoldmostad, I., and Thoresen, L., α-Linolenic acid deficiency in patients on long-term gastric tube feeding, Estimation of linolenic acid and long chain unsaturated *n*-3 fatty acids requirements in man, *Am. J. Clin. Nutr.*, 45, 66, 1987.

12. Anderson, G. J. and Connor, W. E., On the demonstration of ω-3 essential fatty acid deficiency in humans, *Am. J. Clin. Nutr.*, 49, 585, 1989.

13. Sinclair, H. M., Essential fatty acids in perspective, *Human Nutrition: Clinical Nutrition*, 38C, 245, 1984.

14. Hutchinson, M. L. and Clemans, G. G., Essential fatty acids, *Clinics in Lab. Med.*, 1, 665, 1981.

15. Simopoulos, A. P., Omega-3 fatty acids in health and disease, *J. Nutrition, Growth and Cancer*, 3, 69, 1986.

16. Nestel, P. J., Polyunsaturated fatty acids, *Am. J. Clin. Nutr.*, 45, 1161, 1987.

17. Neuringer, M., Anderson, G. J., and Connor, W. E., The essentiality of N-3 fatty acids for the development and function of the retina and brain, *Annu. Rev. Nutr.*, 8, 517, 1988.

18. Ziboh, V. A. and Miller, C. C., Essential fatty acids and polyunsaturated fatty acids, *Annu. Rev. Nutr.*, 10, 433, 1990.

19. Linscheer, W. G. and Vergroesen, A. J., Lipids, in *Modern Nutrition in Health and Disease*, Shils, M. E., Olson, J. A., and Shike, M., Eds., 8th edition, Lea & Febiger, Philadelphia, 1994, 47.

20. Jonnalagadda, S. S., Mustad, V. A., Yu, S., Etherton, T. D., and Kris-Etherton, P. M., Effects of individual fatty acids on chronic diseases, *Nutr. Today*, 31, 90, 1996.

21. Reddy, S., Sanders, T. A. B., and Abeid, O., The influence of maternal vegetarian diet on essential fatty acid status of the newborn, *Eur. J. Clin. Nutr.*, 48, 358, 1994.

22. Innis, S. M., Essential fatty acid requirements in human nutrition, *Can. J. Physiol. Pharmacol.*, 71, 699, 1993.

23. Birch, D. G., Birch, E. E., Hoffman, D. R., and Uaury, R. D., Retinol development in very low-birth-weight infants fed diets differing in omega-3 fatty acids, *Invest. Othalmol. Visual Sci.*, 33, 2365, 1992.

24. Carlson, S. E., Cooke, R. J., Rhodes, P. G., Peeples, J. M., and Werkman, S. H., Effect of vegetable and marine oils in pre-term infant formulas on blood arachidonic and docosahexaenoic acids, *J. Pediatr.*, 120, S159, 1992.

25. Uaury, R. D., Birch, D. G., Birch, E. E., Tyson, J. E., and Hoffman, D. R., Effect of omega-3 fatty acids on retinol functions of very low birth weight neonates, *Pediatr. Res.*, 28, 485, 1990.

26. Conquer, J. A. and Holub, B. J., Supplementation with an algae source of docosahexaenoic acid increases (n-3) fatty acid status and alters selected risk factors for heart disease in vegetarian subjects, *J. Nutr.*, 126, 3032, 1996.

27. Wolff, J. A., Margolis, S., Bujdoso-Walff, K., Matusick, E., and McLean, W. C. Jr., Plasma and red blood cell fatty acid composition in children with protein-calorie malnutrition, *Pediatr. Res.*, 18, 162, 1984.

28. Stevens, L. J., Zentall, S. S., Deck, J. L., Abate, M. L., Watkins, B. A., Lipp, S. R., and Burgess, J. R., Essential fatty acid metabolism in boys with attention-deficient hyperactivity disorder, *Am. J. Clin. Nutr.*, 62, 761, 1995.

29. Holman, R. T., Caster, W. O., and Wiese, H. F., The essential fatty acid requirement of infants and the assessment of their dietary intake of linoleate by serum fatty acid analysis, *Am. J. Clin. Nutr.*, 14, 70, 1964.

30. Holman, R. T., Essential fatty acid deficiency, in *Progress in the Chemistry of Fats and Other Lipids*, Holman, R. T., Ed., Volume 9, Part 2, Pregamon Press, New York, 1971, 275.

31. Holman, R. T., The ratio of trienoic/tetranoic acids in tissue lipids as a measure of essential fatty acid requirement, *J. Nutr.*, 70, 405, 1960.

32. Holman, R. T., Smythe, L., and Johnson, S., Effect of sex and age on fatty acid composition of human serum lipids, *Am. J. Clin. Nutr.*, 32, 2390, 1979.

33. Bivins, B. A., Bell, R. M., Rapp, R. P., and Griffen, W. O., Interrelationships of linoleic acid and linolenic fatty acids in human nutrition, in *Parenteral Nutrition in the Infant Patient*, Files, L. J. and Leathem, W. D., Eds., Abbott Laboratories, North Chicago, IL, 1983, 133.

34. FAO/WHO Expert Consultation: The Role of Dietary Fat and Oils in Human Nutrition, FAO Food and Agriculture Organization, Rome, 1978.

35. Cederholm, T. E., Berg, A. B., Johansson, E. K., Hellstrom, K. H., and Palmblad, J. E. W., Low levels of essential fatty acids are related to impaired delayed skin hypersensitivity in malnourished chronically ill elderly people, *Eur. J. Clin. Invest.*, 24, 615, 1994.

36. Kinsella, J. E., Lokesh, B., Broughton, S., and Whelan, J., Dietary polyunsaturated fatty acids and eicosanoids: potential effects on the modulation of inflammatory and immune cells: an overview, *Nutrition*, 6, 24, 1990.

37. Bjerve, K. S., Fischer, S., and Alme, K., Alpha-linolenic acid deficiency in man: effect of ethyl linolenate on plasma and erythrocyte fatty acid composition and biosynthesis of prostanoids, *Am. J. Clin. Nutr.*, 46, 570, 1987.

38. Alexander, L. R. and Justice, J. B., Fatty acid composition of human erythrocyte membranes by capillary gas chromatography-mass spectrometry, *J. Chromatogr. Biomed. Appl.*, 342, 1, 1985.

39. Fleming, C. R., Smith, L. M., and Hodges, R. E., Essential fatty acid deficiency in adults receiving total parenteral nutrition, *Am. J. Clin. Nutr.*, 29, 976, 1976.

40. Richardson, T. J. and Sgoutas, D., Essential fatty acid deficiency in four adult patients during total parenteral nutrition, *Am. J. Clin. Nutr.*, 28, 258, 1975.

41. Leaf, A., Health claims: Omega-3 fatty acids and cardiovascular disease, *Nutr. Rev.*, 50, 150, 1992.

42. Illingworth, D. R., and Schmidt, E. B., The influence of dietary *n*-3 fatty acids on plasma lipids and lipoproteins, *Ann. N.Y. Acad. Sci.*, 676, 60, 1993.

43. Leaf, A. and Weber, P. C., Cardiovascular effects of *n*-3 fatty acids, *N. Engl. J. Med.*, 318, 549, 1988.

44. Stone, N. J., Fish consumption, fish oil, lipids, and coronary heart disease, *Am. J. Clin. Nutr.*, 65, 1083, 1997.

45. Siguel, E. N., Chee, K. M., Gong, J., and Schaefer, E. J., Criteria for essential fatty acid deficiency in plasma as assessed by capillary column gas-liquid chromatography, *Clin. Chem.*, 33, 1869, 1987.

46. Marin, M. C., DeTomas, M. E., Mercuri, O., Fernadez, A., and de Serres, C. T., Interrelationship between protein-energy malnutrition and essential fatty acid deficiency in nursing infants, *Am. J. Clin. Nutr.*, 53, 466, 1991.

47. Farrell, P. M., Gutcher, G. R., Palta, M., and DeMets, D., Essential fatty acid deficiency in premature infants, *Am. J. Clin. Nutr.*, 48, 220, 1988.

48. Friedman, Z., Polyunsaturated fatty acids in the low-birth-weight infants, *Seminars in Perinatology*, 3, 341, 1979.

49. Cooke, R. J., Zee, P., and Yeh, Y.–Y., Essential fatty acid status of the premature infant during short-term fat-free parenteral nutrition, *J. Pediatric Gastroenterol. Nutr.*, 3, 446, 1984.

50. Gutcher, G. R. and Farrell, P. M., Intravenous infusion of lipid for the prevention of essential fatty acid deficiency in premature infants, *Am. J. Clin. Nutr.*, 54, 1024, 1991.

51. Friedman, Z., Essential fatty acid consideration at birth in the premature neonate and the specific requirement for preformed prostaglandin precursors in the infant, *Prog. Lipid Res.*, 25, 355, 1986.

52. Jeppesen, P. B., Christensen, M. S., Hoy, C.–E., and Mortensen, P. B., Essential fatty acid deficiency in patients with severe fat malabsorption, *Am. J. Clin. Nutr.*, 65, 837, 1997.

53. Perry, D. A., Markin, R. S., Rose, S. G., and Schenken, J. R., Changes in laboratory values in patients receiving total parenteral nutrition, *Lab. Medicine*, 21, 97, 1990.

54. Fulco, A. J. and Mead, J. F., Metabolism of essential fatty acids, VIII. Origins of 5,8,11-eicosatrienoic acid in the fat-deficient rat, *J. Biol. Chem.*, 234, 1411, 1959.

55. Sardesai, V. M., The essential fatty acids, *Nutrition in Clinical Practice*, 7, 179, 1992.

56. Hepburn, F. N., Exler, J., and Weihrauch, J. L., Provisional tables on the content of omega-3 fatty acids and other fat components of selected foods, *J. Am. Diet. Assoc.*, 86, 788, 1986.

57. Hunter, J. E., *n*-3 Fatty acids from vegetable oils, *Am. J. Clin. Nutr.*, 51, 809, 1990.

58. Crawford, M. A., Casteloe, K., Ghebremeskel, K., Phylactos, A., Skirvin, L., and Stacy, F., Are deficits of arachidonic and docosahexaenoic acids responsible for the neural and vascular complications of pre-term babies, *Am. J. Clin. Nutr.*, 66, 1032S, 1997.

59. Lloyd-Still, J. D., Johnson, S. B., and Holman, R. T., Essential fatty acid status and fluidity of plasma phospholipids in cystic fibrosis infants, *Am. J. Clin. Nutr.*, 54, 1029, 1991.

60. Fan, Y.–Y. and Chapkin, R. S., Importance of dietary γ-linolenic acid in human health and nutrition, *J. Nutr.*, 128, 1411, 1998.

61. Jeppesen, P. B., Hoy, C.–E., and Mortensen, Per B., Essential fatty acid deficiency in patients receiving home parenteral nutrition, *Am. J. Clin. Nutr.*, 68, 126, 1998.

62. Raiten, D. J., Talbot, J. M., and Waters, J. H., Assessment of nutrient requirements for infant formulas, *J. Nutr.*, 128, 2059S, 1998.

63. Holman, R. T., The slow discovery of the importance of ω3 essential fatty acids in human health, *J. Nutr.*, 128, 427S, 1998.

Index

Index